INTRODUCTION TO FUNCTIONAL MAGNETIC RESONANCE IMAGING
Principles and Techniques

Functional Magnetic Resonance Imaging (fMRI) is now a standard tool for mapping activation patterns in the human brain. This highly interdisciplinary field involves neuroscientists and physicists as well as clinicians, and the range, flexibility, and sophistication of the techniques being used are increasing rapidly. In this book, Richard Buxton, a leading authority on fMRI, provides an invaluable introduction to how fMRI works, from basic principles and the underlying physics and physiology to newer techniques such as arterial spin labeling and diffusion tensor imaging. The book also includes discussion of how fMRI relates to other imaging techniques (such as positron emission tomography, or PET) and a guide to the statistical analysis of fMRI data. This book will be useful to both the experienced researcher using fMRI and the clinician or researcher with no previous knowledge of the technology.

Richard B. Buxton is Professor of Radiology and Director of Magnetic Resonance Research at the University of California at San Diego. For the past fifteen years he has worked on the development of MRI techniques. His current research is focused on fMRI applications and on the physiological basis of fMRI.

For Lynn

INTRODUCTION TO FUNCTIONAL MAGNETIC RESONANCE IMAGING

Principles and Techniques

RICHARD B. BUXTON

University of California at San Diego

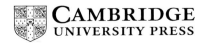

CAMBRIDGE
UNIVERSITY PRESS

PUBLISHED BY THE PRESS SYNDICATE OF THE UNIVERSITY OF CAMBRIDGE
The Pitt Building, Trumpington Street, Cambridge, United Kingdom

CAMBRIDGE UNIVERSITY PRESS
The Edinburgh Building, Cambridge CB2 2RU, UK
40 West 20th Street, New York, NY 10011-4211, USA
10 Stamford Road, Oakleigh, VIC 3166, Australia
Ruiz de Alarcón 13, 28014 Madrid, Spain
Dock House, The Waterfront, Cape Town 8001, South Africa

http://www.cambridge.org

First published 2002

Printed in the United States of America

Typefaces Times Ten 10/13 pt. and Kabel   *System* QuarkXPress™   [HT]

A catalog record for this book is available from the British Library.

Library of Congress Cataloging in Publication Data

Buxton, Richard B., 1954 –
Introduction to functional magnetic resonance imaging: principles
and techniques/Richard B. Buxton.
p. cm.
ISBN 0-521-58113-3 (hardback), ISBN 0-521-00275-3 (supplementary CD-ROM),
ISBN 0-521-00274-5 (hardback plus supplementary CD-ROM)
1. Brain – Magnetic resonance imaging. 2. Magnetic resonance imaging. I. Title.
RC386.6.M34 B895 2001
616'.047548–dc21   00-050235

ISBN   0 521 58113 3   hardback
ISBN   0 521 00275 3   supplementary CD-ROM
ISBN   0 521 00274 5   hardback plus supplementary CD-ROM

Contents

Preface

The field of functional magnetic resonance imaging (fMRI) is intrinsically interdisciplinary, involving neuroscience, psychology, psychiatry, radiology, physics, and mathematics. For me, this is part of the pleasure in working in this area, providing an opportunity to collaborate with scientists and clinicians with a wide range of backgrounds. This book is intended as an introduction to the basic ideas and techniques of fMRI. My goal was to provide a guide to the principles of fMRI with sufficient depth to be useful to the active neuroscience investigator using fMRI in their research, but also to make the material accessible to the new investigator or clinician with no prior knowledge of the field. The viewpoint of the book reflects my own background as a physicist, focusing on how the techniques work. The emphasis is on examples that illustrate the basic principles rather than a more comprehensive review of the field or a more rigorous mathematical treatment of the fundamentals.

This book grew out of courses I taught with my colleagues L. R. Frank and E. C. Wong, and their insights have significantly shaped the way in which the material is presented. Our courses were geared toward graduate students in neuroscience and psychology, but the book should also be useful for clinicians who want to understand the basis of the new fMRI techniques and potential clinical applications, and for physicists and engineers who are looking for an overview of the ideas of fMRI. Some of the techniques described are not yet part of the mainstream of basic neuroscience applications, such as arterial spin labeling, bolus tracking, and diffusion tensor imaging. However, the clinical application of these techniques is rapidly growing, and I think that over the next few years they will become an integral part of many neuroscience fMRI studies. This book should also serve as an introduction to recent excellent multiauthor works that present some of this material in greater depth, such as *Functional MRI* edited by C. T. W. Moonen and P. A. Bandettini (published in 1999 by Springer).

In writing this book, I have benefited from helpful discussions and critical readings from several of my close colleagues, including Eric Wong, Larry Frank, Tom Liu, Karla Miller, Antigona Martinez, and David Dubowitz. I am also fortunate to be able to work with faculty and students in the San Diego neuroscience community, including Geoff Boynton, Greg Brown, Adina Roskies, Marty Sereno, Joan Stiles, Dave Swinney, and many others. Their insights, comments, and questions have stimulated me to think about many of the topics discussed in the book. In addition,

I have also benefited from numerous discussions with colleagues in the field over the years, including Peter Bandettini, Anders Dale, Arno Villringer, Robert Weisskoff, Joe Mandeville, Van Wedeen, Bruce Rosen, Ken Kwong, Robert Turner, Gary Glover, Robert Edelman, Mark Henkelman, and many others. Although these individuals have strongly influenced my own thinking, they are not responsible for what appears here, particularly any errors that may remain.

Finally, this could not have been completed without the loving support of Lynn Hall, and the book is dedicated to her.

Richard B. Buxton

Introduction

Just over 50 years ago, two scientific developments occurred; these advancements are the deep roots of modern functional neuroimaging and the primary role played by functional magnetic resonance imaging (fMRI). In 1948, S. Kety and C. Schmidt described the nitrous oxide technique for measuring cerebral blood flow (CBF). For the first time it was possible to measure CBF in human subjects, providing a new window on the physiological functioning of the human brain. Although the original technique only measured global CBF, subsequent techniques with radioactive tracers ultimately led in the 1970s and 1980s to positron emission tomography (PET) methods, which made possible local measurements of CBF with a spatial resolution better than one cubic centimeter. These techniques were the initial basis for functional neuroimaging to map patterns of activation in the working human brain. Although the sophistication of these techniques has steadily improved, they are all based on the fundamental ideas introduced by Kety and Schmidt.

At about the same time that Kety and Schmidt were working to measure CBF, two physics research groups led by E. Purcell and F. Bloch demonstrated for the first time the phenomenon of nuclear magnetic resonance (NMR). Their seminal work in 1946 provided a sensitive tool for studying subtle magnetic properties of atomic nuclei, but it is unlikely that anyone at the time could have imagined the practical applications of NMR that we have today. From basic physics studies, NMR moved to analytical chemistry applications, and in the 1970s NMR imaging was developed. As clinical applications grew, the N in NMR was dropped in the medical jargon, to avoid confusion with nuclear medicine techniques. Magnetic resonance imaging (MRI) reveals fine details of anatomy without using any ionizing radiation or radioactive tracers and is now an indispensible tool for clinical diagnosis. Most of the clinical MRI studies performed today are essentially studies of anatomy, but MRI is such a flexible technique that it is also possible to measure the physiological functioning of tissue.

In the broadest sense, fMRI refers to any MRI technique that goes beyond anatomy to measure aspects of local physiology. In a more specific sense, the term fMRI refers to techniques that exploit a phenomenon discovered in the early 1990s, now called the Blood Oxygenation Level Dependent (BOLD) effect. With appropriate techniques, the MR signal can be made sensitive to local changes in the oxygenation of blood. Local neural activation increases local CBF more than the local oxygen metabolism rate, so blood oxygenation increases in activated parts of the brain. Activation patterns in the working human brain can be mapped with high temporal and spatial resolution using fMRI based on the BOLD effect.

In addition, other classes of MRI techniques have been developed based on the same ideas of tracer kinetics introduced by Kety and Schmidt that underlie the PET methods. Dynamic contrast agent studies have become routine in clinical applications, and arterial spin labeling (ASL) techniques show great promise for providing local CBF measurements with higher spatial and temporal resolution than any other technique. The ASL techniques are beginning to be used both clinically and for basic studies of brain activation, and will likely be applied more extensively in the future.

Functional neuroimaging with fMRI is a highly interdisciplinary field, involving neuroscientists, psychologists, psychiatrists, radiologists, physicists, and engineers. One of the difficulties in doing fMRI is that the effects being measured are subtle, so the experimental neuroscientist or clinician using fMRI needs to understand in some detail how the techniques work and potential sources of artifacts and errors. The flexibility of MRI is what makes it such a powerful tool, but this also makes it harder for a new investigator to acquire a solid grasp on the fundamentals of fMRI. For example, a computed tomography (CT) x-ray image is relatively easy to understand: the intensity at each point in the image is proportional to the corresponding local x-ray attenuation coefficient. But in MRI the intensity at each point in the image depends not only on the local proton density that generates the MR signal but also on two relaxation times, blood oxygenation, blood flow, the heterogeneous structure of the tissue, and the local diffusion characteristics of water including anisotropic directional properties. The extent to which each of these physical characteristics of the medium affects the MR signal depends on exactly how the image is acquired, so all these aspects are under the control of the experimenter.

This book is organized in three parts, each of which has two subparts. Part I is an introduction to functional neuroimaging in general and to fMRI in particular. All the essential ideas are introduced in this section so that it can serve as an overview of how fMRI works and how it fits into the broader field of functional neuroimaging. Part IA describes energy metabolism in the brain, the nature of cerebral blood flow and oxygen metabolism, and basic nuclear medicine approaches to measuring these quantities. Part IB describes the basic ideas of NMR, how an MR image is made, and how the MR signal can be made to be sensitive to functional activity.

Parts II and III discuss in more depth the basic ideas introduced in Part I. Part II focuses on the principles of MRI. Part IIA describes the nature of the NMR signal, sources of image contrast in MRI, and the sensitivity of the MR signal to local diffusion characteristics of the tissue. The last forms the basis for a potentially powerful technique for mapping the white matter fiber connections between different areas of the brain. Diffusion tensor imaging is a relatively new application of MRI, but it is likely to become a standard adjunct to fMRI studies of brain activation and functional connectivity. Part IIB describes how the local MR signal is imaged, including the basic Fourier transform relationship that lies at the heart of MR imaging, techniques for image acquisition, and noise and artifacts in the images. Because noise is a critical limiting factor in detecting weak signal changes due to subtle brain activation, it is treated in some detail.

Part III deals with the techniques of fMRI in the broader sense. Part IIIA describes the basic principles of tracer kinetic studies, bolus tracking experiments with MR contrast agents, and arterial spin labeling techniques for direct measurement of CBF. Part IIIB focuses on fMRI based on the BOLD effect, including the nature of the hemodynamic response that underlies the BOLD effect, basic techniques for mapping activation patterns with BOLD techniques, the statistical analysis of BOLD data, and the efficient design of BOLD experiments to optimize sensitivity.

Finally, the appendix contains a more thorough discussion of the physics behind NMR. In the main text, the physics is presented from the simpler classical viewpoint, but NMR is in fact a prime example of a quantum phenomenon. For the curious reader, the appendix compares the classical and quantum views of NMR.

IA

Introduction to Functional Neuroimaging

The subject to be observed lay on a delicately balanced table which could tip downwards either at the head or at the foot if the weight of either end were increased. The moment emotional or intellectual activity began in the subject, down went the balance at the head-end, in consequence of the redistribution of blood in his system . . .

We must suppose a very delicate adjustment whereby the circulation follows the needs of the cerebral activity. Blood very likely may rush to each region of the cortex according as it is most active, but of this we know nothing.

William James (1890)

1

Energy Metabolism in the Brain

METABOLIC ACTIVITY ACCOMPANIES NEURAL ACTIVITY

Mapping Brain Activity

The goal of understanding the functional organization of the human brain has motivated neuroscientists for well over 100 years, but the experimental tools to measure and map brain activity have been slow to develop. Neural activity is difficult to localize without placing electrodes directly in the brain. Fluctuating electric and magnetic fields measured at the scalp provide information on electrical events within the brain. From these data the location of a few sources of activity can be estimated, but the information is not sufficient to produce a detailed map of the pattern of activation. However, precise localization of the metabolic activity that follows neural activity is much more feasible and forms the basis for most of the functional neuroimaging techniques is use today, including positron emission tomography (PET) and functional

4

magnetic resonance imaging (fMRI). Although comparatively new, fMRI techniques are now a primary tool for basic studies of the organization of the working human brain, and clinical applications are growing rapidly.

In 1890, William James published *The Principles of Psychology,* a landmark in the development of psychology as a science grounded in physiology (James, 1890). The possibility of measuring changes in brain blood flow associated with mental activity clearly lay behind the experiment performed by Angelo Mosso and recounted by James in the quotation at the beginning of Part IA. By current standards of blood flow measurement, this experiment is quaintly crude, but it indicates that the idea of inferring neural activity in the brain from a measurement of changes in local blood flow long preceded the ability to do such measurements (Raichle, 1998).

In fact, this experiment is unlikely to have worked reliably for an important reason. The motivation for this experiment may have been an analogy with muscle activity. Vigorous exercise produces a substantial muscle swelling due to increased blood volume, and thus a redistribution of weight. But the brain is surrounded by fluid and encased in a hard shell, so the overall fluid volume within the cranium must remain nearly constant. Blood volume changes do occur in the brain, and the brain does move with cardiac pulsations, but these changes most likely involve shifts of cerebrospinal fluid as well. As a result, the weight of the head should remain approximately constant.

Furthermore, this experiment depends on a change in blood volume, rather than blood flow, and blood flow and blood volume are distinct quantities. Blood *flow* refers to the volume per minute moving through the vessels, whereas blood *volume* is the volume occupied by the vessels. In principle, there need be no fixed relation between blood flow and blood volume. Flow through a set of pipes can be increased by increasing the driving pressure without changing the volume of the plumbing. Physiologically, however, experiments typically show a correlation between cerebral blood flow (CBF) and cerebral blood volume (CBV), and functional neuroimaging techniques are now available for measuring both quantities.

The working brain requires a continuous supply of glucose and oxygen, which must be supplied by CBF. The human brain receives 15% of the total cardiac output of blood, about 700 ml/min and yet accounts for only 2% of the total body weight. Within the brain the distribution of blood flow is heterogeneous, with gray matter receiving several times more flow per gram of tissue than white matter. Indeed, the flow per gram of tissue to gray matter is comparable to that in the heart muscle, the most energetic organ in the body. The activity of the brain generates about 11 W/kg of heat, and glucose and oxygen provide the fuel for this energy generation. Yet the brain has virtually no reserve store of oxygen, and thus depends on continuous delivery by cerebral blood flow. If the supply of oxygen to the brain is cut off, unconsciousness results within a few minutes.

The Energy Cost of Neural Activity

As is true for all organs, energy metabolism in the brain is necessary for the basic processes of cellular work, such as chemical synthesis and chemical transport. But the particular work done by the brain, which requires the high level of energy metabolism, is the generation of electrical activity required for neuronal signaling. The connection between neural activity and energy metabolism is the foundation of functional neuroimaging, yet the physiological basis of this connection is still incompletely understood. To explore this connection, we begin by reviewing the basic processes involved in neural activity from the perspective of thermodynamics, in order to emphasize the essential role of energy metabolism. A more complete description can be found in Nicholls, Martin, and Wallace (1992).

The primary example of neural activity is the generation of an action potential and the release of neurotransmitter at a synapse. In the neuron there is an electric potential difference across the cell membrane, with the potential more negative inside. An *action potential* is a transient disturbance of that potential, a rapid depolarization of the membrane. The action potential propagates down the axon until it reaches a junction with another neuron at a *synapse*, and the arrival of the action potential then influences the firing of the second neuron by creating a local fluctuation in the postsynaptic potential. With an *excitatory postsynaptic potential* (EPSP) the potential inside is raised, moving the second neuron closer to firing its own action potential, and for an *inhibitory postsynaptic potential* (IPSP) the potential inside is decreased. Each neuron thus has the capacity to integrate the inputs from many other neurons through their cumulative effect on the postsynaptic potential. From an electrical viewpoint, the working neuron is an intricate pattern of continuously fluctuating membrane potentials punctuated by occasional sharp action potentials.

The resting potential, the action potential, and the fluctuating postsynaptic potentials all depend on maintaining the intracellular and extracellular concentrations of several ions in a state far from chemical equilibrium (Figure 1.1). For example, at rest there is an excess concentration of sodium (Na^+) ions and calcium (Ca^{++}) ions in the extracellular space and an excess concentration of potassium (K^+) in the intracellular space. In the absence of a potential difference across the cell membrane, the natural tendency of this system would be for a net diffusion of each ion species from higher to lower concentration. But because the electric potential inside the cell is negative compared to the outside, an electrical force that favors the motion of positive charges into the cell and negative charges out comes into play. The K^+ distribution is near equilibrium, in the sense that the tendency for the K^+ to diffuse down its concentration gradient and equalize the concentrations is balanced by the opposite tendency for the positive charges to accumulate on the negative potential side of the membrane. But the Na^+ distribution is far from equilibrium, and both the concentration gradient and the potential difference (the electrochemical gradient) across the membrane would tend to drive sodium into the cell. This is prevented at rest because the permeability of the membrane to sodium is very low.

However, the membrane permeability to sodium is sensitive to the voltage across the membrane so that, when the potential difference decreases, the permeability increases. The sodium permeability is a weak function of the potential inside the cell until the protential is raised to a critical threshold. Once this threshold is passed, the permeability increases sharply as the potential increases. The increased sodium flux into the cell raises the potential even more, further increasing the sodium flux. The result is a rapid depolarization of the membrane as the potential

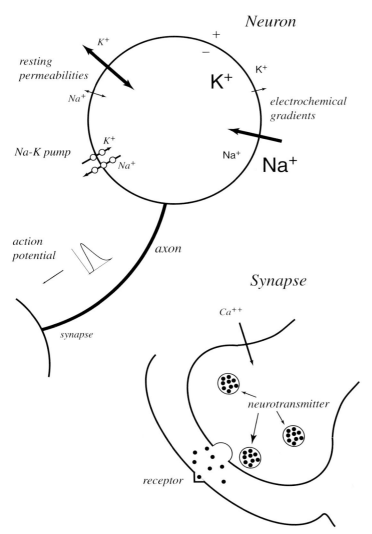

Figure 1.1. Neural activity. The schematic diagram shows the distribution and transport of the key ions, sodium, potassium, and calcium in the brain and the events following the arrival of an action potential at the synapse. The sodium distribution is maintained far from equilibrium by its low resting membrane permeability and by the action of Na-K-ATPase (the Na/K pump), which actively transports potassium into and sodium out of the cell. A transient increase in sodium permeability leads to a sharp depolarization of the membrane (an action potential), which travels down the axon and reaches the synapses with other neurons. The arrival of the action potential triggers an influx of calcium, which causes the prepackaged vesicles containing neurotransmitter to fuse with the membrane and spill into the synaptic cleft. Binding of the neurotransmitter to receptors on the postsynaptic neuron produces a postsynaptic fluctuation in the membrane potential. Recovery from neuronal signaling requires uptake and repackaging of neurotransmitter and restoration of ionic gradients, all uphill reactions that consume ATP.

inside the cell increases toward zero and even briefly becomes positive. The flux of sodium ions across the membrane in generating an action potential is then a passive approach to equilibrium as sodium flows down its electrochemical gradient and requires no driving energy. After a short time, the sodium permeability returns to normal, and the potassium permeability increases to return the potential to its resting value. The result of this process is that there is a net flux of Na^+ into the cell and K^+ out of the cell during the depolarization.

The action potential travels down the axon as the small current through a patch of the membrane triggers a change in the sodium permeability of the next patch. The propagation of the action potential over a long distance would then require a small leak of ions down the entire length of the axon. In longer nerve fibers this leakage is minimized by the myelin sheath that surrounds the axon. Myelin is a poor conductor, so ion currents are small. But for the action potential to be able to propagate, the myelin sheath is periodically interrupted by bare patches called the nodes of Ranvier. At these nodes the sodium and potassium fluxes occur, effectively allowing the action potential to jump from node to node. Although the redistribution of ions in the creation of an action potential is small, it is nevertheless a degradation of the original distribution. Over time the neuron will run down as the ionic concentrations move toward equilibration.

At a synapse with another neuron, the arrival of the action potential triggers an increase of the membrane permeability to calcium, allowing Ca^{++} entry into the presynaptic terminal. Within the presynaptic terminal, neurotransmitter is concentrated in small packages called vesicles. Through mechanisms that are not completely understood, the influx of calcium triggers these vesicles to merge with the cell membrane and spill their contents into the synaptic gap. The neurotransmitter molecules drift across the gap and bind to receptor sites on the postsynaptic terminal. Glutamate is a common excitatory neurotransmitter (Erecinska and Silver, 1990). When the glutamate binds to the receptors, the postsynaptic potential is slightly depolarized, moving the neuron closer to producing an action potential of its own. In contrast, at an inhibitory synapse, the binding of the neurotransmitter causes a change in the postsynaptic potential that opposes depolarization, acting to inhibit the neuron from generating a new action potential. A common inhibitory neurotransmitter is gamma-aminobutyric acid (GABA), which is biochemically derived from glutamate. In each case, the action of the neurotransmitter is to alter the local membrane permeability, and a slight shift in the ionic concentrations then alters the local membrane potential. The effect on the second cell may be excitatory or inhibitory, depending on the type of synapse, but either way a signal has been sent from one neuron to another in the form of a slight shift in the postsynaptic potential.

From a thermodynamic point of view, each of these steps in neuronal signaling is a downhill reaction in which a system held far from equilibrium is allowed to approach closer to equilibrium. The high extracellular sodium concentration leads to a spontaneous inward ion flow after the trigger of a permeability increase occurs. Similarly, the calcium influx occurs spontaneously after its membrane permeability is increased, and the neurotransmitter is already tightly bundled in a small package waiting to disperse freely once the package is opened. We can think of neuronal signaling as a spontaneous, but controlled, process. Nature's trick in each case is to maintain a system away from equilibrium, waiting for the right trigger to allow it to naturally move toward equilibrium.

The production of EPSPs, IPSPs, and action potentials illustrates that the brain, like any physical system, is constrained by thermodynamics. We can think of the set of intracellular and extracellular ionic concentrations as a thermodynamic system whose equilibrium state would be one of zero potential difference across the cell membrane, with equal ionic concentrations on either side. Any chemical system that is removed from equilibrium has the capacity to do useful work, and this capacity is called the free energy of the system. The neuronal system, with its unbalanced ionic concentrations, has the potential to do work in the form of neuronal signaling. But with each action potential and release of neurotransmitter at a synapse, the free energy is reduced. Returning the neurons to their prior state, with the original ion gradients and neurotransmitter distributions, requires energy metabolism.

ATP Is the Common Energy Currency in the Body

Restoring the sodium and potassium gradients requires active transport of each ion against its natural drift direction and is thermodynamically an uphill process increasing the free energy of the system. For such a change to occur, the Na^+/K^+ transport must be coupled to another system whose free energy decreases sufficiently in the process so that the total free energy decreases. The reestablishment of ionic gradients thus requires a source of free energy, and in biological systems free energy is primarily stored in the relative proportions of the three phosphorylated forms of adenosine: adenosine triphosphate (ATP), adenosine diphosphate (ADP), and adenosine monophosphate (AMP) (Siesjo, 1978). Inorganic phosphate can combine with ADP to form ATP, but thermal equilibrium of this system at body temperature strongly favors the ADP form. Yet in the body, the ATP/ADP ratio is maintained at a far higher value, about $10:1$ in the mammalian brain (Erecinska and Silver, 1994). The conversion of ATP to ADP thus involves a large release of free energy, enough to drive other uphill reactions. Despite the large free energy change associated with the reaction ATP to ADP, the ATP form is relatively stable against a spontaneous reaction. To make use of this stored free energy, the conversion of ATP to ADP is coupled to other uphill reactions through the action of an enzyme, generically referred to as an ATPase. The ATP/ADP system is used throughout the body as a common free energy storage system.

The transport of sodium and potassium against their existing gradients is accomplished by coupling the transport of ions to the breakdown of ATP to ADP. The enzyme Na-K-ATPase, also known as the Na/K pump, performs this task by transporting three sodium ions out of the cell and two potassium ions into the cell for each ATP molecule consumed. The Na/K pump is critical not just for energetic recovery from an action potential or a fluctuating postsynaptic potential, but also simply to maintain the cell's resting potential. The resting permeability to sodium is small, but not zero, so there is a constant leak of sodium into the cell. This excess sodium must be pumped out continuously by the Na/K pump, requiring a constant source of ATP. In addition, ATP is the indirect source of free energy for other processes that do not explicitly require ATP. For example, a mechanism exists to move bicarbonate ions into the cell in exchange for movement of chloride ions out of the cell (Thomas, 1977). The process is involved in the control of intracellular pH, and for both ions the direction of transport is against the concentration gradient and so is a thermodynamically uphill process. The free energy for this transport comes from the sodium gradient itself, by coupling the transport to an influx of sodium down its electrochemical gradient. Ultimately, the sodium gradient must be restored by the action of the Na/K pump and the consumption of ATP.

The recovery from neural activity at the synapse similarly requires a number of uphill processes. The excess intracellular calcium is pumped out of the presynaptic terminal by two transport systems (Blaustein, 1988). One mechanism directly involves ATP, transporting one calcium ion out of the cell for each ATP consumed. The second system is driven by the sodium gradient, transporting one calcium ion out in exchange for an inward flux of three sodium ions. Note that by either transport system, one ATP is required to move one calcium ion out of the cell because in the second system the Na/K pump will ultimately be required to consume one ATP to transport the three sodium ions back out of the cell.

At the synapse, the neurotransmitter must be taken up by the presynaptic terminal and repackaged into vesicles. For glutamate the process of reuptake involves a shuttle between the astrocytes and the neurons (Erecinska and Silver, 1990). Astrocytes are one of the most common glial cells in the brain, frequently located in areas of high synaptic density. The glutamate from the synapse is transported into the astrocytes by coupling the passage of one glutamate with the movement of three sodium ions down the sodium gradient. The transport of the sodium back out of the cell requires the action of the Na/K pump and consumption of one ATP. In the astrocyte, the glutamate is converted to glutamine, which requires an additional ATP, and the glutamine is then released back into the synaptic gap. Glutamine does not bind to the glutamate receptors and so is inert as far as neuronal signaling is concerned.

The glutamine is passively taken up by the presynaptic terminal, where it is converted back to glutamate. Repackaging the glutamate into the vesicles then requires transporting the neurotransmitter against a strong concentration gradient, a process that requires more ATP. One proposed mechanism for accomplishing this is first to create a strong concentration gradient of H^+ ions, with the H^+ concentration high inside the vesicle (Erecinska and Silver, 1990). The inward transport of neurotransmitter is then coupled to a degradation of this gradient. The H^+ gradient itself is created by an ATP-powered pump.

In brief, a source of free energy is not required for the production of a neuronal signal but rather for the reestablishment of chemical gradients reduced by the action potential and the release of neurotransmitter at the synapse. Without this replenishment, the system eventually runs down like an old battery in need of charging. The restoration of chemical gradients is driven either directly or indirectly by the conversion of ATP to ADP. To maintain their activity, the cells must restore their supply of ATP by reversing this reaction and converting ADP back to ATP. This requires that the strongly uphill conversion of ADP to ATP must be coupled to an even more strongly downhill reaction. In the brain, virtually all the ATP used to fuel cellular work is derived from the metabolism of glucose and oxygen (Siesjo, 1978). Both oxygen and glucose are in short supply in the brain, and continued brain function requires continuous delivery of these metabolic substrates by CBF.

CEREBRAL GLUCOSE METABOLISM

In the preceding discussion, neural activity was discussed in terms of a thermodynamic framework in which uphill chemical processes are coupled to other, downhill processes. For virtually all cellular processes, this chain of thermodynamic coupling leads to the ATP/ADP system within the body. But the next step in the chain, the restoration of the ATP/ADP ratio, requires coupling the body to the outside world through intake of glucose and oxygen. Despite the fact that a bowl of sugar on the dining room table surrounded by air appears to be quite stable, glucose and oxygen together are far removed from equilibrium. When burned, glucose and oxygen are converted into water and carbon dioxide, releasing a substantial amount of heat. If a more controlled conversion is performed, much of the free energy can be used to drive the conversion of ATP to ADP, with metabolism of one glucose molecule generating enough of a free energy change to convert 38 ADP to ATP. As far as maintaining neural activity is concerned, the chain of thermodynamically coupled systems ends with glucose and oxygen. As long as we eat and breathe, we can continue to think.

But before considering how glucose metabolism works, we can consider how this chain of coupled thermodynamic systems extends to the rest of the world. The supply of glucose and oxygen is maintained by plants, which convert carbon dioxide and water into oxygen and organic compounds including glucose. The source of free energy for this strongly uphill process is sunlight, and the degradation of sunlight is coupled to these chemical reactions in photosynthesis. The source of the free energy of sunlight is that the photons, which started off in thermodynamic equilibrium when they left the sun, are far from equilibrium when they reach the earth. The energy density and the spectrum of photons in thermal equilibrium are determined by temperature, with higher energy photons at higher temperatures. The distribution of photon energies in the light leaving the sun is set by the sun's surface temperature (about 5700 K). As these photons travel away from the sun, they spread out so that the density of photons at the surface of the earth is much reduced. As a result, the photons arriving at earth have a spectrum characteristic of a 5,700 K source but an energy density equivalent to thermodynamic equilibrium at a temperature of only about 300 K. In other words, the photons arriving at the surface of the earth can be thought of as a system far from equilibrium, with the energy concentrated in high energy photons, whereas thermodynamic equilibrium favors more photons with lower energy. The degradation of these high-energy photons to low-energy photons thus releases a tremendous amount of free energy, which plants couple to chemical processes through photosynthesis. Life on earth thus depends on sunlight to drive chemical synthesis. It is interesting to note that it is not primarily the *heat* of the sunlight that is critical but rather the *spectrum* of the photons. Just as glucose and oxygen can combine when burned to produce heat, the free energy of the photons warms the surface of the earth. The same amount of heating could in principle be supplied by a lower temperature source of photons, but these photons would be inadequate to drive photosynthesis. So the existence of life on earth ultimately depends on the fact that the sun is hot enough to produce high-energy photons, but far enough away so that the equilibrium temperature on earth is much lower.

Glycolysis and the TCA Cycle

We now turn to the question of how the combination of glucose and oxygen can be harnessed to produce ATP. The metabolism occurs in two stages: *glycolysis* and the *trans-carboxylic acid* (TCA) cycle (Figure 1.2). Glycolysis does not require oxygen but produces only a small amount of ATP. The further metabolism of glucose through the TCA cycle requires oxygen and produces much more ATP. Oxidative glucose metabolism involves many steps, and the following is a sketch of only a few key features. A more complete discussion can be found in Siesjo (1978).

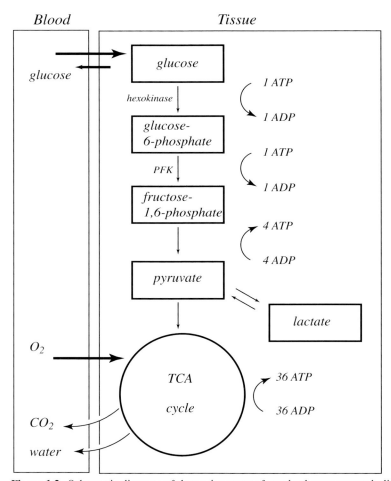

Figure 1.2. Schematic diagram of the major steps of cerebral energy metabolism. Glucose is taken up from blood and first undergoes glycolysis (the steps in boxes) to produce pyruvate, for a net conversion of 2 ADP to ATP. The pyruvate from glycolysis and oxygen extracted from the blood enter the TCA cycle and produce an additional 36 ATP. The waste products carbon dioxide and water are cleared from the tissue by blood flow.

In glycolysis, the breakdown of a glucose molecule into two molecules of pyruvate is coupled to the net conversion of two molecules of ADP to ATP. The process involves several steps, with each step catalyzed by a particular enzyme. The first step in this process is the addition of a phosphate group to the glucose, catalyzed by the enzyme hexokinase. The phosphate group is made available by the conversion of ATP to ADP, so in this stage of glycolysis one ATP is consumed and fructose-6-phosphate is produced. A second phosphorylation stage, catalyzed by phosphofructokinase (PFK), consumes one more ATP molecule. Up to this point two ATP molecules have been consumed, but in the remaining steps the complex is broken down into two pyruvate molecules accompanied by the conversion of four ADP to ATP. The net production of ATP is then two ATP for each glucose molecule undergoing glycolysis.

The possibilities for local control of glycolysis can be appreciated by noting that the activities of the key enzymes are sensitive to the local environment. Hexokinase is inhibited by its own product, so unless the fructose-6-phosphate continues down the metabolic path, the activity of hexokinase is curtailed. The step catalyzed by PFK is the major control point in glycolysis (Bradford, 1986). The enzyme PFK is stimulated by the presence of ADP and inhibited by the presence of ATP. In this way, there is a natural mechanism for increasing glycolysis when the stores of ATP need to be replenished. A number of other factors also influence the activity of PFK, including inhibition when the pH decreases, so it is likely that the cerebral metabolic rate of glucose (CMRGlc) can be adjusted to meet a variety of demands.

If the pyruvate is not further metabolized, it is reversibly converted to lactate through the action of the enzyme lactate dehydrogenase. The end point of glycolysis is then the production of two ATP molecules and two lactate molecules from each glucose molecule. But glycolysis alone taps only a small fraction of the available free energy in the glucose, and utilization of this additional energy requires further metabolism of pyruvate in the TCA cycle. In the healthy brain, nearly all the pyruvate produced by glycolysis is destined for the TCA cycle. The TCA cycle involves many steps, each catalyzed by a different enzyme, and the machinery of the process is housed in the mitochondria. Pyruvate (or lactate) and oxygen (O_2) must enter the mitochondria to become available for metabolism. At the end of the process, carbon dioxide and water are produced, and an additional 36 ATP molecules are created. The full oxidative metabolism of glucose thus produces about 18 times as much ATP as glycolysis alone. The overall metabolism of glucose is then

$$C_6H_{12}O_6 + 6O_2 \rightarrow 6CO_2 + 6H_2O \ (+ \ 38 \ \text{ATP})$$

Blood flow delivers glucose to the brain, but only about 30% or less of the glucose that enters the capillary is extracted from the blood (Oldendorf, 1971). Glucose does not easily cross the blood brain barrier, and a transporter sysem is required (Robinson and Rapoport, 1986). This type of transport is called *facilitated diffusion*, rather than active transport, because no energy metabolism is required to move the glucose out of the blood. Glucose simply diffuses down its gradient from a higher concentration in blood to a lower concentration in tissue through particular channels (transporters) in the capillary wall. The channels have no preference for which way the glucose is transported; consequently, they also transport unmetabolized glucose out of the tissue and back into the blood. Once across the capillary wall, the glucose must diffuse through the interstitial space separating the blood vessels and the cells and enter the intracellular environment. There the glucose enters into the first steps of glycolysis. But not all the glucose that leaves the blood is metabolized. About half of the extracted glucose diffuses back out into the blood and is carried away by venous flow (Gjedde, 1987). That is, glucose is delivered in excess of what is required at rest. The net extraction of glucose, the fraction of glucose delivered to the capillary bed that is actually metabolized, is only about 15%. Carbon dioxide, the end product of glucose metabolism, diffuses out of the cell and into the blood and is carried off to the lungs to be cleared from the body.

The Deoxyglucose Technique for Measuring Glucose Metabolism

The development of the deoxyglucose (DG) technique was a landmark in the evolution of functional neuroimaging techniques (Sokoloff, 1977; Sokoloff et al., 1977) (Figure 1.3 and Box 1). With this method it became possible to map the pattern of glucose utilization in the brain with a radioactive tracer, whose distribution in an animal brain can be measured by a process called autoradiography. In *autoradiography,* a radioactive nucleus is attached to a molecule of interest and injected in an animal. After waiting for a time to allow the tracer to distribute, the animal is sacrificed, and the brain is cut into thin sections. Each section is laid on photographic film to allow the photons produced in the decay of the radioactive nucleus to expose the film. The result is a picture of the distribution of the agent at the time of sacrifice.

However, autoradiography cannot be used with labeled glucose itself because the brain concentration of the tracer at any single time point is never a good reflection of the glucose metabolic rate. Suppose that glucose is labeled with a radioactive isotope of carbon (e.g., ^{14}C). At early times the amount of tracer in the tissue does not reflect the local metabolic rate because some of that tracer will diffuse back out into the blood and will not be metabolized. If we wait a longer time, the unmetabolized tracer may have cleared, but some of the ^{14}C tracer that was attached to the glucose that *was* metabolized has also cleared as carbon dioxide. In short, to measure the glucose metabolic rate with labeled glucose, measurements at multiple time points are required, and this cannot be done with autoradiography. It is this central problem that was solved with the deoxyglucose method. Deoxyglucose differs from glucose only in the removal of one of the oxygen atoms. This analog of glucose is similar enough to glucose that it binds with the enzyme hexokinase catalyzing the first step of glycolysis. But because of the difference between DG and glucose, the DG cannot proceed down the glycolysis pathway, and the process halts after the DG has been converted to fructose-6-phosphate. The result is that the radioactive label on DG essentially sticks in the tissue. It cannot proceed down the metabolic path, and the clearance of the compound from the tissue is very slow. After a sufficient waiting period to allow clearance of the unmetabolized fraction, the tissue concentration of the label is a direct, quantitative reflection of local glucose metabolism (Figure 1.3).

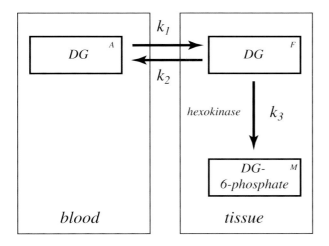

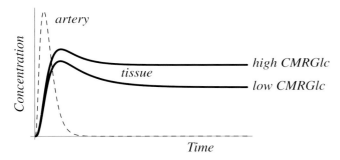

Figure 1.3. The deoxyglucose method for measuring the cerebral metabolic rate of glucose. The DG is metabolized similarly to glucose through the essentially irreversible phosphorylation catalyzed by hexokinase, but it cannot proceed farther and remains trapped in the tissue. The tissue concentration of the DG over time then shows an initial peak because more DG is taken up from the blood than will ultimately be metabolized. After a sufficient time for clearance of this unmetabolized fraction of the tracer, the tissue concentration directly reflects the metabolic rate.

With the adaptation of the DG method to positron emission tomography, studies of glucose metabolism were extended to the working human brain. Carbon-14, the radioactive tracer used in the DG autoradiographic method, cannot be used in humans because the electron emitted in the decay of the nucleus has a very short range in tissue, producing a large radiation dose in the subject but virtually no detectable external signal. In PET the radioactive tracers used are nuclei with an excess ratio of protons to neutrons, and the decay produces a positron. A positron is the antiparticle of an electron, with all the same properties as an electron except for an opposite sign of its charge. Normal matter contains only electrons, so a positron is an exotic particle. Positrons are emitted with substantial kinetic energy, which is dissipated within a few millimeters of travel through the tissue. When the positron has

BOX 1. DEOXYGLUCOSE TRACER KINETICS

In determining metabolic rates or CBF with radioactive tracers, the dynamic quantities that potentially can be measured are the arterial concentration and the tissue concentration curve over time. These time/activity curves are interpreted in terms of underlying physiological processes with a kinetic model, and we can illustrate the general approach with the deoxyglucose method. The uptake and metabolism of DG is modeled as shown in the upper part of Figure 1.3, with three compartments representing arterial blood *(A)*, free unmetabolized tissue DG *(F)*, and metabolized tissue DG *(M)*, with the assumption that the metabolized form remains trapped in the tissue during the experiment. In compartmental modeling such as this, each compartment is assumed to be well mixed and described by an instantaneous uniform concentration *C*. The kinetics of the tracer are then described by

$$\frac{dC_F}{dt} = k_1 C_A(t) - k_2 C_F(t) - k_3 C_F(t)$$

$$\frac{dC_M}{dt} = k_3 C_F(t)$$

The parameters k_1, k_2, and k_3 are first-order rate constants. In the first equation, the three terms on the right describe, respectively, the delivery of DG by arterial flow, clearance of unmetabolized DG passed back to the venous blood, and metabolism of DG. The arterial concentration curve $C_A(t)$ drives the system, and the resulting total tissue concentration $C_T(t) = C_F(t) + C_M(t)$ then depends on the values of k_1, k_2, and k_3.

Ideally, the values of the *k*'s for glucose and DG would be the same (i.e., transport and metabolism of the two molecules would be identical up to the point at which DG stops). Unfortunately, this is not the case, so a correction must be applied. But for now we can assume that glucose and DG behave identically to show how the tracer kinetic curve of DG is quantitatively related to the cerebral metabolic rate of glucose. If glucose metabolism is in a steady state with arterial glucose concentration C_0, then the rate at which glucose is delivered to the tissue is $k_1 C_0$. The fraction of this extracted glucose that continues down the metabolic path, rather than exiting into the blood, is $k_3/(k_2 + k_3)$. The metabolic rate (moles/g-min) is then

$$\text{CMRGlc} = C_0 \frac{k_1 k_3}{k_2 + k_3}$$

Turning now to the dynamic DG curves illustrated in Figure 1.3, there is an initial peak in the concentration, but over time C_T plateaus to a constant level. The peak occurs because more DG enters the tissue than will ultimately be metabolized, and the plateau occurs when the concentration in the first tissue compartment *(F)* has fallen to zero. In other words, by this time all the extracted tracer has either proceeded down the metabolic path or cleared from the tissue by venous flow. The important question is: How is the plateau DG concentration related to the *k*'s? We can answer this question with reasoning similar to that used earlier for glucose, taking into account the dynamic nature of the arterial DG concentration $C_A(t)$. The amount of DG entering the tissue in a short interval dt is $k_1 C_A(t)dt$, and so the total amount delivered during the experiment is the integral of this term. But only a fraction $k_3/(k_2 + k_3)$ of this extracted DG is metabolized and trapped, so the plateau tissue concentration is

$$C_T(\infty) = \frac{k_1 k_3}{k_2 + k_3} \int_0^\infty C_A(t) \, dt$$

This is the same combination of k's needed to measure CMRGlc, so the final expression is

$$CMRGlc = \frac{C_0}{LC} \frac{C_T(\infty)}{\int C_A \, dt}$$

where we have also included the lumped constant LC, which accounts for the fact that the k's are not the same for glucose and DG. The lumped constant is determined empirically by comparing DG measurements with CMRGlc estimates derived with another method (Reivich et al., 1985).

Although one could analyze the entire time/activity curve of DG to make separate estimates of each of the k's, the power of this technique is that the plateau concentration alone directly reflects CMRGlc. (In practice, corrections can be made for residual DG in blood at the time of measurement, and some loss of the metabolized DG, but these are usually small corrections.) The integrated arterial curve and the lumped constant essentially define a global scaling factor that converts measured DG concentrations into units of CMRGlc. For studies of absolute CMRGlc such scaling is necessary, but for comparisons within a study (e.g., comparing CMRGlc in two different brain regions) a map of DG concentration alone is sufficient.

slowed sufficiently, it will annihilate with an electron. In this process the positron and the electron cease to exist, and two high-energy photons are created. In this annihilation process, energy and momentum are conserved, with the energy of each photon equal to the rest mass energy of an electron (511 KeV), and the photons are emitted in two directions close to 180° apart.

The emitted positron thus annihilates within a few millimeters of its origin, but the two photons travel through the tissue and can be measured with external detectors. Furthermore, because two photons traveling in opposite directions are produced, the detectors can be coordinated to count only *coincidence* detections, the arrival of a photon in each of two detectors within a very narrow window of time. The detection of such a coincidence then determines the origin of the photons, the site of the radioactive nucleus, to lie on a line between the two detectors. The total count of photons along a ray is proportional to the sum of all the activity concentrations along the ray. By measuring many of these projections of the radioactivity distribution, an image of that distribution can be reconstructed in an analogous way to x-ray computed tomography (CT) images.

Positron emitting nuclei are particularly useful for human metabolic imaging because the nuclei are biologically interesting (e.g., ^{11}C, ^{15}O), the radioactive half-lives are short, and the decay photons readily pass through the body and so can be detected. A short half-life is important because it reduces the radiation dose to the subject, but this also requires that the isotope be prepared shortly before it is used, typically requiring an on-site cyclotron.

The PET version of the DG techniques uses ^{18}F-fluoro-deoxyglucose (FDG) as the tracer (Phelps and Mazziotta, 1985; Reivich et al., 1979). Fluorine-18 decays by positron emission with a half-life of about 2 hr. The tracer is injected in a subject, and after a waiting period of about 45 min to allow unmetabolized tracer to clear from the tissue, a PET image of the distribution of the label is made. In fact, PET images can be acquired throughout this period to measure the local kinetics of the FDG. Such time/activity curves can be analyzed with a kinetic model to extract estimates of individual rate constants for uptake of glucose from the blood and for the first stage of glycolysis (see Box 1). But the power of the technique is that the distribution of the tracer at a late time point directly reflects the local glucose metabolism.

To derive a quantitative measure of glucose metabolism with either the DG or FDG technique, two other quantities are required (see Box 1 for details). The first is a record of the concentration of the tracer in arterial blood from injection up to the time of the PET image (or the time of sacrifice of the animal in an autoradiographic study). The integrated arterial time/activity curve describes how much of the agent the brain was exposed to and essentially provides a calibration factor for converting the amount of activity measured in the brain into a measure of the local metabolic rate. The second quantity that is needed is a correction factor to account for the fact that it is really the metabolic rate of DG, rather than glucose, that is measured. This correction factor is called the *lumped constant* because it incorporates all the factors that make the uptake and phosphorylation rate of DG differ from glucose. An important question for the interpretation of FDG-PET studies in disease states is whether the lumped constant remains the same, and this question is still being investigated (Reivich et al., 1985).

The Association of Glucose Metabolism with Functional Activity

Over the last two decades numerous animal studies have clearly demonstrated a close link between local functional activity in the brain and local glucose metabolism (Kennedy et al., 1976; Schwartz et al., 1979; Sokoloff, 1981). An early monkey study examining the effects of visual occlusion showed a clear demonstration that the striate cortex is organized in alternating ocular dominance columns. This organizational pattern was known from previous, painstaking recordings from many cells, but the autoradiogram showed the full pattern in one experiment. These experiments also demonstrated that glucose metabolism decreases in association with a decrease of functional activity. When only one eye was patched, the ocular dominance columns associated with the patched eye appeared lighter (less exposed) on the autoradiogram than the columns corresponding to the open eye. With reduced visual input from the patched eye, glucose metabolism was also reduced.

Activation studies, in turn, showed an increase of glucose metabolic rate in the functionally active regions (Schwartz et al., 1979). Furthermore, with functional activity of different degrees, the change in glucose metabolism also showed a graded response (Kadekaro, Crane, and Sokoloff, 1985). The connection between functional activity and glucose metabolism through ATP-dependent processes was demonstrated by an experiment in which the activity of the Na/K pump was blocked by a specific inhibitor, with the result that the increase of glucose metabolism with electrical stimulation was suppressed (Mata et al., 1980). In short, animal studies with DG and autoradiography, and human studies with FDG and PET (Phelps and Mazziotta, 1985), have found a close correspondence between local neural activity and local glucose metabolism.

The Location of Glucose Metabolism in the Brain

In the brain, the consumption of glucose is heterogeneous. The metabolic rate in gray matter is three to four times higher than that in white matter. The low metabolic rate in white matter suggests that the energy cost of sending an action potential down an axon is small, most likely because of the efficient propagation along myelinated fibers. Instead, the energy metabolism is more closely associated with the synapses. Within the layers that make up cortical gray matter, the glucose metabolic rate is highest in layer IV, an area rich in synaptic connections. This area also shows the largest changes in CMRGlc with activation. High-resolution studies of the precise location of the increased glucose metabolism suggest that it is not the cell body of the neuron, but rather these areas of dense synaptic connections that show the largest increase in metabolic rate (Sokoloff, 1991).

The regions exhibiting high glucose metabolic rates also contain high concentrations of astrocytes, one of the nonneuronal cell types that make up about half of the brain. A recent theory proposes that glycolysis occurs preferentially in the astrocytes, and the resulting lactate is shuttled to the neurons for further metabolism by the TCA cycle in the mitochondria. Based primarily on work with cultures of astrocytes and neurons from mouse cerebral cortex and the retina of the honeybee drone (Magistretti and Pellerin, 1996; Tsacopoulos and Magistretti, 1996), the theory presents an appealing picture (Figure 1.4). Astrocytes are closely connected to the blood supply, with projecting endfeet that surround the capillary, so they are well positioned for uptake of glucose from the blood. Furthermore, glycolysis in astrocytes is stimulated by glutamate, a common neurotransmitter, and astrocytes are intimately involved in the uptake and reprocessing of this neurotransmitter. Glutamate released at the synapse is taken up by the astrocyte, converted to glutamine, and returned to the extracellular space where it is taken up by the neurons and converted back to glutamate, as described earlier. This suggests a possible mechanism for coupling neural activity to energy metabolism: the release of glutamate at the synapse stimulates glycolysis and lactate production, and the lactate is then transported to the neurons for oxidative metabolism and the further generation of ATP. In addition, the energy cost to the astrocyte of taking up one glutamate and converting it to glutamine is two ATP, which can be precisely met with the glycolysis of one glucose molecule. Additional support for this hypothesis was recently presented based on NMR studies of the metabolism of glucose labeled with ^{13}C (Sibson et al., 1998). With NMR it is possible to follow the chemical fate of the labeled carbon as it enters the brain as glucose and enters the glutamate pool through the TCA cycle. These studies in the rat cerebral cortex in vivo found that

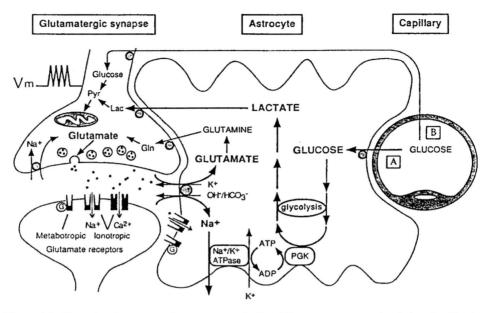

Figure 1.4. The role of astrocytes in energy metabolism. The astrocytes are closely involved in the uptake of the neurotransmitter glutamate from the synaptic cleft, and the conversion of it to glutamine, which then is taken up by the neuron and converted back to glutamate. By a current theory of energy metabolism in the brain, glycolysis occurs primarily in the astrocytes, and the lactate produced is then shuttled to the neurons for further oxidative metabolism. (Reprinted with permission from Magistretti and Pellerin, *Cerebral Cortex* **6**:50–61, 1996; copyright 1996 by Oxford University Press.)

the rate of glutamate-neurotransmitter cycling was closely matched to the rate of oxidative glucose metabolism. This model directly illustrates the close integration of neural activity and energy metabolism.

REFERENCES

Blaustein, M. P. (1988) Calcium transport and buffering in neurons. *Trends Neurosci.* **11**, 438–43.

Bradford, H. F. (1986) *Chemical Neurobiology.* W. H. Freeman and Co.: New York.

Erecinska, M., and Silver, I. A. (1990) Metabolism and role of glutamate in mammalian brain. *Prog. Neurobiol.* **35**, 245–96.

Erecinska, M., and Silver, I. A. (1994) Ions and energy in mammalian brain. *Prog. Neurobiol.* **43**, 37–71.

Gjedde, A. (1987) Does deoxyglucose uptake in the brain reflect energy metabolism? *Biochem. Pharmacol.* **36**, 1853–61.

James, W. (1890) *The Principles of Psychology.* Harvard: Cambridge, MA.

Kadekaro, M., Crane, A. M., and Sokoloff, L. (1985) Differential effects of electrical stimulation of sciatic nerve on metabolic activity in spinal cord and dorsal root ganglion in the rat. *Proc. Natl. Acad. Sci. USA* **82**, 6010–13.

Kennedy, C., Rosiers, M. H. D., Sakurada, O., Shinohara, M., Reivich, M., Jehle, J. W., and Sokoloff, L. (1976) Metabolic mapping of the primary visual system of the monkey by means of the autoradiographic [14C]deoxyhemoglobin technique. *Proc. Natl. Acad. Sci. USA* **73,** 4230–4.

Magistretti, P. J., and Pellerin, L. (1996) Cellular bases of brain energy metabolism and their relevance to functional brain imaging: evidence for a primary role of astrocytes. *Cerebral Cortex* **6,** 50–61.

Mata, M., Fink, D. J., Gainer, H., Smith, C. B., Davidsen, L., Svaki, H., Schwartz, W. J., and Sokoloff, L. (1980) Activity-dependent energy metabolism in rat posterior pituitary primarily reflects sodium pump activity. *J. Neurochem.* **34,** 213–15.

Nicholls, J. G., Martin, A. R., and Wallace, B. G. (1992) *From Neuron to Brain.* Sinauer: Sunderland, MA.

Oldendorf, W. H. (1971) Brain uptake of radiolabeled amino acids, amines, and hexoses after arterial injection. *Am. J. Physiol.* **221,** 1629–39.

Phelps, M. E., and Mazziotta, J. C. (1985) Positron emission tomography: Human brain function and biochemistry. *Science* **228,** 799–809.

Raichle, M. E. (1998) Behind the scenes of functional brain imaging: A historical and physiological perspective. *Proc. Natl. Acad. Sci., USA* **95,** 765–72.

Reivich, M., Alavi, A., Wolf, A., Fowler, J., Russell, J., Arnett, C., MacGregor, R. R., Shiue, C. Y., Atkins, H., and Anand, A. (1985) Glucose metabolic rate kinetic model parameter determination in humans: The lumped constants and rate constants for [18F]-fluorodeoxyglucose and [11C]-deoxyglucose. *J. Cereb. Blood Flow Metabol.* **5,** 179–92.

Reivich, M., Kuhl, D., Wolf, A., Greenberg, J., Phelps, M., Ido, T., Cassella, V., Fowler, J., Hoffman, E., Alavi, A., Som, P., and Sokoloff, L. (1979) The [18F]-fluoro-deoxyglucose method for the measurement of local cerebral glucose measurement in man. *Circulation Res.* **44,** 127–37.

Robinson, P., and Rapoport, S. I. (1986) Glucose transport and metabolism in the brain. *Am. J. Physiol.* **250,** R127–36.

Schwartz, W. J., Smith, C. B., Davidsen, L., Savaki, H., Sokoloff, L., Mata, M., Fink, D. J., and Gainer, H. (1979) Metabolic mapping of functional activity in the hypothalamo-neurohypophysial system of the rat. *Science* **205,** 723–5.

Sibson, N. R., Dhankhar, A., Mason, G. F., Rothman, D. L., Behar, K. L., and Shulman, R. G. (1998) Stoichiometric coupling of brain glucose metabolism and glutamatergic neuronal activity. *Proc. Natl. Acad. Sci., USA* **95,** 316–21.

Siesjo, B. K. (1978) *Brain Energy Metabolism.* Wiley: New York.

Sokoloff, L. (1977) Relation between physiological function and energy metabolism in the central nervous system. *J. Neurochem.* **29,** 13–26.

Sokoloff, L. (1981) The relation between function and energy metabolism: its use in the localization of functional activity in the nervous system. *Neurosci. Res. Prog. Bull.* **19,** 159–210.

Sokoloff, L. (1991) Relationship between functional activity and energy metabolism in the nervous system: Whether, where and why? In: *Brain Work and Mental Activity: Quantitative Studies with Radioactive Tracers,* pp. 52–67. Eds. N. A. Lassen, D. H. Ingvar, M. E. Raichle, and L. Friberg. Munksgaard: Copenhagen.

Sokoloff, L., Reivich, M., Kennedy, C., Rosiers, M. H. D., Patlak, C. S., Pettigrew, K. D., Sakurada, O., and Shinohara, M. (1977) The [14-C]deoxyglucose method for the measurement of local cerebral glucose utilization: Theory, procedure, and normal values in the conscious and anesthetized albino rat. *J. Neurochem.* **28,** 897–916.

Thomas, R. C. (1977) The role of bicarbonate, chloride and sodium ions in the regulation of intracellular pH in snail neurones. *J. Physiol.* **273,** 317–38.

Tsacopoulos, M., and Magistretti, P. J. (1996) Metabolic coupling between glia and neurons. *J. Neurosci.* **16,** 877–85.

2

Cerebral Blood Flow

THE BLOOD SUPPLY OF THE BRAIN

The Vascular System

Cerebral blood flow (CBF) delivers glucose and oxygen to the brain, so it is natural to suppose that local CBF varies with neural activity, as suggested by James in the second quote at the beginning of Part IA. Although we certainly know more about the changes in CBF with activation and in disease states than was known in James' time, a full understanding is still lacking, and some basic questions are still unanswered.

The vascular system that supplies blood to the brain is organized on spatial scales that span a size range of four orders of magnitude, from the diameter of a capillary (about 10 μm) to the size of a distribution volume of a major artery (about 10 cm). The complexity of the vascular system of the brain can be appreciated from

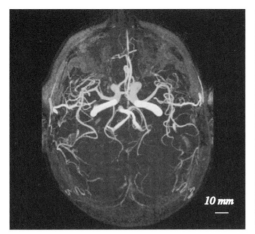
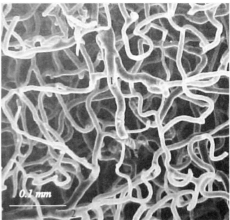
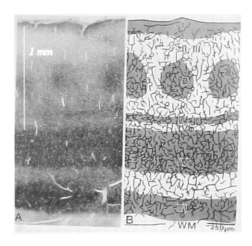

Figure 2.1. The vascular system of the brain. On the top left is a magnetic resonance angiogram showing the major vessels. On the right is a microscopic view showing the multidirectional orientation of the capillary mesh, taken from a cast of a human brain (Duvernoy et al., 1981). On the bottom left is a photomicrograph of a stained section through the lamina of the primary visual cortex of a monkey (Zheng et al., 1991). The staining indicates areas with high concentrations of cytochrome oxidase, an enzyme involved in oxidative metabolism, and highlights layers IV and VI and also blobs in layer II. The bottom right shows a camera lucida drawing of the vessels in the stained section, showing higher capillary densities in the stained areas. (Top right figure reproduced with permission from Duvernoy et al., *Brain Research Bulletin* **7:**519–579, 1981; copyright 1981 by Elsevier Science. Bottom figures reproduced with permission from Zheng et al., *J. Neuroscience* **11:**2622–2629, 1991; copyright 1991 by the Society for Neuroscience.)

Figure 2.1. On the top left is a magnetic resonance angiogram, showing the major arteries delivering blood to the tissue, and the veins carrying it back toward the heart. This angiogram shows vessels down to a few millimeters in diameter. On the top right is a microscopic view, showing the complex geometry of the smallest vessels, the arterioles, capillaries, and venules. This image was created from a cast of the microvasculature of a human brain (Duvernoy, Delon, and Vannson, 1981). The smallest capillaries have a diameter of about 6–8 µm, comparable to the size of a red blood cell. The bottom of Figure 2.1 shows images illustrating the distribution of capillary density within the layers of the cortex (Zheng, LaMantia, and Purves, 1991). On the left is a photomicrograph of a 1-mm wide strip from a cytochrome oxidase-stained section of a slice through the primary visual cortex (Area 17) of a squirrel monkey, and on the right is a camera lucida tracing of the blood vessels (mostly capillaries). Cytochrome oxidase is one of the enzymes involved in oxidative metabolism, and the uneven distribution of the enzyme in the brain suggests a heterogenous distribution of oxygen metabolism. In this study the microvessel density, as measured by the total length of vessels visible in the slice, showed a close correspondence with the cytochrome oxidase stained areas. The peak density in the cortex was in layer IV, where the density was about 1.5 to 3 times higher than that of white matter.

This study also shows how the functional organization of the brain is at least partially reflected in the blood vessel density. The border between the primary and secondary visual cortex (Areas 17 and 18) is distinguished by changes in the laminar structure, and the microvessel density correspondingly was found to be about 25% higher in the primary visual cortex. On an even smaller scale, in the primary visual cortex of primates, functional units called blobs have been identified based on their higher concentration of cytochrome oxidase. The blobs are located in layers II and III of the cortex and are about 250 µm in extent in the images in Figure 2.1. The capillary density in the blobs was about 40% higher than that in the interblob regions. In short, the architecture of the vascular tree shows distinct organization on a spatial scale as small as a few hundred micrometers.

The Meaning of Perfusion

Because many functional imaging techniques, including functional magnetic resonance imaging (fMRI), depend on changes in CBF, it is important to understand precisely what CBF is and how it can be measured. The term *perfusion* is used in a general way to describe the process of nutritive delivery of arterial blood to a capillary bed in the tissue. Because functional neuroimaging is potentially sensitive to several aspects of the perfusion state of tissue, it is important to clarify exactly what is meant by several terms. The *cerebral blood flow* is the rate of delivery of arterial blood to the capillary beds of a particular mass of tissue, as illustrated in Figure 2.2. For convenience, a common unit for CBF is milliliters of blood per 100 grams of tissue per minute, and a typical average value in the human brain is 60 ml/100 g-min. In some circumstances it is convenient to express this as flow delivered to a unit volume of tissue rather than a unit mass of tissue. In imaging applications a signal is measured from a particular volume in the brain, and the actual mass of tissue within that volume is not known. Because the density of brain is close to 1 g/ml, CBF values expressed in these units are similar. Note, however, that the units of CBF are then ml/ml-min, which are essentially units of inverse time. For this reason, it is sometimes useful to think of CBF as having the same units as a rate constant (e.g., 60 ml/100 g-min is equivalent to 0.01 s^{-1}).

The cerebral blood volume (CBV) is the fraction of the tissue volume occupied by blood vessels, and a typical value for the brain is 4% (CBV = 0.04). The CBV is a

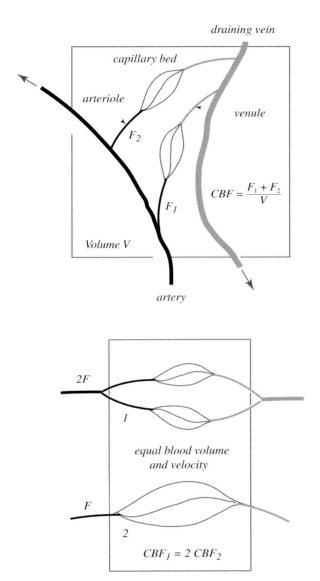

Figure 2.2. The meaning of perfusion. The top figure illustrates the blood vessels within a small element of tissue. Cerebral blood flow is the delivery of arterial blood to the capillary beds ($F_1 + F_2$), and so is not directly related to the local blood volume, which also includes arterial blood destined for a more distal tissue element and venous blood draining more distal tissues. The bottom figure shows that measurement of blood volume and blood velocity is not sufficient to measure CBF. In the lower capillary bed, the vessels are twice as long, so the blood volume and blood velocity are the same, yet the CBF is twice as large in the upper capillary bed.

dimensionless number (milliliters of blood vessel per milliliter of tissue), and usually refers to the entire vascular volume within the tissue. In some applications, however, it is important to subdivide total CBV into arterial, capillary, and venous volumes. Estimates of the relative sizes of these volumes vary, but typical numbers are 5% for the arterial volume, with the rest divided about equally between capillaries and veins (Pawlik, Rackl, and Bing, 1981). The blood volume can change in several distinct ways. The dilation of the arterioles that leads to an increase in flow is a volume increase on the arterial side, but this change is likely to be a small fraction of the total blood volume. Some data have suggested that at rest only a fraction of the tissue capillaries are open channels and that capillary recruitment (i.e., opening the previously collapsed capillaries) is involved in increasing CBF (Frankel et al., 1992; Shockley and LaManna, 1988; Weiss, 1988). However, the issue of whether capillary recruitment occurs in the brain is still being debated, and questions have been raised about the accuracy of the techniques used in these studies (Gobel, Theilen, and Kuschinsky, 1990). A number of recent studies have concluded that capillary recruitment is a small effect, if it occurs at all (Bereczki et al., 1993; Gobel et al., 1989; Klein et al., 1986; Pawlik et al., 1981; Vetterlein et al., 1990; Villringer et al., 1994; Wei et al., 1993). Finally, the venous vessels may expand in response to pressure changes, and because the venous side of the vasculature is a large fraction of the total blood volume, the venous volume change may make a large contribution to overall CBV change.

The velocity of blood in the vessels is also an important physiological parameter. Blood velocity varies from tens of centimeters per second in large arteries to as slow as 1 mm/s in the capillaries. At the capillary level, the pulsatility seen in the arterial vessels is largely damped out. But studies of the passage of red blood cells through individual capillaries have found that the flow is often irregular, rather than a smooth constant velocity (Villringer et al., 1994). This is likely due to the fact that the red cell diameter is about the same as the capillary diameter, and the red cells are deformable. One way to increase CBF is to increase the capillary blood velocity, and studies in rats have found such increases during hypoxia (Bereczki et al., 1993) and decreases with pentobarbitol (Wei et al., 1993).

Although CBF, CBV, and blood velocity are all important aspects of the perfusion state of tissue, they are distinct physiological quantities. With the preceding definitions, CBF does not explicitly depend on either blood volume or the velocity of blood in the vessels. An increase in CBF with brain activation could occur through a number of different changes in blood volume or blood velocity. For example, an increase of blood velocity in a fixed capillary bed or an increase in the number of open capillaries but with blood moving at the same velocity in each capillary would both lead to an increase of CBF. In both cases more arterial blood flows through the capillary bed. Furthermore, even specification of capillary velocity and capillary volume is not sufficient to determine CBF, as illustrated in the lower part of Figure 2.2. Two idealized capillary beds are shown, one with two sets of shorter capillaries, and one with a single set of capillaries twice as long. In both beds the blood velocity is the same, and we have constructed them to have the same capillary blood volume. But the CBF is twice as large in the upper bed with two sets of shorter capillaries because the volume of arterial blood delivered to the bed per minute is twice as great.

Intuitively, it seems that specification of the blood volume and blood velocity ought to determine CBF, but the preceding example shows that they do not. The missing piece that *does* differ between the two scenarios is the capillary transit time. In the capillary bed with the longer capillaries, the capillary transit time is twice as long. And it is transit time, rather than blood velocity, that is directly connected to CBV and CBF. The important relationship, known as the *central volume principle*, has been recognized for a long time (Stewart, 1894):

$$\tau = CBV/CBF \tag{2.1}$$

where τ is the mean transit time through the volume defined by CBV. For a CBF of 60 ml/100 g-min ($0.01\ s^{-1}$) and a typical CBV of 4%, the vascular transit time is about 4 s from this equation. By restricting the volume to a subset of the entire blood volume, such as the capillary volume, the relation still holds with τ defined as the mean transit time through the capillary volume.

In summary, the definition of CBF involves some subtleties that can be appreciated from Figure 2.2 In this idealized tissue vasculature, the flow rates through the two capillary beds are designated F_1 and F_2 (expressed in milliliters per minute), and if these beds feed a volume of tissue V, then CBF is simply $(F_1 + F_2)/V$. But an element of tissue will also contain in larger arteries arterial blood that is just passing through, destined for a capillary bed in another location. The tissue element may also contain venous blood passing through as it drains another tissue element. For these reasons it is difficult to make reliable measurements of CBF by looking at the blood itself within a tissue element, although such techniques are in use. For example, laser Doppler flowmetry (LDF) measures a frequency shift in light reflected from moving red blood cells (RBCs) (Dirnagl et al., 1989; Stern, 1975). The proportion of the reflected light that is Doppler-shifted is a measure of the number of moving RBCs, the total blood volume, and the average frequency shift is a measure of the average RBC velocity. Taken together, these data provide a measure of blood motion within an element of tissue. But this general motion of the blood does not necessarily reflect CBF, the flow of arterial blood into the capillary beds. For example, an element of tissue could have no change in CBF (e.g., F_1 and F_2 remain constant in Figure 2.2) but show increased RBC motion if CBF increases in a distal tissue element with a corresponding increase in speed of the arteries and draining veins that also happen to pass through the first element. The LDF technique is useful for studies of the microvasculature in animal models, but estimates of CBF with these techniques should be interpreted with caution. The central problem is that the defining characteristic of CBF is not blood motion *within* the tissue element but rather delivery of arterial blood *to* the capillary bed. For this reason, a more accurate approach for estimating CBF is to measure the rate of delivery of an agent carried to the tissue by flow.

MEASURING CEREBRAL BLOOD FLOW

The Microsphere Technique

The most direct way to measure CBF is to inject labeled microspheres into the arterial system. If these microspheres are carefully designed to be small enough to pass through the arterioles but large enough that they will not fit through the capillaries, then they will be trapped in the capillary bed. After injection in a large artery, the bolus of microspheres will be delivered to each of the tissue elements served by that artery in proportion to their respective local CBF. The number of microspheres lodged in an element of tissue is then a direct measure of the local CBF. Typically, this method uses radioactive microspheres, sectioning of the tissue, and then counting the radioactivity in each sample. For measurements at multiple time points, micropheres labeled with different radioactive nuclei can be used and then distinguished later based on differences in the energies of the radioactive decay photons (Yang and Krasny, 1995). Although widely regarded as the gold standard for perfusion measurements, microspheres are not appropriate for human subjects. However, a number of the techniques we will discuss are closely related, to the extent that they use a tracer that stays in the tissue during the experiment, like a microsphere, and can be measured externally and noninvasively.

The Nitrous Oxide Technique

A milestone in the development of techniques for measuring CBF in humans was the nitrous oxide technique (Kety and Schmidt, 1948). This was the first technique capable of producing quantitative measurements of global brain blood flow in humans, and it was quickly applied to investigate perfusion changes in a number of conditions. In this technique, the subject breathes NO_2 continuously for several minutes. During this time the arterial and venous concentrations of NO_2 are sampled frequently (e.g., from the carotid artery and jugular vein). The NO_2 diffuses freely from blood into tissue, and if the arterial concentration remains elevated for a sufficiently long time, the arterial, venous, and tissue concentrations of NO_2 will come into equilibrium. In this equilibrium state the concentrations in tissue, arterial blood, and venous blood are equal, and so this equilibrium condition carries no information about the flow. But the time required to reach this equilibrium is strongly sensitive to flow.

As an analogy, consider a large, well-mixed tank of water (the tissue) fed by an inlet pipe (arterial flow) and drained by an outlet pipe (venous flow), as illustrated in Figure 2.3. If dye is now introduced into the inlet side at a constant concentration, the concentration of dye in the tank will gradually increase until it comes into equilibrium with the inlet concentration. If the tank is well mixed at all times, the outlet concentration will approach the inlet concentration in an exponential fashion. The larger the rate of inflow, the more quickly the concentration in the tank will reach equilibrium. By observing only the inlet and outlet concentrations, the time constant τ for the outlet concentration to equilibrate with the inlet concentration can be measured. And this time constant is $\tau = V/F$, where F is the flow rate into the tank (ml/min) and V is the volume of the tank (ml). To generalize this idea to brain studies with an exogenous agent, the volume V is more precisely defined as the *volume of distribution* of the agent, the volume to which the agent has access and will eventually fill over time. Nitrous oxide freely diffuses throughout the brain, and so the volume of distribution is approximately the volume of the brain itself.

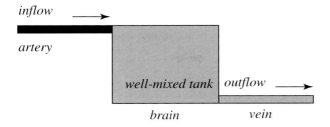

NO₂ Time/Concentration Curves

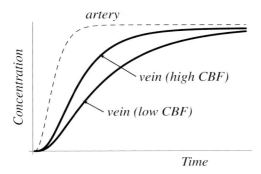

Figure 2.3. The nitrous oxide technique for measuring global cerebral blood flow. A subject breathes NO_2 continuously while the blood concentration of the agent is sampled in the carotid artery and jugular vein. Over time, the NO_2 will distribute throughout the brain, like a well-mixed tank being filled with fluid containing a dye, and the venous concentration will approach the arterial concentration. The time constant for reaching this equilibrium is inversely proportional to the global CBF.

Diffusible vs. Intravascular Tracers

Brain studies use a number of different tracers, but most of them fall into one of two basic classes, *diffusible* tracers or *intravascular* tracers, which differ in their volumes of distribution. Nitrous oxide freely diffuses out of the capillary bed and fills the entire tissue space, so its volume of distribution is essentially the whole brain volume. In contrast, an agent that remains in the blood has a volume of distribution that is much smaller, only about 4% of the total brain volume. For such an intravascular agent, the time constant for the venous blood to equilibrate with the arterial blood is correspondingly shorter. In other words, for the same flow the volume of distribution of an intravascular agent is quickly filled because the blood volume is only a small fraction of the total tissue volume.

For the nitrous oxide studies described earlier, the time constant τ was defined in terms of the global flow rate F, measured in milliliters per minute, and the volume of distribution V in milliliters. But for local measurements it is useful to define these quantities for a unit mass of tissue and to adopt the more standard definition of CBF as flow per gram of tissue, as discussed earlier, and the volume of distribution as volume per gram of tissue. In this book, we will use f to indicate CBF defined in this way, and the symbol λ to indicate the volume of distribution. Because both F and V are simply divided by a unit mass of tissue, the time constant for the local concentration of the agent to equilibrate with the arterial concentration is still $\tau = \lambda/f$. The standard units of f are then milliliters of blood per minute per gram of tissue, and the units of λ are milliliters per gram of tissue. However, in imaging studies a unit block of tissue is defined as a unit volume, rather than a unit mass, and it is often convenient to describe f and λ in units of milliliters per minute per milliliter of tissue and milliliter per milliliter of tissue, respectively. This definition has the advantage of simplifying the dimensions as well: the dimensions of f are simply inverse time, and λ is then dimensionless. For the human brain a typical value of f is 0.01 s^{-1}, corresponding to a CBF of 60 ml/min/100 g of tissue. For a diffusible tracer λ is approximately 1, and for an intravascular tracer λ is about 0.04, the typical blood volume fraction in the human brain. The time required for a diffusible agent to equilibrate in the brain is then on the order of 100 s, whereas τ for an intravascular agent is only about 4 s.

This difference in the equilibration times directly affects what can be measured with diffusible and intravascular tracers. Imagine that an agent is injected into the blood, and the tissue concentration of the agent is measured over time. After the agent has equilibrated within its volume of distribution, the tissue concentration of the agent is independent of flow but provides a robust measure of the volume of distribution. Just as with nitrous oxide, flow affects the kinetics of the agent only during its approach to this equilibrium. So an intravascular agent provides a robust measurement of CBV because that is its volume of distribution but a poor measurement of flow because it equilibrates so quickly. On the other hand, a diffusible tracer provides a robust measurement of flow because the flow-dependent part of the tissue concentration curve is much longer. With these basic ideas in mind, we can consider the development of techniques to measure local CBF with diffusible tracers.

The Radioactive Xenon Technique

The nitrous oxide technique made possible a measurement of global blood flow from measurements of the arterial and venous concentrations of the agent over time. However, this technique provides no way to determine local blood flow to a particular region of the brain. In principle, the flow to a smaller subregion of the brain could be determined by collecting the venous samples from a smaller vein that only drains that subregion, but this is not practical in human studies. An alternative approach measures the local tissue concentration of the agent itself. From the preceding arguments, each local element of tissue should come into equilibrium with the arterial concentration with a local time constant that depends directly on the local blood flow and volume of distribution of the agent. This type of measurement became possible with the introduction of radioactive tracers and external detectors for measuring regional concentrations of the agents. The use of diffusible radioactive tracers to measure CBF is illustrated in Figure 2.4 and described in more detail in Box 2.

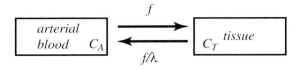

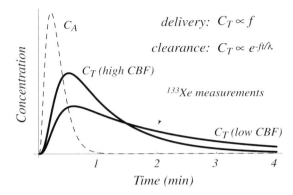

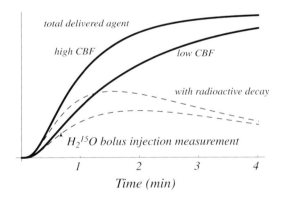

Figure 2.4. Measurement of CBF with diffusible radioactive tracers. The tissue concentration $C_T(t)$ of the agent is modeled in terms of the arterial concentration $C_A(t)$, the driving function of the system, and the local flow f and volume of distribution λ using the compartmental model shown at the top. Local flow affects both delivery and clearance of the agent. With the ^{133}Xe method, flow is estimated from the time constant for clearance, and with the PET $H_2^{15}O$ bolus injection method flow is estimated from the integrated activity delivered during the first 40 s.

In the 1960s, regional measurements of CBF in humans became possible with the introduction of radioactive inert gases (Ingvar and Lassen, 1963), most notably the ^{133}Xe technique (Obrist et al., 1967). Xenon is an inert gas that freely diffuses throughout the brain. The radioactive isotope ^{133}Xe decays with the emission of a photon that can be captured by an external detector on the surface of the head. The agent typically is administered by inhalation, entering the bloodstream in the lungs

BOX 2. MEASUREMENT OF CBF WITH A DIFFUSIBLE TRACER

A diffusible tracer is one that freely leaves the blood and enters the tissue so that its extraction E during passage through the capillary bed is near 100% and its volume of distribution λ is near 1. For any agent the volume of distribution is the fraction of the total tissue volume to which the agent has access. Inert gases, such as xenon, and water have volumes of distribution of approximately 1. The extraction of water in the capillary bed, particularly at high flows, is likely less than 100% (Herscovitch et al., 1987), but PET studies using water labeled with ^{15}O for many years have been the standard technique for quantitative CBF measurements. In studies with radioactive tracers, the time/activity curves in arterial blood and brain tissue are measured and related to the local value of CBF with the help of a tracer kinetic model (Lassen and Perl, 1979). The model most often used is shown at the top of Figure 2.4, and the corresponding equation for the tissue concentration C_T in terms of the arterial concentration C_A, the local cerebral blood flow f, and the volume of distribution λ is

$$\frac{dC_T}{dt} = f\, C_A - \frac{f}{\lambda}\, C_T$$

As in the deoxyglucose technique (Box 1), the arterial concentration of the tracer drives the system. The resulting tissue curve from this equation is

$$C(t) = f \int_0^t C_A(t')\, e^{-(t-t')f/\lambda}\, dt'$$

Representative curves for a bolus administration of the agent for two values of flow are illustrated in Figure 2.4. Note that because the arterial concentration is high for only a brief period (about 10–20 s), there is insufficient time for the tissue concentration to come into equilibrium with the arterial concentration, unlike the case for the nitrous oxide experiment.

The tissue curves in Figure 2.4 show that flow affects both the delivery and the clearance of the agent. With higher flow, more of the agent is delivered during the bolus, so the peak concentration is larger, and the subsequent clearance is more rapid. During the delivery portion the tissue concentration is proportional to f, and PET studies with a bolus injection of $H_2^{15}O$ measure the integrated activity over the first 40 s following injection of the tracer (illustrated in the lower part of Figure 2.4). By looking at the integrated activity, this technique overcomes a basic problem in the interpretation of time/activity curves of diffusible tracers: measurement of the tissue concentration at any one time point is not necessarily a good indicator of relative CBF. For the two flow values illustrated, the two curves cross during the clearance portion so that at later times the tissue concentration is higher for the lower flow. This ambiguity is eliminated by looking at the integrated activity over the early part of the curve, which is approximately proportional to f. The solid curves in the lower part of Figure 2.4 represent the tissue concentration of agent without taking into account radioactive decay, and the dashed curves show the true concentration of the radioactive label including decay with a 2-min half-life.

During the clearance of the agent after the arterial bolus, the tissue concentration decreases exponentially with a time constant λ/f. In ^{133}Xe studies this clearance portion of the curve is measured with external detectors registering regional activity. Unlike the measurements with tomographic techniques, this is not a true measurement of the tissue concentration of the agent but rather a measurement proportional to C_T. Nevertheless, the rate constant for clearance can be calculated from such measurements over time.

The $H_2^{15}O$ method and the ^{133}Xe method illustrate two broad classes of techniques for measuring CBF: those that measure delivery of an agent and those that measure clearance of an agent from tissue. In general, the methods based on delivery are more robust because they depend less on the details of the kinetic model used to interpret the data. This can be seen from the two ways in which f enters the equation for the tissue concentration. It appears in front as a multiplicative factor because of its role in delivery, and by looking only at the early portions of the tissue curve the subsequent fate of the agent is unimportant. If most of the delivered agent is still in the tissue at the time of measurement, then it is acting essentially like a microsphere, and the tissue concentration is a robust measure of CBF. In contrast, measuring CBF from the clearance portion of the curve is based on the second appearance of f in the equation, in the exponential decay term. But the mathematical form of this equation is valid only for the simplest compartmental model. For a more complex tissue (e.g., a sampled mixture of gray and white matter with different flows), a more complex model is required to model the clearance of the agent accurately. As discussed in Part III, the distinction between techniques designed to measure delivery and those designed to measure clearance also carries over to NMR techniques.

and traveling throughout the body in the arterial flow. After allowing sufficient time for the xenon to equilibrate in the brain, the supply of xenon is cut off, and the clearance of the agent from the brain is monitored. An array of detectors is arranged around the head, with each detector most sensitive to the nearest regions of the brain. Each detector then measures a regional level of radioactivity, which decreases over time. Clearance is accomplished by CBF, so the larger the CBF the faster the radioactive xenon clears from the tissue. The time constant for clearance is λ/f, where λ, the volume of distribution of xenon, is about 1 because xenon is a diffusible tracer.

PET Techniques

Radioactive xenon studies only allow measurement of regional flows because of the limited spatial selectivity of the detectors. But with positron emission tomography (PET), an image of the concentration of radioactivity in a brain section can be measured with a spatial resolution of about 1 cm^3. With dynamic measurements the concentration is measured as a function of time, referred to as a tissue time/activity curve. (Note that *activity* here refers to radioactivity, the number of measured radioactive decays per second, and not to neural activity in the brain.) The ability to measure the distribution of a radioactive tracer tomographically with spatial resolution on the order of 1 cm^3 made possible a much more detailed study of local CBF changes.

For blood flow studies with PET, the most common agent used is water labeled with ^{15}O, which has a radioactive half-life of about 2 minutes (Frackowiak et al., 1980; Raichle, 1983). Water is a diffusible tracer with λ near 1. There are two standard methods for measuring CBF with $H_2^{15}O$. In the first, the labeled water is injected and image data are acquired for the first 40 s after injection. Such a measurement is thus an integration over 40 s of the tissue concentration curve during the early phase as the tracer is delivered to the brain. The second method takes advantage of the short half-life of ^{15}O. Because the label is decaying away, there is another way for the agent to "clear" from the voxel in addition to venous flow. The water itself does not clear any faster, but the radioactive tracer marking the water disappears by radioactive decay, so for practical purposes the agent can be cleared from the tissue by two mechanisms. If the ^{15}O is delivered continuously from the arterial flow, a steady state will be reached in which delivery by flow and clearance by flow plus radioactive decay are balanced. At this steady state the tissue concentration provides a measurement of CBF, with a higher concentration when the flow is higher. Continuous delivery of the tracer is accomplished by having the subject breath $C^{15}O_2$. When the labeled CO_2 enters the blood through the lungs, the ^{15}O quickly exchanges with the oxygen of water to produce $H_2^{15}O$.

CONTROL OF CEREBRAL BLOOD FLOW

Vasodilatory Agents

Over 100 years ago, Roy and Sherrington described the basic principle that, at least in a general sense, has motivated thinking about the local control of CBF:

We conclude then, that the chemical products of cerebral metabolism contained in the lymph which bathes the walls of the arterioles of the brain can cause variations of the calibre of the cerebral vessels: that in this re-action the brain possesses an intrinsic mechanism by which its vascular supply can be varied locally in correspondence with local variations of functional activity (Roy and Sherrington, 1890).

The increased flow supports the delivery of glucose and oxygen, the substrates for local energy metabolism. In this way there is a natural balance between the energy demands of neural activity and the local energy supply, which depends on blood flow. If we broaden this proposal to include direct and indirect products of neural activity, this view is still widely held today, although the details are likely more complex than Roy and Sherrington imagined (Villringer and Dirnagle, 1995). A number of chemical agents have been found to have a vasodilatory effect on cerebral vessels, and several mechanisms for local control of flow have been suggested. Given the fact that CBF serves several functions, including delivery of glucose and oxygen and clearance of CO_2 and heat, it should not be surprising if several mechanisms exist for its control. Different conditions may trigger CBF responses in different ways to satisfy particular demands.

The rate of delivery of arterial blood to a small element of tissue depends on the pressure driving the blood through the vascular tree and the resistance that must be overcome along the way. Specifically, blood flow can be taken to be the ratio of the arterial pressure (P_a) to the cerebrovascular resistance (CVR): $CBF = P_a/CVR$ (this is essentially the definition of CVR). The arterioles are the smallest of the arterial branches, located just prior to the capillaries. Although they account for only a few percent of the vascular volume of tissue, they account for most of the resistance to flow in the vascular tree. In the healthy body, autoregulation operates to maintain CBF at a nearly constant value despite alterations in arterial pressure over a range from about 75 to 175 mmHg (Guyton, 1981). As pressure changes, CVR changes in a compensatory way by dilating or constricting the arterioles.

During brain activation the arterial pressure remains constant, but the resistance decreases due to dilation of the arterioles to increase local CBF. In fact, resistance is likely to be a steep function of arteriolar diameter. For laminar flow of a simple fluid, the resistance is proportional to $1/r^4$, where r is the radius of the vessel. Thus, to decrease the resistance of the arterioles by 100%, the radius of the arteriole need increase only 19%. Blood is not a simple fluid, and the flow is not likely to be purely laminar; nevertheless, this argument suggests a sensitive mechanism to control blood flow.

The diameter change of the arteriole is accomplished by a coat of smooth muscle surrounding the vessel, which contracts to constrict the vessel and relaxes to dilate it. Since smooth muscle requires oxygen to remain contracted, we might imagine that as oxygen is depleted by increased metabolism, the muscle relaxes, and CBF is increased to supply more oxygen. However, this hypoxia theory is almost certainly wrong (Lassen, 1991). Direct measurements of tissue oxygen tension, the partial pressure of oxygen (pO_2), showed two interesting facts. At rest, the pO_2 is already low, and with activation the pO_2 *increases*, opposite to what this theory would predict (Leniger-Follert and Lubbers, 1976). As discussed later, this occurs because the flow change with activation is much larger than the change in the cerebral metabolic rate of oxygen ($CMRO_2$), so the capillary and venous blood have a higher oxygen content, and the oxygen content of tissue is correspondingly increased.

One of the first chemical agents found to have a strong effect on CBF was carbon dioxide, which fits in nicely with Roy and Sherrington's original proposal because CO_2 is the natural end product of oxidative glucose metabolism. Carbon dioxide is a gas that readily dissolves in water; it combines with water to form bicarbonate ions (HCO^-_3) and H^+. This has two important consequences: the high solubility of CO_2 allows blood to carry it away efficiently from the tissue, and the amount of CO_2 present directly affects the pH. In fact, CO_2 has a potent effect on the intracellular pH of the brain because it passes easily across the blood brain barrier (BBB) and cellular membranes (Siesjo, 1978). In contrast, charged molecules do not easily cross the BBB, so a change in the pH of blood at a constant CO_2 level has little effect on the intracellular pH of brain. But raising the arterial pCO_2 from its normal resting value of about 40 mmHg to 60 mmHg by breathing a gas mixture enriched with CO_2 nearly doubles the global cerebral blood flow in monkeys (Grubb et al., 1974). The brain is evidently very sensitive to pH changes, and the large CBF response may serve to increase the clearance rate of CO_2 and provide some control over pH changes.

The global response to altered arterial CO_2 content is most likely a nervous response initiated by CO_2 receptors in the large vessels, but the evident importance of maintaining a constant pH in the brain suggests that H^+ may also exert a local control over CBF (Lassen, 1991). Numerous studies have shown that local acidosis causes dilitation and alkalosis constriction of the brain arterioles. Furthermore, animal studies have shown decreases in pH associated with the large flow changes accompanying induced seizures, consistent with the idea that increased H^+ produces an increase in CBF (Kuschinsky and Wahl, 1979).

In addition to H^+, other positively charged ions (cations) exhibit a strong vasodilatory effect. Increased potassium (K^+) and decreased calcium (Ca^{++}) in the fluid space around the cerebral arterioles both produce dilitation. And because neural activity involves an increase of extracellular K^+ and a decrease of extracellular Ca^{++}, there is a natural mechanism for increasing CBF in response to neural activity. This is known as the *cation hypothesis* for CBF regulation (Lassen, 1991). The role of potassium in stimulating blood flow may also involve the astrocytes. As noted in Chapter 1, astrocytes have endfeet that surround the capillaries, and increased potassium in the extracellular space causes the astrocytes to release potassium from their endfeet. This could provide a rapid mechanism for communicating K^+ concentration changes to the blood vessels (Paulson and Newman, 1987).

Another molecule with a demonstrated vasodilatory effect is adenosine (Dirnagl et al., 1994; Winn, Ngai, and Ko, 1991). Adenosine likely plays several roles in neurotransmission. It acts as a neuromodulator, and adenosine receptors are found on neurons, astrocytes, and the endothelial cells of blood vessels (Villringer and Dirnagle, 1995). The proposal for a direct role of adenosine in regulating blood flow is based on the idea that during activation the increased dephosphorylation of ATP (and ADP and AMP) leads to an increase in adenosine in the cells and extracellular space, which then triggers an increase in CBF to supply the needed oxygen and glucose.

Recently, the importance of nitric oxide (NO) in regulating cerebral blood flow has been recognized (Iadecola, 1993; Watkins, 1995). It diffuses rapidly through the tissue, is short-lived, and is a potent vasodilator (Villringer and Dirnagle, 1995). Furthermore, NO is produced locally from neurons and astrocytes following glutamate receptor activity, and it has been implicated in modulating the vasodilatory effects of virtually all the potential mediators of CBF control discussed earlier: CO_2, H^+, K^+, and adenosine. Thus, the full picture of the control of cerebral blood flow may involve complicated interrelationships between NO and other mediators.

A recent study demonstrates some of the complexities involved in sorting out the roles of different mediators of CBF control (Akgoren et al., 1997). In the rat cerebellar cortex, the activity of the large neurons, called Purkinje cells, is determined by two excitatory inputs, from axons called parallel and climbing fibers. These separate fibers make synapses on different parts of the Purkinje cells, and the synapses have different strengths, with the climbing fibers creating stronger excitatory postsynaptic potentials. By separately stimulating these fibers and recording the CBF change with laser Doppler flowmetry, these investigators could compare the mechanisms of regulation of the CBF response due to activity in synapses with different strengths in the same target cell. They concluded that the CBF response to both types of stimulus was reduced by 40–50% when local NO synthase activity was blocked, indicating an important role of NO. But they also found that the response to the climbing fibers, but not the response to the parallel fibers, was reduced with blockade of adenosine receptors, suggesting a role for adenosine in one type of synapse but not the other.

Finally, the principle of metabolic control may not tell the full story of local control of cerebral blood flow. There is a rich innervation of cerebral vessels which are active in cerebral autoregulation (Branston, 1995). This suggests the possibility that such mechanisms may be involved in local control of CBF during activation as well (Cohen et al., 1996).

Changes in Cerebral Blood Volume

Cerebral blood volume, although closely related to cerebral blood flow, is a distinctly different physiological quantity, as discussed earlier in the chapter. However, at some level, changes in CBF and CBV are linked because the change in CBF is accomplished by a change in the cerebrovascular resistance, and this is accomplished by dilating the arterioles. For example, consider the simple example of laminar flow in a straight cylindrical vessel introduced earlier. The resistance is proportional to $1/r^4$, where r is the vessel radius, and the volume for a fixed length is proportional to r^2. Suppose now that the vessel dilates so that the radius doubles to reduce the resistance and increase the flow. For a constant driving pressure, the flow increases by a factor of $2^4 = 16$, and the volume increases by a factor of 4. More generally, the relationship between the change in blood flow and blood volume for this example is that the volume change is proportional to the square root of the flow change. If the diameter of every vessel in the vascular tree is increased by the same factor, and the resistance to flow follows the $1/r^4$ law for every vessel, then the changes in CBF and CBV would follow this square root relation.

In a more general way, we can describe this type of relationship as

$$\frac{V}{V_0} = \left(\frac{F}{F_0}\right)^\alpha \qquad\qquad [2.2]$$

where F_0 is the resting flow, V_0 is the resting blood volume, and α is a numerical exponent. For this simple example, $\alpha = 0.5$. But in a real vascular tree, we would expect that the volume change necessary to produce a CBF change is much smaller because the cerebrovascular resistance is concentrated in the arterioles. Dilating the arterioles does increase CBV, but because the arterioles are a small fraction of the total blood volume ($< 5\%$), the net change in CBV is small. For example, suppose that the arterioles account for 5% of the blood volume but 50% of the cerebrovascular resistance at rest. Then, if the cross-sectional area of the arteriole doubles, with no change in the rest of the vascular tree, CBF increases by 60% due to a change of only 5% in CBV.

This argument suggests that the blood volume change *required* to produce a large flow change may be quite small. But a much larger volume change may accompany the flow change due to the distensibility of the vessels. The veins are described as the capacitance vessels in the vascular tree (Guyton, 1981). They are the most distensible and account for most of the total blood volume. Because of their distensibility, it is possible that large changes in the local venous blood volume may accompany CBF changes. When the resistance of the arterioles is reduced and flow increases, the pressure drop across the arteriolar segment is also reduced. This will increase the pressure in all later segments of the vascular tree, and depending on the distensibility of the vessels, this pressure increase can dilate the veins and possibly the capillaries as well. Changing the diameter of these vessels will also decrease the total resistance, but with less of an effect on flow than would be caused by dilating the arterioles. The result is that changes in blood volume are not likely to be evenly distributed along the entire vascular tree, and the veins, because they are the most distensible, may account for the majority of the volume change.

From these arguments, we can conclude that the CBV change required to increase CBF may be quite small, but that a much larger change in CBV, dominated by changes on the venous side, could occur as a passive response to the decreased arteriolar resistance. With these theoretical considerations in mind, we can examine the available data on blood volume changes in the brain with activation. Unfortunately, there have been far fewer studies of blood volume change than blood flow change. The classic paper of Grubb et al. (1974) is still the primary reference for the quantitative relationship between CBF and CBV changes. These investigators altered the inspired pCO_2 in monkeys and measured global changes in blood flow and blood volume. They then fit the measured pairs of CBF and CBV values to Equation [2.2] and found that the data were best described by $\alpha = 0.38$. In this experiment the total CBV was measured, so it was not possible to isolate the contributions of changes in the arterial, capillary, and venous blood volumes.

The relationship measured by Grubb and co-workers is really a steady-state relationship that results after the pCO_2 has been stable long enough for CBF and CBV to adjust to their new levels. But an important question is: how long does it take to reach these new levels? If the CBV changes are the *cause* of the CBF change (i.e., necessary to lower the resistance), then we would expect the two quantities to approach their new steady-state levels with the same time constant. On the other hand, if the CBV change is a passive response of the veins, the volume change may lag behind the flow change. The technology for measuring the dynamics of changes in CBV has only recently become available. Using a paramagnetic intravascular contrast agent, Mandeville and co-workers (1998) were able to monitor the local blood volume in rat brain with magnetic resonance imaging and a time resolution of a few seconds. They found that the blood volume change associated with stimulating one forepaw had a time constant of about 18 s to reach a new value, and a similar time was required for the volume to return to baseline at the end of the stimulus. This time constant is longer than has been observed for the flow response, which is typically a few seconds, suggesting that the major part of the volume change follows the flow change rather than causes it.

REFERENCES

Akgoren, N., Mathiesen, C., Rubin, I., and Lauritzen, M. (1997) Laminar analysis of activity-dependent increases of CBF in rat cerebellar cortex: Dependence on synaptic strength. *Am. J. Physiol.* **273,** H1166–76.

Bereczki, D., Wei, L., Otsuka, T., Acuff, V., Pettigrew, K., Patlak, C., and Fenstermacher, J. (1993) Hypoxia increases velocity of blood flow through parenchymal microvascular systems in rat brain. *J Cereb. Blood Flow Metabol.* **13,** 475–86.

Branston, N. M. (1995) Neurogenic control of the cerebral circulation. *Cerebrovascular and Brain Metabolism Reviews* **7,** 338–49.

Cohen, Z., Bonvento, G., Lacombe, P., and Hamel, E. (1996) Serotonin in the regulation of brain microcirculation. *Prog. Neurobiol.* **50,** 335–62.

Dirnagl, U., Kaplan, B., Jacewicz, M., and Pulsinelli, W. (1989) Continuous measurement of cerebral cortical blood flow by laser-Doppler flowmetry in a rat stroke model. *J. Cereb. Blood Flow Metabol.* **9,** 589–96.

Dirnagl, U., Niwa, K., Lindauer, U., and Villringer, A. (1994) Coupling of cerebral blood flow to neuronal activation: Role of adenosine and nitric oxide. *Am. J. Physiol.* **267,** H296–301.

Duvernoy, H. M., Delon, S., and Vannson, J. L. (1981) Cortical blood vessels of the human brain. *Brain Res. Bull.* **7,** 519–79.

Frackowiak, R. S. J., Lenzi, G. L., Jones, T., and Heather, J. D. (1980) Quantitative measurement of cerebral blood flow and oxygen metabolism in man using 15O and PET: Theory, procedure and normal values. *J. Comput. Assist. Tomogr.* **4,** 727–36.

Frankel, H. M., Garcia, E., Malik, F., Weiss, J. K., and Weiss, H. R. (1992) Effect of acetazolamide on cerebral blood flow and capillary patency. *J. Appl. Physiol.* **73,** 1756.

Gobel, U., Klein, B., Schrock, H., and Kuschinsky, W. (1989) Lack of capillary recruitment in the brains of awake rats during hypercapnia. *J. Cereb. Blood Flow Metab.* **9,** 491–9.

Gobel, U., Theilen, H., and Kuschinsky, W. (1990) Congruence of total and perfused capillary network in rat brains. *Circulation Res.* **66,** 271–81.

Grubb, R. L., Raichle, M. E., Eichling, J. O., and Ter-Pogossian, M. M. (1974) The effects of changes in PCO_2 on cerebral blood volume, blood flow, and vascular mean transit time. *Stroke* **5,** 630–9.

Guyton, A. C. (1981) *Textbook of Medical Physiology.* W. B. Saunders: Philadelphia.

Herscovitch, P., Raichle, M. E., Kilbourn, M. R., and Welch, M. J. (1987) PET measurement of cerebral blood flow and permeability-surface-area-product of water using [O-15]water and [C-11]butanol. *J. Cereb. Blood Flow Metabol.* **7,** 527–42.

Iadecola, C. (1993) Regulation of cerebral microcirculation during neural activity: is nitric oxide the missing link? *TINS* **16,** 206–14.

Ingvar, D. H., and Lassen, N. H. (1963) Regional blood flow of the cerebral cortex determined by 85-krypton. *Acta Physiol. Scand.* **54,** 325–38.

Kety, S. S., and Schmidt, C. F. (1948) Nitrous oxide method for quantitative determination of cerebral blood flow in man: Theory, procedure and normal values. *J. Clin. Invest.* **27,** 475–83.

Klein, B., Kuschinsky, W., Schrock, H., and Vetterlein, F. (1986) Interdependency of local capillary density, blood flow, and metabolism in rat brains. *Am. J. Physiol.* **251,** H1330–40.

Kuschinsky, W., and Wahl, M. (1979) Perivascular pH and pial arterial diameter during bicuculline induced seizures in cats. *Pflugers Arch.* **382,** 81–5.

Lassen, N. A. (1991) Cations as mediators of functional hyperemia in the brain. In: *Brain Work and Mental Activity: Quantitative Studies with Radioactive Tracers,* pp. 68–77. Eds. N. A. Lassen, D. H. Ingvar, M. E. Raichle, and L. Friberg. Munksgaard: Copenhagen.

Lassen, N. A., and Perl, W. (1979) *Tracer Kinetic Methods in Medical Physiology.* Raven Press: New York.

Leniger-Follert, E., and Lubbers, D. W. (1976) Behavior of microflow and PO_2 of the brain cortex during and after direct electrical stimulation. *Pflugers Arch.* **366,** 39–44.

Mandeville, J. B., Marota, J. J. A., Kosofsky, B. E., Keltner, J. R., Weissleder, R., Rosen, B. R., and Weisskoff, R. M. (1998) Dynamic functional imaging of relative cerebral blood volume during rat forepaw stimulation. *Magn. Reson. Med.* **39,** 615–24.

Obrist, W. D., Thompson, H. K., King, C. H., and Wang, H. S. (1967) Determination of regional cerebral blood flow by inhalation of 133-xenon. *Circulation Res.* **20,** 124–35.

Paulson, O. B., and Newman, E. A. (1987) Does the release of potassium from astrocyte endfeet regulate cerebral blood flow? *Science* **237,** 896–8.

Pawlik, G., Rackl, A., and Bing, R. J. (1981) Quantitative capillary topography and blood flow in the cerebral cortex of cats: An in vivo microscopic study. *Brain Res.* **208,** 35–58.

Raichle, M. E. (1983) Brain blood flow measured with intravenous $H_2^{15}O$: Implementation and validation. *J. Nucl. Med.* **24,** 790–8.

Roy, C. S., and Sherrington, C. S. (1890) On the regulation of the blood-supply of the brain. *J. Physiol.* **11,** 85–108.

Shockley, R. P., and LaManna, J. C. (1988) Determination of rat cerebral cortical blood volume changes by capillary mean transit time analysis during hypoxia, hypercapnia and hyperventilation. *Brain Res.* **454,** 170–8.

Siesjo, B. K. (1978) *Brain Energy Metabolism.* Wiley: New York.

Stern, M. D. (1975) In vivo evaluation of microcirculation by coherent light scattering. *Nature* **254,** 56–8.

Stewart, G. N. (1894) Researches on the circulation time in organs and on the influences which affect it. *J. Physiol. (London)* **15,** Parts I–III.

Vetterlein, F., Demmerle, B., Bardosi, A., Gobel, U., and Schmidt, G. (1990) Determination of capillary perfusion pattern in rat brain by timed plasma labeling. *Am. J. Physiol.* **258,** H80–4.

Villringer, A., and Dirnagle, U. (1995) Coupling of brain activity and cerebral blood flow: Basis of functional neuroimaging. *Cerebrovascular and Brain Metabolism Reviews* **7,** 240–76.

Villringer, A., Them, A., Lindauer, U., Einhaupl, K., and Dirnagl, U. (1994) Capillary perfusion of the rat brain cortex: An in vivo confocal microscopy study. *Circ. Res.* **75,** 55–62.

Watkins, L. D. (1995) Nitric oxide and cerebral blood flow: An update. *Cerebrovascular and Brain Metabolism Reviews* **7,** 324–37.

Wei, L., Otsuka, T., Acuff, V., Bereczki, D., Pettigrew, K., Patlak, C., and Fenstermacher, J. (1993) The velocities of red cell and plasma flows through parenchymal microvessels of rat brain are decreased by pentobarbital. *J. Cereb. Blood Flow Metab.* **13,** 487–97.

Weiss, H. R. (1988) Measurement of cerebral capillary perfusion with a fluorescent label. *Microvasc. Res.* **36,** 172–80.

Winn, H. R., Ngai, A. C., and Ko, K. R. (1991) Role of adenosine in regulating microvascular CBF in activated sensory cortex. In: *Brain work and mental activity: Quantitative studies with radioactive tracers.* Eds. N. A. Lassen, D. H. Ingvar, M. E. Raichle, and L. Friberg. Munksgaard: Copenhagen.

Yang, S. P., and Krasny, J. A. (1995) Cerebral blood flow and metabolic responses to sustained hypercapnia in awake sheep. *J. Cereb. Blood Flow Metabol.* **15,** 115–23.

Zheng, D., LaMantia, A. S., and Purves, D. (1991) Specialized vascularization of the primate visual cortex. *J. Neuroscience* **11,** 2622–9.

3

Brain Activation

PHYSIOLOGICAL CHANGES DURING BRAIN ACTIVATION

Blood Flow and Glucose Metabolism Increase with Functional Activity

In the second quote from William James that opened Part IA, he speculated that "Blood very likely may rush to each region of the cortex according as it is most active." With the development of tomographic techniques for measuring local cerebral blood flow (CBF) and the cerebral metabolic rate for glucose (CMRGlc), we now know that he was right. This rush of blood to activated areas is the physiological basis for most of the modern techniques of functional neuroimaging. Comparisons of CBF and CMRGlc changes have consistently found good agreement in the locations of the activation (Ginsberg, Dietrich, and Prusto, 1987; Yarowsky and Ingvar, 1981). With the development of positron emission tomography (PET), these types of experiments were extended to human subjects. For example, in a sensori-motor activation task, subjects were asked to discriminate between three classes of mah-jongg tiles by touch (Ginsberg et al., 1988). Four sequential PET scans were conducted on each subject to measure glucose metabolism with ^{18}F-Fluoro-deoxyglucose (FDG) and CBF using $H_2^{15}O$ in the resting and activated states. On average, in the area of the sensorimotor cortex associated with the task, the glucose metabolic rate increased by 17%, and the CBF increased by 26%. In another human study with PET and a sensorimotor task, changes of 50% in CMRGlc and 50% in CBF were found (Fox et al., 1988).

There is ample evidence that both flow and glucose metabolism increase substantially in activated areas of the brain. However, the observed correlation between changes in CBF and glucose metabolism does not necessarily imply a link between the two. Even though it is tempting to suppose that the flow increases to support the change in glucose metabolism, this is likely not the case. Several lines of evidence suggest that an increase in CBF is not required to increase CMRGlc. The first is the observation that at rest glucose is delivered in excess of what is required (Gjedde, 1987). That is, about half of the glucose that crosses the capillary wall is not metabolized and is eventually cleared from the tissue in the venous flow. This means that from the point of view of glucose delivery, CMRGlc could in principle increase by about a factor of 2 with no increase in CBF.

The second piece of evidence suggesting that glucose delivery is relatively independent of flow comes from a study in which the change in CBF with activation was measured at several levels of hypoglycemia (Powers, Hirsch, and Cryer, 1996). Despite the changes in glucose delivery to the capillary bed, there was no change in the CBF response. These investigators concluded that the CBF change is not regulated to match glucose supply with glucose demand. Finally, a recent study showed that blocking the production of nitric oxide in the neurons suppresses the CBF change during activation but does not affect the glucose metabolism change (Cholet et al., 1997), demonstrating that CMRGlc can increase without a change in CBF. These arguments taken together suggest that the CBF change is not *required* to support the CMRGlc change, even though the two physiological changes are closely correlated.

Oxygen Metabolism Increases Much Less Than Blood Flow

The cerebral metabolic rate of oxygen (CMRO$_2$) also can be measured with PET, but it is more difficult to measure than either CBF or CMRGlc because three different tracers are required to account for blood flow and blood volume effects properly (Frackowiak et al., 1980; Mintun et al., 1984). As a result, less data are available on CMRO$_2$ changes during activation. Studies of the *resting* distribution of CMRO$_2$ in the brain have found a rather uniform O$_2$ extraction fraction of about 40% (Marchal et al., 1992). The ratio of oxygen consumption to glucose consumption at rest is usually about 5 : 1, which approaches the ratio for complete oxidative metabolism of glucose (6 : 1). These data describe a simple and expected picture of coupled flow and metabolism at rest.

This close coupling of flow and metabolism also was supported by the CBF and CMRGlc measurements during brain activation described earlier, suggesting a straightforward picture of a localized, balanced increase in flow and metabolism with activation. This simple picture was challenged when Fox and Raichle (1986) measured the change in $CMRO_2$ associated with brain activation and made a surprising discovery. In a somatosensory stimulation experiment they found a focal CBF increase of 29% in the appropriate area of the brain, but only a 5% increase in $CMRO_2$. In a later visual stimulation study they again found a large imbalance in the CBF and $CMRO_2$ changes and confirmed that the CMRGlc change was indeed large and comparable to the CBF change (Fox et al., 1988). The large imbalance in the changes in CBF and $CMRO_2$ was described as an uncoupling of flow and oxygen metabolism during activation, in the sense that the large change in CBF seemed to serve some need other than increased oxygen metabolism. This finding focused attention on a fundamental question: why does flow increase so much with activation? From the arguments made earlier, the large change in CBF is not required to support the CMRGlc change, and the magnitude of the change is out of proportion to the small change in $CMRO_2$.

We will return to this question later and consider the hypotheses that have been offered. But first, it is important to consider the consequences of this experimental result. The finding that glucose metabolism increases much more than oxygen metabolism has immediate implications for the magnitude of the energy metabolism changes during activation. Most of the increase in the metabolic rate of glucose is glycolysis, and not full oxidative metabolism. This means that the actual change in energy metabolism is much less than would have been assumed from the increase in CMRGlc alone because glycolysis is much less efficient in generating ATP. The observed imbalance also implies that there should be a substantial production of lactate. This finding was confirmed with direct measurements of lactate accumulation in human subjects measured with spectroscopic NMR studies (Prichard et al., 1991; Sappey-Marinier et al., 1992).

In recent years functional magnetic resonance imaging (fMRI) has provided ample confirmation that the imbalance of flow and oxygen metabolism changes is not an artifact of the PET techniques but is instead a widespread physiological phenomenon (Prichard and Rosen, 1994). The Blood Oxygenation Level Dependent (BOLD) signal changes measured with fMRI result from this imbalance. If flow increases more than O_2 metabolism, less O_2 is removed from the blood and the venous blood oxygenation must increase. The magnetic resonance (MR) signal is sensitive to this change because deoxyhemoglobin (dHb) is paramagnetic, and the presence of dHb reduces the MR signal at rest. In the resting state the normal brain extracts about 40% of the O_2 delivered to it. Taking the average numbers measured by Fox and Raichle, if the flow then increases by 30% and the O_2 metabolism only increases by 5%, the O_2 extraction fraction must drop to about 32%. The deoxyhemoglobin concentration will then be reduced in the capillary and venous blood, and the MR signal will increase slightly. This MR signal increase during brain activation has now been measured during a wide range of sensory, motor, and cognitive tasks. Although the underlying reasons are still unclear, it appears that a strong imbalance in blood flow and O_2 metabolism is a common occurrence during brain activation.

Given the small observed change in $CMRO_2$, and the limited sensitivity of the techniques used to measure such changes, it is reasonable to ask whether there is any change at all with activation. In recent years, investigators attempting to model the BOLD effect have often adopted the simplifying assumption that there is no change in $CMRO_2$ with activation. But PET studies, with the exception of one (Gjedde et al., 1991), have consistently found changes in $CMRO_2$ that, although smaller than the changes in CBF, are nevertheless measurable (Fox and Raichle, 1986; Fox et al., 1988; Marrett and Gjedde, 1997; Roland et al., 1987, 1989; Seitz and Roland, 1992; Vafaee et al., 1998, 1999). Additional evidence for an increase in $CMRO_2$ with activation comes from an elegant experiment using MRI techniques for direct measurement of perfusion in conjunction with BOLD signal measurements (Davis et al., 1998). In these experiments, flow and BOLD signal changes were compared between two paradigms that both increase CBF: a sensory activation experiment and a paradigm that altered the CO_2 content of the subject's inspired air. Both activation and increased CO_2 are expected to alter CBF, but altered CO_2 has been found to have no effect on $CMRO_2$. In this way, the CO_2 experiment provides a calibration of the degree of BOLD signal change for a given flow change when there is no change in $CMRO_2$. The experimental result was that, for the same change in flow, the activation experiment showed a smaller BOLD signal change, consistent with a larger concentration of deoxyhemoglobin resulting from increased $CMRO_2$ during activation. In other words, the dHb production by increased $CMRO_2$ partially offset the dHb dilution due to the increased CBF. In short, although the change in $CMRO_2$ during activation is small, it is not zero.

WHY IS THE CBF INCREASE DURING ACTIVATION SO LARGE?

The Significance of Large Flow Changes with Activation

The question of why the CBF change is much larger than the $CMRO_2$ change remains the central question at the heart of functional neuroimaging. Most of the techniques in use today depend on large changes in CBF. If the change in CBF were smaller, matched to the change in $CMRO_2$, fMRI based on the BOLD effect would not be possible because there would be no shifts in blood oxygenation with activation. Recent optical and near-infrared techniques are also on detecting shifts in the deoxy- and oxyhemoglobin concentrations (Grinvald et al., 1991; Villringer et al., 1993). PET techniques using $H_2{}^{15}O$ would be hard pressed to detect the weaker signal changes due to smaller changes in CBF. Furthermore, if CBF changes are truly uncoupled from the metabolic changes, is it possible to interpret maps of CBF change in any quantitative way as a map of neural activity? That is, if the CBF change in one area of the brain is twice as large as in another area, are we justified in concluding that the change in neural activity was twice as great in the first area?

Empirically, the coupling between CBF change and functional activity is reasonably tight, both in location and in degree of change. For example, the human visual cortex has been a prime testing ground for exploring the connections between brain activity and metabolic changes. An early PET study measured the blood flow response of the visual cortex to photic stimuli of different frequencies (Fox and Raichle, 1984). The subjects wore goggles flashing a 5×6 rectangular grid of red light-emitting diodes with an adjustable flashing rate. The CBF response showed a consistent variation with stimulus rate, characterized by a roughly linear increase up to 8 Hz, followed by a gradual decline for higher flashing frequencies. At 8-Hz flicker rate the CBF increased by about 30%. In their original paper describing the BOLD signal changes with brain activation, Kwong and co-workers repeated this experiment and found that the BOLD signal showed the same pattern, increasing to a peak around 8 Hz and then decreasing slightly with higher flashing rates (Kwong et al., 1992). In this experiment, the BOLD signal closely followed the CBF change, suggesting that the change in blood oxygenation was altered in parallel with the CBF change. More recently, $CMRO_2$ was measured with PET using a different stimulus but again investigating the response to different stimulus frequencies (Vafaee et al., 1999). The visual stimulus consisted of a blue and yellow radial checkerboard, with the colors reversing at the different frequencies. In this experiment, the $CMRO_2$ change peaked at about 18% with a 4-Hz flicker rate, and at 8 Hz the $CMRO_2$ change was much less. Comparing these data with the earlier CBF data, the different responses at 8 Hz could be taken as evidence for an uncoupling of CBF and $CMRO_2$. However, these data should be compared with caution because of the different stimuli used. It is possible that a checkerboard reversing at a rate of 4 Hz is more similar to a flashing light at 8 Hz, because in both cases a new visual pattern is presented at a rate of 8 Hz.

Recently Hoge and colleagues reported the most convincing evidence to date for a close relationship between the CBF and $CMRO_2$ changes in the visual cortex (Hoge et al., 1999a, 1999b). Their data, based on the calibrated BOLD technique, showed a linear variation of CBF with $CMRO_2$, with the CBF change about twice as large as the $CMRO_2$ change. This technique and their data are discussed more fully in Chapter 16. Taken together, the available PET and fMRI data suggest that both CBF and $CMRO_2$ increase in a graded fashion with increasing neural activity, arguing against an uncoupling of flow and metabolism. However, the basic question of why the change in CBF is so much larger than the change in $CMRO_2$ still remains.

Several possible explanations for the small $CMRO_2$ changes have been proposed. An early suggestion was that oxidative metabolism at rest is already operating at the maximal rate possible (Berg, 1986). This was based on observations of tissue slices, which suggested that at normal tissue oxygen tensions the rate of oxygen metabolism was limited by the enzyme concentration rather than the O_2 concentration. A further need for energy metabolism associated with activation then must be met by glycolysis alone. However, large increases in $CMRO_2$ have been observed in seizures (Katsura et al., 1994), and although this represents an extreme form of activation, it does argue against enzymatic limitation of $CMRO_2$. Furthermore, this scenario only explains why the $CMRO_2$ change is small and the CMRGlc change is large, and the reason or reasons for the large change in CBF are unexplained.

Coarse Spatial Control of CBF?

Another hypothesis is that CBF is controlled on a coarse spatial scale, with areas of increased $CMRO_2$ occurring on a finer spatial scale. In studies of the cortical columns of the cat, the blood flow response was not as tightly localized to a column as was a brief initial *increase* in deoxyhemoglobin following a visual stimulus (Malonek and Grinvald, 1996). In these studies, the brain of a cat is exposed, and the reflectance spectrum of light off the surface is measured. Because oxyhemoglobin and deoxyhemoglobin have different reflectance spectra, it is possible to decompose the measured spectrum into contributions from oxyhemoglobin, deoxyhemoglobin, and a less specific scattered component. The spectra can be measured rapidly, and with high spatial resolution, so this technique provides a way to measure the dynamics of oxy- and deoxyhemolobin changes. The stimulus in these experiments was 2 s of either horizontal or vertical lines, which have been shown to stimulate distinct columns. The experimental finding was that there was a widespread decrease in deoxyhemoglobin that peaked several seconds after the beginning of the stimulus, consistent with a flow change much larger than the $CMRO_2$ change, but the spatial map of this flow change did not reveal the cortical column structure. However, an early initial *increase* in deoxyhemoglobin, prior to the larger decrease, provided a more robust map of the columns. The interpretation of this result was that this early increase in deoxyhemoglobin is due to a highly localized increase in $CMRO_2$ prior to the flow increase, and that the later flow increase occurs over a wider spatial area to support this small region of $CMRO_2$ change. In other words, the argument is that CBF is only controlled on a coarse spatial scale. This hypothesis has been poetically described as "watering the garden for the sake of one thirsty flower" (Malonek and Grinvald, 1996).

If confirmed, this model has important consequences for the ultimate spatial resolution obtainable with functional neuroimaging techniques that either directly or indirectly reflect blood flow changes. The limitation on spatial resolution may then be physiological, rather than technological, determined by the minimum volume of tissue over which CBF can be controlled. This model of highly focal $CMRO_2$ changes coupled with broader flow changes also suggests an interpretation of the imbalance of the flow and oxygen metabolism changes observed during activation. With spatial resolution typical of noninvasive functional neuroimaging, the average $CMRO_2$ change is diluted, but the average flow change is not, resulting in an apparent imbalance of average CBF and $CMRO_2$ changes.

The optical imaging results described are intriguing, and such studies will undoubtedly be important for achieving an understanding of the metabolic changes associated with activation. But it is not yet clear how specific these results are to the columnar architecture of the visual cortex, and whether coarse control of CBF can provide a general explanation for the observed low $CMRO_2$ changes accompanied by large CBF changes. The fact that fMRI studies have been successful in mapping activations in many areas of the brain suggests that the imbalance between CBF and $CMRO_2$ changes is widespread. One would expect that for some activation paradigms the region of activation would be sufficiently large that measured $CMRO_2$ changes and CBF changes would appear to be comparable. Such an experiment would then show a large CBF change, but little or no activation in a BOLD fMRI study. No such activations have been reported, although to our knowledge this has not been investigated systematically.

A counterexample to the idea of coarse control of blood flow is illustrated by experiments on the whisker barrel of the rat. Each whisker projects to a grouping of cortical neurons in the somatosensory cortex called a barrel, and deoxyglucose studies show a focal glucose metabolism increase in the appropriate barrel when a single whisker is stimulated (McCasland and Woolsey, 1988). In addition, studies of the angioarchitecture of the barrels indicates a separate arteriolar supply for each, making possible a highly focal blood flow response (Woolsey and Rovainen, 1991). Visual cortex columns and whisker barrels both may represent highly specialized metabolic architectures that are not representative of the rest of the brain. Further studies will be required to demonstrate that tissue heterogeneity of $CMRO_2$ changes and coarse control of CBF can provide a general explanation for the widely observed imbalance of CBF and $CMRO_2$ changes. Even if this explanation cannot account for the full observed imbalance of CBF and $CMRO_2$ changes, it likely will be a part of the explanation, particularly in experiments that activate small volumes of tissue. The issue of the extent of spatial control of CBF is critical for setting the ultimate limits on spatial resolution with fMRI, and further studies in other regions of the brain will be important.

Limited Oxygen Delivery?

An alternative hypothesis is that the observed imbalance of flow and oxygen metabolism changes, instead of being evidence for an uncoupling of the two, is a natural result of tight coupling of flow and metabolism in the face of limited oxygen delivery at rest (Buxton and Frank, 1997). Within the context of this *oxygen limitation model,* a large flow change is required to support a small increase in oxygen metabolism. The argument is based on two assumptions. The first is that oxygen delivery to tissue is "barrier-limited," which was suggested by Gjedde et al. (1991) and experimentally confirmed in a canine model more recently (Kassissia et al., 1995). The effect of this limitation is that only a fraction of the oxygen delivered to the capillary bed manages to leave the capillary and become available for metabolism, and the extraction fraction becomes dependent on the capillary transit time. The second assumption is that a CBF increase is accomplished by increasing the velocity of capillary blood rather than by capillary recruitment (Bereczki et al., 1993; Gobel, Therlen, and Kuschinsky, 1990). Then a CBF increase leads to a decreased capillary transit time and a reduced extraction of oxygen. The oxygen metabolic rate is proportional to the product of CBF and the oxygen extraction fraction *E.* The essential problem involved in increasing $CMRO_2$ is then that increasing CBF *decreases E,* and so the flow must be increased substantially to produce a small increase in their product. When this model is put on a firmer mathematical footing (Buxton and Frank, 1997), the prediction is that for a resting oxygen extraction fraction of 40% the flow must increase by 30% to support a 5% increase in oxygen metabolism, which is in good agreement with the PET results of Fox and Raichle. The oxygen limitation model is described in more detail in Box 3 and illustrated in Figure 3.1.

The picture of brain activation portrayed in the oxygen limitation model is then that flow increases substantially during activation to support a small increase in the

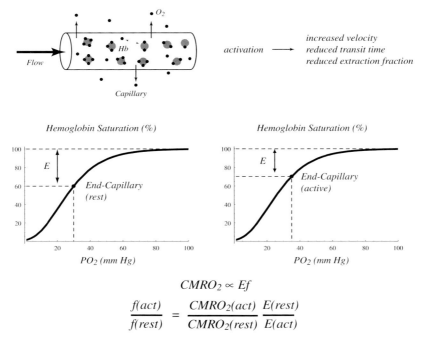

Figure 3.1. The oxygen limitation model for the coupling of flow and metabolism during brain activation. The basic idea of the model can be viewed in two ways (Buxton and Frank, 1997). If the extraction of O_2 is limited at rest and blood flow increases by increasing capillary velocity, then the capillary transit time drops, and the O_2 extraction is reduced (top). The average capillary plasma O_2 concentration drives the diffusion of O_2 into the tissue, so to increase $CMRO_2$ the average capillary pO_2 must increase, so the O_2 extraction must drop (middle). If the O_2 extraction fraction is reduced in activation, then flow must increase more than $CMRO_2$.

oxygen metabolic rate. But the change in the glucose metabolic rate is relatively independent of the flow change, in the sense that an increase of CMRGlc does not need to be supported by a flow change. In other words, despite the fact that the magnitude of the CBF and CMRGlc changes are similar and large, so that the $CMRO_2$ change appears to be the odd one out, by this model CBF and $CMRO_2$ are tightly coupled, and CMRGlc varies independently. This is consistent with the earlier arguments suggesting that CMRGlc can change independently of blood flow so that the primary regulation of blood flow during activation is not governed by the need for glucose delivery. Furthermore, because oxidative metabolism is so much more efficient at generating ATP, most of the additional ATP production occurs by oxidative metabolism even when the change in $CMRO_2$ is much smaller than the change in CMRGlc. For example, we can take the change in CBF to be 30% and the change in $CMRO_2$ to be 5%, as found by Fox and Raichle, and further assume that the change in CMRGlc is also 30%, the same as the change in flow. Then, assuming that all this increased metabolism is used to generate ATP, the ATP production rate increases by 7%, but 75% of this increase comes from the increase in oxidative metabolism (Buxton and Frank, 1997).

BOX 3. THE OXYGEN LIMITATION MODEL

The oxygen limitation model offers a relatively simple hypothesis for the uptake and metabolism of O_2 in the brain (Buxton and Frank, 1997). The essence of the model is that a large increase in CBF is required to support a small increase in $CMRO_2$, so that the observed imbalance of these changes with activation is nevertheless consistent with tight coupling of flow and oxygen metabolism. The model is based on two assumptions: (1) blood flow increases by increased capillary blood velocity rather than capillary recruitment, and (2) oxygen delivery is limited at rest, so that only a fraction of the O_2 molecules delivered to the capillary bed are extracted from the blood and become available for metabolism. To understand the significance of these assumptions, it is helpful to review the process of oxygen delivery to tissue.

Local cellular metabolism requires constant delivery of oxygen and constant clearance of CO_2, since one CO_2 is produced for each O_2 metabolized. The essential problem in transporting O_2 through the body is that it has a low solubility in water. Carbon dioxide, in contrast, readily dissolves by chemically combining with water to form bicarbonate ions. If O_2 and CO_2 as gases are maintained at the same partial pressure above a surface of water, the concentration of dissolved CO_2 in the water is about 30 times higher than that of O_2. The clearance of CO_2 by blood flow is then relatively simple, and the delivery of O_2 is the difficult task. Nature's solution has been to develop carrier molecules that readily bind oxygen in the lung and then release it in the capillary. In mammals this molecule is the hemoglobin (Hb) contained in the red blood cells, and it increases the O_2 carrying capacity of blood by about a factor of 30–50.

The O_2-Hb binding curve, the fractional saturation of the Hb as a function of the plasma partial pressure of O_2, has a sigmoidal shape. Figure 3.1 shows the Hb-O_2 saturation curve calculated with an algorithm developed by Buerk and Bridges (1986). In the lungs the plasma partial pressure of oxygen (pO_2) comes into equilibrium with that of the inspired air (about 150 mmHg). As long as that pO_2 is above about 80 mmHg, the arterial Hb is nearly fully loaded with oxygen. When the blood reaches the capillary bed, the O_2 diffuses into the tissue at a rate proportional to the plasma pO_2. Oxygen diffuses from capillary plasma to the mitochondria, driven by the gradient of pO_2 between the capillary and the tissue. If the pO_2 in the mitochondria is very low, then the flux down this gradient is approximately proportional to the pO_2 of plasma. By the time the blood reaches the venous end of the capillary, the resting brain has extracted about 40% of the O_2 that entered the arterial end.

Based on the foregoing arguments, we can describe the transport and metabolism of O_2 as a diffusive flux down an O_2 gradient from the capillaries to the mitochondria. If R is the average distance from a capillary to a mitochondrion, C_{cap} is the average O_2 concentration in capillary plasma, and C_{mit} is the average O_2 concentration in the mitochondria, then

$$CMRO_2 \propto \frac{C_{cap} - C_{mit}}{R} \qquad [B3.1]$$

because the net O_2 flux into the mitochondria (which is the metabolic rate of O_2) is proportional to the O_2 gradient.

(continued)

BOX 3, continued

This approach takes an essentially passive view, describing O_2 metabolism as a flux down a constant gradient. However, we also could take a more dynamic view in terms of the delivery of O_2 to the capillary bed by flow and the subsequent extraction of O_2 into the tissue space. Both views are important for understanding the oxygen limitation model. The rate of delivery of oxygen to the capillary bed is proportional to the local CBF. But for the oxygen to be of use for metabolism, it must pass through the capillary wall and enter the extravascular space. The important flux of O_2 for metabolism is then the rate at which O_2 enters the extravascular space, not the rate at which it enters the arterial end of the capillary. We can describe this by defining the unidirectional extraction fraction, E, as the fraction of the molecules entering the arterial end of the capillary that cross the capillary wall before exiting out the venous end of the capillary. Some of the extracted O_2 will reenter the capillary without being metabolized and clear by venous flow, so the net extraction fraction E_n will be less than E. Because the flux of O_2 into the capillary is proportional to CBF (which we will call simply f), and the fraction of that delivered O_2 that is metabolized is E_n,

$$CMRO_2 \propto fE_n \qquad\qquad [B3.2]$$

As we will see, a key question affecting O_2 transport is whether E_n is close to E or much smaller than E. An early proposed explanation for the much larger increase in CBF than $CMRO_2$ during activation was that the imbalance stems from the limited delivery of O_2 (Gjedde et al., 1991). Gjedde and co-workers suggested that the hemoglobin binding increased the apparent volume of distribution of O_2 in the blood so much that the effective permeability was greatly reduced so that virtually all the O_2 that is extracted is metabolized ($E_n \cong E$). They concluded that increases in $CMRO_2$ may be impossible unless the intercapillary distance is decreased or the capillary surface area is increased, and they found no evidence of a change in the permeability/surface area product in their studies of glucose metabolism. The idea that O_2 delivery is limited at rest, in the sense that a large fraction of the O_2 arriving in blood does not enter the tissue, is a central idea of the oxygen limitation model.

Recently, it was experimentally confirmed in a canine model that about half of the O_2 delivered to the cerebral capillaries never leaves the capillary, indicating a limitation on the delivery of O_2 (Kassissia et al., 1995). Although this is described as barrier-limited, or diffusion-limited, behavior, it is important to note that the terms are misleading when applied to oxygen. The capillary wall does not present an appreciable barrier to the diffusion of oxygen. In fact, O_2 is more soluble in lipid membranes than it is in water, so the permeability of the capillary wall is not the source of the limitation on delivery. Furthermore, the diffusion coefficient for O_2 is high, comparable to that of water, and so the time required for an oxygen molecule to diffuse across the width of the capillary is very short. Instead, the source of the limitation on delivery is that most of the O_2 is bound to hemoglobin (Hb) and the plasma concentration is low. The problem is not that the rate of exchange of O_2 between Hb and plasma is slow, because it is in fact quite fast (Groebe and Thews, 1992). It is simply that the equilibrium of this exchange strongly favors the Hb-bound form so that the plasma concentration of O_2 is only a few percent of the total O_2 concentration because most of it is bound. The O_2 must diffuse out of the capillary as dissolved gas in plasma, so the flux of O_2 across the capillary wall is proportional to the plasma concentration. In other words, the transport rate of O_2 across the capillary wall is much lower than it would be if all the blood oxygen were dissolved in plasma (i.e., the plasma concentration corresponds to a very large effective volume of distribution of oxygen in blood, as suggested by Gjedde and co-workers).

The effect of limited O_2 extraction at rest on the requirements for increasing $CMRO_2$ depends on exactly *how* blood flow increases. The first possibility is that new capillaries, identical to the original capillaries, open up to increase flow (capillary recruitment). The extraction fraction from each capillary is the same, and so E does not change. Then the increase in the rate of delivery of O_2 to tissue increases in proportion to the increase in flow because E is constant. The second possibility is that capillary blood velocity increases without capillary recruitment so that CBF then is proportional to capillary velocity. In this case, the capillary transit time will decrease, and so the extraction fraction will also decrease. Then the increase in the rate of delivery of O_2 to tissue is much less than the rate of increase of CBF because E is reduced. Although early animal studies suggested that capillary recruitment could be an important effect in the brain (Shockley and LaManna, 1988; Weiss, 1988), more recent studies have argued strongly against capillary recruitment (Bereczki et al., 1993; Gobel et al., 1989, 1990; Wei et al., 1993).

With these ideas of a diffusive O_2 flux (Equation [B3.1]) and dynamic extraction of O_2 (Equation [B3.2]), we can return to the question of how $CMRO_2$ can be increased. From Equation [B3.1], the flux from capillary to mitochondrion could be increased in three ways: (1) decrease R, the distance over which diffusion takes place; (2) decrease C_{mit}, the mitochondrial O_2 concentration; or (3) increase C_{cap}, the capillary plasma O_2 concentration. The central argument of the oxygen limitation model is that although all three of these options are in principle possible, the first two options are ineffective in the brain. Then the only way to increase $CMRO_2$ is to increase C_{cap}. The arterial O_2 concentration is fixed; to increase C_{cap}, the venous O_2 concentration must be increased, and this requires a *decrease* of the net O_2 extraction E_n. Then Equation [B3.2] can be satisfied only if f increases substantially more than $CMRO_2$ to overcome the reduction in E_n.

The ineffectiveness of the first two options for increasing $CMRO_2$ stems from the two assumptions of the oxygen limitation model given at the beginning of this box. Both assumptions are motivated by experimental results. To begin with, the O_2 flux could be increased by reducing R through capillary recruitment, the opening of previously closed capillaries during activation. However, the weight of evidence to date suggests that capillary recruitment does not occur (Bereczki et al., 1993; Gobel et al., 1989, 1990; Wei et al., 1993). The second assumption is that O_2 delivery is limited at rest. In terms of O_2 extraction, this means that the net extraction E_n is close to the unidirectional extraction E, and as described earlier, this is supported by experimental data (Kassissia et al., 1995). The OEF (oxygen extraction fraction) measured with PET is really E_n, the net extraction, and typical experimental values for human brain are in the range 30–50% (Fox and Raichle, 1986; Marchal et al., 1992).

Returning now to the more static view of O_2 flux down a gradient from capillary to mitochondrion, how do E and E_n relate to tissue O_2 concentrations? The difference between E and E_n is due to back-flux of O_2 from tissue to the capillary, which is driven

(continued)

BOX 3, continued

by the average O_2 concentration in tissue. In the limit $E \cong E_n$, there is little back-flux so the tissue O_2 concentration must be near zero. In this case, $C_{mit} \ll C_{cap}$, so the O_2 gradient cannot be adjusted by decreasing C_{mit} because it is already so low that the difference $C_{cap} - C_{mit}$ cannot be appreciably increased. If instead $E \cong 100\%$ (with $E_n \cong 40\%$), then C_{mit} would be closer to C_{cap}, and there would be more room to increase the O_2 gradient by decreasing C_{mit}. Or, to describe it in a different but equivalent way, if O_2 were delivered in large excess over what is needed at rest ($E \gg E_n$), then the need for increased $CMRO_2$ could be met by more efficiently utilizing the O_2 that is already extracted by increasing E_n (which is the same as reducing C_{mit}). But the experimental data indicate that E is close to E_n, and direct measurements of tissue pO_2 also suggest that mitochondrial pO_2 is much less than capillary pO_2 (Lubbers, Baumgertl, and Zimelka, 1994).

The basic argument of the O_2 limitation model thus can be stated in two equivalent ways. From the dynamic view, if extraction of O_2 is limited at rest and flow increases by increasing capillary blood velocity, then the transit time necessarily decreases and E is reduced. From the static view of O_2 flux down a gradient, because of the low tissue O_2 concentration and the fixed geometry of the capillary bed, the O_2 gradient can be increased only by increasing the average capillary pO_2, which requires a decrease of E_n. By both arguments the extraction of O_2 must be reduced to increase $CMRO_2$, so f must increase much more than $CMRO_2$ in order to increase the net delivery of oxygen, $E_n f$.

The assumptions of the oxygen limitation model are really a limiting form, meant to illustrate why a much larger change in CBF than $CMRO_2$ should be expected as a natural result of the tight coupling of the two. In reality, there is likely some room for adjusting the other physiological parameters affecting O_2 delivery as well so that the imbalance of the flow and metabolism changes would not be as large as the predictions of the model. Assuming the limiting case $E = E_n = 40\%$, the model predicts that the required fractional flow change is about six times the fractional $CMRO_2$ change (Buxton and Frank, 1997). This number is in good agreement with the original data (Fox and Raichle, 1986), but more recent studies have found ratios in the range of 2–3 in humans (Davis et al., 1998; Hoge et al., 1999b; Kim et al., 1999; Marrett and Gjedde, 1997). Such results are consistent with an increase of the effective O_2 diffusivity with activation (Hyder, Shulman, and Rothman, 1998). Capillary dilitation would provide some reduction in R, and C_{mit} is not zero, so there is likely some room for increasing the O_2 gradient by decreasing C_{mit}. Finally, animal studies in different levels of anesthesia have found ratios of CBF change to $CMRO_2$ change closer to 1 (Hyder et al., 1998). This result could be due to major modifications of the parameters affecting O_2 delivery, or it could be that the need to supply O_2 is not the controlling factor in these lowered activity states.

More detailed modeling of O_2 transport (Hudetz, 1999) and direct measurements of capillary flow dynamics (Kleinfeld et al., 1998) will be important for refining the oxygen limitation model.

Slow Changes in CMRO$_2$?

Finally, another hypothesis has been proposed for the coupling of CBF and CMRO$_2$ changes during activation based on the observed dynamics of the BOLD signal change (Frahm et al., 1996). In studies with sustained visual stimuli lasting several minutes, these investigators found that the BOLD signal change was initially strong but settled down to a much reduced plateau after about 1 min. At the end of the stimulus, the BOLD signal dipped substantially below the baseline level and required several minutes to return to the baseline (Figure 3.2). Although a strong initial overshoot of the BOLD signal has not been widely reported from other BOLD studies, the presence of a strong poststimulus undershoot is a common occurrence in BOLD data. These investigators proposed that this dynamic pattern is evidence that CMRO$_2$ changes are slow to follow CBF changes. The initial overshoot then results when CBF increases without a corresponding increase in CMRO$_2$, the plateau near zero occurs after the CMRO$_2$ has risen to its activated level matched to CBF, and the poststimulus undershoot occurs when CBF has returned to normal but CMRO$_2$ remains elevated and only slowly returns to baseline. This picture then involves an initial uncoupling of flow and oxygen metabolism, a recoupling after a few minutes of sustained activation, and a second uncoupling at the end of the stimulus. This hypothesis, based on observations of the transient features in the BOLD signal response, provides a consistent picture of the data.

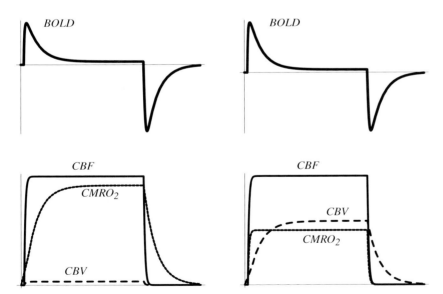

Figure 3.2. BOLD signal transients. Frahm and co-workers found BOLD signal time courses similar to the ones shown here with sustained visual stimuli (10 min or more) (Frahm et al., 1996). These BOLD transients are consistent with a CMRO$_2$ change that lags behind the CBF change so that the apparent uncoupling of CBF and CMRO$_2$ is only transient (left). However, such BOLD curves are also consistent with a CBV change that lags behind the CBF change (right). (BOLD curves were simulated using Equation [B16.4] in Box 16.)

But another interpretation also is consistent with these data. The BOLD effect depends approximately just on the total amount of deoxyhemoglobin within an imaging voxel, and this depends both on changes in the oxygen saturation of the blood and on changes in the blood volume itself. In other words, the BOLD signal change depends not only on the balance of changes in CBF and $CMRO_2$ but also on the change in cerebral blood volume (CBV). A large CBF increase with a small $CMRO_2$ increase lowers the fraction of the blood that is deoxygenated, and so would tend to produce a positive BOLD signal change. But an increase of CBV increases the amount of blood, and thus increases the amount of deoxyhemoglobin, and so would tend to produce a negative BOLD signal change. In other words, the large CBF change and the large CBV change have competitive effects on the BOLD signal change. Indeed, if the $CMRO_2$ change is as large as the CBF change, so that there is no change in the oxygen saturation of the blood, the CBV change would induce a negative BOLD change with activation (i.e., a signal drop in the activated state). Normally, however, the weak $CMRO_2$ change means that the BOLD change at the peak of the BOLD response is dominated by the flow change, so there is a strong positive BOLD signal.

But if the CBV change lags behind the flow change, there can be pronounced transient effects of the form reported by Frahm et al. (1996), as illustrated in Figure 3.2. A slow rise in CBV after the onset of activation will produce an initial overshoot of the BOLD signal because the blood volume has not yet reached its full steady-state value. Once that steady-state level is reached, the plateau BOLD signal is reduced. At the end of the stimulus, if flow returns quickly to baseline but blood volume returns more slowly, there will be a poststimulus undershoot. In the recent work of Mandeville et al. (1998), in which they measured a slow return to baseline of CBV in a rat model, they also measured the BOLD signal response to the same stimulation. They observed a poststimulus undershoot in the BOLD signal, and the time required for the undershoot to resolve was closely matched with the time required for the blood volume to return to baseline. Furthermore, with a calibrated BOLD experiment that allowed dynamic measurements of the $CMRO_2$ change as well, they found that the dynamic $CMRO_2$ change closely followed the CBF change (Mandeville et al., 1999a). Although the time constant for the poststimulus undershoot in these rat experiments was shorter than the very long time constants observed by Frahm and colleagues in human studies with visual stimulation, these data nevertheless provide support for the idea that blood volume changes lag behind blood flow changes and can create strong transients in the BOLD signal.

Recently, two similar biomechanical models were proposed to describe a lagging blood volume change: the delayed compliance model (Mandeville et al., 1999b) and the balloon model (Buxton, Wong, and Frank, 1998). Both models attempt to include mechanical properties of the vessels to account for the dynamic changes in blood volume following pressure changes induced by the change in arteriolar resistance. These models produce dynamic BOLD response curves with a poststimulus undershoot due just to the lagging volume change, even though CBF and $CMRO_2$ remain tightly coupled throughout.

SUMMARY OF PHYSIOLOGICAL CHANGES IN THE BRAIN PERFUSION STATE DURING ACTIVATION

The introduction to studies of brain metabolism in these first three chapters should indicate that much has been learned since James' day, but a number of fundamental questions remain unanswered. What is the function served by the large increase in CBF during activation? Are CBF and $CMRO_2$ coupled during activation? Are CBF and CMRGlc uncoupled? Is the relation between the changes in CBF and CBV uniform, or does it vary across the brain? Is there one primary mechanism for regulating CBF, or several? Is NO the primary mediator of CBF changes? These are areas of intense active research. Nevertheless, from the experimental data we can piece together an empirical picture of the physiological changes that accompany brain activation and form the basis for functional neuroimaging (Figure 3.3).

The primary finding, which makes possible PET and fMRI studies of brain activation, is that CBF increases substantially. The increase is localized, but the fineness of the spatial control of CBF is still debated. The flow change is a graded response in

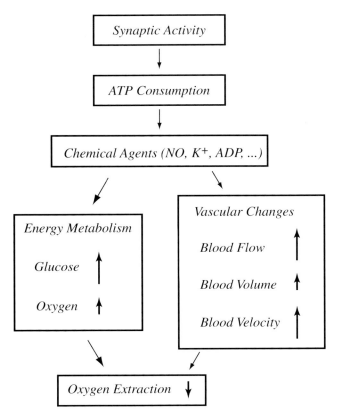

Figure 3.3. Physiological changes accompanying brain activation. Functional neuroimaging is largely based on the metabolism and flow changes in the lower three blocks. The drop in oxygen extraction is the basis of the BOLD signal changes measured with fMRI, but the MR signal is potentially sensitive to blood flow, volume, and velocity as well.

the sense that the magnitude of the flow change is often correlated with other measures of the degree of neural activity. For example, the flow response in the visual cortex to a flashing checkerboard pattern increases as the flicker rate is increased up to about 8 Hz and then slowly declines (Fox and Raichle, 1991), and in the auditory cortex the flow response increases with stimulus rate (Binder et al., 1994). Experimental results such as this support the idea that CBF change reflects not just the location of the activated area but also the degree of activation.

The second finding, which is essential for fMRI sensitivity to brain activation, is that $CMRO_2$ increases much less than CBF. The ratio of percent change in CBF to percent change in $CMRO_2$ has been found to be in the range of 3–6 in PET studies (Fox and Raichle, 1986; Seitz and Roland, 1992) and in the range 2–3 in fMRI studies using hypercapnia to calibrate the BOLD effect (Davis et al., 1998; Hoge et al., 1999b; Kim et al., 1999). The result of this imbalance in the changes of CBF and $CMRO_2$ is a substantial drop in oxygen extraction and a corresponding drop in the deoxyhemoglobin content of the venous blood. This produces the BOLD change in the MR signal.

Even though PET techniques directly measure CBF, the BOLD signal change depends on the combined changes in CBF, $CMRO_2$, and CBV, which complicates interpretation of the BOLD signal in terms of physiological variables. Animal and human studies using radioactive tracers and altered pCO_2 as a means of changing global brain perfusion have found an increase in cerebral blood volume accompanying increased flow (Greenberg et al., 1978; Grubb et al., 1974; Sakai et al., 1985; Smith et al., 1971). The BOLD effect essentially depends on the total amount of deoxyhemoglobin within an image voxel. Assuming that the CBV change is primarily on the venous side, increased CBV tends to increase local deoxyhemoglobin content simply because the volume of venous blood increases. This increase tends to counteract the effects of altered blood oxygenation, which decreases the deoxyhemoglobin content. Under normal circumstances the blood oxygenation effect dominates the blood volume effect, so the BOLD signal change is positive with activation, corresponding to a net decrease in the local deoxyhemoglobin content. This decrease of deoxyhemoglobin has been measured directly with optical (Malonek and Grinvald, 1996) and near-infrared techniques (Villringer et al., 1993). Studies in adult humans have consistently found a decrease in deoxyhemoglobin with activation; however, a recent intriguing report showed an *increase* in deoxyhemoglobin in infants aged 3 days to 14 weeks (Meek et al., 1998). If confirmed, this result could be due to a smaller increase in CBF, a larger increase in $CMRO_2$, or a larger increase in CBV in infants.

The physiological mechanism by which perfusion increases has been controversial. We can imagine two distinct scenarios that bracket a range of possibilities, and evidence has been presented for both views. The first is *capillary recruitment,* in which the flow characteristics within a capillary (velocity, size, etc.) remain constant but more capillaries open up. The second is *increased velocity* through a fixed capillary bed. Although some studies have indicated that at rest as few as 60% of available capillaries are perfused and that this fraction then increases when perfusion increases (Frankel et al., 1992; Shockley and LaManna, 1988; Weiss, 1988), a number of other studies have found that at least 90% of capillaries are open at rest so that perfusion must increase by increased capillary velocity (Bereczki et al., 1993; Gobel et al., 1989, 1990; Pawlik, Rackl, and Bing, 1981; Wei et al., 1993). Note that the observation of increased total blood volume is consistent with either mechanism because the methods used cannot distinguish between capillary, venous, or arterial volume change. Even with a completely fixed capillary bed, the veins may swell as a passive response to a local pressure increase, which might be expected after the arterioles dilate to reduce the local vascular resistance. Although capillary recruitment now seems unlikely, the capillary volume may increase by dilitation (Atkinson, Anderson, and Anderson, 1990; Duelli and Kuschinsky, 1993).

The physiological picture of what happens during brain activation is thus still incomplete. The evidence to date suggests the following scenario: cerebral blood flow increases substantially, cerebral blood volume increases moderately, the O_2 metabolic rate increases slightly, the O_2 extraction fraction drops substantially, and the local blood velocity in the arterioles, capillaries, and venules increases with an accompanying drop in the blood transit time, while the capillary density probably stays about the same (but may increase). With these changes in mind, we can begin to explore the ways in which MRI can be made sensitive to these effects so that we can map patterns of brain activation. Chapter 4–6 give an overview of how MRI works and how different fMRI techniques are sensitive to these physiological changes during activation.

REFERENCES

Atkinson, J. L. D., Anderson, R. E., and Anderson, Jr., T. M. S. (1990) The effect of carbon dioxide on the diameter of brain capillaries. *Brain Res.* **517,** 333–40.

Bereczki, D., Wei, L., Otsuka, T., Acuff, V., Pettigrew, K., Patlak, C., and Fenstermacher, J. (1993) Hypoxia increases velocity of blood flow through parenchymal microvascular systems in rat brain. *J. Cereb. Blood Flow Metabol.* **13,** 475–86.

Berg, C. V. d. (1986) On the relation between energy transformations in the brain and mental activities. In: *Energetics and Human Information Processing,* pp. 131–5. Eds. G. R. J. Hockey, M. G. Gaillard, and H. Coles. Nijhoff: Boston.

Binder, J. R., Rao, S. M., Hammeke, T. A., Frost, J. A., Bandettini, P. A., and Hyde, J. S. (1994) Effects of stimulus rate on signal response during functional magnetic resonance imaging of auditory cortex. *Cognitive Brain Res.* **2,** 31–8.

Buerk, D. G., and Bridges, E. W. (1986) A simplified algorithm for computing the variation in oxyhemoglobin saturation with pH, PCO_2, T and DPG. *Chem. Eng. Commun.* **47,** 113–24.

Buxton, R. B., and Frank, L. R. (1997) A model for the coupling between cerebral blood flow and oxygen metabolism during neural stimulation. *J. Cereb. Blood Flow Metabol.* **17,** 64–72.

Buxton, R. B., Wong, E. C., and Frank, L. R. (1998) Dynamics of blood flow and oxygenation changes during brain activation: the balloon model. *Magn. Reson. Med.* **39,** 855–64.

Cholet, N., Seylaz, J., Lacombe, P., and Bonvento, G. (1997) Local uncoupling of the cerebrovascular and metabolic responses to somatosensory stimulation after neuronal nitric oxide synthase inhibition. *J. Cereb. Blood Flow Metabol.* **17,** 1191–201.

Davis, T. L., Kwong, K. K., Weisskoff, R. M., and Rosen, B. R. (1998) Calibrated functional MRI: Mapping the dynamics of oxidative metabolism. *Proc. Natl. Acad. Sci. USA* **95,** 1834–9.

Duelli, R., and Kuschinsky, W. (1993) Changes in brain capillary diameter during hypocapnia and hypercapnia. *J. Cereb. Blood Flow Metabol.* **13,** 1025–8.

Fox, P. T., and Raichle, M. E. (1984) Stimulus rate dependence of regional cerebral blood flow in human striate cortex, demonstrated by positron emission tomography. *J. Neurophysiol.* **51,** 1109–20.

Fox, P. T., and Raichle, M. E. (1986) Focal physiological uncoupling of cerebral blood flow and oxidative metabolism during somatosensory stimulation in human subjects. *Proc. Natl. Acad. Sci. USA* **83,** 1140–4.

Fox, P. T., and Raichle, M. E. (1991) Stimulus rate dependence of regional cerebral blood flow in human striate cortex, demonstrated by positron emission tomography. *J. Neurophysiol.* **51,** 1109–20.

Fox, P. T., Raichle, M. E., Mintun, M. A., and Dence, C. (1988) Nonoxidative glucose consumption during focal physiologic neural activity. *Science* **241,** 462–4.

Frackowiak, R. S. J., Lenzi, G. L., Jones, T., and Heather, J. D. (1980) Quantitative measurement of cerebral blood flow and oxygen metabolism in man using 15O and PET: Theory, procedure and normal values. *J. Comput. Assist. Tomogr.* **4,** 727–36.

Frahm, J., Krüger, G., Merboldt, K.-D., and Kleinschmidt, A. (1996) Dynamic uncoupling and recoupling of perfusion and oxidative metabolism during focal activation in man. *Magn. Reson. Med.* **35,** 143–8.

Frankel, H. M., Garcia, E., Malik, F., Weiss, J. K., and Weiss, H. R. (1992) Effect of acetazolamide on cerebral blood flow and capillary patency. *J. Appl. Physiol.* **73,** 1756.

Ginsberg, M. D., Chang, J. Y., Kelly, R. E., Yoshii, F., Barker, W. W., Ingenito, G., and Boothe, T. E. (1988) Increases in both cerebral glucose utilization and blood flow during execution of a somatosensory task. *Ann. Neurol.* **23,** 152–60.

Ginsberg, M. D., Dietrich, W. D., and Busto, R. (1987) Coupled forebrain increases of local cerebral glucose utilization and blood flow during physiologic stimulation of a somatosensory pathway in the rat. *Neurology* **37,** 11–19.

Gjedde, A. (1987) Does deoxyglucose uptake in the brain reflect energy metabolism? *Biochem. Pharmacol.* **36,** 1853–61.

Gjedde, A., Ohta, S., Kuwabara, H., and Meyer, E. (1991) Is oxygen diffusion limiting for blood-brain transfer of oxygen? In: *Brain Work and Mental Activity,* pp. 177–84. Eds N. A. Lassen, D. H. Ingvar, M. E. Raichle, and L. Friberg. Alfred Benzon Symposium: Copenhagen.

Gobel, U., Klein, B., Schrock, H., and Kuschinsky, W. (1989) Lack of capillary recruitment in the brains of awake rats during hypercapnia. *J. Cereb. Blood Flow Metabol.* **9,** 491–9.

Gobel, U., Theilen, H., and Kuschinsky, W. (1990) Congruence of total and perfused capillary network in rat brains. *Circulation Res.* **66,** 271–81.

Greenberg, J. H., Alavi, A., Reivich, M., Kuhl, D. and Uzzell, B. (1978) Local cerebral blood volume response to carbon dioxide in man. *Circulation Res.* **43,** 324–31.

Grinvald, A., Frostig, R. D., Siegel, R. M., and Bratfeld, E. (1991) High-resolution optical imaging of functional brain architecture in the awake monkey. *Proc. Natl. Acad. Sci. USA* **88,** 11559–63.

Groebe, K., and Thewes, G. (1992) Basic mechanisms of diffusive and diffusion-related oxygen transport in biological systems: A review. *Adv. Exp. Med. Biol.* **317,** 21–33.

Grubb, R. L., Raichle, M. E., Eichling, J. O., and Ter-Pogossian, M. M. (1974) The effects of changes in PCO_2 on cerebral blood volume, blood flow, and vascular mean transit time. *Stroke* **5,** 630–9.

Hoge, R. D., Atkinson, J., Gill, B., Crelier, G. R., Marrett, S., and Pike, G. B. (1999a) Investigation of BOLD signal dependence on cerebral blood flow and oxygen consumption: The deoxyhemoglobin dilution model. *Magn. Reson. Med.* **42,** 849–63.

Hoge, R. D., Atkinson, J., Gill, B., Crelier, G. R., Marrett, S., and Pike, G. B. (1999b) Linear coupling between cerebral blood flow and oxygen consumption in activated human cortex. *Proc. Natl. Acad. Sci., USA* **96,** 9403–8.

Hudetz, A. G. (1999) Mathematical model of oxygen transport in the cerebral cortex. *Brain Res.* **817,** 75–83.

Hyder, F., Shulman, R. G., and Rothman, D. L. (1998) A model for the regulation of cerebral oxygen delivery. *J. Appl. Physiol.* **85,** 554–64.

Kassissia, I. G., Goresky, C. A., Rose, C. P., Schwab, A. J., Simard, A., Huet, P. M., and Bach, G. G. (1995) Tracer oxygen distribution is barrier-limited in the cerebral microcirculation. *Circulation Res.* **77,** 1201–11.

Katsura, K., Folbergrova, J., Gido, G., and Siesjo, B. K. (1994) Functional, metabolic, and circulatory changes associated with seizure activity in the postischemic brain. *J. Neurochem.* **62,** 1511–15.

Kim, S. G., Rostrup, E., Larsson, H. B. W., Ogawa, S., and Paulson, O. B. (1999) Determination of relative $CMRO_2$ from CBF and BOLD changes: Significant increase of oxygen consumption rate during visual stimulation. *Magn. Reson. Med.* **41,** 1152–61.

Kleinfeld, D., Mitra, P. P., Helmchen, F., and Denk, W. (1998) Fluctuations and stimulus induced changes in blood flow observed in individual capillaries in layers 2 through 4 of rat neocortex. *Proc. Natl. Acad. Sci., USA* **95,** 15741–6.

Kwong, K. K., Belliveau, J. W., Chesler, D. A., Goldberg, I. E., Weisskoff, R. M., Poncelet, B. P., Kennedy, D. N., Hoppel, B. E., Cohen, M. S., Turner, R., Cheng, H.-M., Brady, T. J., and Rosen, B. R. (1992) Dynamic magnetic resonance imaging of human brain activity during primary sensory stimulation. *Proc. Natl. Acad. Sci. USA.* **89,** 5675–9.

Lubbers, D. W., Baumgartl, H., and Zimelka, W. (1994) Heterogeneity and stability of local PO_2 distribution within the brain tissue. *Adv. Exp. Med. Biol.* **345,** 567–74.

Malonek, D., and Grinvald, A. (1996) Interactions between electrical activity and cortical microcirculation revealed by imaging spectroscopy: Implications for functional brain mapping. *Science* **272,** 551–4.

Mandeville, J. B., Marota, J. J. A., Ayata, C., Moskowitz, M. A., Weisskoff, R. M., and Rosen, B. R. (1999a) MRI measurement of the temporal evolution of relative $CMRO_2$ during rat forepaw stimulation. *Magn. Reson. Med.* **42,** 944–51.

Mandeville, J. B., Marota, J. J. A., Ayata, C., Zaharchuk, G., Moskowitz, M. A., Rosen, B. R., and Weisskoff, R. M. (1999b) Evidence of a cerebrovascular post-arteriole Windkessel with delayed compliance. *J. Cereb. Blood Flow Metabol.* **19,** 679–89.

Mandeville, J. B., Marota, J. J. A., Kosofsky, B. E., Keltner, J. R., Weissleder, R., Rosen, B. R., and Weisskoff, R. M. (1998) Dynamic functional imaging of relative cerebral blood volume during rat forepaw stimulation. *Magn. Reson. Med.* **39,** 615–24.

Marchal, G., Rioux, P., Petit-Taboue, M.-C., Sette, G., Travere, J.-M., LePoec, C., Courtheoux, P., Derlon, J.-M., and Baron, J.-C. (1992) Regional cerebral oxygen consumption, blood flow, and blood volume in healthy human aging. *Arch. Neurol.* **49,** 1013–20.

Marrett, S., and Gjedde, A. (1997) Changes of blood flow and oxygen consumption in visual cortex of living humans. *Adv. Exp. Med. Biol.* **413,** 205–8.

McCasland, J. S., and Woolsey, T. A. (1988) High resolution 2DG mapping of functional cortical columns in mouse barrel cortex. *J. Comp. Neurol.* **278**, 555–69.

Meek, J. H., Firbank, M., Elwell, C. E., Atkinson, J., Braddock, O., and Wyatt, J. S. (1998) Regional hemodynamic response to visual stimulation in awake infants. *Pediatric Res.* **43**, 840–3.

Mintun, M. A., Raichle, M. E., Martin, W. R. W., and Herscovitch, P. (1984) Brain oxygen utilization measured with O-15 radiotracers and positron emission tomography. *J. Nucl. Med.* **25**, 177–87.

Pawlik, G., Rackl, A., and Bing, R. J. (1981) Quantitative capillary topography and blood flow in the cerbral cortex of cats: An in vivo microscopic study. *Brain Res.* **208**, 35–58.

Powers, W. J., Hirsch, I. B., and Cryer, P. E. (1996) Hypoglycemia. *Am. J. Physiol.* **270**, H554–9.

Prichard, J., Rothman, D., Novotny, E., Petroff, O., Kuwabara, T., Avison, M., Howseman, A., Hanstock, C., and Shulman, R. (1991) Lactate rise detected by ^{1}H NMR in human visual cortex during physiologic stimulation. *Proc. Natl. Acad. Sci. USA* **88**, 5829–31.

Prichard, J. W., and Rosen, B. R. (1994) Functional Study of the Brain by NMR. *J. Cereb. Blood Flow Metabol.* **14**, 365–72.

Roland, P. E., Eriksson, L., Stone-Elander, S., and Widen, L. (1987) Does mental activity change the oxidative metabolism of the brain? *J. Neurosci.* **7**, 2373–89.

Roland, P. E., Eriksson, L., Widen, L., and Stone-Elander, S. (1989) Changes in regional cerebral oxidative metabolism induced by tactile learning and recognition in man. *Eur. J. Neurosci.* **1**, 3–18.

Sakai, F., Nakazawa, K., Tazaki, Y., Ishii, K., Hino, H., Igarashi, H., and Kanda, T. (1985) Regional cerebral blood volume and hematocrit measured in normal human volunteers by single-photon emission computed tomography. *J. Cereb. Blood Flow Metabol.* **5**, 207–13.

Sappey-Marinier, D., Calabrese, G., Fein, G., Hugg, J. W., Biggins, C., and Weiner, M. W. (1992) Effect of photic stimulation on human visual cortex lactate and phosphates using ^{1}H and ^{31}P magnetic resonance spectroscopy. *J. Cereb. Blood Flow Metabol.* **12**, 584–92.

Seitz, R. J., and Roland, P. E. (1992) Vibratory stimulation increases and decreases the regional cerebral blood flow and oxidative metabolism: a positron emission tomography (PET) study. *Acta Neurol. Scand.* **86**, 60–7.

Shockley, R. P., and LaManna, J. C. (1988) Determination of rat cerebral cortical blood volume changes by capillary mean transit time analysis during hypoxia, hypercapnia and hyperventilation. *Brain Res.* **454**, 170–8.

Smith, A. L., Neufeld, G. R., Ominsky, A. J., and Wollman, H. (1971) Effect of arterial CO_2 tension on cerebral blood flow, mean transit time, and vascular volume. *J. Appl. Physiol.* **31**, 701–7.

Vafaee, M., Marrett, S., Meyer, E., Evans, A., and Gjedde, A. (1998) Increased oxygen consumption in human visual cortex: response to visual stimulation. *Acta Neurol. Scand.* **98**, 85–9.

Vafaee, M. S., Meyer, E., Marrett, S., Paus, T., Evans, A. C., and Gjedde, A. (1999) Frequency-dependent changes in cerebral metabolic rate of oxygen during activation of human visual cortex. *J. Cereb. Blood Flow Metabol.* **19**, 272–7.

Villringer, A., Planck, J., Hock, C., Scheinkofer, L., and Dirnagl, U. (1993) Near infrared spectroscopy (NIRS): a new tool to study hemodynamic changes during activation of brain function in human adults. *Neurosci. Lett.* **154**, 101–4.

Wei, L., Otsuka, T., Acuff, V., Bereczki, D., Pettigrew, K., Patlak, C., and Fenstermacher, J. (1993) The velocities of red cell and plasma flows through parenchymal microvessels of rat brain are decreased by pentobarbital. *J. Cereb. Blood Flow Metabol.* **13,** 487–97.

Weiss, H. R. (1988) Measurement of cerebral capillary perfusion with a fluorescent label. *Microvasc. Res.* **36,** 172–80.

Woolsey, T. A., and Rovainen, C. M. (1991) Whisker barrels: A model for direct observation of changes in the cerebral microcirculation with neuronal activity. In: *Brain Work and Mental Activity: Quantitative Studies with Radioactive Tracers,* pp. 189–98. Eds. N. A. Lassen, D. H. Ingvar, M. E. Raichle, and L. Friberg. Munksgaard: Copenhagen.

Yarowsky, P. J., and Ingvar, D. H. (1981) Neuronal activity and energy metabolism. *Fed. Proc.* **40,** 2353–362.

IB

Introduction to Functional Magnetic Resonance Imaging

Commonplace as such [NMR] experiments have become in our laboratories, I have not yet lost a feeling of wonder, and of delight, that this delicate motion should reside in all the ordinary things around us, revealing itself only to him who looks for it. I remember, in the winter of our first experiments, just seven years ago, looking on snow with new eyes. There the snow lay around my doorstep – great heaps of protons quietly precessing in the earth's magnetic field. To see the world for a moment as something rich and strange is the private reward of many a discovery.

Edward M. Purcell (1953, Nobel Lecture)

4

Nuclear Magnetic Resonance

INTRODUCTION

The field of nuclear magnetic resonance (NMR) began in 1946 with the independent and simultaneous work of two physics groups: Purcell, Torrey, and Pound (1946) and Bloch, Hansen, and Packard (1946). Building on earlier work in nuclear magnetism, these groups performed the first successful experiments demonstrating the phenomenon of NMR. Certain nuclei (including hydrogen) possess an intrinsic magnetic moment, and when placed in a magnetic field, they rotate with a frequency proportional to the field. This "delicate motion" first detected by Purcell and Bloch has proved to have far-reaching applications in fields they could hardly have imagined (see Box 4). In this chapter and the next the basic concepts and techniques of MRI are described. In Chapter 6, the different approaches to functional magnetic resonance imaging (fMRI) are described, including contrast agent and arterial spin

BOX 4. THE HISTORICAL DEVELOPMENT OF NMR AND MRI

In the early part of the twentieth century, it became clear that classical physics could not account for the world of atoms and subatomic particles. Experiments showed that the light emitted from excited atoms consisted of discrete frequencies, suggesting that only certain energy states could exist rather than a continuum of states. To explain subtle but distinct splittings of some of these spectral lines, called the hyperfine structure, Pauli proposed in 1924 that atomic nuclei possess an intrinsic angular momentum (spin) and an associated magnetic moment. The interaction of the electrons in the atom with the magnetic field of the nucleus creates a slight shift in the energy levels and a splitting of the spectral lines. The significance of these small effects is that they provide a window to investigate the basic properties of matter. From the magnitude of this hyperfine structure one could estimate the magnitude of the nuclear magnetic moment, but the precision of these experiments was poor. In the 1930s new techniques were developed based on the deflection of molecular beams in an inhomogeneous magnetic field (Bloch, 1953), but these techniques were still inadequate for precision measurements.

The second world war brought a stop to all basic physics research and perhaps explains the burst in creative activity just after the war that led to the seminal work of Purcell and Bloch. During the war Purcell worked at the Massachusetts Institute of Technology on radar development and Bloch worked at Harvard on radar countermeasures, and their experience with radiofrequency techniques and measurements may have contributed to the success of their NMR studies (Vleck, 1970). In fact, the experiments performed by Purcell and Bloch were rather different, but it was quickly realized that they were looking at two different aspects of the same phenomenon: in a magnetic field nuclei precess at a rate proportional to the field, with the spin axis rotating at a characteristic frequency. Purcell showed that electromagnetic energy is absorbed by a material at this resonant frequency, and Bloch showed that the precessing nuclei induce a detectable oscillating signal in a nearby detector coil. In both experiments, magnetic properties of the nucleus are manifested in terms of a frequency of electromagnetic oscillations, which can be measured with very high precision. In the next few years NMR became a key tool for investigating atomic and nuclear properties based on these small effects of nuclear magnetization. In 1952 Purcell and Bloch were awarded the Nobel Prize for the development of NMR techniques and the contributions to basic physics made possible by NMR.

In Purcell's Nobel award lecture, quoted at the beginning of the chapter, he eloquently describes the feelings of a basic scientist who has discovered a previously unappreciated aspect of the world (Purcell, 1953). At this time NMR was valued as a tool for fundamental physics research, but the remarkable applications of NMR in other fields were still unimagined. In fact, much of the subsequent development of the field of NMR can be viewed as turning artifacts in the original techniques into powerful tools for measuring other properties of matter. The original application of NMR was to measure magnetic moments of nuclei based on their resonant frequencies. But as experimenters moved up the periodic table, it became clear that additional corrections were necessary to take into account shielding of the nucleus by atomic electrons. Electron orbitals create magnetic fields that alter the field felt by the nucleus, and the result is that the reso-

(continued)

nant frequency is shifted slightly depending on the chemical form of the nucleus. In time this chemical shift artifact in the nuclear magnetic moment measurements became the basis for applications of NMR in analytical chemistry, and NMR spectroscopy has now become an enormously powerful tool for chemical analysis. For example, the ^{1}H NMR spectrum of a sample of tissue from the brain is split into numerous lines corresponding to the different chemical forms of hydrogen. By far the most dominant line is due to water, but if this strong signal is suppressed, many other lines appear. Although the frequency differences are small, only a few parts per million, they are nevertheless readily measurable. The relative intensities of the different lines directly reflect the proportion of the corresponding chemical in the sample.

Because the resonant frequency of a nucleus is directly proportional to the magnetic field, any inhomogeneities of the magnet translate into an unwanted broadening of the spectral lines. In 1973 Lauterbur proposed that NMR techniques could also be used for imaging by deliberately altering the magnetic field homogeneity in a controlled way (Lauterbur, 1973). By applying a linear gradient field to a sample, the NMR signals from different locations are spread out in frequency, analogous to the way the signals from different chemical forms of the nucleus are spread in frequency. Measuring the distribution of frequencies in the presence of a field gradient then provides a direct measure of the distribution of signals within the sample: an image. The first commercial magnetic resonance imagers were built in the early 1980s, and magnetic resonance imaging is now an essential part of clinical radiology.

Even with a perfectly homogeneous magnet, the heterogeneity of the human body itself leads to local variations in the magnetic field. These field inhomogeneities first appeared in images as artifacts, either a distortion of the image or a reduction of the local signal because nuclear spins precessing at different rates become out of phase with each other, reducing the net signal. In the early 1990s it was demonstrated that the oxygenation state of hemoglobin has a measurable effect on the signal measured with MR imaging (Ogawa et al., 1990), and this soon led to the capability of mapping brain activity based on blood oxygenation changes accompanying neural activation (Kwong et al., 1992). This technique of functional MRI (fMRI) has become a standard tool for functional neuroimaging and is now widely used for mapping the working human brain.

---

labeling techniques in addition to the intrinsic blood oxygenation level dependent (BOLD) signal changes introduced in earlier chapters. Because these techniques depend on subtle properties of the NMR signal, it is necessary to understand in some detail how magnetic resonance imaging (MRI) works.

Magnetic resonance imaging has become an indispensable tool in diagnostic radiology. MRI reveals fine details of anatomy, and yet is noninvasive and does not require ionizing radiation such as x-rays. MRI is a highly flexible technique so that contrast between one tissue and another in an image can be varied simply by varying the way the image is made. Figure 4.1 shows three magnetic resonance (MR) images of the same anatomical section, exhibiting radically different patterns of

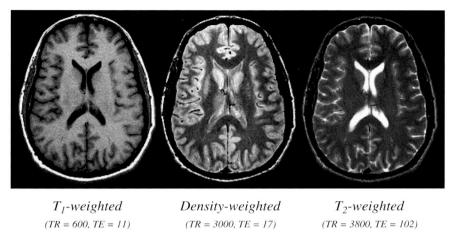

T_1-weighted	Density-weighted	T_2-weighted
(TR = 600, TE = 11)	*(TR = 3000, TE = 17)*	*(TR = 3800, TE = 102)*

Figure 4.1. MR images of the same anatomical section showing a range of tissue contrasts. In the first image, cerebrospinal fluid is black, whereas in the last image it is bright. Contrast is manipulated during image acquisition by adjusting several parameters, such as the repetition time TR and the echo time TE (times given in milliseconds), which control the sensitivity of the signal to the local tissue relaxation times T_1 and T_2 and the local proton density.

contrast. These three images are described as T_1-weighted, density-weighted, and T_2-weighted (the meaning of these technical terms will be made clear shortly). The source of the flexibility of MRI is the fact that the measured signal depends on several properties of the tissue, as suggested by these descriptions. This is distinctly different from other types of radiologic imaging. For example, in computed tomography (CT) the image is a map of one local property of the tissue: the x-ray absorption coefficient. Similarly, with nuclear medicine studies the image is a map of the radioactive tracer concentration. But with MRI, the image is a map of the *local transverse magnetization of the hydrogen nuclei*. This transverse magnetization in turn depends on several intrinsic properties of the tissue. In fact, the transverse magnetization is a transient phenomenon; it does not exist until we start the MRI process.

The fact that the MR signal depends on a number of tissue properties is the source of its flexibility, but it is also a source of difficulty in developing a solid grasp on MRI. To understand the full range of MRI applications, it is necessary to understand the basic physics of NMR and how the MR signal can be manipulated experimentally.

THE NMR SIGNAL

The Basic NMR Experiment

The phenomenon of NMR is not part of everyday experience, so it is helpful to set the stage by considering a purely empirical description of the basic experiment. Every time an MR image is made, it is a variation on this basic experiment. For the

Transmit

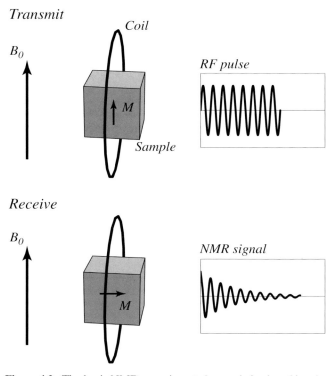

Figure 4.2. The basic NMR experiment. A sample is placed in a large magnetic field B_0, and hydrogen nuclei partially align with the field creating a net magnetization M. In the transmit part of the experiment, an oscillating current in a nearby coil creates an oscillating RF magnetic field in the sample, which causes M to tip over and precess around B_0. In the receive part of the experiment, the precessing magnetization creates a transient oscillating current (the NMR signal) in the coil.

moment we are only concerned with how the MR signal is generated; how that signal is mapped to create an image is taken up in Chapter 5.

The basic experimental setup is illustrated in Figure 4.2. A sample is placed in a large magnetic field, and a coil of wire is placed near the sample oriented such that the axis of the coil is perpendicular to the magnetic field. The coil is used as both a transmitter and a receiver. During the *transmit* phase of the experiment, an oscillating current is applied to the coil for a brief time (a few milliseconds), which produces an oscillating magnetic field in the sample. The oscillations are in the radio frequency (RF) range, so the coil is often referred to as an *RF coil,* and the brief oscillating magnetic field is referred to as an *RF pulse.* For example, for clinical imaging systems with a magnetic field of 1.5 Tesla (about 30,000 times stronger than the natural magnetic field at the surface of the earth), the oscillating field has a magnitude of only a few microteslas, and the oscillations are at a frequency of 64 MHz. During the *receive* phase of the experiment, the coil is connected to a detector circuit that senses small oscillating currents in the coil.

The basic experiment consists of applying a brief RF pulse to the sample and then monitoring the current in the coil to see if there is a signal returned from the sample. If one were to try this experiment naively, with an arbitrary RF frequency, the result would usually be that there is no returned signal. But for a few specific frequencies there would be a weak, transient oscillating current detected in the coil. This current, oscillating at the same frequency as the RF pulse, is the NMR signal. The particular frequencies where it occurs are the resonant frequencies of particular nuclei. At its resonant frequency a nucleus is able to absorb electromagnetic energy from the RF pulse during the transmit phase and return a small portion of that energy back to the coil during the receive phase. Only particular nuclei, those with either an odd number of neutrons or protons, exhibit NMR. For example, ^{12}C with six protons and six neutrons does not show the NMR effect, whereas ^{13}C with seven neutrons does have a resonance. In MRI studies the nucleus of interest is almost always hydrogen.

As an analogy to the NMR experiment, imagine that we are sitting in a quiet room and have a tuning fork with a precise resonant frequency. Our "coil" is a speaker/microphone that can be used either for broadcasting a pure tone into the room or listening for a weak tone coming back from the room. For most frequencies broadcast into the room, there will be no return signal because the tuning fork is unaffected. But when the broadcast frequency matches the resonant frequency of the tuning fork, the fork will begin to vibrate, absorbing acoustic energy. Afterward, the microphone will pick up a weak sound coming back from the vibrating tuning fork.

Precession

The source of the resonance in an NMR experiment is that the protons and neutrons that make up a nucleus possess an intrinsic angular momentum called spin. The word *spin* immediately brings to mind examples of our classical concept of angular momentum: spinning tops, the spin of a curving baseball, and planets spinning on their axes. But the physical concept of nuclear spin is a purely quantum mechanical phenomenon and is fundamentally different from these classical examples. For a spinning top, the "spin" is not an intrinsic feature of the top. The top can be spun faster or slower or stopped altogether. But for a proton, angular momentum is an intrinsic part of being a proton. All protons, neutrons, and electrons have the same magnitude of angular momentum, and it cannot be increased or decreased. The only feature that can change is the *axis of spin,* the direction of the angular momentum. When protons combine to form a nucleus, they combine in pairs with oppositely oriented spins, and neutrons behave similarly. The result is that nuclei with an even number of protons and an even number of neutrons, such as ^{12}C, have no net spin, whereas nuclei with an odd number, such as ^{13}C, do have a net spin. Hydrogen (H), with only a single proton as its nucleus, has a net spin, and because it is far more abundant in the body than any other nucleus, it is the primary focus of MRI.

Associated with the spin of the proton is a *magnetic dipole moment.* That is, the H nucleus behaves like a tiny magnet, with the north/south axis parallel to the spin axis. Now consider a proton placed in a magnetic field. Because of its magnetic dipole moment, the magnetic field exerts a torque on the proton that, in the absence of other effects, would rotate the dipole into alignment with the field, like a compass needle in the earth's magnetic field. But because the proton also possesses angular momentum, this alignment does not happen immediately. Instead, the spin axis of the proton *precesses* around the field axis rather than aligning with it (Figure 4.3). This is an example of the peculiar nature of angular momentum: if one tries to twist a spinning object, the change in the spin axis is at right angles to both the original spin axis and the twisting axis. For example, the wheel of a moving bicycle has an angular momentum around a horizontal axis perpendicular to the bike. If the bike starts to tip to the left it can be righted by twisting the handle bars to the left. That is, applying a torque around a vertical axis (twisting the handle bars) causes the wheel to rotate around a horizontal axis along the length of the bike.

A more direct analogy is a spinning top whose axis is tilted from the vertical. Gravity applies a torque that would tend to make the top fall over. But instead the top precesses around the vertical, maintaining a constant tip angle. In thinking about this process, we must be clear about the distinction between the direction of the field and the axis of the torque the field creates. The gravitational field is vertical, but the torque it creates is around a horizontal axis because it would tend to rotate the top away from vertical, pivoting around the point of contact with the table.

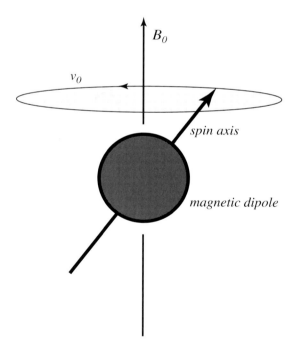

Figure 4.3. Precession of a magnetic dipole in a magnetic field. The magnetic field B_0 exerts a torque on a nuclear magnetic dipole that would tend to make it align with B_0. However, because the nucleus also has angular momentum (spin), it instead precesses like a spinning top at an angle to the gravitational field. The precession frequency v_0 is proportional to the magnetic field and is the resonant frequency of NMR.

TABLE 4.1. Gyromagnetic Ratios of Some Nuclei of Biological Interest

Nucleus	γ (MHz/T)
^{1}H	42.58
^{13}C	10.71
^{19}F	40.08
^{23}Na	11.27
^{31}P	17.25

Thus, when placed in a magnetic field, a proton with its magnetic dipole moment precesses around the field axis. The frequency of this precession, v_0, is the resonant frequency of nuclear magnetic resonance, and is often called the Larmor frequency after the nineteenth century physicist who investigated the classical physics of precession in a magnetic field. The precession frequency is directly proportional to the strength of the magnetic field because the torque applied to the dipole is proportional to the field. The fundamental equation of magnetic resonance is then

$$v_0 = \gamma B_0 \qquad [4.1]$$

where B_0 is the main magnetic field strength and γ is a constant called the gyromagnetic ratio. The factor γ is different for each nucleus and is usually expressed in units of MHz/T (see Table 4.1). Equation [4.1] is the fundamental basis of MRI, which uses subtle manipulations of the resonant frequency to map the location of the signal.

Relaxation

The second important process that affects the orientation of the proton's spin in addition to precession is *relaxation*. If we place a proton in a large magnetic field, the precession rate is very fast: $v_0 = 64$ MHz in a 1.5 T-field. If we could observe the angle of the dipole axis for a few rotations, we would see no change; it would appear as a pure precession with no apparent tendency for the dipole to align with the field. But if we observed the precession for millions of cycles, we would see that the dipole gradually tends to align with the magnetic field. The time constant for this relaxation process is called T_1, and after a time several times longer than T_1 the dipole is essentially aligned with the magnetic field B_0.

Relaxation is an example of energy equilibration. A dipole in a magnetic field is at its lowest energy when it is aligned with the field and at its highest energy when it is aligned opposite to the field. As the dipole changes orientation from its initial angle to alignment with the field, this orientational magnetic energy must be converted into other forms of energy, such as the random thermal motions of the molecules. In other words, the initial orientational magnetic energy must be dissipated as heat. The time required for this energy equilibration depends on how tightly coupled the random thermal motions are to the orientation of the dipole. For H nuclei in water molecules, this coupling is very weak, so T_1 is long. A typical value for T_1 in the human body is about 1 s, eight orders of magnitude longer than the precession period in a 1.5-T magnet.

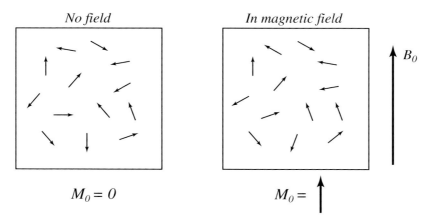

Figure 4.4. Formation of an equilibrium magnetization M_0 due to partial alignment of nuclear magnetic dipoles. In the absence of a magnetic field, the spins are randomly oriented, and there is no net magnetization. When placed in a magnetic field B_0, the spins partly align with the field, a relaxation process with a time constant T_1 of about 1 s, creating a net local magnetization.

Equilibrium Magnetization

Now consider a collection of magnetic dipoles, a sample of water, in a magnetic field. Each hydrogen nucleus is a magnetic dipole; the oxygen nucleus (^{16}O) contains an even number of protons and neutrons and so has no net angular momentum nor a net magnetic moment. The spin axes of the individual H nuclei precess around the field, and over time they tend to align with the field. However, this alignment is far from complete. Exchanges of energy between the orientation of the dipole and thermal motions prevent the dipoles from settling into their lowest energy state. In fact, the energy difference between a hydrogen nucleus aligned with the field and one opposed to the field at 1.5 T is only about 1% of the random thermal energy of the water molecule. The result is that at equilibrium the difference between the number of spins aligned with the field and the number opposed to the field is only about 1 part in 10^5. Nevertheless, this creates a weak *equilibrium magnetization* M_0 aligned with the field (Figure 4.4). M_0 is the net dipole moment per cubic centimeter, and one can think of it loosely as a weak, but macroscopic, local magnetic field that is the net result of summing up the magnetic fields due to each of the H nuclei. That is, each cubic centimeter of a uniformly magnetized sample carries a net dipole moment M_0. The magnitude of M_0 is directly proportional to the local *proton density* (or *spin density*).

The RF Pulse

The local equilibrium magnetization M_0 is the net difference between dipoles aligned with the field and opposite to the field, but it is not directly observable because it is many orders of magnitude weaker than B_0. However, if all the dipoles that contribute to M_0 could be tipped 90°, they would all precess around the field at the same rate. Thus, the magnetization M_0 would also tip 90° and begin to precess around the main field. Tipping over the magnetization produces a measurable, transient signal, and the tipping is accomplished by the RF pulse. During the transmit part of the basic NMR experiment, the oscillating RF current in the coil creates in the sample an oscillating magnetic field B_1 perpendicular to B_0. The field B_1 is in general several orders of magnitude smaller than B_0. Nevertheless, this causes the net magnetic field, the vector sum of B_1 and B_0, to wobble slightly around the B_0 direction. Initially M_0 is aligned with B_0, but when the net field is tipped slightly away from B_0, the magnetization M_0 begins to precess around the new net field. If the oscillation frequency of B_1 is different from the precession frequency v_0, not much happens to M_0 except a little wobbling around B_0. But if the RF frequency matches the precession frequency, a resonance phenomenon occurs. As the net magnetic field wobbles back and forth, the magnetization precesses around it in synchrony. The effect is that with each precessional rotation M_0 tips farther away from B_0, tracing out a growing spiral (Figure 4.5). After a time, the RF field is turned off, and M_0 then continues to precess around B_0. The net effect of the RF pulse is thus to tip M_0 away from B_0, and such pulses are usually described by the flip angle they produce (e.g., a 90° pulse or a 30° pulse). The flip angle can be increased either by increasing the amplitude of B_1 or by leaving B_1 on for a longer time.

It is remarkable that a magnetic field as weak as B_1 can produce arbitrarily large flip angles. From an energetics point of view, tipping the net magnetization away from B_0 increases the orientational energy of the dipoles: the nuclei absorb energy from the RF pulse. This transfer of energy is possible even with small B_1 fields because B_1 oscillates at the resonant frequency of the nuclei, the precession frequency. This is much like pushing a child on a swing. The swing has a natural resonant frequency, and giving very small pushes at that frequency produces a large amplitude of motion. That is, the swing efficiently absorbs the energy provided by the pusher when it is applied at the resonant frequency.

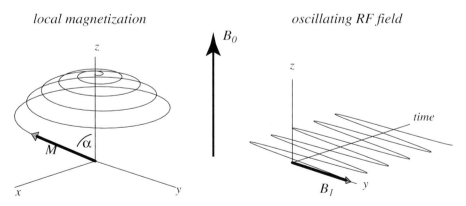

local magnetization   *oscillating RF field*

Figure 4.5. Tipping over the magnetization with an RF pulse. The RF pulse is a small oscillating field B_1 perpendicular to B_0 that causes the net magnetic field to wobble slightly around the z-axis. As the magnetization M precesses around the net field, it traces out a widening spiral. M is tipped away from the longitudinal axis, and the final *tip angle* (or *flip angle*) α is controlled by the strength and duration of the RF pulse.

The Free Induction Decay Signal

A precessing macroscopic magnetization produces a magnetic field that is changing with time. This will induce a current in a nearby coil, creating a measurable NMR signal that is proportional to the magnitude of the precessing magnetization. This detected signal is called a *free induction decay (FID)* and is illustrated in Figure 4.6. *Free* refers to free precession of the nuclei, *induction* is the electromagnetic process by which a changing magnetic field induces a current in the coil, and *decay* describes the fact that the signal is transient. The signal decays away because the precessing component of the magnetization itself decays away. The reason for this is that the individual dipoles that sum to produce the magnetization are not precessing at precisely the same rate. As a water molecule tumbles due to thermal motions, each H nucleus feels a small, randomly varying magnetic field in addition to B_0, due primarily to the other H nucleus in the molecule. When the random field adds to B_0, the dipole precesses a little faster, and when it subtracts from B_0, it precesses a little slower. For each nucleus the pattern of random fields is different, so as time goes on the dipoles get progressively more out of phase with one another, and as a result no longer add coherently. The net precessing magnetization then decays away exponentially, and the time constant for this decay is called T_2.

Let's examine a few characteristic tissues in the human brain; for white matter $T_2 \approx 70$ ms, for gray matter $T_2 \approx 90$ ms, and for cerebrospinal fluid (CSF) $T_2 \approx 400$ ms. From this we can begin to see how tissue contrast can be produced in an MR image. By delaying measurement of the signal for 100 ms or so, the CSF signal will be much larger than the brain parenchyma signal, and an image of the signal distribution at that time will show CSF as bright and the rest of the brain as dark. The image on the right in Figure 4.1 is an example of such a T_2-weighted image.

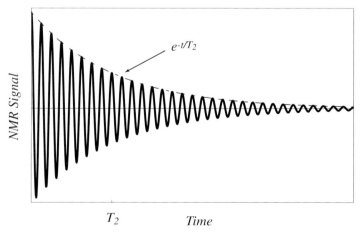

Figure 4.6. The free induction decay. After a 90° RF pulse tips the longitudinal magnetization into the transverse plane, a detector coil measures an oscillating signal, which decays in amplitude with a time constant T_2 in a perfectly homogeneous magnetic field. (In an inhomogeneous field the signal decays more quickly, with a time constant $T_2^* < T_2$.) The plot is not to scale; typically the signal will oscillate more than a million times during the interval T_2.

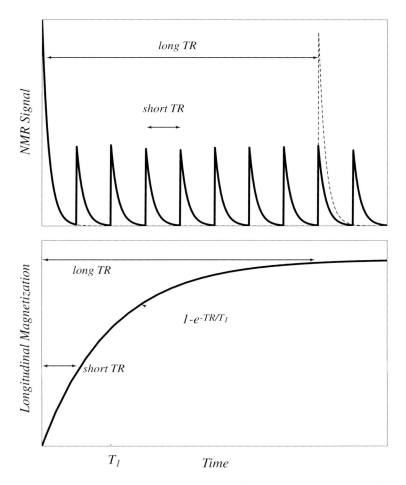

Figure 4.7. Effect of repetition time. Repeated RF pulses generate repeated FID signals, but if TR is short, each repeated signal will be weaker than the first (top). The magnitude of the signal with a 90° RF pulse is proportional to the magnitude of the longitudinal magnetization just prior to the RF pulse. After a 90° RF pulse the longitudinal magnetization recovers toward equilibrium with a relaxation time T_1 (bottom). If this recovery is incomplete because TR < T_1, the next FID signal is reduced.

Now imagine repeating the experiment, after the signal has decayed away, to generate a new signal. How does this new signal compare with the first? The answer depends on the time between RF pulses, called the *repetition time* TR. When TR is very long (say 20 s), the signal generated by the second RF pulse is equal in magnitude to that generated by the first RF pulse. But as TR is shortened, the signal generated by the second RF pulse becomes weaker (see Figure 4.7). To generate a second full amplitude signal, a recovery time of several times longer than T_1 is required to allow the spins to relax back to equilibrium. The recovery process is also exponential, described by the time constant T_1. This relaxation time also varies among tissues: at a magnetic field of 1.5 T, for gray matter $T_1 \approx 900$ ms, for white matter $T_1 \approx 700$ ms, and for CSF $T_1 \approx 4000$ ms. Here we can see another way to produce contrast between tissues in an MR image. If the repetition time is short (say, 600 ms), the signal from white matter will recover more fully than that of CSF, so white matter will appear bright and CSF dark in an image, as illustrated in the first image of Figure 4.1. This is described as a T_1-weighted image.

The Basic NMR Experiment Again

We can now return to the basic NMR experiment and describe it in terms of the basic physics (Figure 4.8). A sample of water is placed in a magnetic field B_0. Over an interval of time several times longer than T_1, the magnetic dipole moments of the H nuclei tend to align with B_0, creating a local macroscopic magnetization M_0 aligned with B_0. An RF pulse is applied that tips M_0 away from B_0, creating a transverse magnetization M_T. The newly created transverse magnetization precesses around B_0, generating a detectable signal in the coil (the FID) with an amplitude proportional to M_T. Over time the precessing magnetization, and thus the signal, decreases exponentially, and after a time several times longer than T_2 the signal is

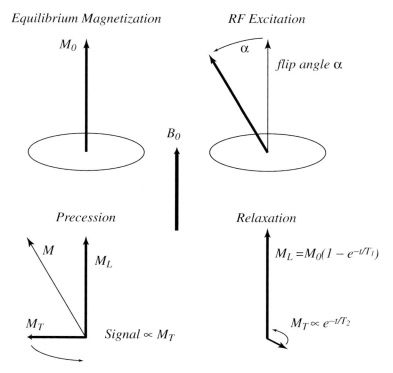

Figure 4.8. The basic physics of the NMR experiment. In a magnetic field B_0, an equilibrium magnetization M_0 forms due to the alignment of nuclear dipoles (top left). An RF pulse tips over M_0 (top right), creating a longitudinal component M_L and a transverse component M_T (bottom left). M_T precesses around the direction of B_0, generating a detectable NMR signal. Over time M_T decays to zero with a relaxation time T_2, and M_L recovers to M_0 with a relaxation time T_1 (bottom right).

essentially gone. Meanwhile, the longitudinal magnetization along B_0 slowly reforms, so that after several T_1 times we are back to where we started, with an equilibrium magnetization M_0 aligned with B_0.

However, if another RF pulse is applied before this recovery is complete, the longitudinal magnetization will be less than M_0. When this partially recovered magnetization is tipped over, the transverse magnetization will be smaller, and thus the detected MR signal will also be smaller. Again the longitudinal magnetization regrows from zero, and if another RF pulse is applied after the same interval TR, another FID will be created. However, if the RF flip angle is 90°, the amount of recovery during each successive TR period is the same: the longitudinal magnetization is reduced to zero after each 90° pulse and then relaxes for a time TR before the next RF pulse. So the signal generated after each subsequent RF pulse is the same as that after the second pulse. This signal, regenerated with each RF pulse, is described as the *steady-state* signal. Nearly all MR imaging applications involve applying a series of RF pulses at a fixed repetition time, so the steady-state signal typically is measured. In fact, the signals from the first few pulses are usually discarded to allow the magnetization to reach a steady state. In this example with 90° pulses, the steady state is reached after one RF pulse, but for other flip angles several pulses are necessary. Thus, the equilibrium magnetization M_0 determines the maximum signal that can be generated; however, unless TR is much longer than T_1, the measured steady-state signal is less than this maximum.

A quantitative description of the MR signal produced by a particular tissue thus depends on at least three intrinsic tissue parameters: the proton density, which determines M_0, and the relaxation times T_1 and T_2. Note that for each of the brain tissues, T_1 is on the order of ten times larger than T_2, which is usually the case with biological specimens. This means that the processes that lead to recovery are much slower than those that lead to signal decay.

We have just described a simple *pulse sequence:* an RF pulse is applied to the sample, and after a repetition time TR the same RF pulse is applied again. The signal generated after the second pulse depends on a pulse sequence parameter (TR) but also on properties of the sample (e.g., T_1). This basic theme runs throughout MRI. A particular pulse sequence will involve several parameters that can be adjusted in making the image, and these parameters interact with intrinsic parameters of the tissue to affect the measured signal. This dependence of the signal on multiple parameters gives MRI its unique flexibility.

At this point it is helpful to review some of the standard terminology used in NMR. We are always dealing with a local three-dimensional magnetization vector M. M is taken to have a *longitudinal* component parallel to B_0 and a *transverse* component perpendicular to B_0. The longitudinal axis is usually designated z, and the transverse plane is then the x-y plane. The transverse component of M (M_{xy} or M_T) is the part that precesses, so the detected signal is always proportional to the transverse component. The transverse component decays away with a time constant T_2, called the *transverse relaxation time*. At equilibrium the longitudinal magnetization has the value M_0, and there is no transverse magnetization. The time constant for the longitudinal magnetization M_z to grow to its equilibrium value is T_1, the *longitudinal relaxation time.*

BASIC PULSE SEQUENCES

Pulse Sequence Parameters and Image Contrast

In the preceding sections we considered how an MR signal is generated in a small volume of tissue. In MRI, the intensity of each pixel in the image is directly proportional to this local MR signal. That is, every MR image is a picture of the local transverse magnetization at the time the image data were collected. And because the transverse magnetization is intrinsically a transient phenomenon, each MR image is a snapshot of a dynamic process at a particular time. Indeed, before the first excitation pulse there is no transverse magnetization at all, and the RF pulse sequence itself creates the quantity that is imaged. The MR signal depends on several intrinsic properties of the tissue (proton density and tissue relaxation times) and also on particular parameters of the pulse sequence used (e.g., repetition time). The power and flexibility of MRI derives from the fact that many pulse sequences are possible, and by adjusting pulse sequence parameters such as TR, the sensitivity of the MR signal to different tissue parameters can be adjusted to alter contrast in the image. For example, when TR is longer than any of the tissue T_1s, each local magnetization recovers completely between RF pulses, so the local magnetization is insensitive to the local T_1. But if TR is shorter than the tissue T_1s, recovery is incomplete, and the local magnetization depends strongly on the local T_1, creating a T_1-weighted signal.

At first glance it might appear that the optimal choice of pulse sequence parameters would be those that maximize the signal. The MR signal is intrinsically weak, and noise in the images is the essential limitation on spatial resolution. But in fact, maximum signal to noise ratio (SNR) is not optimal for anatomical imaging. A high SNR image that is uniformly gray is not of much use. Instead, the contrast to noise ratio (CNR) is what determines whether one tissue can be distinguished from another in the image. It is often useful for comparing different pulse sequences to evaluate the CNR between standard tissues such as gray matter, white matter, and CSF. In the following section we will consider the most commonly used pulse sequences and how they generate image contrast.

Gradient Echo Pulse Sequence

The simplest pulse sequence is the free induction decay described earlier: a series of RF pulses creates a precessing transverse magnetization and a measurable signal. When an FID pulse sequence is used for imaging, it is called a *gradient echo (GRE) pulse sequence,* for reasons that will be explained in Chapter 5. In its basic form the pulse sequence depends on just two parameters: the repetition time TR and the flip angle α. The strength of the signal depends on a combination of these adjustable parameters and the intrinsic tissue parameters S_0, the proton density, and the longitudinal relaxation time T_1. (If the signal is measured soon after the RF pulse, there will be little time for the signal to decay away, and so it will not depend strongly on T_2.) The local MR signal is always proportional to the proton density because the proton density determines the equilibrium magnetization M_0 and thus sets the maximum transverse magnetization that could be produced. If TR is much longer than T_1, the longitudinal magnetization will fully recover during TR. Because the signal does not depend on T_1, but only on the proton density (M_0), the contrast with such a pulse sequence is described as *density-weighted*. The fraction of the longitudinal magnetization that is tipped into the transverse plane is sin α, so a 90° RF pulse puts all the magnetization into the transverse plane and generates the largest signal. Thus, for long TR the signal is density-weighted and proportional to sin α.

But with short TR, the signal depends on TR, T_1, and α in a more interesting way (Figure 4.9). In fact, the signal and contrast characteristics depend on precisely how the pulse sequence is constructed, which is discussed in Chapter 7. In anticipation of the terminology introduced there, the following discussion applies to a *spoiled GRE pulse sequence*. With $\alpha = 90°$, all the longitudinal magnetization is tipped over on each pulse, and there is little time for it to recover before the next pulse if TR < T_1. As a result, the steady-state magnetization created after each RF pulse is weak. The degree of recovery during TR depends strongly on T_1, so the resulting signal is strongly T_1-weighted. Note that the signal is still proportional to M_0, and so is also density-weighted, but the popular terminology is to describe such a pulse sequence as simply T_1-weighted. But the density-weighting is important for determining tissue contrast. For most tissues in the body, a larger proton density is associated with a longer T_1, and this produces an essential conflict for achieving a good CNR between tissues: the density-weighting would tend to make the tissue with the larger M_0 brighter, but the T_1 weighting would tend to make the same tissue darker

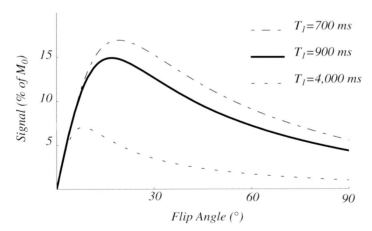

Figure 4.9. Gradient echo signal. The dependence of the signal on flip angle for a spoiled GRE pulse sequence is illustrated for three values of T_1. For small flip angles the signal is insensitive to T_1 (density-weighted), but it is strongly T_1-weighted for larger flip angles. The flip angle for peak signal is substantially smaller than 90° and depends on T_1.

because there is less recovery for a longer T_1. The two sources of contrast thus conflict with each other. Nevertheless, T_1-weighted imaging is very common because the variability of T_1 between tissues is much greater than the variability of proton density, and so T_1-weighting usually dominates the contrast.

Alternatively, to produce a proton density-weighted image, the sensitivity to T_1 must be reduced. As already discussed, this can be done simply by using a long TR so that tissues with different T_1s all recover to their equilibrium values. But a long TR is a disadvantage in conventional MRI. To collect sufficient data to reconstruct an image, the pulse sequence usually must be repeated many times, and so the total imaging time is proportional to TR. With a GRE pulse sequence there is another, somewhat surprising way to reduce the T_1 sensitivity while keeping TR short: the flip angle can be reduced (Buxton et al., 1987). At first glance, this would seem to just reduce the transverse magnetization (and thus the signal) by tipping only a part of the longitudinal magnetization into the transverse plane. But this also modifies the steady-state amplitude of the longitudinal magnetization in a way that reduces the sensitivity to T_1. Consider the steady-state signal generated when TR $<< T_1$. For a 90° pulse the recovery during TR is very small, and so the signal is weak (often described as *saturated*). But if the flip angle is small, the longitudinal magnetization is hardly disturbed by the RF pulse. As a result, there is very little relaxation to do; the longitudinal magnetization is already near its equilibrium value. The sensitivity of the resulting signal to differences in T_1 is then greatly reduced. In summary, for short TR the signal is T_1 weighted for large flip angles but only proton density weighted for small flip angles. Figure 4.9 illustrates how the tissue contrast in an image can be manipulated by adjusting the flip angle.

The simple GRE pulse sequence described earlier illustrates how pulse sequence parameters and intrinsic tissue parameters interact to produce the MR signal. But one important tissue parameter did not enter into the discussion: T_2, the transverse relaxation time. The reason T_2 was left out was that we assumed that the signal was measured immediately after the RF pulse. But we can modify the GRE sequence to insert a delay after the RF pulse before data acquisition begins. During this delay the transverse magnetization, and thus the signal, would be expected to decrease exponentially with a time constant T_2 due to transverse relaxation. If we performed this experiment, we would indeed find that the signal decreased, but typically by much more than we would expect for a known T_2. This enhanced decay is described in terms of an apparent transverse relaxation time T_2^* (read as "T_2 star") that is less than T_2.

The source of this T_2^* effect is magnetic field inhomogeneity. Because the precession frequency of the local transverse magnetization is proportional to the local magnetic field, any field inhomogeneity will lead to a range of precession rates. Over time the precessing magnetization vectors will get out of phase with one another so that they no longer add coherently to form the net magnetization. As a result, the net signal is reduced because of this destructive interference. At first glance this seems similar to the argument for T_2 relaxation itself. Earlier we argued that the net transverse magnetization would decrease over time because each spin feels a random fluctuating magnetic field in addition to the main magnetic field B_0. Because each spin feels a different pattern of fluctuating fields, the spins gradually become out of phase with one another (the phase dispersion increases) so that the net transverse magnetization is reduced. The T_2^* effect, however, is due to *constant* field offsets rather than fluctuating fields. And because these field offsets are static, there is a clever way to correct for these inhomogeneity effects.

Spin Echo Pulse Sequence

In 1950 Hahn showed that a remarkable phenomenon occurs when a second RF pulse is applied following a delay after the first RF pulse (Hahn, 1950). After the first RF pulse an FID signal is generated that decays away quickly due to a short T_2^*. But a second RF pulse applied after a delay TE/2 creates an echo (a *spin echo*) of the original FID signal at a time TE, the *echo time*. This effect can be quite dramatic. The original FID signal can be reduced to an undetectable level, but the second pulse will create a strong echo. However, the echo is reduced in intensity from the original full FID due to true T_2 decay. As soon as the echo forms, it will again decay quickly due to T_2^* effects, but another RF pulse will create another echo. This can be carried on indefinitely, but each echo is weaker than the last due to T_2 decay (see Figure 4.10).

The phenomenon of echo formation due to a second RF pulse is very general and occurs for any flip angle, although for small flip angles the echo is weak. Hahn's original demonstration used 90° flip angles, but in most applications a 180° pulse is used because it creates the strongest echo. The effect of a 180° pulse is illustrated in

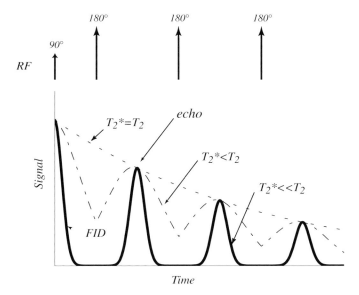

Figure 4.10. Spin echoes. In an inhomogeneous field, spins precess at different rates, and the FID signal created after a 90° excitation pulse decays with a time constant T_2^* less than T_2. A 180° RF pulse refocuses this signal loss due to static field offsets and creates a transient spin echo. The SE signal decays with the true T_2 of the sample. Repeated 180° pulses generate repeated spin echoes.

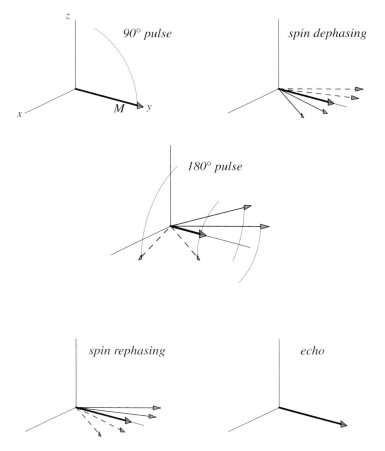

Figure 4.11. Formation of a spin echo. After tipping the magnetization into the transverse plane (top left), spins in different fields precess at different rates (top right). Individual magnetization vectors begin to fan out, reducing the net signal. The 180° pulse at time TE/2 flips the transverse plane like a pancake (middle), and each magnetization vector continues to precess in the same direction (bottom left), so that they realign to form a spin echo at TE (bottom right).

Figure 4.11. After the initial 90° pulse the individual magnetization vectors corresponding to different parts of the sample are in-phase and so add coherently. But due to field inhomogeneity, each precesses at a slightly different rate. The growing phase dispersion can be visualized by imagining that we ourselves are precessing at the average rate. That is, we plot how these vectors evolve in time in a rotating reference frame rotating at the average precession rate. Then a magnetization vector precessing at precisely the average rate appears stationary, whereas vectors precessing faster rotate in one direction and vectors precessing more slowly rotate in the other direction. Over time the vectors spread into a fan in the transverse plane, and the net signal is reduced. However, if we now apply a 180° RF pulse, the fan of vectors is rotated through 180°, so that whatever phase φ was acquired by a particular vector is converted into a negative phase: φ → – φ. After the 180° pulse, each vector will again precess at the same rate as before. But at the echo time TE, each spin will have acquired the same additional phase that it acquired during the interval between the 90° and 180° pulses (TE/2), and the net acquired phase is thus precisely zero. That is, all vectors come back in-phase and create an echo. This effect works because the phase accumulated by a particular vector is simply proportional to elapsed time so that the phase acquired during the first half of the echo time is identical to that acquired during the second half. Because the 180° pulse reverses the sign of the phase halfway through, the net phase for each vector is zero at the echo time. Because of this effect, a 180° RF pulse is often called a *refocusing pulse.* However, a 180° pulse does not refocus true T_2 effects because the additional phase acquired due to random fluctuations is not the same in the first and second halves of the echo time. A multiecho pulse sequence using a string of 180° pulses thus will create a chain of echoes with the peak of each echo falling on the true T_2 exponential decay curve.

The *spin echo (SE) pulse sequence* is the workhorse of clinical MRI. Field inhomogeneity is difficult to eliminate, particularly because the head itself is inhomogeneous, and T_2^* effects lead to signal loss in areas near air/tissue and bone/tissue interfaces (discussed in more detail later). The particular advantage of the SE pulse sequence is that it is insensitive to these inhomogeneities, so that the local signal and the tissue contrast reflect only the interaction of the pulse sequence parameters with the intrinsic tissue parameters. The SE sequence is nearly always used with a 90°–180° combination of RF pulses, so the flip angles usually are not adjusted to control image contrast. That leaves TR and TE as the adjustable pulse sequence parameters, and three tissue parameters affect the signal: M_0, T_1, and T_2. The dependence of the SE signal on proton density and T_1 is similar to that of the GRE sequence with a 90° pulse. The dependence on T_2 is simply an exponential decrease of the signal with increasing TE. When TE is much shorter than T_2, there is little decay, so the signal is insensitive to T_2. For TE much longer than T_2, there is substantial decay and thus very little signal left to measure. But when TE is comparable to T_2, the signal is strongly sensitive to the local T_2, and the signal is described as T_2-weighted.

In an SE pulse sequence the signal is measured at the peak of the echo, where the effects of field inhomogeneities are refocused, and this is the standard implementation for clinical imaging. But in applications such as fMRI based on the BOLD effect, the microscopic field variations induced by changes in blood oxygenation make the MR signal sensitive to brain activation. Some sensitivity to field variations can be retained by shifting the time of data collection away from the echo peak. In such an *asymmetric spin echo (ASE) pulse sequence* the data acquisition occurs at a fixed time τ after the RF pulse, but the time of the 180° pulse is shifted so that the spin echo occurs at a time TE different from τ. Then in addition to T_2 decay for a time τ, there will also be an additional decay due to the phase dispersion resulting from evolution in the inhomogeneous field for a time τ-TE.

Inversion Recovery Pulse Sequence

A third widely used pulse sequence is *inversion recovery (IR),* illustrated in Figure 4.12. This sequence begins with a 180° pulse, then after a delay TI, called the

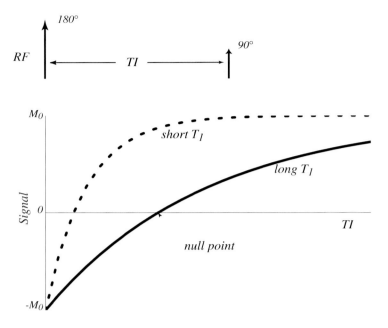

Figure 4.12. Inversion recovery. In an IR pulse sequence an initial 180° RF pulse flips the magnetization from $+z$ to $-z$, and it then relaxes back toward equilibrium. After an inversion time TI, a 90° excitation pulse tips the current longitudinal magnetization into the transverse plane to generate a signal. The signal is strongly T_1-weighted, and for a particular TI exhibits a null point where no signal is generated because the longitudinal magnetization is passing through zero.

inversion time a regular SE or GRE pulse sequence is started. The initial 180° pulse is called an inversion pulse, and can be thought of as a preparation pulse that affects the longitudinal magnetization before it is tipped over to generate a signal. For the IR sequence, the preparation pulse enhances the T_1-weighting of the signal. The effect of the initial 180° pulse is to invert the longitudinal magnetization so that it points along $-z$ instead of $+z$. Note that this does not yet create a signal, because there is no transverse magnetization. After the inversion pulse the longitudinal magnetization begins to re-grow toward its equilibrium value along $+z$. After a delay TI a 90° pulse is applied; this pulse tips whatever longitudinal magnetization exists at that time into the transverse plane. The resulting signal thus reflects the degree of recovery during the time TI. If TI is much longer than T_1, the longitudinal magnetization recovers completely, and the inversion has no effect on the resulting signal. But if TI is comparable to T_1, the recovery is incomplete, and the signal is strongly T_1-weighted. The T_1-weighting is more pronounced than in a typical T_1-weighted GRE or SE pulse sequence because the longitudinal magnetization is recovering over a wider dynamic range, from $-M_0$ to M_0 instead of from 0 to M_0. This is the essential difference between an inversion recovery experiment (following a 180° pulse) and a saturation recovery experiment (following a 90° pulse). Indeed, because the longitudinal magnetization in an IR experiment is recovering from a negative value to a positive value, there is a particular value of TI, called the *null point,* when the longitudinal magnetization is zero, and for this TI no signal is generated. A typical set of parameters for T_1-weighted IR is TI approximately equal to T_1 and TR several times longer than T_1 to allow recovery before the pulse sequence is repeated, beginning with another inversion pulse.

The SE and IR pulse sequences illustrate two different uses of a 180° RF pulse, as reflected in the descriptive terms: it is a "refocusing" pulse in the SE sequence and an "inversion" pulse in the IR sequence. In both cases it is the same RF pulse. The difference is whether we are concerned with its effect on transverse magnetization or on longitudinal magnetization. A 180° pulse flips the transverse plane like a pancake, reversing the phase of the transverse magnetization and producing an echo, but the same flip sends the longitudinal magnetization from +z to –z. In the SE experiment the inversion effect of the 180° pulse is small because the longitudinal magnetization was reduced to zero by the initial 90° pulse, so it has only recovered a small amount during the time TE/2 between the 90° and 180° pulses. In the IR experiment there is no transverse magnetization to refocus at the time of the 180° pulse, and we are interested only in its inversion effect on the longitudinal magnetization.

REFERENCES

Bloch, F. (1953) The principle of nuclear induction. *Science* **118,** 425–30.

Bloch, F., Hansen, W. W., and Packard, M. (1946) Nuclear induction. *Phys. Rev.* **69,** 127.

Buxton, R. B., Edelman, R. R., Rosen, B. R., Wismer, G. L., and Brady, T. J. (1987) Contrast in rapid MR imaging: T_1- and T_2-weighted imaging. *J. Comput. Assist. Tomogr.* **11,** 7–16.

Hahn, E. L. (1950) Spin echoes. *Phys. Rev.* **80,** 580–93.

Kwong, K. K., Belliveau, J. W., Chesler, D. A., Goldberg, I. E., Weisskoff, R. M., Poncelet, B. P., Kennedy, D. N., Hoppel, B. E., Cohen, M. S., Turner, R., Cheng, H.-M., Brady, T. J., and Rosen, B. R. (1992) Dynamic magnetic resonance imaging of human brain activity during primary sensory stimulation. *Proc. Natl. Acad. Sci. USA.* **89,** 5675–9.

Lauterbur, P. C. (1973) Image formation by induced local interactions: Examples employing nuclear magnetic resonance. *Nature* **242,** 190–1.

Ogawa, S., Lee, T.-M., Nayak, A. S., and Glynn, P. (1990) Oxygenation – Sensitive contrast in magnetic resonance image of rodent brain at high magnetic fields. *Magn. Reson. Med.* **14,** 68–78.

Purcell, E. M. (1953) Research in nuclear magnetism. *Science* **118,** 431–6.

Purcell, E. M., Torrey, H. C., and Pound, R. V. (1946) *Phys. Rev.* **69,** 37.

Vleck, J. H. V. (1970) A third of a century of paramagnetic relaxation and resonance. In: *International Symposium on Electron and Nuclear Magnetic Resonance,* pp. 1–10. Eds. C. K. Coogan, N. S. Ham, S. N. Stuart, J. R. Pilbrow, and G. V. H. Wilson. Plenum Press: Melbourne.

5

Magnetic Resonance Imaging

PRINCIPLES OF MAGNETIC RESONANCE IMAGING

In Chapter 4 we discussed how the local magnetic resonance (MR) signal is produced as a result of the interaction of the particular pulse sequence parameters with local tissue properties. The pulse sequence produces a transient pattern of transverse magnetization across the brain. How do we map that pattern? It is remarkable that magnetic resonance imaging (MRI) is able to image the distribution of transverse magnetization in the human brain with a spatial resolution of better than 1 mm, even though the coils used for generating the RF pulses and detecting the signal are much larger. The heart of MRI can be stated in a beautifully simple way: *the phase of the local signal is manipulated in such a way that the net signal traces out the spatial Fourier transform of the distribution of transverse magnetization.* A full interpretation of what this statement means is developed in Chapter 10, but the basic concepts involved in making an MR image are described here.

RF Coils

In an MRI scanner the radiofrequency (RF) coil used to detect the MR signal is sensitive to a large volume of tissue. For example, in brain imaging studies the subject is placed in a cylindrical coil that surrounds the head, and typically this coil is used both for the transmit and receive parts of the experiment. When one of the simple pulse sequences described earlier is applied, the entire head will be exposed to the RF pulses, and the resulting signal produced in the coil will be the sum of the signals from each tissue element in the head. In some studies the transmit and receive functions are accomplished with separate coils: a large uniform coil to produce the RF pulses and a smaller receive coil placed near the part of the head of interest. A separate receive coil is referred to as a *surface coil*. The advantage of using a surface coil is that the signal-to-noise ratio is improved because the coil is nearer to the source of the signal to be detected. The cost of this, though, is that the coil is sensitive to only a small volume of tissue rather than to the whole brain. Use of a surface coil thus achieves some degree of volume localization because of its limited spatial sensitivity. But this level of localization is much coarser than what is required for imaging.

Magnetic Field Gradients and Gradient Echoes

In MRI, spatial localization of the signal is not dependent on the size of the coils used. Instead, localization is based on the fundamental relationship of nuclear magnetic resonance (NMR) (Equation [4.1]): the resonant frequency is directly proportional to the magnetic field at the location of the nucleus. MRI is based on manipulations of the local resonant frequency through control of the local magnetic field by applying *magnetic field gradients*. In an MR scanner there are three gradient coils in addition to the RF coils and the coils of the magnet itself. Each gradient coil produces a magnetic field that varies linearly along a particular axis. For example, a z-gradient coil produces a magnetic field that is zero at the center of the magnet and becomes more positive moving along the $+z$ direction and more negative moving along the $-z$ direction. The three gradient coils are designed to produce field gradients along three orthogonal directions (x, y, and z) so that a field gradient along any arbitrary direction can be produced by turning them on in appropriate combinations. The fields produced by the gradient coils add to the main magnetic field B_0 but are much weaker. Nevertheless, these gradients have a pronounced effect on the MR signal.

A key concept in MRI is the phenomenon of a gradient echo (Figure 5.1). The idea of a gradient echo occurs often, and we have already noted that a simple free induction decay (FID) imaging sequence is referred to as a gradient echo pulse sequence. As we will see, this terminology is somewhat unfortunate, but it is now standard usage. To understand what a gradient echo is, consider a simple FID experiment in which a signal is generated, and suppose that a field gradient in x is then turned on for a few milliseconds (described as a gradient pulse). How does this affect the signal? Prior to the field gradient there is a strong coherent signal, as long as T_2^* is not too short. Each spin precesses at the same rate, so at any instant of time the

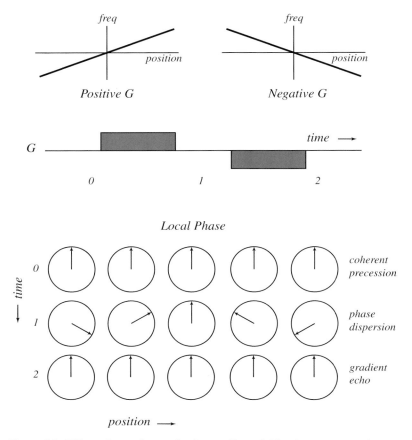

Figure 5.1. Effect of a gradient pulse. In a uniform field, spins precess at the same rate and remain in phase (time point 0). A gradient field produces a linear variation of the precession rate with position (top). At the end of the first gradient pulse (time point 1), the local phase angle varies linearly across the object (phase dispersion). A gradient pulse of opposite sign and equal area reverses these phase offsets and creates a gradient echo when the spins are back in phase (time point 2).

angle that each magnetization vector makes in the transverse plane (the phase angle) is the same. But with the field gradient on, the magnetization vectors of the spins at different x-positions precess at different rates. As the magnetization vectors get out of phase with each other, the net signal drops to near zero. The gradient pulse thus acts as a spoiler pulse, destroying the coherence of the transverse magnetization. After the gradient is turned off, the spins again precess at the same rate, but the phase differences induced by the gradient remain locked in. Now suppose that another gradient pulse with the same amplitude is applied, but this time with opposite sign to the first one. By opposite sign, we mean that the gradient runs in the opposite direction. If the first gradient increases the precession rate at positive x-positions, the second decreases it. If this gradient pulse is left on for the same amount of time as the first, it will precisely unwind the phase offsets produced by the first gradient pulse. The result is that the signals arising from different x-positions come back into phase, creating a gradient echo at the end of the second gradient pulse. A gradient echo can occur even when the second pulse has a different amplitude or duration provided that the area under the two pulses is the same. Or, put another way, a gradient echo occurs whenever the net area under the gradient waveform is zero.

A gradient echo can also occur in a spin echo (SE) experiment. Suppose in the experiment above that a 180° RF pulse is inserted after the first gradient pulse. This will change the sign of each of the phases acquired during the first pulse, so now to unwind them the second gradient pulse should have the *same* sign as the first. Again the gradient echo occurs when the spins are back in phase after the second gradient pulse. The rule for an SE pulse sequence is that a gradient echo occurs when the areas under the gradient pulses are equal on the two sides of the 180° pulse.

The phenomenon of a gradient echo is reminiscent of the process of a spin echo. The spin echo refocuses phase offsets due to static field inhomogeneities, and the gradient echo refocuses phase offsets produced by a gradient pulse. This was the original motivation for calling an FID pulse sequence a gradient echo (GRE) imaging sequence (i.e., that an SE pulse sequence uses an RF echo, and a GRE sequence uses a gradient echo). But this is highly misleading. All imaging pulse sequences, including SE, use gradient echoes as a basic part of the imaging process. In fact, the spin echo is not directly involved in image formation at all; it simply improves the local signal that is being mapped by refocusing the effects of inhomogeneities. But this terminology is now ubiquitous: any imaging pulse sequence that lacks a 180° refocusing pulse is called a gradient echo pulse sequence.

Localization

The central task of MRI is to extract information about the spatial distribution of the MR signal. This is a three-dimensional problem: the source of each component of the signal must be isolated to a particular location *(x, y, z)*. Any spatial localization method has resolution limits, so the imaging process will lead to some degree of uncertainty about the precise location of the source of the signal. We can express this uncertainty in terms of a volume resolution element (voxel) with dimensions $(\Delta x, \Delta y, \Delta z)$. Each of these numbers characterizes the uncertainty of the localization along a particular spatial axis, and the product $\Delta V = \Delta x \Delta y \Delta z$ is called the voxel volume. It is often convenient to think of a voxel as a rectangular block, but it is important to remember that the localization is never that precise. The quantitative meaning of resolution will be discussed in greater detail in Chapter 10.

In MRI, localization is done in three ways corresponding to the three spatial directions: *slice selection, frequency encoding,* and *phase encoding.* The gradient pulses used to accomplish this encoding are diagrammed in Figure 5.2. The usual terminology is to describe the slice selection axis as *z,* the frequency-encoded axis as *x,* and the phase-encoded axis as *y.* However, the actual orientation of this coordinate system in space is arbitrary. In particular, this imaging coordinate system does not have any fixed relationship to the coordinate system used to describe the magnetic field, in which the longitudinal axis along the direction of B_0 was called *z* and the transverse plane was called the *x-y* plane. The imaging coordinate system can have any orientation relative to the magnetic field, even though both the direction of B_0 and the axis perpendicular to the image plane are usually referred to as the *z*-axis. In

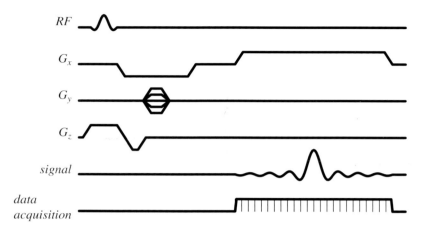

Figure 5.2. A basic imaging pulse sequence. During the RF excitation pulse a gradient in z is applied (slice selection), and during read-out of the signal a gradient in x is applied (frequency encoding). Between these gradient pulses, a gradient pulse in y is applied, and the amplitude of this pulse is stepped through a different value each time the pulse sequence is repeated (phase encoding). Typically 128 or 256 phase-encoding steps (repeats of the pulse sequence) are required to collect sufficient information to reconstruct an image.

transverse (or axial) images the slice selection axis *is* along the magnetic field direction in most scanners, but in coronal images the two directions are perpendicular.

Slice Selection

With slice selection the effect of the RF pulse is limited to a single thin slice, typically 1–10 mm thick (Figure 5.3). This is accomplished by turning on a gradient field along the slice selection axis (z, perpendicular to the desired slice) while the RF pulse is applied. While the gradient field is on, the resonant frequency will vary linearly along the z-axis. The RF pulse is tailored so that it contains only a narrow range of frequencies, centered on a frequency v_0. Then because of the presence of the gradient field, only a narrow spatial band in the body will have a resonant frequency within the bandwidth of the RF pulse. On one side of the slice, the local resonant frequency will be too high, and on the other side, too low. When the frequency of the RF pulse differs from the local resonant frequency, the pulse has little effect on the local longitudinal magnetization. Thus, the effect of a slice selective RF pulse is to tip over the magnetization only in a restricted slice. The location of the slice can be varied by changing the center frequency v_0 of the RF pulse, and the spatial thickness of the excited slice depends on the ratio of the frequency width of the RF pulse to the strength of the field gradient. If the gradient is increased, the resonant frequency becomes a steeper function of position along the z-axis, and so the same RF frequency band corresponds to a thinner slice. Similarly, reducing the bandwidth of the RF pulse with the same gradient strength excites a thinner slice. In practice, the slice width typically is adjusted by changing the gradient strength, and on most MR imagers the maximum available gradient strength limits the thinness of selected slices to 1–2 mm.

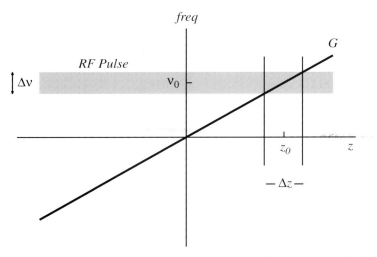

Figure 5.3. Slice selection. An RF excitation pulse with a narrow bandwidth (Δv) is applied in the presence of a z-gradient. The RF pulse centered on frequency v_0 is on-resonance only for spins within a narrow band of positions Δz centered on z_0 so that only these spins are tipped over.

Frequency Encoding

Slice selection limits the effects of the RF excitation pulse so that transverse magnetization is created only in one slice. However, the net signal still reflects the sum of all the signals generated across the slice, and the remaining localization in the x-y plane is done with frequency encoding and phase encoding. These two methods are closely related, and both have the remarkable effect of encoding information about the spatial location of the signal into the signal itself. For frequency encoding, a negative field gradient pulse along the x-axis is turned on after the excitation RF pulse. Following this pulse, a positive x-gradient is turned on so that a gradient echo occurs halfway through the second gradient pulse. The data collection window is typically centered on this gradient echo (Figure 5.2). Because the gradient is turned on during data collection, the precession frequency of the local magnetization varies linearly along the x-axis. The net signal is thus transformed from a sum of signals all at the same frequency to a sum of signals covering a range of frequencies (Figure 5.4), and the signals corresponding to each frequency can be readily separated. Any signal measured as a series of amplitudes over time can be converted to a series of amplitudes corresponding to different frequencies (v) by calculating the Fourier transform (FT). Thus, the measured signal $S(t)$ is mathematically transformed to $S(v)$ and because of the field gradient, frequency corresponds directly with spatial position along the x-axis.

Phase Encoding

Slice selection limits the signal generated to one slice, and frequency encoding separates the signals arising from different positions along the x-axis. But each of these separated signals is still a sum of all the signals arising from different y-positions at

Without gradient

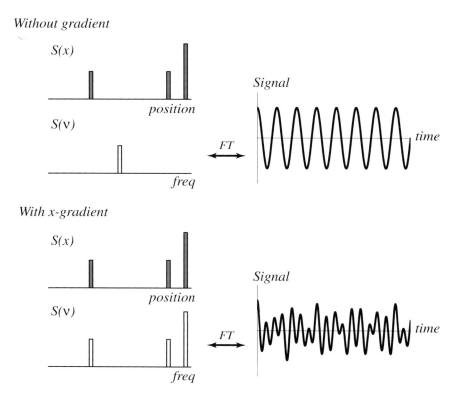

Figure 5.4. Frequency encoding. Three small signal sources are shown at different locations on the *x*-axis. During data collection, with no field gradient all spins precess at the same rate, but with a gradient field in *x* the frequencies of the three sources are spread out, and this is reflected in the interference of these signals in the net signal. From the net signal the frequency spectrum is calculated with the Fourier transform, and the spectrum provides a direct measure of the spatial distribution of the signal along *x*.

a single *x*-position. That is, frequency encoding measures a one-dimensional (1D) projection of the image onto the *x*-axis. This suggests a way to make a full two-dimensional (2D) image that is directly analogous to x-ray computed tomography (CT). The pulse sequence is repeated, exciting a new signal pattern across the slice, but the *x*-axis is rotated slightly so that a new projection of the 2D image is acquired. By continuing to repeat the pulse sequence, each time measuring a different projection, sufficient information can be gathered to reconstruct the 2D image. (This typically requires 128 or more different projection angles.) The rotation of the *x*-axis is accomplished by turning on two of the gradient coils at once, varying the relative current applied to each one. The first demonstration of MR imaging by Lauterbur used this *projection reconstruction* (PR) technique (Lauterbur, 1973). PR techniques are still used in some specialized MRI applications, but conventional MRI uses phase encoding to collect equivalent information.

Phase encoding is a more subtle technique, but it is closely related to frequency encoding. During the interval between the RF pulse and the data acquisition, a gradient field along the y-axis is applied for a short interval (Figure 5.2). While the y-gradient is on, the transverse magnetization at different y-positions precesses at different rates, so the phase difference between the signals at two positions increases linearly with time. After the gradient is turned off, all spins again precess at the same rate, but with the y-dependent phase differences locked in. The effect is then that prior to frequency encoding and data acquisition, each local precessing magnetization is marked with a phase offset proportional to its y-position. The frequency-encoding process then produces further phase evolution of the signal from a voxel with the rate of change of the phase (i.e., the frequency) proportional to the x-position. Data acquisition completes one phase-encoding step. The full image acquisition requires collection of many steps, typically 128 or 256. For each phase-encoding step the pulse sequence is repeated exactly the same except that the amplitude of the y-gradient is increased in a regular fashion. The effect of the increased gradient amplitude is that the y-dependent phase acquired by the magnetization at a particular y-position will also increase. Thus, with each repetition the phase of the magnetization at position y will increase at a rate proportional to y. But these phase increases with each phase-encoding step are precisely analogous to the phase increases with time during frequency encoding: the rate at which phase increases with time is the definition of frequency.

We can thus summarize the imaging process as follows. The local transverse magnetization of a small volume of tissue is a precessing vector, so at any point in time it can be described by two numbers: a magnitude, which depends on the local relaxation times and the pulse sequence parameters described earlier, and a phase angle that describes how much the magnetization has precessed up to that time. The application of field gradient pulses alters the local phase by speeding up or slowing down the precession in a position-dependent way. Then in MRI an image of the magnitude of the local transverse magnetization is created by encoding the location of the signal in the phase of the magnetization. The x-position of a local signal is encoded in the rate of change of the phase of the signal with time during each data acquisition window, and the y-position is encoded in the rate of change of the local phase between one phase-encoding step and the next. Although these two processes both manipulate the phase of the signal, they do not interfere with one another.

We can picture this imaging process as measuring a data matrix in which the signals measured for one phase-encoding step constitute one line in the matrix (Figure 5.5). Stepping through all the phase-encoding steps fills in the data matrix, and the image is calculated by applying the 2D Fourier transform to the data. Just as a time series can be represented as a sum of pure frequencies with different amplitudes, a distribution in space can be represented in terms of amplitudes of different spatial frequencies k. The 2D Fourier transform of the image relates the image to this k-space representation, and so MR imaging directly maps k-space. The spatial resolution of the image depends on the range of spatial frequencies measured (i.e., the largest values of k that are sampled). Resolution in x can be improved by using a stronger read-out gradient or by extending the data collection time. Resolution in y can be improved by increasing the strength of the maximum phase-encoding gradient. Viewing the MRI process as a sampling of the k-space representation of the

Fourier Imaging

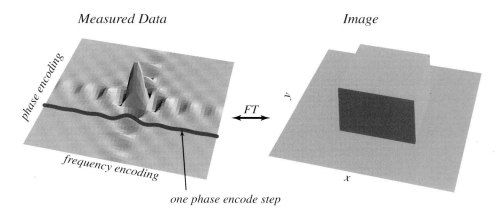

Figure 5.5. Basic Fourier imaging. The measured data is the 2D Fourier transform of the spatial distribution of transverse magnetization (pictured as a square on the right). Each time the pulse sequence in Figure 5.2 is repeated one line is measured, and the phase-encoding step moves the sampling to a new line. Applying the FT along both directions yields the image. The representation of the image in terms of spatial frequencies (left) is described as k-space, where k is a spatial frequency (inverse wavelength).

image is a powerful tool for understanding many aspects of MRI, and this approach is developed in detail in Chapter 10.

MRI TECHNIQUES

Fast Imaging

In the conventional imaging scheme just described, the data corresponding to one phase-encoding step are acquired each time the pulse sequence is repeated. With each repetition, another excitation pulse is applied, generating a new signal that is then position encoded. The total imaging time depends on the total number of phase-encoding steps and the repetition time TR. For example, for a resolution of 128 pixels across the field of view in the y-direction, 128 phase-encoding steps are required. A T_1-weighted spin echo image, with a TR of 500 ms, would thus require about 1 min of imaging time. But a T_2-weighted SE image, with a TR of 3,000 ms, would require about 6 min. One approach to faster imaging is to use a GRE pulse sequence and simply reduce the TR, using the flip angle to adjust the contrast. For example, with TR = 7 ms, a 128×128 image can be collected in less than 1 s.

Another approach to reducing the imaging time is to collect the data corresponding to more than one phase-encoding step from each excitation, and there are a number of schemes for doing this (Figure 5.6 shows some examples). In echo planar imaging (EPI), the gradients are oscillated so rapidly that sufficient gradient echoes are created to allow measurement of all the phase-encoding steps required for an image (Mansfield, 1977). In this single-shot imaging, the full data for a low-resolution image are acquired from the signal generated by one RF pulse. EPI requires strong gradients and puts more demands on the imaging hardware than does conventional imaging. Single-shot images can also be collected with pulse sequences that generate a string of spin echoes, a technique originally called rapid acquisition with relaxation enhancement (RARE) (Hennig, Nauerth, and Friedburg, 1986). A more recent descendent of RARE is HASTE, which is also a single-shot technique, and fast spin echo (FSE), which uses multiple excitations but a train of spin echoes following each one, with each spin echo phase encoded differently. For example, if an echo train of eight echoes is used, the imaging time is reduced by a factor of eight from that of a conventional image. This reduction is not as dramatic as with the single-shot techniques, but single-shot images are also low resolution. FSE techniques are widely used in clinical imaging because they greatly reduce the imaging time for T_2-weighted imaging without sacrificing resolution or signal-to-noise ratio.

Although BOLD activations have been demonstrated with many different imaging schemes, most fMRI work is done with single-shot EPI. The image matrix is typically 64×64, so the spatial resolution is poorer than with standard MR images, but the temporal resolution is far better. The entire data collection window for the image is only 30–100 ms. Spatial resolution can be improved by using multishot EPI, in which a few RF pulses are used to collect data for more phase-encoding steps, but at the expense of more imaging time. One of the key advantages of single-shot imaging is that the data collection is so short that the images are insensitive to motions that would create artifacts in standard images, such as pulsatile flow, swallowing, and other patient motions.

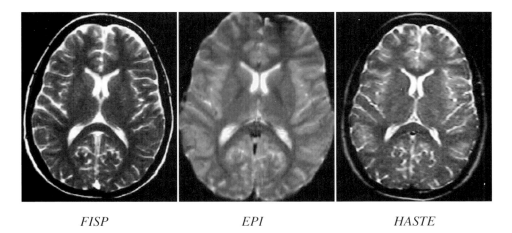

FISP   *EPI*   *HASTE*

Figure 5.6. Examples of techniques for fast MRI. The fast imaging with steady-state precession (FISP) pulse sequence collects one phase-encoding step after each RF excitation, but the TR is very short (7 ms), so the total data collection time is about 900 ms. The EPI and HASTE sequences are examples of single-shot imaging, in which all the phase-encoding lines following one RF pulse are collected in fewer than 100 ms with a series of gradient echoes (EPI) or collected in fewer than 300 ms with a series of spin echoes (HASTE). (Images courtesy of D. Atkinson.)

Volume Imaging

The techniques just described are all examples of 2D planar imaging. Only one slice is acquired at a time by selectively exciting just that one slice. With these techniques a volume can be imaged by simply imaging many slices in succession. For example, with EPI, as soon as the acquisition is completed on one slice, another slice can be excited and imaged. With more conventional imaging, requiring many RF pulses, the multiple slices can be interleaved in an efficient way. A *multislice interleaved* acquisition takes advantage of the fact that the data acquisition on one slice requires only a small fraction of TR because the TR is chosen to produce a desired tissue contrast. For example, with a T_1-weighted SE sequence (TR = 500 ms, TE = 20 ms), the pulse sequence has completely played out after about 25 ms. During the long dead time between repetitions, data for other slices are acquired sequentially until it is time to return to the original slice after a delay TR and acquire data for another phase-encoding step. In this interleaved multislice acquisition, there is no time cost for imaging multiple slices; the scanner is simply acquiring data more efficiently by using the dead time. But for EPI, multiple slices are acquired sequentially, so the time required to cover a volume is directly proportional to the number of slices needed. On most scanners equipped with EPI, the maximum image acquisition rate is in the range of 4 to 12 images per second.

The methods described so far are all intrinsically 2D methods, but true three-dimensional (3D) imaging also can be done. The slice selective pulse is eliminated, so that the whole volume of tissue within the RF coil is excited, or reduced so that only a thick slab is excited. Spatial information in the third *(z)* dimension is then encoded by phase encoding that axis in addition to the *y*-axis. This means that data must be collected for every possible pairing of phase-encoding steps in *y* and *z*. That is, for each of the phase-encoding steps in *y*, the full range of phase-encoding steps in *z* must be measured. Compared to a single slice acquisition, the total imaging time is then increased by a factor equal to the number of phase-encoding steps in *z*. This makes for a prohibitively long acquisition time unless the TR is very short. But with GRE acquisitions the TR can be shorter than 10 ms, so volume acquisitions with high spatial resolution are possible in a few minutes.

The advantage of a 3D acquisition is a large improvement in the signal-to-noise ratio (SNR). The SNR in an image depends on two factors: the voxel volume, which determines the raw signal contributing to each voxel, and the number of times the signal from a voxel is measured, which helps to beat down the noise. For the same repetition time TR and echo time TE, the SNR is then proportional to $\Delta V \sqrt{n}$, where ΔV is the voxel volume (the product of the resolution in each direction: $\Delta x \Delta y \Delta z$) and n is the total number of measurements made of the signal from a voxel. For a standard 2D aquisition, with n_x samples collected during frequency encoding on each of n_y phase-encoding steps, $n = n_x n_y$. If each phase-encoding step is averaged n_{av} times, $n = n_{av} n_x n_y$. For a multislice interleaved acquisition, the data collected on subsequent slices does not contribute to the SNR of a voxel in the first slice. In a 3D acquisition, however, the signal from each voxel contributes to every measurement, so $n = n_{av} n_x n_y n_z$. With this boost in SNR, it is possible to reduce the voxel volume

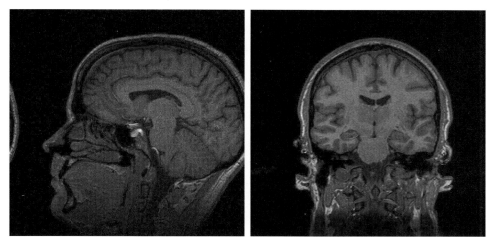

Figure 5.7. High-spatial-resolution images collected with a volume-imaging pulse sequence. On the left is a sagittal section 1 mm thick from a volume collected in about 8 min, and on the right is a coronal section 3 mm thick from a volume collected in about 12 min. Note the improved SNR in the image on the right with the larger voxel and longer acquisition time.

and acquire high-resolution images with a voxel volume of 1 mm^3 while maintaining reasonable SNR. The factors that affect image SNR are discussed more fully in Chapter 10.

A commonly used volume-imaging sequence is MP-RAGE, which combines a periodic inversion pulse to enhance the T_1-weighting in the image with a rapid GRE acquisition to produce high-spatial-resolution images with good contrast between gray matter and white matter (Figure 5.7).

BEYOND ANATOMY

In MRI as previously described, contrast in an image is due to the interplay of a few adjustable pulse sequence parameters (e.g., TR and TE) and physical properties of the local tissue (e.g., proton density, T_1, and T_2). Because these physical quantities vary between tissues, the resulting images provide a sensitive map of anatomy. However, MRI is such a flexible technique that it is possible to make the MR signal sensitive to several other physiological parameters that carry MRI beyond anatomical imaging. These techniques open the door to functional MRI (fMRI) and the mapping of physiological activity as well as anatomy. It is interesting to note that the physical effects that underlie these fMRI techniques first appeared as artifacts in conventional anatomical MRI: sensitivity to motion and magnetic field inhomogeneities.

Motion Sensitivity: Flow and Diffusion Imaging

Sensitivity to bulk motion makes possible direct imaging of blood flowing in large vessels and the construction of MR angiograms for visualizing the vascular tree (Anderson, Edelman, and Turshi, et al, 1993). These magnetic resonance angiography (MRA) techniques are noninvasive and do not require administration of a contrast agent; the intrinsic motion of the blood distinguishes it from the surrounding tissue. Sensitivity to motion also can be pushed to the microscopic scale with diffusion-weighted imaging, which is sensitive to the intrinsic random thermal motions of the water molecules (LeBihan, 1991). Recent work in diffusion imaging has shown that the local diffusion of water is altered in stroke and that this alteration is detectable before there are changes in the MR relaxation times (Baird and Warach, 1998). In addition, diffusion is not always isotropic. In white matter, water diffuses more readily along the fiber tracts, and this effect can be used to map fiber orientations (Moseley, Cohen, and Kucharczyk, 1990).

Two effects of motion on the MR signal underlie MRA techniques. The *time-of-flight (TOF) effect* results from refreshment of blood in the imaging slice due to flow. Imagine an image plane cutting through a blood vessel with fast flow. In the imaging process the pulse sequence is repeated with a repetition time TR. For a static tissue, if TR is shorter than T_1, the longitudinal magnetization will not fully recover, so the steady-state magnetization is reduced or partly saturated. With a short TR gradient echo pulse sequence with a large flip angle, the tissue signal is usually substantially reduced by this saturation. But if the flow in the blood vessel is fast enough, the blood in the imaging plane will be replaced by fresh blood carrying a fully relaxed magnetization during each TR interval. As a result, the blood signal when this magnetization is tipped over will be much stronger than the signal of the surrounding tissue, creating strong image contrast. In this way, the MR image shows bright focal spots where the image plane cuts through blood vessels (Figure 5.8).

A common way to view this data, that brings out the structure of the vascular tree, is to take a stack of such images and view them with a maximum intensity projection (MIP). The projection image is constructed by viewing the three-dimensional data set along a chosen axis, and for each ray through the data taking the maximum intensity encountered along the ray as the intensity in the projection image (Figure 5.8). Typically a series of projections from different angles are calculated and viewed as a cine loop.

The second effect of motion on the MR signal is a phase effect, and this is the basis of the *phase contrast MRA techniques*. The phase of the local MR signal is altered whenever a bipolar gradient pulse is applied in the presence of motion. A bipolar pulse consists of a gradient pulse followed by another of opposite sign and forms the basis of the idea of a gradient echo (Figure 5.1). For static spins the first lobe of the gradient pulse creates a phase offset that depends on the spins' position. The second lobe with opposite sign reverses that phase offset and brings all the spins back in phase. But if the spin moves along the gradient axis during the interval between the two lobes, then the phase acquired during the second lobe will not be precisely the opposite of the phase acquired during the first lobe. The signal from moving spins will thus acquire a phase offset. This offset is proportional to the distance moved and so is proportional to the spins' velocity. This has two important results. First, this effect provides a way to measure quantitatively the velocity of flowing blood by measuring the phase of the local signal. Second, any dispersion of

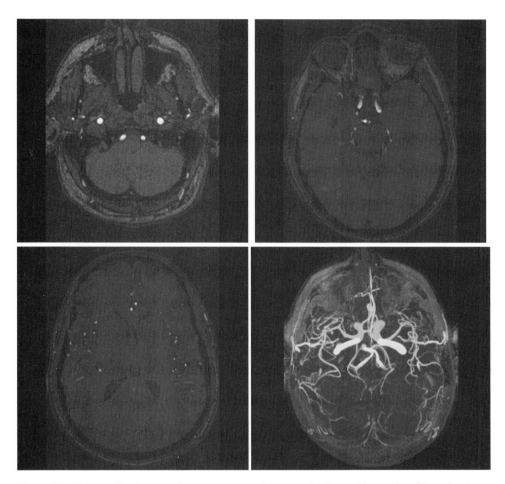

Figure 5.8. Time-of-flight magnetic resonance angiography. In these thin-section (1-mm) volume acquisitions the signal of flowing blood is refreshed, but the signal of static tissue is saturated, creating strong contrast between blood and tissue in the images. Data were collected as six slabs, with a saturation pulse applied above each slab to reduce the refreshment effect for veins, so the visible vessels are primarily arteries. The sections shown illustrate cuts through carotid and vertebral arteries in the neck (top left), major cerebral arteries near the circle of Willis (top right), and smaller arteries (bottom left). The maximum intensity projection through the full stack of 135 images (bottom right) reveals the arterial vascular tree.

velocities within an imaging voxel will lead to a range of phase angles and attenuation of the net signal. Thus, in areas where the flow pattern is reasonably uniform on the scale of a voxel, the phase effect can be used to map flow velocity, but in areas of complex flow the signal may be destroyed due to phase dispersion. Figure 5.9 shows an example of phase contrast MRA.

The sensitivity of the MR signal to motion can also be extended to microscopic scales with *diffusion-weighted imaging*. These methods are also based on the effect of motion on the phase of the MR signal. Because of their intrinsic thermal energy, water molecules are in constant random motion so that over time each molecule

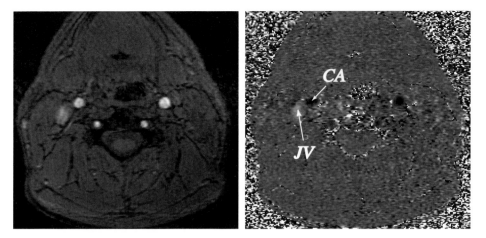

Figure 5.9. Phase contrast magnetic resonance angiography. Phase contrast MRA differs from TOF MRA by the addition of bipolar gradient pulses along one of the spatial axes. The result is that the phase of the local signal (right) is proportional to the velocity along the axis of the bipolar gradient. The magnitude image (left) shows some TOF contrast enhancement in both the carotid artery (CA) and the jugular vein (JV), indicating flow refreshment in both vessels, but the phase image also reveals the magnitude and direction of the flow (note the opposite phase offsets in the artery and vein, indicated by arrows).

tends to drift away from its starting location. As a result of this self-diffusion, a molecule moves only about 20 μm during a 100-ms interval, but this small displacement is sufficient to have a measurable effect on the MR signal with appropriate pulse sequences. With a sufficiently strong bipolar gradient pulse, even these small displacements can create significant phase offsets, and because the motions are random a range of phase offsets is produced. The net signal from the voxel is attenuated due to the phase dispersion, and the degree of attenuation depends on the magnitude of the diffusional motions. In tissues the diffusional motions of water are often restricted by the presence of membranes and large protein molecules so that the magnitude of the diffusion varies among tissues and sometimes along different directions within one tissue, such as white matter.

Magnetic Susceptibility Effects

When a body is placed in a magnetic field B_0 created by the magnet, the local field at a particular location is not just B_0. All materials become partly magnetized as magnetic moments within the body tend to align with the field, and the net field at any location is then B_0 plus the field due to the magnetized body itself. Magnetic susceptibility is a measure of the degree to which a material becomes magnetized when placed in a magnetic field. Whenever dissimilar materials are in close proximity, there are likely to be magnetic field distortions due to different magnetic susceptibilities. This is often seen at interfaces of air, bone, and other tissues, as illustrated in Figure 5.10. This figure shows the magnitude and phase of a coronal GRE image of the brain. Because each local spin precesses at a rate proportional to the local field, an image of the phase of the signal is a map of the field offset. The phase of a

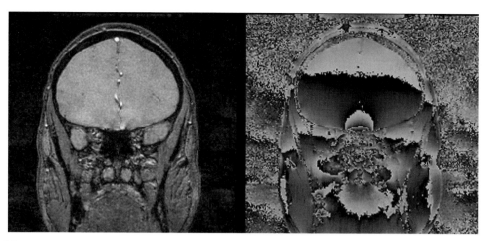

Figure 5.10. Mapping the local magnetic field with gradient echo phase images. The local precession frequency is proportional to the local magnetic field offset, so the local phase of the signal at the time of data collection is proportional to the field offset. The abrupt changes from black to white in the phase image (right) are due to the cyclic nature of the phase angle and can be interpreted as contour lines of the magnetic field. The field offset resembles a dipole field centered on the sinus cavity.

GRE image is thus a useful way to map the distortions of the magnetic field. Because the phase angle is cyclic, the phase image shows abrupt transitions from black to white as the phase changes from 359° to 0°. These transitions are thus an artifact of the display but can be thought of as contours of equal field offset. Figure 5.10 shows substantial field variation due in large part to the susceptibility difference between the sinus cavities and the brain tissue.

Furthermore, the pattern of field distortion depends strongly on the geometry of the tissues. A very simple field distortion is illustrated in Figure 5.11. Each image shows a cross section through two concentric cylinders. Both cylinders contain water, but the inner cylinder was doped with gadolinium (Gd-DTPA), a commonly used MR contrast agent, which has the effect of altering the magnetic susceptibility. (Gadolinium also alters the relaxation times, but that is not the effect we are after here.) Gradient echo MRI was used to map the field offsets. The field offset pattern is a dipole field, and it becomes more pronounced as the susceptibility difference between the inner cylinder and the surrounding medium is increased by increasing the concentration of Gd-DTPA. The field distortion around a magnetized cylinder is a useful model for thinking about field distortions around blood vessels. Susceptibility differences between blood and the surrounding tissue, due either to injected contrast agents or to intrinsic changes in blood oxygenation, are at the heart of most fMRI techniques.

The MR signal is sensitive to magnetic field variations within a voxel produced by magnetic susceptibility variations. Spins precess at a rate determined by the local magnetic field, so with a gradient echo sequence the individual signals that make up the net voxel signal become steadily more and more out of phase, and the signal is strongly attenuated. One remedy for this T_2^* effect is to use a spin echo sequence to

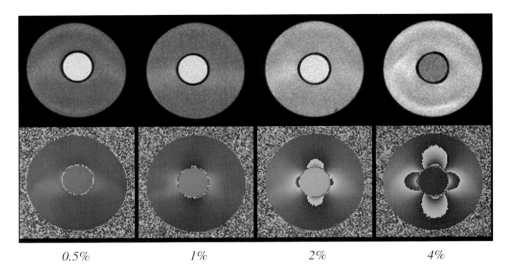

0.5%   *1%*   *2%*   *4%*

Gd-DTPA Concentration

Figure 5.11. Field distortions around a magnetized cylinder. Cylinders filled with different concentrations of Gd-DTPA, a common MR contrast agent, were imaged with a GRE pulse sequence. These phantoms consist of concentric cylinders with the Gd-DTPA in the inner cylinder and water in the outer cylinder. The top row of magnitude images illustrates the *relaxivity* effect of gadolinium: in low concentrations the signal is increased on these T_1-weighted images because T_1 is reduced, and with a high concentration the shortening of T_2 becomes important and the signal is reduced. The phase images (bottom) show the dipole field distortion due to the magnetic susceptibility effect of gadolinium, creating field gradients around the cylinder. Similar field distortions occur around magnetized blood vessels containing deoxyhemoglobin.

refocus the phase dispersion; this will restore signal dropouts due to large-scale field variations such as those produced by the sinus cavities. But when the spatial scale of the field variations is much smaller, comparable to the distance a water molecule diffuses during the echo time TE, a spin echo is less effective at refocusing because of the diffusional motions. A spin echo works only if the phase acquired by a spin during the first half of the echo is the same as that acquired during the second half, and motion through spatially varying magnetic fields will change this. The effect is analogous to that of a bipolar gradient pulse described earlier, except that now the effect is due to intrinsic field variations within the tissue rather than applied gradients.

REFERENCES

Anderson, C. M., Edelman, R. R., and Turski, P. A. (1993) *Clinical Magnetic Resonance Angiography.* Raven Press: New York.

Baird, A. E., and Warach, S. (1998) Magnetic resonance imaging of acute stroke. *J. Cereb. Blood Flow Metabol.* **18,** 583–609.

Hennig, J., Nauerth, A., and Friedburg, H. (1986) RARE imaging: A fast imaging method for clinical MR. *Magn. Reson. Med.* **3,** 823–33.

Lauterbur, P. C. (1973) Image formation by induced local interactions: examples employing nuclear magnetic resonance. *Nature* **242,** 190–1.

LeBihan, D. (1991) Molecular diffusion nuclear magnetic resonance imaging. *Magn. Reson. Quart.* **7,** 1–30.

Mansfield, P. (1977) Multi-planar image formation using NMR spin echoes. *J. Phys.* **C10,** L55–8.

Moseley, M. E., Cohen, T., and Kucharczyk, J. (1990) Diffusion weighted MR imaging of anisotropic water diffusion in cat central nervous system. *Radiology* **176,** 439–46.

Imaging Functional Activity

MR EFFECTS OF BRAIN ACTIVATION

In Chapter 3 the basic physiological changes accompanying brain activation were described. Cerebral blood flow (CBF) increases dramatically, and the metabolic rate of oxygen consumption increases by a smaller amount. As a result, the oxygen content of the capillary and venous blood is increased. In addition, the blood volume and blood velocity increase. With this picture of brain activation in mind, what are the possible observable effects these physiological changes might have on the magnetic resonance signal that could form the basis for measuring activation with magnetic resonance imaging?

The first potential effect is due to increased velocity of the blood. By applying bipolar gradient pulses, the intrinsic flow sensitivity of the magnetic resonance (MR) signal can be exploited. Individual capillaries cannot be resolved, so the flow effect is more analogous to diffusion imaging than to MR angiography. An early conceptual model for functional imaging is to imagine that a capillary bed consists of randomly oriented cylinders. Then the uniform motion of the blood, but in random directions, is similar to the random walk of freely diffusing water molecules (LeBihan et al., 1988). The effect on the MR signal of this *IntraVoxel Incoherent Motion (IVIM)* is qualitatively similar to the effect of diffusion: when a bipolar gradient is applied, the signal is reduced because the spins move during the interval between the two lobes of the gradient pulse so that refocusing is incomplete. Quantitatively, the IVIM effect is much larger than diffusion because the spins are carried farther by capillary flow than by diffusional motions.

If the bipolar gradient pulse is sufficiently strong so that the signal from moving blood is completely destroyed, rather than just attenuated, the blood volume can be measured by subtracting the signals measured with and without diffusion weighting. However, this approach involves some complications. The total signal is viewed as the sum of the signals from two pools: the intravascular spins and the extravascular spins. Ideally, we would manipulate only the intravascular signal by applying the bipolar gradient pulse, so that the extravascular signal would subtract out, leaving just a measure of the intrinsic intravascular signal. But the extravascular signal is also affected by the gradient pulse due to true diffusion of the spins in the tissue. The attenuation of the extravascular signal due to diffusion is much less than the attenuation of the blood signal due to flow, but the absolute signal change associated with the two effects is similar because the intravascular signal is such a small fraction of the total signal. For example, the net signal change due to a gradient pulse that attenuates the tissue signal by 5% by diffusion is comparable to complete attenuation of a blood signal that makes up 4% of the total signal. This approach thus requires accurate measurements of small signal changes, and careful corrections for confounding effects such as diffusional attenuation of the tissue signal.

An alternative approach to measuring blood volume is to use intravascular contrast agents, such as gadolinium-DTPA (Gd-DTPA) (Rosen, Belliveau, and Chien, 1989; Villringer et al., 1988). As described in Chapter 5, gadolinium has a large magnetic moment and so alters the magnetic susceptibility of the blood. The altered susceptibility in turn creates field gradients within and around the vessels, leading to attenuation of the MR signal. Although the agent is confined to the intravascular space, the total MR signal is affected because the microscopic field gradients penetrate into the extravascular space. As a result, the signal changes can be quite large (30–50%), much larger than the small changes associated with the IVIM effect. And the larger the blood volume, the larger the effect on the MR signal. Following a bolus injection of the agent, the local MR signal in the brain drops transiently as the agent passes through the vasculature. This effect lasts only a brief time (10 s or so) and fast dynamic imaging is required to measure it. For the same bolus, the signal dip will be more pronounced in areas with a larger blood volume.

With contrast agents, a susceptibility difference between the intravascular and extravascular space is induced by the experimenter. But there is also a natural physiological mechanism for producing a susceptibility difference: deoxyhemoglobin is paramagnetic, but oxyhemoglobin is not. As a result, the magnetic susceptibility of the blood is altered depending on the blood concentration of deoxyhemoglobin (Ogawa et al., 1990a). At rest, arterial blood arrives at the brain fully oxygenated, and about 40% of the oxygen is extracted in passing through the capillary bed. The venous blood, and to a lesser extent the capillary blood, thus contains a significant concentration of deoxyhemoglobin. The susceptibility change due to this amount of deoxyhemoglobin is about an order of magnitude smaller than that due to a concentrated bolus of Gd, so the signal attenuation is weaker. In the resting brain the gradient echo (GRE) signal attenuation is estimated to be about 8% at a field strength of 1.5 T compared to what the signal would be if the blood remained fully oxygenated (i.e., no oxygen metabolism) (Davis et al., 1998). This signal attenuation is called a Blood Oxygenation Level Dependent (BOLD) effect (Ogawa et al., 1990b).

However, the existence of a BOLD effect on the MR signal does not necessarily lead to a way of measuring brain activation. If blood flow and oxygen metabolism increase in a matched way (e.g., a 20% increase in both), then the blood oxygenation remains the same and the signal attenuation due to the BOLD effect would also remain the same. But the nature of brain activation is that CBF increases much more than the cerebral metabolic rate of oxygen ($CMRO_2$) (see Chapter 3), leading to increased venous blood oxygenation and a reduced concentration of deoxyhemoglobin. As a result, the degree of attenuation due to the BOLD effect is reduced, and the MR signal increases. In a typical study to map patterns of brain activation based on the BOLD effect, a series of dynamic images is acquired while the subject alternates between periods of performing a task and periods of rest. The time series of images is then analyzed to identify individual pixel time courses that show a significant correlation with the stimulus pattern (i.e., a signal increase during performance of the task) (Bandettini et al., 1993). These pixels are then colored to produce a map of the pattern of brain activation and overlayed on a gray-scale image of the anatomy.

The MR methods described so far all yield information about the perfusion state of the brain, but none of them provides a direct measure of the perfusion itself: cerebral blood flow (CBF). One approach to measurement of CBF is to look more closely at the dynamic signal change curves measured with contrast agents such as Gd-DTPA (Østergaard et al., 1996a, 1996b). With such curves the magnitude of the transient signal change is determined by the blood volume, and so these data yield a robust measurement of cerebral blood volume (CBV). But the *duration* of the signal dip depends on the vascular transit time, which in turn depends on the CBF. The lower the CBF, the longer the transit time. However, pulling out a quantitative measurement of CBF from such data is difficult because CBF is not the only factor that affects the width of the signal dip. The dominant contribution to the width is the width of the bolus itself. The agent is injected into a vein, and so must pass through the heart before being delivered to the brain in arterial blood. As a result, even if the injected bolus is sharply defined in time, the delivered bolus to the brain is substantially broadened. To derive a measurement of CBF from contrast agent data, an estimate of the natural width of the bolus in the arterial blood arriving at the brain tissue is required, and this usually involves imaging of the blood signal in a large artery. The calculation of CBF is then more involved mathematically than computing a map of CBV and is likely more prone to error.

An alternative approach to measuring CBF directly is related to the idea of the time-of-flight effects that are the basis of the MR angiography techniques described in Chapter 5. In arterial spin labeling (ASL) techniques, the magnetization of the arterial blood is manipulated before it reaches the slice of interest (Detre et al., 1992). In a typical ASL experiment the arterial blood is tagged by inverting the magnetization, and after a delay this tagged blood arrives at the image plane and an image is acquired. A control measurement is then made without tagging the arterial blood. If the tag and control images are carefully adjusted so that the signal from the static spins is the same in both, then the difference signal will be proportional to the amount of arterial blood delivered, and thus proportional to CBF. Like other functional magnetic resonance imaging (fMRI) techniques, the signal change associated with tagging the blood is small. A rough estimate can be made by considering how much tagged water can enter the brain during the experiment. The essential limitation on this is the short longitudinal relaxation time, which is on the order of 1 s. One can think of this as analogous to dealing with a tracer with a very short half-life. The arterial inversion creates labeled water that can be measured, but after a few seconds the label has disappeared. The amount of label that can be delivered into a tissue voxel is then on the order of fT_1, where f is the local CBF and T_1 is the longitudinal relaxation time. For the human brain f is about 0.01 s^{-1}, and T_1 is about 1 s, so the fractional change in the total signal due to arterial tagging is only about 1%. Nevertheless, these small signal changes can be measured reliably, and ASL techniques can produce quantitative maps of perfusion with high temporal and spatial resolution.

At first glance, the IVIM and ASL methods sound somewhat similar. In both cases the MR signal of blood is selectively manipulated so that a difference image isolates the signal of blood from the net MR signal. And yet the IVIM method yields a measurement of blood volume, and the ASL method yields a measurement of blood flow, a very different quantity. The key difference between these methods is which pool of blood is manipulated. With the IVIM method, all the blood in the voxel is affected, and so the method provides a measure of how much blood is there. But this tells us nothing about how fast that blood is being replaced by fresh arterial blood. In contrast, with the ASL methods only the arterial blood is manipulated before it arrives in the voxel. This gives a direct measure of how much blood is delivered during the experiment and is independent of how much blood is within the voxel.

These changes in the MR signal induced by changes in blood velocity, volume, flow, and oxygenation are the basis for all the functional imaging methods to follow. Historically, the IVIM methods were the first MR methods for examining the perfusion state of tissue, but they have largely been superceded by the other methods. The first demonstration of brain activation was done with two bolus injections of Gd-DTPA, with and without a visual stimulus (Belliveau et al., 1991). However, because of the requirement for multiple injections, contrast agent methods are not routinely used for brain activation studies. But such techniques have become an important clinical tool for evaluating brain pathology associated with altered blood volume, such as tumors and stroke. (Such studies are often described as "perfusion" studies, even though blood volume, rather than blood flow, is usually measured.) It was the discovery of the BOLD effect that significantly broadened the field of functional neuroimaging (Bandettini et al., 1992; Frahm et al., 1992; Kwong et al., 1992; Ogawa et al., 1992). Virtually all the fMRI studies performed to map patterns of brain activation are based on the BOLD effect. However, the BOLD effect has an important drawback for clinical applications: all that can be measured is a change in the perfusion state. That is, BOLD studies tell us nothing about the resting perfusion, only which areas change when the subject performs a different task. For clinical applications such as stroke, the important measurement is the resting CBF, and so for this reason clinical fMRI studies are likely to require ASL techniques. The various fMRI techniques are described in more detail in the following sections.

CONTRAST AGENT METHODS

Contrast Agents Alter the Local Relaxation Times

Most MRI is done completely noninvasively, in the sense that nothing is injected into the subject. Detailed anatomic images can be created based solely on intrinsic properties of the tissues. But the use of a contrast agent can further enhance the contrast in an image. The most commonly used contrast agent in clinical studies is gadolinium-DTPA. The gadolinium is the active part of the agent, and the DTPA is a chelating agent. Gadolinium has several unpaired electrons, and the interaction of the large magnetic dipole moments of these electrons with the water molecules leads to a decrease in the local relaxation times. In describing the effects of a contrast agent, it is convenient to talk of the effect on the relaxation *rate constant R,* the inverse of the relaxation time. In brain tissues the transverse relaxation rate R_2 ($= 1/T_2$) is about ten times larger than the longitudinal relaxation rate R_1 ($= 1/T_1$). The effect of gadolinium is to add to each of these rates a change ΔR that is proportional to the concentration of gadolinium. But because R_2 is much larger than R_1, for moderate concentrations of gadolinium the effect is a large change in R_1, but only a minor change in R_2. For this reason, gadolinium acts primarily as a T_1-agent, altering the T_1 of spins that come into contact with the gadolinium.

The relaxivity effect of gadolinium is exploited in clinical studies to enhance the signal of particular tissues in T_1-weighted images, with the primary application being in brain tumor imaging. An important criterion for evaluating brain masses is whether they have an intact blood brain barrier (BBB), and this can be directly assessed with Gd-DTPA. The relaxivity effect of gadolinium only operates when the water comes into contact with the agent. With an intact BBB, the gadolinium cannot cross into the extravascular space and so remains confined in the blood. The relaxation time of the blood is reduced, but because the blood contributes only a few percent of the net signal, there is little enhancement in a T_1-weighted image. In contrast, if the BBB is leaky, the gadolinium enters the tissue and reduces the T_1. The result is a significant enhancement of the tumor in a T_1-weighted image.

More recently, Gd-DTPA-enhanced angiography has become a useful tool for visualizing the large blood vessels. After a rapid injection of the agent, dynamic imaging is used to capture the passage of the agent through the major vessels. Because the T_1 of the blood is greatly reduced, the blood signal relaxes quickly and so produces a strong signal and high contrast between the vessels and the surrounding tissues.

Signal Drop Due to Contrast Agent in the Vasculature

The possibility of using Gd-DTPA to assess aspects of microvascular flow in the brain began with the observation that a bolus of Gd-DTPA creates a transient *drop* in the MR signal as it passes through the brain (Villringer et al., 1988) (illustrated in Figure 6.1). This clearly suggested that dynamic measurement of the kinetics of Gd-DTPA could provide information on the perfusion state of the tissue. However, the observed effect was rather surprising given the preceding discussion because Gd-

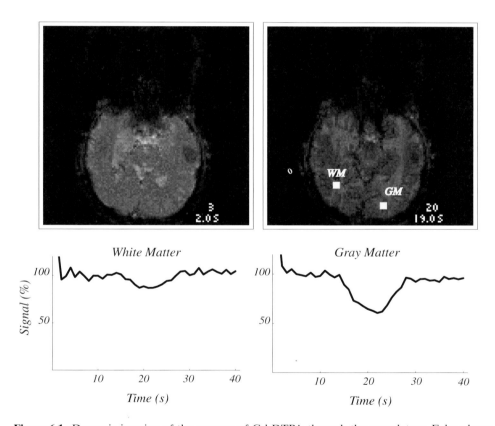

Figure 6.1. Dynamic imaging of the passage of Gd-DTPA through the vasculature. Echo planar single-shot images are collected every second for 40 s following injection of the contrast agent (top). Gadolinium alters the magnetic susceptibility of the blood, creating field gradients around the vessels and a transient drop in the signal (bottom). The magnitude of the signal drop reflects the local blood volume. The third image in the series (top left) shows little contrast between gray and white matter, whereas the image at 20 s (top right) shows a deeper signal reduction in gray matter due to the larger blood volume. The signal variations over time are plotted for a region of white matter (WM) and gray matter (GM). (Data courtesy of B. Georgi.)

DTPA is commonly used to *enhance* the MR signal by reducing the T_1. In a normal brain with an intact BBB, the Gd remains confined to the vascular space, so there should be no effect on the T_1 of tissue. This, combined with the fact that the signal change is in the wrong direction for a T_1 shortening effect, suggests that the observed signal drop is due to an effect of gadolinium different from its effect on the longitudinal relaxation.

As described earlier, gadolinium possesses an additional physical property with magnetic effects: a large magnetic dipole moment. The large magnetic moment of gadolinium alters the magnetic susceptibility of the blood, creating a large susceptibility difference between the vessels and the extravascular space. Field gradients are produced throughout the tissue, and these field gradients lead to signal loss. Note that this susceptibility effect occurs for precisely the same reason that the relaxivity effects of gadolinium are minor: the agent is confined to the vascular space. If, instead, the gadolinium freely diffused into the extravascular space, the intra- and extravascular concentrations would be about the same, and there would be no susceptibility difference and no signal loss. The fact that there is a strong susceptibility effect has been demonstrated by using a different contrast agent, dysprosium. Dysprosium also has a large magnetic moment, even larger than gadolinium, but has essentially no effect on relaxivity. Experiments with dysprosium show an even larger signal drop for the same dose, as would be expected for a larger change in magnetic susceptibility (Villringer et al., 1988).

The signal drop as gadolinium passes through the microvasculature is transient but can be measured with fast imaging techniques such as echo planar imaging (EPI). In qualitative terms, we expect that the larger the amount of the agent within the voxel, the larger the signal dip will be. Because the agent is confined to the blood vessels, the total amount present is directly proportional to the local cerebral blood volume. A full quantitative analysis of the kinetic curves of Gd-DTPA is somewhat more involved and is discussed in Chapter 14, but the basic idea is that the magnitude of the signal drop reflects local blood volume.

Brain Activation Measured with Contrast Agents

The first measurement of brain activation with MRI used this basic analysis to measure CBV in two states (Belliveau et al., 1991). In the resting state, the subject lay quietly in the dark. In the active state, the subject viewed a flashing grid of red lights through a goggle system. In each state Gd-DTPA was injected, and the kinetic curves were measured in a slice through the visual cortex along the calcarine fissure. The dynamic curve for each voxel was analyzed to produce a map of CBV, and image voxels showing a significant change in CBV were highlighted. The results were that CBV increased on average by 24% in the visual cortex.

For studies of brain activation, contrast agent techniques are technically demanding. A separate injection is required for each measurement of CBV. The gadolinium quickly spreads to other parts of the body, so it is present in the blood in sufficient concentration to produce the desired susceptibility effect only in its first pass through the vasculature. Because multiple injections are required, only a few states of activation can be examined in one subject. Also, the dose and rate of injection must be carefully controlled to ensure that each injection is identical. The administered dose, and even the rate of injection, directly affect the shape of the tissue curve, so any difference in the injections could produce an artifactual difference in the CBV measured in two states. Furthermore, the gadolinium bolus injection technique cannot measure the dynamics of a changing CBV. In each measurement we assume that the CBV is constant, and the changing MR signal then reflects the changing concentration of gadolinium in this fixed volume.

These technical problems could be alleviated if the susceptibility agent remained in the blood for a sufficiently long time so that the blood concentration remains constant during a study. For a fixed CBV the signal would be offset from the signal without the agent but would be constant once the agent had equilibrated in the blood. Dynamic changes in the signal then would reflect changes in CBV. Experimental paradigms like those used for BOLD studies could be used, and because the signal changes produced by contrast agents can be substantially larger than BOLD signal changes due to oxygenation changes, these techniques could be quite sensitive to subtle brain activations. Such agents have been developed for animal studies and used to measure dynamic CBV changes during activation (Mandeville et al., 1998). If such agents are approved for human studies, they will provide a powerful tool for investigating brain activation. For now, though, contrast agent methods for fMRI have been superceded for activation studies in humans by the methods based on intrinsic blood oxygenation changes. However, blood volume measurements with Gd-DTPA have become a standard clinical tool for the evaluation of stroke and other brain lesions.

ARTERIAL SPIN LABELING

Imaging Cerebral Blood Flow

The goal with arterial spin labeling is to map cerebral blood flow directly. The contrast agent methods described earlier are primarily sensitive to cerebral blood volume, and it is difficult to extract a CBF measurement from observations of the kinetics of an intravascular tracer. The BOLD methods are sensitive to changes in blood oxygenation, which depend on the combined effect of changes in CBF, CBV, and $CMRO_2$. Even though the BOLD effect correlates strongly with changes in CBF, it does not provide a direct quantitative measurement of CBF alone. In nuclear medicine studies, CBF is measured with a diffusible tracer that readily leaves the capillary and diffuses throughout the tissue volume. The tracer is delivered to different brain areas in proportion to the local CBF, and so the amount delivered to a tissue element directly reflects the perfusion of that element. Over time the tracer will clear from the tissue element, and the rate of clearance is also proportional to local CBF. Blood flow can be found by measuring the tissue concentration over time, monitoring either the delivery or the clearance of the tracer. In PET studies with $H_2{}^{15}O$, the tissue concentration of ^{15}O is imaged to determine the rate of delivery of the tracer to each image voxel, and in ^{133}Xe studies the rate of clearance of the tracer from different brain regions is monitored with external detectors (see Chapter 2).

In recent years, several MRI techniques which are similar in principle to these nuclear medicine techniques, have been developed (Detre et al., 1992; Edelman et al., 1994; Kim, 1995; Wong, Buxton, and Frank, 1998). With these ASL techniques, the water of arterial blood is labeled before it is delivered to the imaging plane, and so these methods are similar in many respects to tracer studies with $H_2^{15}O$. Although the basic principles and approach to quantifying CBF carry over from nuclear medicine techniques to MRI, a crucial difference between ASL methods and radioactive tracer methods is that in ASL no tracer is injected. Instead, the arterial blood is tagged magnetically with MR techniques, and the delivery of this tagged water to each image voxel is measured. Because these techniques are completely noninvasive, the tagging can be repeated many times for averaging to produce perfusion maps with a high signal-to-noise ratio (SNR). ASL, thus, has the potential to produce maps of perfusion in the human brain with higher spatial and temporal resolution than any other existing technique.

Principles of Arterial Spin Labeling

Arterial spin labeling is based on a simple idea, but in practice using this idea to create quantitative perfusion maps requires careful attention to several sources of systematic error. For this reason, dealing with these technical difficulties is a critical aspect of ASL methods, and the implementation of these methods involves some subtle, but important, features. To begin with, though, we will ignore these difficulties to clarify the basic idea behind the method. The practical problems are discussed in Chapter 15.

Suppose that the goal is to measure the perfusion in each voxel of a transverse slice through the brain. The ASL experiment involves making two images of this slice, referred to as the tag and control images. For the tag image, the magnetization of the water in the arterial blood is inverted before it reaches the slice. For example, a 180° RF pulse applied in a slice-selective fashion to a thick slab below the imaging slice will invert all the spins, including those of arterial blood that will eventually be delivered to the slice of interest. After a delay inversion time TI (typically about 1 s) to allow inverted blood to flow into the slice, an image of the slice itself is collected, creating the tag image. The control image is acquired in exactly the same way but with one exception: the arterial magnetization is not inverted. If this is done carefully, any difference in the signal of a voxel between the tag and control images should be due only to the difference in the signal of arterial blood delivered during the interval TI. Specifically, in each image the voxel signal is proportional to the longitudinal magnetization of the voxel at the time of the image. If no arterial blood is delivered, the signals measured in the tag and control images should be the same, and so the difference image should be zero. But if arterial blood is delivered to a voxel it will carry an inverted magnetization in the tag image but a fully relaxed magnetization in the control image, and so the signals of blood will not cancel in the subtraction image.

The ASL difference image is then proportional to how much arterial blood has entered the slice during the interval TI. If the local CBF is denoted by f (milliliters of blood per milliliter of tissue per second), and the volume of a voxel is V (ml), then the total rate of arterial flow (ml/s) into the voxel is fV, and the volume of arterial blood delivered during TI is fVTI. Or, more simply, the fraction of the voxel volume that is replaced with incoming arterial blood during the interval TI is fTI. For example, for a typical CBF in the human brain, $f = 0.01$ s^{-1}, and so for a typical delay of TI = 1 s, the delivered volume of arterial water is only 1% of the volume of the voxel. If CBF increases by 50%, the amount of arterial water delivered will also increase by 50%, so the ASL difference signal is directly proportional to CBF.

In practice, to make this a quantitatively accurate measurement, several confounding factors must be taken into account. Probably the most important correction that must be included accounts for the fact that the blood requires some time to travel from the inversion band to the imaging voxel (Alsop and Detre, 1996; Buxton et al., 1998). This transit delay not only varies across the brain but also changes in the same brain region with activation. If the transit delay effect is not taken into account, the ASL image is only a semiquantitative map of perfusion because the measured signal will reflect the transit delay as well. Another problem is that some of the tagged arterial blood present in the slice when the image is acquired may be in large vessels and destined to perfuse a more distal capillary bed, rather than the capillary bed of the voxel in which it appears. This can lead to an overestimate of local perfusion.

The magnetization of the tagged blood decays in the time between the inversion pulse and the measurement, reducing the ASL signal. This decay is analogous to radioactive decay of a tracer, and a correction must be made to account for it. But this is complicated because the decay rate initially is governed by the T_1 of arterial blood, but after the water molecule has left the capillary and entered the extravascular space, the decay is governed by the T_1 of tissue. This correction thus depends on the time of exchange of water from the blood to the tissue. Finally, an absolute calibration of the ASL difference signal in terms of CBF units requires information about the M_0 of blood. All these factors must be taken into account to produce a quantitative map of CBF, and much of the current research in this area focuses on how to deal with these problems. But when these effects are carefully controlled, ASL can produce accurate maps of CBF.

There are several versions of ASL techniques, differing in how the tagging is done, the nature of the control image, whether they are compatible with multislice imaging, and sensitivity to the various confounding factors that complicate the determination of a quantitative CBF map. These techniques are discussed in detail in Chapter 15. But for now, we can illustrate the potential of ASL imaging of perfusion with a set of images made with a technique called QUIPSS II (Quantitative Imaging of Perfusion with a Single Subtraction, version II) (Wong et al., 1998). The images in Figure 6.2 show five slices with the T_1-weighted anatomical images on the bottom and the ASL perfusion images on the top. The perfusion images were acquired in a total imaging time of 3 min by alternating between tag and control images every 2 s and constructing the average difference map. Because the ASL signal change is so small, averaging is necessary to improve the SNR. The areas of highest perfusion closely follow the gray matter.

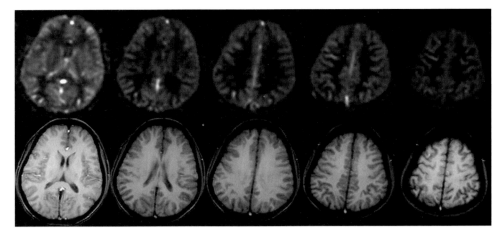

Figure 6.2. Arterial spin labeling images of cerebral blood flow. The top row shows five contiguous 8-mm sections through the brain collected with the QUIPSS II pulse sequence, and the bottom row shows conventional anatomical images for comparison. Note that the CBF is highest in gray matter, as would be expected. Averaging for the ASL images required 3 min of data acquisition. (Data courtesy of E. Wong.)

BLOOD OXYGENATION LEVEL DEPENDENT fMRI

Blood Susceptibility Depends on Deoxyhemoglobin Content

In contrast agent studies the susceptibility of the blood is manipulated by the experimenter. But nature has also provided an intrinsic physiological agent that alters blood susceptibility: deoxyhemoglobin. Fully oxygenated blood has about the same susceptibility as other brain tissues, but deoxyhemoglobin is paramagnetic and changes the susceptibility of the blood. As capillary and venous blood become more deoxygenated, field distortions around the vessels are increased, and the local signal decreases. And in a complementary fashion, if blood oxygenation increases the local MR signal also increases. This BOLD contrast is the basis of most of the fMRI studies of brain activation performed today.

The phenomenon of changes in blood oxygenation producing a measurable effect on MR images was first observed by Ogawa and co-workers (1990a). In this pioneering study they imaged the brain of a mouse breathing different levels of O_2, using a 9-T system with strong gradients to produce a voxel resolution of 65 μm in plane and a slice thickness of 700 μm. They found that when the mouse breathed 100% oxygen, the brain image was rather uniform and featureless. But when the animal breathed only 20% oxygen there was a dramatic change. Many dark lines appeared, outlining the major structures in the brain. The dark lines corresponded to the locations of blood vessels, and when the oxygenation of the blood was increased back to 100%, the lines reversibly disappeared. These investigators also noted that the signal loss around the vessels was greater with increased TE, and that the width of some of the lines grew larger as TE was increased, suggesting that the presence of the deoxygenated blood in the vessels affected the transverse relaxation outside as well as within the vessels. The observed signal loss was interpreted to be a result of the change in the magnetic susceptibility of the blood vessel compared to its surroundings due to an increase in deoxyhemoglobin.

The fact that deoxyhemoglobin is paramagnetic, and that this creates magnetic field gradients inside and around the red blood cells, was well known (Thulborn et al., 1982), but this was the first demonstration that this phenomenon could produce a measurable effect in an MR image following a physiological manipulation. Subsequent studies in a cat model at 4 T using EPI further demonstrated that changes in brain oxygenation following respiratory challenges could be followed with GRE imaging (Turner et al., 1991).

These animal studies in which blood oxygenation was manipulated by the experimenter suggested that natural physiological processes that alter the oxygenation of blood also might be detectable with MRI. Kwong and co-workers reported a demonstration of mapping activation in the human brain using gradient echo MR imaging during visual stimulation and a simple motor task (Kwong et al., 1992). In these experiments a 1-min stimulus period alternated with a 1-min rest period, and EPI images were collected throughout several periods of stimulus and rest. The GRE signal in the visual cortex increased by about 3–4% during the photic stimulation, and a similar increase was observed in the hand motor area during a hand-squeezing task. This report, and several others published shortly afterward (Bandettini et al., 1992; Frahm et al., 1992; Ogawa et al., 1992), marked the beginning of functional human brain mapping based on the BOLD effect.

At first glance, the observation of a signal increase during activation seems somewhat surprising because it implies that the blood is more oxygenated in areas of focal brain activation. Ogawa et al. (1990a) in their original paper had earlier speculated that the deoxyhemoglobin effect could be used to monitor regional oxygen usage, suggesting that more active regions would appear darker because of increased deoxyhemoglobin resulting from higher oxygen consumption. However, this plausible prediction turned out to be wrong because of the nature of the physiological changes that occur during brain activation. As discussed in Chapter 3, earlier positron emission tomography studies by Fox and co-workers (Fox and Raichle, 1986; Fox et al., 1988) had found a pronounced mismatch between the increases in blood flow and oxygen metabolism during brain activation: CBF increases much more than $CMRO_2$. As a result, the delivery of oxygen to the capillary bed is substantially increased, but less is removed from the blood, so the blood is more oxygenated.

Our picture of the BOLD effect is then as follows. In the normal awake human brain about 40% of the oxygen delivered to the capillary bed in arterial blood is extracted and metabolized. There is thus a substantial amount of deoxyhemoglobin in the venous vessels, and so the MR signal is attenuated from what it would be if there were no deoxyhemoglobin. When the brain is activated, the local flow increases substantially, but oxygen metabolism increases only a small amount. As a result, the oxygen extraction is reduced, and the venous blood is more oxygenated. The fall in deoxyhemoglobin concentration leads to a signal increase. At 1.5 T the increase is typically small (a few percent or less). Nevertheless, with careful statistical analysis such small changes can be reliably detected. At higher fields, such as 4 T, the signal changes are much larger, in the range of 5–15%.

Mapping Brain Activation with BOLD Signal Changes

Since the discovery that brain activation creates small changes in the local MR signal through the BOLD effect, a number of imaging approaches have been used to measure it. The prototype brain mapping experiment consists of alternating periods of a stimulus task and a control task (Bandettini et al., 1993). For example, in one of the most often repeated experiments, a subject rapidly taps the fingers of one hand against the thumb for a short period (e.g., 30 s) and then rests for the same period. This cycle is repeated several times. Throughout these stimulus/control cycles dynamic echo planar images are collected covering all or part of the brain. For a typical implementation the EPI images are acquired rapidly in a single-shot mode, requiring 100 ms or less for each image acquisition, and the spatial resolution is low compared to conventional MR images (e.g., $3 \times 3 \times 5$ mm). In this multislice dynamic imaging, images of each of the chosen slices are acquired in rapid succession, and after a repetition time TR this set of images is acquired again. The image acquisition is repeated at regular intervals of TR throughout the experiment, while the subject alternates between stimulus and control tasks.

This set of images can be thought of as a four-dimensional data set: three spatial dimensions plus time. For example, Figure 6.3 shows a single slice through the motor area from such a study in which eight cycles of 16 s of finger tapping were alternated with 16 s of rest. With TR = 2 s, 128 images were collected covering the eight cycles. The figure shows a high-resolution anatomical image and one image from the dynamic EPI series. The signal time courses for a block of 3×3 pixels of the dynamic images are also shown. These data are analyzed to identify areas of activation by examining the signal time course for each individual pixel with the goal of identifying pixels in which the signal shows a significant change between the stimulus and control periods. In Figure 6.3 the eight-cycle pattern is clearly evident in a few pixels, but often changes that are not apparent to the eye are nevertheless statistically significant. Because the signal changes due to the BOLD effect are small (only a few percent at 1.5 T), this statistical analysis is a critical aspect of interpreting BOLD data and is described in more detail in Chapter 18. The end result of the statistical analysis is a decision for each voxel of whether or not there was a significantly detectable activation, based on whether a calculated statistic, such as the t-statistic or the correlation coefficient, passed a chosen threshold.

An important factor to include in the statistical analysis of BOLD data is that the metabolic activity producing the change in blood oxygenation and the BOLD effect lags behind the stimulus itself. That is, one must assume some model for the hemodynamic response to stimulation, and a typical assumed form is a delayed trapezoid. Figure 6.4 illustrates a correlation analysis of the dynamic BOLD data in Figure 6.3. The hemodynamic response (i.e., the BOLD signal change) is modeled as a trapezoid with 6-s ramps and a delay of 2 s after the start of the stimulus, and the

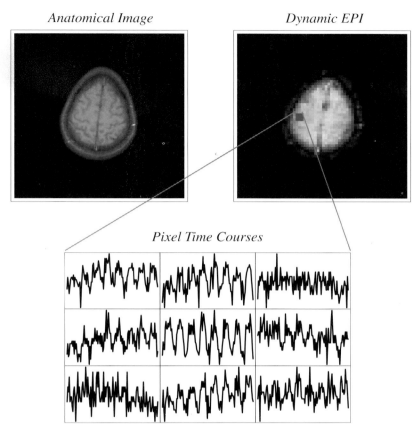

Figure 6.3. BOLD signal changes. On the left is a high-resolution anatomical image (256×256 matrix) cutting through the central sulci and the hand motor and sensory areas. On the right is one image from a series of 128 low-resolution dynamic images (64×64 matrix) collected every 2 s with EPI. The signal time courses from a 3×3 block of pixels is shown at the bottom. During the data acquisition the subject performed eight cycles of a bilateral finger tapping task, with one cycle consisting of 16 s of tapping followed by 16 s of rest. Several pixels show clear patterns of signal variation that correlate with the task. (Data courtesy of L. Frank.)

correlation of this model function with the measured pixel time course is calculated for each pixel. Those pixels that show a correlation coefficient greater than a chosen threshold value are designated as activated pixels and are then displayed in color overlayed on a gray scale image of the underlying anatomy. The gray scale image could be one of the EPI images from the dynamic time series or a higher resolution structural image acquired separately, such as a volume acquisition. Only the pixels that pass the chosen statistical threshold are colored, and for these pixels the color used typically reflects either the value of the statistic (e.g., the correlation coefficient) or a measure of the degree of signal change (e.g., percent signal change) (Bandettini et al., 1993).

This basic paradigm is widely used, but there are many variations. Single-shot EPI is the most commonly used image acquisition technique because it has desir-

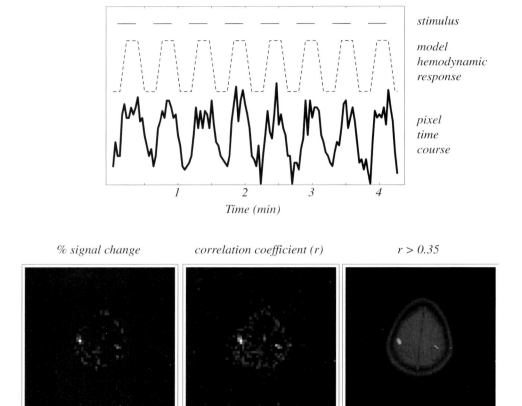

Figure 6.4. Correlation analysis of dynamic EPI data to identify pixels showing evidence of activity. The hemodynamic response is modeled as a trapezoid, with 6-s ramps and a delay of 2 s from the beginning of the stimulus (top). By correlating the model function with a pixel time course, the signal change (left image) and the correlation coefficient r can be calculated (middle image). The pixels passing a threshold of $r > 0.35$ are highlighted on the anatomical image (right image). For this final display the 64×64 calculated image of r was interpolated up to 256×256 to match the high-resolution image.

able features of rapid data acquisition and a high SNR. But multishot EPI and conventional 2D and 3D GRE imaging also are used. Both GRE and SE images exhibit BOLD effects, although the GRE signal is more sensitive because the signal changes produced by activation are larger. However, because the SE signal changes are more likely to reflect microvascular changes, they may give a more precise spatial map of the areas of activation. In addition, asymmetric spin echoes (ASE) are sometimes used because the ASE signal is intermediate between the GRE and SE signals in terms of both overall sensitivity and sensitivity to the microvasculature. The basic block design of stimulus trials is often used, but single-trial (Dale and Buckner, 1997) and continuously varying (Sereno et al., 1995) stimulus paradigms have also been developed.

REFERENCES

Alsop, D. C., and Detre, J. A. (1996) Reduced transit-time sensitivity in noninvasive magnetic resonance imaging of human cerebral blood flow. *J. Cereb. Blood Flow Metabal.* **16,** 1236–49.

Bandettini, P. A., Jesmanowicz, A., Wong, E. C., and Hyde, J. S. (1993) Processing strategies for time-course data sets in functional MRI of the human brain. *Magn. Reson. Med.* **30,** 161–73.

Bandettini, P. A., Wong, E. C., Hinks, R. S., Tikofsky, R. S., and Hyde, J. S. (1992) Time course EPI of human brain function during task activation. *Magn. Reson. Med.* **25,** 390–7.

Belliveau, J. W., Kennedy, D. N., McKinstry, R. C., Buchbinder, B. R., Weisskoff, R. M., Cohen, M. S., Vevea, J. M., Brady, T. J., and Rosen, B. R. (1991) Functional mapping of the human visual cortex by magnetic resonance imaging. *Science* **254,** 716–19.

Buxton, R. B., Frank, L. R., Wong, E. C., Siewert, B., Warach, S., and Edelman, R. R. (1998) A general kinetic model for quantitative perfusion imaging with arterial spin labeling. *Magn. Reson. Med.* **40,** 383–96.

Dale, A. M., and Buckner, R. L. (1997) Selective averaging of rapidly presented individual trials using fMRI. *Human Brain Mapping* **5,** 329–40.

Davis, T. L., Kwong, K. K., Weisskoff, R. M., and Rosen, B. R. (1998) Calibrated functional MRI: Mapping the dynamics of oxidative metabolism. *Proc. Natl. Acad. Sci. USA* **95,** 1834–9.

Detre, J. A., Leigh, J. S., WIlliams, D. S., and Koretsky, A. P. (1992) Perfusion imaging. *Magn. Reson. Med.* **23,** 37–45.

Edelman, R. R., Siewert, B., Darby, D. G., Thangaraj, V., Nobre, A. C., Mesulam, M. M., and Warach, S. (1994) Qualitative mapping of cerebral blood flow and functional localization with echo-planar MR imaging and signal targeting with alternating radio frequency (STAR) sequences: Applications to MR angiography. *Radiology* **192,** 513–20.

Fox, P. T., and Raichle, M. E. (1986) Focal physiological uncoupling of cerebral blood flow and oxidative metabolism during somatosensory stimulation in human subjects. *Proc. Natl. Acad. Sci. USA* **83,** 1140–4.

Fox, P. T., Raichle, M. E., Mintun, M. A., and Dence, C. (1988) Nonoxidative glucose consumption during focal physiologic neural activity. *Science* **241,** 462–4.

Frahm, J., Bruhn, H., Merboldt, K.-D., Hanicke, W., and Math, D. (1992) Dynamic MR imaging of human brain oxygenation during rest and photic stimulation. *J. Magn. Reson. Imag.* **2,** 501–5.

Kim, S.-G. (1995) Quantification of regional cerebral blood flow change by flow-sensitive alternating inversion recovery (FAIR) technique: Application to functional mapping. *Magn. Reson. Med.* **34,** 293–301.

Kwong, K. K., Belliveau, J. W., Chesler, D. A., Goldberg, I. E., Weisskoff, R. M., Poncelet, B. P., Kennedy, D. N., Hoppel, B. E., Cohen, M. S., Turner, R., Cheng, H.-M., Brady, T. J., and Rosen, B. R. (1992) Dynamic magnetic resonance imaging of human brain activity during primary sensory stimulation. *Proc. Natl. Acad. Sci. USA* **89,** 5675–9.

LeBihan, D., Breton, E., Lallemand, D., Aubin, M.-L., Vignaud, J., and Laval-Jeantet, M. (1988) Separation of diffusion and perfusion in intravoxel incoherent motion MR imaging. *Radiology* **168,** 497–505.

Mandeville, J. B., Marota, J. J. A., Kosofsky, B. E., Keltner, J. R., Weissleder, R., Rosen, B. R., and Weisskoff, R. M. (1998) Dynamic functional imaging of relative cerebral blood volume during rat forepaw stimulation. *Magn. Reson. Med.* **39,** 615–24.

Ogawa, S., Lee, T.-M., Nayak, A. S., and Glynn, P. (1990a) Oxygenation – Sensitive contrast in magnetic resonance image of rodent brain at high magnetic fields. *Magn. Reson. Med.* **14,** 68–78.

Ogawa, S., Lee, T. M., Kay, A. R., and Tank, D. W. (1990b) Brain magnetic resonance imaging with contrast dependent on blood oxygenation. *Proc. Natl. Acad. Sci. USA* **87,** 9868–72.

Ogawa, S., Tank, D. W., Menon, R., Ellermann, J. M., Kim, S.-G., Merkle, H., and Ugurbil, K. (1992) Intrinsic signal changes accompanying sensory stimulation: functional brain mapping with magnetic resonance imaging. *Proc. Natl. Acad. Sci. USA.* **89,** 5951–5.

Østergaard, L., Sorensen, A. G., Kwong, K. K., Weisskoff, R. M., Gyldensted, C., and Rosen, B. R. (1996a) High resolution measurement of cerebral blood flow using intravascular tracer bolus passages. Part II: Experimental comparison and preliminary results. *Magn. Reson. Med.* **36,** 726–36.

Østergaard, L., Weisskoff, R. M., Chesler, D. A., Gyldensted, C., and Rosen, B. R. (1996b) High resolution measurement of cerebral blood flow using intravascular tracer bolus passages. Part I: Mathematical approach and statistical analysis. *Magn. Reson. Med.* **36,** 715–25.

Rosen, B. R., Belliveau, J. W., and Chien, D. (1989) Perfusion imaging by nuclear magnetic resonance. *Magn. Reson. Quart.* **5,** 263–81.

Sereno, M. I., Dale, A. M., Reppas, J. R., Kwong, K. K., Belliveau, J. W., Brady, T. J., Rosen, B. R., and Tootell, R. B. H. (1995) Functional MRI reveals borders of multiple visual areas in humans. *Science* **268,** 889–93.

Thulborn, K. R., Waterton, J. C., Matthews, P. M., and Radda, G. K. (1982) Oxygenation dependence of the transverse relaxation time of water protons in whole blood at high field. *Biochim. Biophys. Acta* **714,** 265–70.

Turner, R., LeBihan, D., Moonen, C. T. W., Despres, D., and Frank, J. (1991) Echo-planar time course MRI of cat brain oxygenation changes. *Magn. Reson. Med.* **27,** 159–66.

Villringer, A., Rosen, B. R., Belliveau, J. W., Ackerman, J. L., Lauffer, R. B., Buxton, R. B., Chao, Y.-S., Wedeen, V. J., and Brady, T. J. (1988) Dynamic imaging with lanthanide chelates in normal brain: contrast due to magnetic susceptibility effects. *Magn. Reson. Med.* **6,** 164–74.

Wong, E. C., Buxton, R. B., and Frank, L. R. (1998) Quantitative imaging of perfusion using a single subtraction (QUIPSS and QUIPSS II). *Magn. Reson. Med.* **39,** 702–8.

Part Two

PRINCIPLES OF MAGNETIC RESONANCE IMAGING

IIA

The Nature of the Magnetic Resonance Signal

7

Basic Physics of Magnetism and NMR

INTRODUCTION

In Chapter 4 the basic features of the nuclear magnetic resonance (NMR) experiment were introduced, and in this chapter the basic physics underlying NMR is presented in more detail. We begin with a review of the basic physics of magnetic fields, including how coils are used to detect the NMR signal and how gradient fields are produced for imaging. The dynamics of a magnetic dipole in a magnetic field, which is the central physics underlying NMR, is considered next in terms of the two important physical processes of precession and relaxation. Precession and relaxation have quite different characteristics; precession is a rotation of the magnetization without changing its magnitude, whereas relaxation creates and destroys magnetization. The interplay of these two processes leads to a rich variety of dynamical behavior of the magnetization. In the final section the magnetic properties of matter are considered in terms of how the partial alignment of dipoles with the magnetic field creates additional fields in the body. These field variations due to magnetic susceptibility differences between tissues lead to unwanted distortions in magnetic resonance (MR) images, but such effects are also the basis for most of the functional magnetic resonance imaging (fMRI) techniques.

In trying to understand how NMR works, it is helpful to have an easily visualized model for the process. The physical picture presented here is a classical physics view, and yet the physics of a proton in a magnetic field is correctly described only by quantum mechanics. The source of the NMR phenomenon is that the proton possesses spin, and spin is intrinsically a quantum mechanical property. Despite the familiar sounding name, spin is fundamentally different from the angular momentum of more familiar terrestrial scale objects. For example, a spinning baseball possesses angular momentum, and yet we can easily imagine changing that angular momentum by spinning it faster or stopping it altogether. In other words, the spin is not an intrinsic part of the baseball. But for a proton, the spin *is* an intrinsic part of being a proton. It never speeds up and never slows down, and the only aspect of the spin that can be changed is the orientation of the spin axis. Neutrons also possess spin, and protons and neutrons combine to form a nucleus such that their spins mutually cancel (opposite spin axes), so that the nucleus has no net spin unless there are an odd number of protons or neutrons. Thus, the nuclei of ^1H (1 proton) and ^{13}C (6 protons and 7 neutrons) have a net spin, but ^{12}C does not.

Furthermore, the quantum view is still stranger, with only certain states allowed, and even the definition of a state is rather different from the classical view. At first glance, the quantum view seems to simplify the picture of the NMR phenomenon. The centerpiece of the quantum view is that any measurement of one component of the spin of a proton will yield only one of two possible values of the spin orientation: spin up or spin down. It seems as if this two-state system ought to be easier to think about than magnetic moment vectors that can point in any direction. However, this sort of partial introduction of quantum ideas into the description of NMR often leads to confusion. After all, if the spin can only be up or down in a magnetic field, how do we ever get transverse magnetization, precession, and the NMR signal? In short, the quantum view is correct, but it is difficult to think about the wide range of phenomena involved in NMR from a purely quantum viewpoint. Fortunately, however, the classical view, although totally incorrect in its description of the behavior of a single proton, nevertheless gives the correct physics for the *average* behavior of many protons, and accurately describes most of the physics encountered in magnetic resonance imaging (MRI). For this reason, we will develop a physical picture of NMR based on a classical view, and the only feature from quantum mechanics that is essential is the existence of spin itself. For the interested reader, the appendix contains a sketch of the quantum mechanical view of NMR.

ELECTROMAGNETIC FIELDS

The Field Concept

Nearly every aspect of the world around us is the result of the interactions of charged particles. Electrons in an atom are bound to the nucleus by the electric force between the charges, and light, and other forms of electromagnetic radiation, can be understood as the cooperative interplay among changing electric and magnetic fields. The phenomenon of NMR is, of course, deeply connected to magnetic field interactions, in particular the behavior of a magnetic dipole in a magnetic field. In addition, a recurring theme in MRI is the geometrical shape of the magnetic field, which underlies the design of coils for MRI, distortions in fast MRI, and the microscopic field variations that are the basis for the Blood Oxygenation Level Dependent (BOLD) signal changes measured during brain activation. To begin with, we consider the nature of magnetic fields. (Excellent introductions to electromagnetic fields are Purcell, 1965, and Feynman, Leighton, and Sands, 1965.)

The concept of a field is a useful way of visualizing physical interactions, and the simplest example is a gravitational field. In comparison with the complex interactions of charged particles, the gravitational interaction of two massive bodies is relatively simple. The two bodies attract each other with a force that is proportional to the product of their masses and inversely proportional to the square of the distance between them. We describe this interaction in terms of a field by saying that the second body interacts with the gravitational field created by the first body. The field extends through all of space, and the strength of the field at any point is proportional to the mass of the body and falls off with distance from the body with an inverse square law.

The gravitational field is a vector field in which each point in space has a vector arrow attached that describes the local strength and direction of the field. For visualizing a field, the most direct way is to imagine such arrows at every point in space, but this is difficult to draw. Instead, the usual way to show fields is to draw continuous *field lines*. A field line is an imagined line running through space such that the direction of the local field at any point on the line is tangent to the line. Each point in space has a field line running through it, but the field pattern can be graphically depicted by showing only selected field lines. Field lines naturally show the local field direction, but the magnitude of the local field is shown in a more subtle way. The stronger the field, the more closely spaced the field lines are drawn. Thus, for the gravitational field around a spherical body, the field is drawn as radial lines pointed inward.

The electric field is in some ways analogous to the gravitational field, with electric charge playing the role of mass. The electric force between two charged bodies is proportional to the product of their charges and falls off with the square of the distance between them. However, there are two important differences between the electric field and the gravitational field: (1) the electric force between two like charges is repulsive, rather than attractive, and (2) charges can be either positive or negative, and the force between opposite charges is attractive. Because mass is

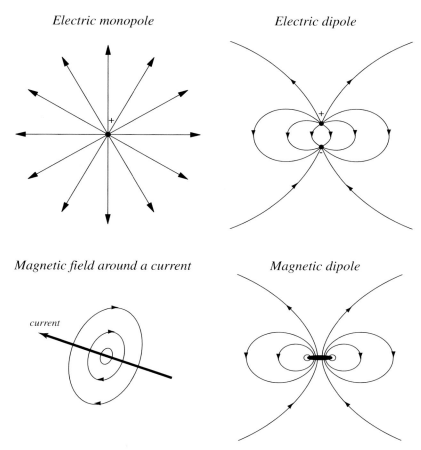

Figure 7.1. Basic electric and magnetic field patterns. The simplest electric fields are the monopole field produced by a single charge (top left) and the dipole field produced by two opposite and slightly displaced charges (top right). There are no magnetic monopoles, and the simplest source of a magnetic field is a straight wire carrying a current (bottom left). If the wire is bent into a small loop of current, the field is a magnetic dipole field (bottom right). The electric and magnetic dipole fields are identical far from the source but are quite different near the source.

always positive, gravity is always attractive and tends to pull matter into large massive bodies such as stars and planets. And because charges can be positive or negative, the electric force tends to group matter into smaller stable structures with no net charge, such as atoms and molecules.

The electric field can be represented graphically in the same way as the gravitational field, with the local vector arrows indicating the direction of the force on a positively charged particle (a negatively charged particle would feel a force in the opposite direction). For example, Figure 7.1 (top left) shows the electric field around a positive charge, a *monopole field*. The field lines are radial and point outward, indicating that the force on another positive charge is repulsive. If the central charge were negative, the field lines would point inward like a gravitational field. However, because there are both positive and negative charges, there are electric field configurations that have no counterpart in a gravitational field. For example, Figure 7.1 (top right) shows the field around two charges with equal magnitude but opposite sign, a pattern known as an *electric dipole field*. There is no corresponding dipole gravitational field.

Magnetic Fields

The existence of both positive and negative charges introduces some complexities into the interaction of charged particles, but the electric field is only a part of the picture. In addition to the electric interactions, there are additional forces generated due to the motions of the charges. When a charged particle moves through a region where a magnetic field is present, the particle will feel a force in addition to that due to any electric field that may be present. For example, consider two parallel wires carrying currents in the same direction. The positive and negative charges in each wire are balanced, so there is no electric force between the two wires. Yet experiments show that with parallel currents there is an attractive force between the two wires. If the current in one wire is reversed, the force becomes repulsive, and if the current in one wire is reduced to zero, the force disappears. This additional force is a result of the interaction of the moving charges in one wire interacting with the magnetic field created by the current in the other wire.

The force on a wire carrying a current in a magnetic field is the basis for a loudspeaker system, making possible the conversion of electrical signals into mechanical vibrations. It is also the source of the loud acoustic noise in an MR scanner. Imaging depends on applying pulsed gradient fields to the sample, which means that strong current pulses are applied to the gradient coils. These wires carry substantial current and are in a large magnetic field, so there are large forces produced, creating a sharp tapping sound when the gradients are pulsed. The sound can be quite loud, particularly when strong gradients are used, and subjects to be scanned must wear ear protection.

Magnetic fields are produced whenever there is a flow of electric charge creating a current. Figure 7.1 (bottom left) shows the magnetic field around a long straight wire. The field lines for this simple current are concentric circles in the plane perpendicular to the wire and centered on the wire. The direction of the field lines depends on the direction of the current, following a right-hand rule: with your right thumb pointing along the direction of the current, your fingers curl in the direction of the magnetic field. The magnetic field strength diminishes as the distance from the wire increases.

If a wire carrying a current is bent into a small circular loop, the magnetic field is distorted as shown in Figure 7.1 (bottom right). Near the wire the concentric field lines are similar to the straight wire. That is, if one is close enough to the current loop so that the curvature is not apparent, the magnetic field is similar to that of a straight wire. However, far from the source this magnetic field pattern is identical to the electric dipole field, and correspondingly, this pattern is called a *magnetic dipole field*. In general, the term *dipole field* refers to the pattern far from the source, and so two fields can be quite different near the source but still be described as dipole fields. For the electric field, all the field lines end on one or the other of the two

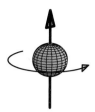

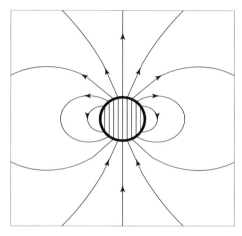

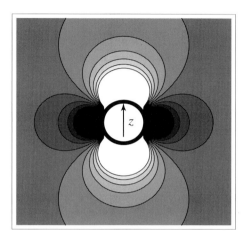

Magnetic Field Lines   *Contours of B_z*

Figure 7.2. The dipole field of a spinning, charged sphere. A charged sphere rotating around the z-axis produces a magnetic dipole field outside. The field lines themselves are shown on the left, but usually just the z-component of the field is of interest. Contours of equal B_z are shown on the right.

charges that make up the dipole. In contrast, the magnetic dipole field is composed of continuous loops that pass through the ring of current. This is a general and important difference in the geometry of electric and magnetic fields: magnetic field lines always form closed loops.

A small ring of current is the prototype of a magnetic dipole, but another classical example of a magnetic dipole is a spinning, charged sphere (Figure 7.2). This is the basic picture of an atomic nucleus (e.g., the proton, the nucleus of hydrogen) often used for visualizing NMR. For simplicity, assume that the charge is uniformly distributed over the surface of the sphere. This rotating sphere can be viewed as a stack of current loops, with the largest loop area and highest current at the equator of the sphere. When these loops are summed, the net magnetic dipole moment of the sphere turns out to be identical to that of a single current loop at the center of the sphere. Figure 7.2 illustrates the magnetic dipole field by plotting both the field lines (left) and a contour map of just the z-component. (For most NMR applications the z-component of additional fields are important because this is what adds to B_0 to create field variations.)

Induction and NMR Signal Detection

Our picture of electromagnetic fields so far is that charges create electric fields, and charges in motion (currents) create magnetic fields. In the first half of the nineteenth century, Faraday unraveled an additional feature: *changing* magnetic fields create electric fields. This phenomenon, called electromagnetic induction, is at the heart of many examples of electrical technology. For example, induction makes possible the generation of electricity from a mechanical energy source, such as hydroelectric power, and the conversion of acoustic signals into electrical signals in a microphone.

In NMR, induction is the process that generates a measurable signal in a detector coil. Imagine a small dipole moment, a spinning charged sphere, rotating around an axis perpendicular to its spin axis. The spinning sphere creates a dipole magnetic field in its vicinity, and as the magnet rotates the dipole field sweeps around as well. As a result, at any fixed point in space near the magnetic dipole, the magnetic field changes cyclically with time. If we now place a loop of wire, a detector coil, near the spinning dipole, the changing magnetic field will create a current in the wire through the process of induction (Figure 7.3).

The strength of the induced current in the coil depends on both the proximity and orientation of the coil with respect to the magnetic dipole. The quantitative relation is that the induced current is proportional to the rate of change of the *flux* of the magnetic field through the coil. For example, consider a circular coil and imagine

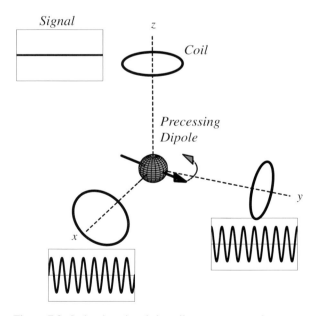

Figure 7.3. Induction signals in coils near a precessing magnetic dipole. For a dipole rotating in the x-y plane, coils along the x- and y-axis show oscillating signals with a relative phase shift of 90° as the magnetic flux of the dipole sweeps across the coils. For the coil along the z-axis, the flux is constant, and so no current is induced.

the disklike surface enclosed by the wire. The net flux of the magnetic field is calculated by adding up the perpendicular components of the magnetic field lines at each point on this surface. Or, more qualitatively, the flux is proportional to the number of field lines enclosed by the coil.

The somewhat abstract concept of magnetic flux suggests a flow of something through the coil, but the thing "flowing" is the magnetic field. The source of the terminology is a close analogy between magnetic fields and velocity fields in a fluid. Velocity is also a vector, and the velocity field within a fluid can be plotted as a field with the same conventions that we use for the magnetic field. Velocity field lines in an incompressible fluid also form closed loops, like magnetic field lines. Placing our coil in the fluid, the calculated flux is simply the volume flow rate through the coil. When the coil is perpendicular to the local flow direction, the flux is high; if the coil is placed so that the flow passes over it rather than through it, the flux is zero.

Figure 7.3 illustrates a spinning magnetic dipole inducing currents in several nearby coils. Note that when the coil is oriented such that the axis of the coil is the same as the axis of rotation of the dipole, the flux is constant so there is no induced current. For other orientations, though, a cyclic signal is generated in the coil with the same frequency as the frequency of rotation of the dipole. The maximum signal is produced when the axis of the coil is perpendicular to the axis of rotation of the dipole because this orientation creates the largest change in flux as the dipole field sweeps past the coil. When the coil is moved farther from the source, the flux is diminished, and so the change in flux also is diminished, and the signal created in the coil is weaker.

The two coils oriented 90° from each other, but with the axis of each coil perpendicular to the rotation axis, show the same strength of induced current, but the signals are shifted in time. This time shift of the signal is described as a *phase shift,* and in this case it is a phase shift of 90°. For any periodic signal with a period *T,* a shift in time can be described as an angular phase shift in analogy with circular motion. A phase shift of one full period *T* corresponds to one complete cycle, a phase shift of 360°, and a time shift of *T*/4 corresponds to a phase shift of 90°. Sometimes phase shifts are expressed in radians rather than degrees, where 360° = 2π radians.

The concept of phase recurs often in MRI. In particular, the concept of phase dispersion and a resulting loss in signal is important in virtually all MRI techniques. Imagine a coil detecting the signal from several rotating dipoles. If the dipoles are all rotating in phase with one another, so that at any instant they are all pointing in the same direction, then the signals induced by each in the coil add coherently and create a strong net signal. However, if there is phase dispersion, so that at any instant the dipoles are not aligned, then there is destructive interference when the signals from each dipole are added together in the coil, and the net signal is reduced.

The configuration of two coils perpendicular to each other is an example of a *quadrature detector.* Each coil is sensitive to the component of the magnetization perpendicular to the coil because that is the component that creates a changing flux through the coil. Because of their orientation, the signal measured in the second coil is phase-shifted 90° from the signal in the first coil. By electronically delaying the second signal for one quarter of a cycle, the two signals are brought back in phase and can be averaged to improve the signal-to-noise ratio (SNR) before being sent to the amplifier. Noise comes about primarily from fluctuating stray currents in the sample, which create random currents in the detector coil. Because the two coils of a quadrature detector are oriented perpendicular to each other, the fluctuating fields that cause noise in one coil have no effect on the other coil. If the fluctuating fields along these two directions are statistically independent, the noise signals measured in the two coils will also be independent. Then when the signals from the two coils are combined the incoherent averaging of the noise improves the SNR by $\sqrt{2}$ compared with a single-coil measurement.

In a *phased array coil arrangement,* two or more coils send signals to separate amplifiers, with the result that the two detected signals are analyzed individually. Phased array coils are useful for imaging as a way of improving the SNR beyond what can be achieved by quadrature detection alone (Grant, Vigneron, and Barkovich, 1998). The noise picked up by a coil is proportional to its sensitive volume, which is on the order of the size of the coil. Thus, a small coil has a higher SNR, but the drawback of a small coil is that only a small region can be imaged. With a phased array system several small coils can be used to achieve the coverage of a large coil but with the SNR of a small coil. Each coil is sensitive to a different location and so provides a high SNR measurement of the signal from that location. Note that this requires separate amplifier channels for each coil. If the signals from the different coils were combined before being sent to a single amplifier, the noise from each coil would contaminate the signals from the other coils, destroying the SNR advantage.

Gradient and Radiofrequency Coils

Any configuration of wires carrying a current creates a magnetic field in the vicinity of the wires. We will refer to any such arrangement as a coil, even if it is not a simple loop or helical configuration. In MRI, coils are used for generating the main magnetic field, for generating the oscillating RF field used to tip over the local magnetization, and for detecting the NMR signal. A surface coil for detecting the signal may be as simple as a single loop of wire, but the designs of more complex RF and gradient coils are much more sophisticated. Nevertheless, we can appreciate how different field patterns can be created by considering two prototype coil configurations produced by combining two circular coils carrying a current. The field of each coil separately was shown in Figure 7.1, and the net fields for two coil arrangements are illustrated in Figure 7.4. Each set consists of two circular coils oriented on a common axis, with the currents parallel in the first set and opposite in the second set. On the top of the figure, the magnetic field lines are shown for each configuration, in the middle are contour plots of just the z-component of the field, and plots of B_z along the coil axis are shown on the bottom.

The first arrangement, called a Maxwell pair, produces a rather uniform field between the two coils, with the field diverging and weakening at the two ends. If many such coils are stacked together, the result is a solenoid with a very uniform field inside. This is the basic coil design used for creating the main magnetic field of an MRI sys-

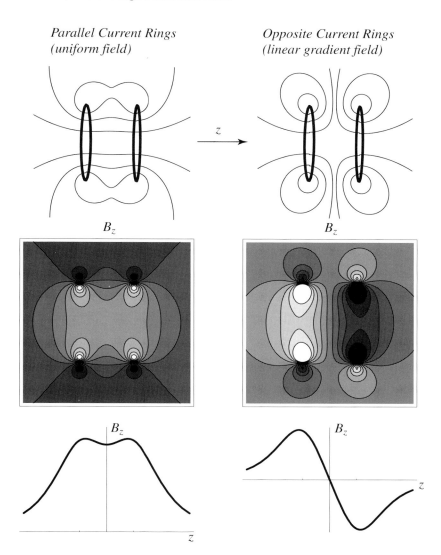

Figure 7.4. Two simple coil configurations suggest how the geometry of magnetic fields can be manipulated. Two circular coils with parallel currents (left column) create a roughly uniform field between them, a prototype for the solenoid current arrangement that generates a uniform B_0. Two circular coils with opposite currents (right column) generate a linear gradient field in the region between them, a prototype for the gradient coils used for imaging. The top row shows the field lines, the middle row shows contour plots of the z-component of the magnetic field, and the bottom row shows plots of B_z vs. z along the axis of the coils.

tem, and in a commercial scanner the field variation over a central region of about 20 cm is less than a few tenths of a part per million. The field strength depends on the total current flowing through the coil, and large, uniform magnetic fields can be created when superconducting (zero resistance) coils are used.

The arrangement of two coils with currents running in opposite directions is known as a Helmholtz pair. The effect of this arrangement is that the fields created by the two loops tend to cancel in the region halfway between them. Moving off center along the coil axis, the field increases in one direction and decreases in the other direction. This type of field is called a *gradient field,* and gradient fields are a critical part of MRI. In an MR imager the gradient coils produce additional fields, which add to the main field B_0. The direction of B_0 is usually defined as the z-axis, and the goal with a gradient coil is to produce an additional field along z such that B_z varies linearly along one axis. In practice the designs for linear imaging gradients are more sophisticated than this simple Helmholtz pair to improve the linearity and homogeneity of the field. That is, for an ideal linear gradient coil the field component B_z varies linearly moving along the coil axis but is uniform moving perpendicular to the coil axis.

In imaging applications we are interested in just the z-component of the field offset because that is the only component that will make a significant change in the net field amplitude and so affect the resonant frequency. A weak field component, on the order of a few parts per million, perpendicular to B_0 will produce a change in the total field magnitude on the order of 10^{-12}, a negligible amount. But an offset in B_z itself of a few parts per million will directly alter the total field strength, and thus the resonant frequency, by a few parts per million. Offsets of this magnitude are comparable to the field offsets between one voxel and its neighbor during frequency encoding in MRI. The important effect of gradient fields for imaging is thus that they modify the z-component, producing a gradient of B_z.

The preceding discussion suggests how different coil configurations can be used to generate different patterns of magnetic field. However, when a coil is used for signal *detection,* the physics at first glance seems to be rather different. As described in the previous section, the current induced in a coil by a local precessing magnetization is proportional to the changing magnetic flux through the coil. Fortunately, it turns out that there is a simple relation between the magnetic field *produced* by a coil when a current is run through it and the current *induced* in the coil by an external changing magnetic field. For any coil used as a detector, an associated *sensitivity* pattern describes the strength of the signal produced in the coil by sources at different locations in space. One could calculate the sensitivity map by placing rotating dipoles at many positions relative to the coil and using the changing magnetic flux rule to determine the induced current. However, this sensitivity pattern also can be calculated from a useful rule called the *principle of reciprocity:* the sensitivity of any coil to a rotating magnetic dipole at any point in space is directly proportional to the magnetic field that would be produced at that point in space by running a current through the coil. Specifically, imagine a precessing magnetic dipole M sitting near a coil, and consider the magnetic field vector **b** that would be produced at the location of the dipole by running a unit current through the coil. The signal produced in the coil by the dipole depends directly on the vector **b**: the signal is proportional to the product of the magnitude of **b** and the component of M that lies along **b** (i.e., the scalar product of **b** and M). For example, if the arrangement of the coil is such that **b** is perpendicular to M (such as a circular coil with its axis along z), no signal is generated. For any orientation, the magnitude of **b** is small far from the coil, so the sensitivity of the coil is weak. Thus, an RF coil can be thought of as having two roles: a producer of magnetic fields and a detector of changing magnetic fields. The geometrical pattern associated with each is the same.

DYNAMICS OF THE NUCLEAR MAGNETIZATION

Interaction of a Magnetic Dipole with a Magnetic Field

In the previous sections the discussion focused on the magnetic field created by a magnetic dipole. In NMR the fundamental interaction is between the magnetic dipole moment of the atomic nucleus and the local external magnetic field, which is characterized by two basic effects. The first is that the field exerts a torque on the dipole that tends to twist it into alignment with the field, and the second is that in a nonuniform field there is a force on the dipole pulling it toward the region of stronger field. These effects are most easily understood by considering an electric dipole in an electric field. A magnetic dipole in a magnetic field behaves in the same way as the electric dipole, but the physical arguments that demonstrate this are more subtle (details are given in the appendix).

An electric dipole can be thought of as two opposite charges attached to a rod of fixed length, with the direction of the dipole vector running from the negative to the positive charge. When the dipole is placed at an angle to a uniform electric field (Figure 7.5), there is a moment arm between the points where the two forces are applied, and the result is a torque on the dipole. One end is pulled up, the other is pushed down, and the dipole pivots around the center. The only stable configuration for the dipole is when it is aligned with the field. When the dipole is placed in a nonuniform electric field, again the field will produce a torque that will align the dipole with the field. However, because the field is not uniform, the forces on the

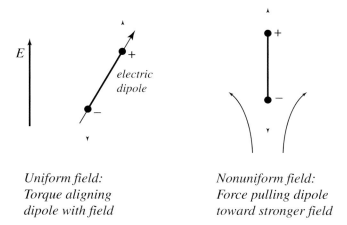

Uniform field:
Torque aligning
dipole with field

Nonuniform field:
Force pulling dipole
toward stronger field

Figure 7.5. Dipole interactions with a field. The nature of the forces are most easily illustrated by an electric dipole placed in an electric field E. An electric dipole consists of two opposite charges separated by a short distance and an external field, which exerts a torque acting to align the dipole with the field and a force drawing the aligned dipole into regions of stronger field. (Forces are shown as thin arrows.)

positive and negative charges do not balance even when the dipole is aligned with
the field; the force down on the lower charge is stronger than the force up on the
positive charge. The result is that there is a net force downward on the dipole,
pulling the dipole toward the region of stronger field. If the dipole is aligned opposite to the field, the force also is opposite, pushing the dipole toward the region of
weaker field. However, such an alignment would be unstable for an electric dipole:
the torque would twist it 180°, and it would be pulled toward the region with a
stronger field.

Both of these effects can be described in an equivalent way in terms of the
energy of a dipole in a field. The dipole has the lowest energy when it is aligned
with the field, and the energy progressively increases as the dipole is tipped away
from the field. The highest energy configuration is when the dipole is aligned opposite to the field. Similarly, the energy of the dipole is lower when it is in a stronger
field, so it is drawn toward regions with a larger field. Both alignment with the field
and moving toward stronger fields are then examples of the system seeking a lower
energy state.

Precession

A magnetic dipole placed in a magnetic field experiences the same two effects: a
torque tending to align the dipole with the field and a force drawing it toward
regions of stronger field. However, for a nuclear magnetic dipole the intrinsic angular momentum of the nucleus changes the dynamics in a critical way. Viewing a magnetic dipole as a rotating charged sphere brings out the close connection between
the magnetic moment and the angular momentum. Both the angular momentum
and the magnetic dipole moment are proportional to the rate of spin of the sphere.
Faster rotation increases the angular momentum as well as the current produced by
the charges on the surface, and so also increases the magnetic moment. Because of
this intimate link between angular momentum and the magnetic dipole moment, the
ratio of the two is a constant called the *gyromagnetic ratio,* γ. Each nucleus that
exhibits NMR has a unique value of γ.

The presence of angular momentum makes the dynamics of a magnetic dipole in
a magnetic field distinctly different from the dynamics of an electric dipole in an
electric field. As already described, the effect of the field is to exert on the dipole a
torque that would tend to twist it into alignment. Physically, torque is the rate of
change of angular momentum, analogous to Newton's first law that force is the rate
of change of momentum. Precession comes about because the torque axis is perpendicular to the existing angular momentum around the spin axis. The *change* in angular momentum then is along the direction of the torque and so is always
perpendicular to the existing angular momentum. In other words, the change in
angular momentum produced by the torque is a change in the *direction* of spin, not
the magnitude. Thus, the angular momentum (and the spin axis) precess around the
field. (A more mathematical derivation of precession is given in the appendix.)

This is an example of the peculiar nature of angular momentum and is exactly
analogous to the behavior of a spinning top or bicycle wheel. A spinning top tipped
at an angle to the vertical would be in a lower energy state if it simply fell over;

instead, the rotation axis precesses around a vertical line. For a nucleus in a magnetic field, the frequency of precession, called the *Larmor frequency,* is $\omega_0 = \gamma B_0$; the stronger the field, the stronger the torque on the dipole and the faster the precession. We will use the convention that when frequency is represented by ω, it is expressed as angular frequency (radians per second), and when it is represented by ν, it is expressed as cycles per second (Hz), with the relation $\omega = 2\pi\nu$. The equation for the Larmor frequency holds regardless of whether we are using angular frequency or cycles per second, with a suitable adjustment in the magnitude of γ. The precession frequency ω_0 is the resonant frequency of NMR.

Relaxation

The foregoing considerations apply to a single nucleus in a magnetic field. From the precession arguments alone, one might conclude that a proton would never align with the main field, despite the fact that the energy is lower. But in a real sample, B_0 is not the only source of magnetic field. The magnetic moments of other nuclei produce additional, fluctuating magnetic fields. For example, in a water molecule, a hydrogen (H) nucleus feels the field produced by the other H in the molecule. Because the molecules are rapidly tumbling due to their thermal motions, the total field felt by a particular nucleus fluctuates around the mean field B_0. These fluctuations alter both the total magnetic field magnitude and the direction. As a result, the proton's precession is more irregular, and the axis of precession fluctuates. Over time, the protons gradually tend to align more with B_0, through the process called *relaxation.*

Because the energy associated with the orientation of the magnetic dipole moment of a hydrogen nucleus in a magnetic field is small compared with the thermal energy of a water molecule, the average degree of alignment with the field is small, corresponding to a difference of only about one part in 10^5 between those nuclei aligned with the field and those opposite. However, this is sufficient to produce a slight net magnetization M_0 of the water. The creation of M_0 can be understood as a relaxation toward thermal equilibrium. When a sample is first placed in a magnetic field, the magnetic dipoles are randomly oriented so that the net magnetization is zero. This means that the dipoles possess a higher energy due to their orientation than they would if they were partly aligned with the field. (The lowest possible energy would correspond to complete alignment.) As the system relaxes, this excess energy is dissipated as heat, the dipoles align more with the field, and the longitudinal magnetization M grows toward its equilibrium value M_0.

In a pure water sample the main source of a fluctuating magnetic field that produces relaxation is the field produced by the other H nucleus in the same water molecule. But the presence of other molecules in the liquid (protein, etc.) can alter the relaxation rate by changing either the magnitude or the frequency of the fluctuating fields. A large molecule will tumble more slowly than a water molecule so that a water molecule that transiently binds to the large molecule will experience more slowly fluctuating fields. The magnitude of the fluctuating fields can be increased significantly in the presence of paramagnetic compounds. Paramagnetic compounds have unpaired electrons, and electrons have magnetic moments more than a thousand times larger than a proton. This is the basis for the use of paramagnetic contrast agents, such as Gd-DTPA, as a way of reducing the local relaxation time. The physical sources of the relaxation times are discussed more fully in Chapter 8.

The time constant for relaxation is T_1 and varies from about 0.2 to 4.0 s in the body. The fact that T_1 varies by an order of magnitude between different tissues is important because this is the source of most of the contrast differences between tissues in MR images. The T_1 variations are due to differences in the local environment (e.g., chemical composition or biological structures). In general, the higher the water content of a tissue, the longer the T_1. The strong dependence of the relaxation time on the local environment is exactly analogous to everyday experiences of relaxation phenomena. A cup of hot coffee sitting in a cool room is not in thermal equilibrium. Over time, the coffee will cool to room temperature (thermal equilibrium), but the time constant for this relaxation depends strongly on the local environment. If the coffee is in a thin-walled open cup, it may cool in a few minutes, whereas if it is in a covered, insulated vessel, it may take hours to cool. Regardless of how long it takes to get there, the final equilibrium state (cold coffee) is the same. Similarly with NMR relaxation, the equilibrium magnetization M_0 depends on the density of dipoles and the magnetic field, but the relaxation time required to reach this equilibrium depends on the environment of the spins.

The relaxation time T_1 is called the *longitudinal* relaxation time because it describes the relaxation of the component of the magnetization that lies along the direction of B_0. Two other relaxation times, T_2 and T_2^*, describe the decay of the *transverse* component of the magnetization. At equilibrium the magnetization is aligned with B_0, so there is no transverse component. Application of a 90° radio frequency (RF) pulse tips the magnetization into the transverse plane, where it precesses and generates a signal in a detector coil by induction. In a homogeneous field, the transverse component, and thus also the NMR signal, decays away with a time constant T_2, and this process often is abbreviated as transverse relaxation. In the human body at field strengths typical of MR imagers, T_1 is about eight to ten times larger than T_2.

In practice, one finds experimentally that the NMR signal often decays more quickly than would be expected for the T_2 of the sample. This is qualitatively described by saying that the decay time is T_2^*, with T_2^* less than T_2. The reason for this is simply inhomogeneity of the magnetic field. If two regions of the sample feel different magnetic fields, the precession rates will differ, the local transverse magnetization vectors will quickly get out of phase with each other, and the net magnetization will decrease due to *phase dispersion*. However, this signal decay is due to constant field offsets within the sample and not to the fluctuating fields that produce T_2 decay. Because of this, the additional decay due to inhomogeneity is reversible with a spin echo, introduced in Chapter 4 and discussed in more detail in Chapter 8.

The combined processes of precession and relaxation are mathematically described by the Bloch equations, a set of differential equations for the three components of the magnetization (see Box 7). These are the basic dynamical equations of NMR and are used frequently to describe the behavior of the magnetization.

BOX 7. THE BLOCH EQUATIONS

Early in the development of NMR, Bloch proposed a set of differential equations to model the dynamics of the magnetization produced by nuclear magnetic dipoles in a magnetic field. The equations include precession, as derived above, and also exponential relaxation with relaxation times T_1 and T_2. The representation of relaxation is essentially empirical, designed to reproduce the experimentally observed dynamics. The Bloch equations are still the basic equations used to understand the magnitude of the NMR signal. The equations are written separately for the three components of the magnetization, M_x, M_y and M_z:

$$\frac{dM_x}{dt} = \gamma B_0 M_y - \frac{M_x}{T_2}$$

$$\frac{dM_y}{dt} = -\gamma B_0 M_x - \frac{M_y}{T_2}$$

$$\frac{dM_z}{dt} = -\frac{M_z - M_0}{T_1}$$

Precession is incorporated into the equations in the way that the rates of change of the two transverse components, M_x and M_y, depend on the current values because precession rotates M_x partly into M_y, and vice versa. Relaxation is described by a steady decrease of the transverse component by the transverse relaxation rate, $1/T_2$, and relaxation with a rate $1/T_1$ of the M_z component toward the equilibrium magnetization M_0. If we start with an arbitrary magnetization vector, with a transverse component $M_{xy}(0)$ and a longitudinal component $M_z(0)$, the magnitudes of these components at later times given by the solution of the Bloch equations are

$$M_{xy} = M_{xy}(0)e^{-t/T_2}$$

$$M_z = M_0 - [M_0 - M_z(0)]\, e^{-t/T_1}$$

In addition to these magnitude changes, the full solution also includes precession of the transverse component with frequency γB_0. The transverse component decays exponentially with time constant T_2. The relaxation of the longitudinal component can be described as an exponential decay with time constant T_1 of the *difference* between the starting value $M_z(0)$ and the equilibrium value M_0. In fact, we could describe both decay processes as an exponential decay of the difference between the initial state and the equilibrium state, and the equilibrium state is M_0 along M_z and a transverse component of zero.

The preceding equations describe relaxation and free precession when the only magnetic field acting on the magnetization is B_0. To describe what happens during the RF pulse, we must also include the effects of an oscillating field B_1. This is most easily represented in a frame of reference rotating at the frequency of B_1 oscillations, ω. This transformation essentially takes out the basic precession and simplifies the equations. In this rotating frame, B_1 appears to be constant, and we can take it to lie along the x-axis.

(continued)

BOX 7, continued

Also, the apparent precession rate of M due to B_0 in this rotating frame is reduced to ω_{rot} $= \omega_0 - \omega$, and so it appears as if the magnetic field in the z-direction has been reduced to $B_z = B_0 - \omega_1/\gamma$. The effective magnetic field in the rotating frame then has two components, B_1 along the x-axis and B_z along the z-axis, and the dynamics of M is then precession around B_{eff} plus relaxation. If we represent the amplitude of B_1 as an equivalent precession frequency $\omega_1 = \gamma B_1$ (the rate at which M would precess around B_1), the Bloch equations in the rotating frame take the form

$$\frac{dM_x}{dt} = \omega_{rot}M_y - \frac{M_x}{T_2}$$

$$\frac{dM_y}{dt} = -\omega_{rot}M_x - \frac{M_y}{T_2} + \omega_1 M_z$$

$$\frac{dM_z}{dt} = -\frac{M_z - M_0}{T_1} - \omega_1 M_y$$

This form of the equations clearly shows how the dynamics of the magnetization depend on four distinct rate constants: the off-resonance frequency of B_1, ω_{rot}; the amplitude of B_1 expressed as a precession frequency, ω_1; and the two relaxation rates, $1/T_2$, and $1/T_1$. Different proportions of these parameters produce a wide range of dynamics. Furthermore, in a tailored RF pulse the amplitude of B_1 is a function of time, and in an adiabatic pulse the off-resonance frequency is also a function of time.

RF Excitation

Nuclear magnetic resonance is a transient phenomenon. The fact that the magnetic dipole moments of protons tend to align with the field, producing a net magnetization M_0, does not lead to any measurable signal (a constant magnetic field produces no currents). However, if M_0 is tipped away from the direction of B_0, it will precess; all the nuclear dipoles will precess together if they are tipped over, so the net magnetization M_0 also will precess at the same frequency. The transverse component of M_0 then produces a changing magnetic field and will generate a transient NMR signal in a nearby detector coil by induction.

The tipping of the magnetization is accomplished by the RF pulse, an oscillating magnetic field B_1 perpendicular to B_0 and oscillating at the proton precession frequency. It is simplest to picture B_1 as a small magnetic field with constant amplitude in the transverse plane that rotates at a rate matched to the proton precession rate. Such a field is described as a *circularly polarized* oscillating field. When B_1 is turned on, the net field, the vector sum of B_0 and B_1, is tipped slightly away from the z-axis and rotates over time. Because the magnetization M_0 along the z-axis is no longer aligned with the net magnetic field, it begins to precess around the net field even as that field itself rotates. In other words, the basic physical process involved with the RF pulse is still just precession of M_0 around a magnetic field, but it is now more difficult to picture because the magnetic field itself is also rotating as the magnetization tries to precess around it. To understand the complexity of this process, a useful conceptual tool is the rotating frame of reference.

To introduce the rotating frame, forget B_1 for the moment and picture a magnetization vector M tipped away from the z-axis (Figure 7.6). We know that in the laboratory frame of reference the magnetization will simply precess around the field B_0 lying along the z-axis. We will ignore relaxation effects for now as well and assume that we are watching the magnetization for a short enough time that relaxation effects are negligible. Because the time scale for precession is so much shorter than that for relaxation, we could observe the precession for thousands of cycles with no detectable effects from relaxation. Now imagine that we observe this precession from a frame of reference that is itself rotating at the Larmor frequency, $\omega_0 = \gamma B_0$. In this frame we are carried around at the same rate as the precession, as though we were riding on a turntable, and so in the rotating frame the magnetization appears to be stationary. Because there appears to be no precession in the rotating frame, it appears as if there is no magnetic field (i.e., as if B_0 is zero). Now suppose that we are in a rotating frame rotating with an arbitrary angular frequency ω. In this new rotating frame the magnetization precesses around the z-axis, but with an effective

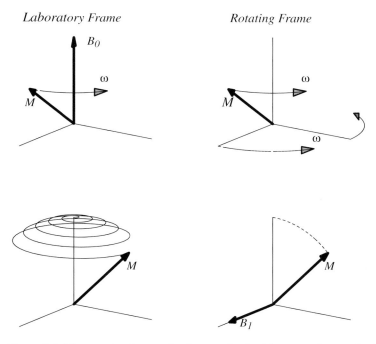

Laboratory Frame   *Rotating Frame*

Figure 7.6. The rotating frame of reference. In the laboratory frame of reference the magnetization precesses around the magnetic field with a frequency ω. In a frame of reference rotating at the same rate, the magnetization appears to be stationary, so in this frame there appears to be no magnetic field. An RF field B_1 rotating at the resonant frequency appears stationary in the rotating frame, and RF excitation is then a simple precession of M around B_1 in the rotating frame. In the laboratory frame this motion is a slowly widening spiral.

angular frequency $\omega_0 - \omega$. In other words, the magnetization behaves in this rotating frame exactly as it would in a stationary frame if the magnetic field were reduced from B_0 to $B_0 - \omega/\gamma$. This is the power of the rotating frame as a conceptual tool: the physics of precession is the same in a rotating frame as in a stationary frame, but the apparent magnetic field in the rotating frame is changed.

We can now return to the RF pulse and look at B_1 in the frame rotating with angular velocity ω, the oscillation frequency of B_1. To begin with, we will assume that B_1 is oscillating on resonance with the protons ($\omega = \omega_0$), and we will return to consider off-resonance effects later. In the rotating frame, B_1 is constant, and we will call its direction the x-axis of the rotating frame. When B_1 is on-resonance, the apparent field along the z-axis is zero in the rotating frame. This means that from this perspective there is only the field B_1 along x, so M_0 begins to process around the x-axis in the rotating frame. The RF field B_1 is much weaker than B_0, so the rate of precession around B_1 is correspondingly slower. But if we wait long enough (perhaps a few milliseconds for the RF pulses used in imaging), the magnetization will rotate around B_1, tipping away from the z-axis and toward the y-axis of the rotating frame. If B_1 is left on long enough to tip M_0 fully onto the y-axis, the RF pulse is called a 90° pulse. If left on longer, or if the amplitude of B_1 is increased, the flip angle can be increased to 180° or even 360°, which would leave M_0 where it started along the z-axis. Thus, the complex picture of precession around a time-varying magnetic field in the laboratory frame is reduced to a simple precession around B_1 in the rotating frame. To picture the full dynamics of the magnetization as it would appear in the laboratory frame, this slow precession around B_1 must be added to a rapid precession of the rotating frame itself around the z-axis. The net result in the laboratory frame is a tight spiral that slowly increases the angle between M_0 and B_0 (Figure 7.6).

After B_1 is turned off, M_0 continues to precess around B_0 and generates a signal in the detector coil. The signal is called a free induction decay (FID), where *free* relates to free precession, '*induction*' is the physical process described earlier in which a varying magnetic field (the precessing magnetization) produces a current in a coil, and *decay* indicates that the signal eventually dies out. Over time, M_0 will relax until it is again aligned with B_0. Because the action of an RF pulse is to tip M_0 away from B_0, such pulses usually are described by the *flip angle* (or *tip angle*) they produce (e.g., a 90° RF pulse or a 180° RF pulse). The flip angle is adjusted by changing either the duration or the amplitude of B_1.

From the thermodynamic point of view, the process of tipping M_0 can be interpreted as the system of magnetic dipoles absorbing energy from the RF field because the alignment of M_0 is changing and then dissipating this energy over time as heat as the system relaxes back to equilibrium. For this reason, the RF pulse is often described as an *excitation pulse* because it raises the system to an excited (higher energy) state.

Frequency Selective RF Pulses: Slice Selection

In the previous description of the RF pulse, we assumed that B_1 was oscillating at precisely the resonant frequency of the protons, ω_0. What happens if the RF pulse is off-resonance? This is an important question for imaging applications because the process of slice selection, which limits the effects of the excitation pulse to just a thin slice through the body, is based on the idea that an RF pulse far off-resonance should have a negligible effect on the magnetization. Slice selection is accomplished by turning on a magnetic field gradient during the RF pulse so that the resonant frequency of spins above the desired slice will be higher, and that of spins below the slice will be lower, than the frequency of the RF pulse. The RF pulse will then be on-resonance for the spins at the center of the slice, and only these will be tipped over. However, for spins slightly removed from the central slice plane, the RF pulse will only be a little off-resonance, so we would expect that these spins will be partly flipped, but not as much as those at the center. The slice profile, the response of spins through the thickness of the slice, will then depend on the degree of tipping produced by a slightly off-resonance RF pulse. The most desirable slice profile is a perfect rectangle because this means that the slice has a well-defined slice thickness and a sharp edge. In practice, this cannot be achieved, but with carefully tailored RF pulses the slice profile approaches a rectangle.

We can understand the physics of off-resonance excitation by returning to the frame of reference rotating at the oscillation frequency ω of B_1, and we will now relax our earlier assumption that ω is equal to ω_0, the Larmor frequency (Figure 7.7). If ω and ω_0 are different, then in the rotating frame the magnetization behaves as though there were an apparent field along the z-axis of $B_z = B_0 - \omega/\gamma$. In other words, in the absence of B_1, the magnetization would precess around the z-axis with an angular frequency $\omega_0 - \omega$. When B_1 is turned on along the x-axis in the rotating frame, the effective field B_{eff} is the vector sum of B_z and B_1, and so is a vector lying somewhere in the x-z plane. If B_1 is nearly on-resonance, then $\omega_0 - \omega$ is small and B_z is small, so B_{eff} points only slightly away from the x-axis. But if the frequency of B_1 is far off-resonance, B_{eff} points nearly along the z-axis. The effective field is constant in the rotating frame, so the motion of M_0 is simply a precession around B_{eff} with angular frequency γB_{eff} for the duration of the B_1 pulse.

Qualitatively, then, we can see why a far off-resonance pulse does little tipping of the magnetization because, with B_{eff} nearly aligned with the z-axis, the precession around B_{eff} leaves M_0 very near to its original orientation along the z-axis (Figure 7.7). More quantitatively, this picture can be used to calculate the effects of off-resonance excitation, and thus the slice profile in an imaging experiment. Figure 7.8 (top) shows M_z after an RF pulse with an amplitude and duration matched to give a 90° flip angle on-resonance. Two curves are shown, one for a constant amplitude B_1 throughout the RF pulse and one for a tailored RF pulse in which the amplitude of B_1 is modulated. By modulating the amplitude of B_1, the frequency selectivity of the pulse, and thus the slice profile, can be improved considerably. The cost of using a shaped pulse, however, is that the duration of the RF pulse is increased. The on-resonance flip angle is proportional to the area under the RF pulse profile, so a constant amplitude pulse is the most compact in time. To create a shaped RF pulse profile with the same duration and flip angle, the peak amplitude of B_1 would have to be significantly increased, but hardware limitations set the maximum peak ampli-

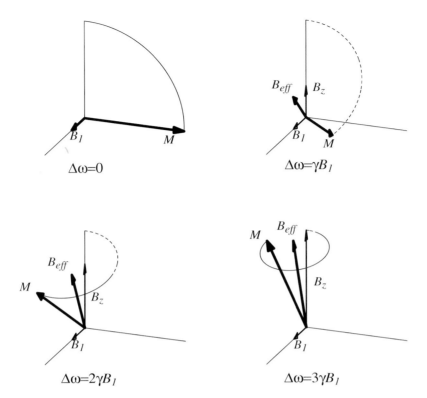

Figure 7.7. Off-resonance excitation. The effect of an off-resonance RF pulse (B_1) can be understood as precession around the effective field in the rotating frame. Because the rotation of the frame differs from the precession frequency of M, the precession of M in the rotating frame is equivalent to precession in a magnetic field B_z. The vector sum of B_1 and B_z is the effective field B_{eff}. When B_1 is on-resonance (top left) the effect is a simple 90° flip of M, but as the off-resonance frequency $\Delta\omega$ is increased, the RF pulse is less effective in tipping over M.

tude. So it is usually necessary to extend the duration of the RF pulse to produce a cleaner slice profile.

The slice profile can be further improved by allowing B_1 to vary in frequency as well as amplitude. An *adiabatic* RF pulse is an example that produces a particularly clean slice profile (Frank, Wong, and Buxton, 1997; Silver, Joseph, and Hoult, 1985). In an adiabatic pulse, the magnetization is not so much precessing around the effective field as following it as it slowly rotates. To see how this works, imagine starting B_1 far off-resonance. Then B_{eff} is nearly along the z-axis, and the magnetization will precess around it, while remaining nearly parallel to B_{eff}. If we now slowly change the frequency of B_1, moving it closer to resonance, the effective field will slowly tip toward the x-axis. If this is done slowly enough, so that the magnetization precesses many times around B_{eff} during the process, then M_0 will follow B_{eff}, precessing in a tight cone around it, as B_{eff} slowly tips toward the x-axis. As soon as the frequency of B_1 reaches ω_0, the effective field and M_0 will lie along the x-axis, and the net effect will be a 90° pulse. If the pulse is continued,

Slice Selection

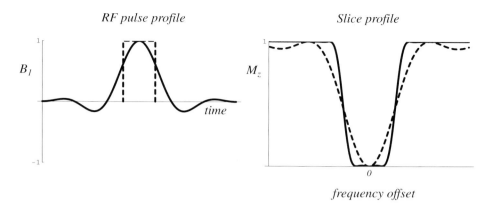

Adiabatic Inversion Pulse

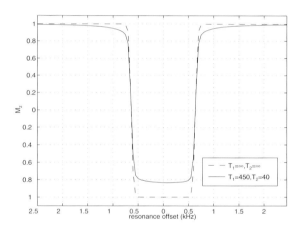

Figure 7.8. Slice selection with frequency selective RF pulses. Slice selection in MRI uses RF pulses with a narrow bandwidth in combination with a magnetic field gradient to tip over spins within a narrow range of positions. For two RF pulse shapes (top left) the resulting slice profiles are shown by plotting the remaining z-magnetization after the pulse (top right). A simple rectangular RF pulse produces a poor slice profile, but a longer, shaped RF pulse produces a profile closer to a rectangle. With even longer, adiabatic pulses, the profile is even better, as illustrated by the inversion profile on the bottom. With the adiabatic pulse the duration is long enough for relaxation to begin to have an effect. (Adiabatic inversion plot courtesy of L. Frank.)

moving beyond the resonance condition until M_0 is rotated onto the $-z$-axis, the net effect is a 180° inversion pulse. As shown in Figure 7.8 (bottom), the slice profile can be quite good. The cost of this, however, is that such RF pulses take a long time to play out because of the need to sweep slowly through frequency. In imaging applications, a standard slice selection pulse may take 3 ms, whereas a good adiabatic pulse may require 20 ms or more.

Finally, an ingenious application of the idea of an adiabatic pulse is the selective inversion of flowing blood using a continuous RF pulse. Calling something a continuous pulse sounds like an oxymoron, but it is actually fairly descriptive: no RF field lasts forever, so really any applied RF field is a pulse, and *continuous* just indicates that it is on for a much longer time (e.g., several seconds) than is typical for a standard excitation pulse. Such pulses are often used in arterial spin labeling (ASL) methods for measuring cerebral blood flow (Alsop and Detre, 1996). The goal in such experiments is to invert the magnetization of arterial blood (i.e., flip it 180°) before the blood reaches the tissue of interest and then subtract this tagged image from a control image in which the blood was not inverted. This ASL difference signal is then directly proportional to the amount of blood delivered to the tissue. Continuous inversion works on the same principle as an adiabatic RF pulse, except that B_1 is constant; it is the resonant frequency of the moving spins that is varied. This is accomplished by turning on a gradient in the superior/inferior direction so that, as an element of blood moves up the artery toward the head, its resonant frequency changes because its position in the gradient field changes. The frequency of the RF pulse is set to correspond to the resonant frequency in a particular transverse plane in the neck. When an element of blood is far from this zero plane, B_1 is off-resonance, and so the effective field is nearly along the z-axis. As the blood approaches the zero plane, the z-component of the effective field diminishes as the resonant frequency approaches the RF frequency. When the blood crosses the zero plane B_{eff} is entirely along x, and as the blood continues, moving off-resonance in the other direction, B_{eff} tips down toward the negative z-axis. If this sweep of B_{eff} is slow enough, the magnetization will follow B_{eff} and end up inverted. This continuous labeling technique produces a steady stream of inverted blood as long as the RF is turned on. Arterial spin labeling techniques are discussed in greater detail in Chapter 15.

MAGNETIC PROPERTIES OF MATTER

Paramagnetism, Diamagnetism, and Ferromagnetism

Matter contains several components that possess magnetic dipole moments, and the nuclear spins that give rise to NMR are actually among the weakest. Far more important in determining the magnetic properties of materials are the magnetic dipole moments of unpaired electrons. The dipole moment of an electron is three orders of magnitude larger than that of a proton, and so the alignment of electron magnetic moments in a magnetic field leads to much larger effects. Based on our preceding arguments about the interactions of a magnetic dipole with a magnetic field, we would expect that when a sample is placed in a magnetic field B_0, the dipole moments in the sample would tend to align with the field, creating a net dipole moment parallel to the field. If the magnetic field is nonuniform, we would expect there to be a net force on the sample drawing it toward the region of higher field.

To test this prediction, that materials should feel a force in a nonuniform field, we could perform an experiment using a standard magnetic resonance imager. The magnet is typically oriented horizontally, with a uniform magnetic field in the center but a diverging and weakening field near the ends of the bore. Then we would expect that, as a sample of a particular material is brought near to the bore, it would feel a force pulling it into the magnet. Because the magnetization associated with the intrinsic magnetic dipoles is weak, the force on most materials should also be weak so that a sensitive measuring system is required. When this experiment is performed on a variety of materials, some, such as aluminum, are pulled toward the bore with a force on the order of 1% of the weight of the sample, and these materials are described as *paramagnetic*. However, many other materials, such as water, are weakly *repulsed* by the magnetic field and pushed away from the bore with weaker forces, and these materials are described as *diamagnetic*. Finally, a third class of materials, including iron and magnetite, are strongly attracted toward the magnet, with forces orders of magnitude larger than those of paramagnetic materials. These materials are described as *ferromagnetic*.

From our foregoing arguments about the forces on dipoles in a field, paramagnetism is easily understood and expected. Paramagnetism arises primarily from the effects of unpaired electrons aligning with the magnetic field, with a small additional component from the alignment of nuclear dipoles (Figure 7.9). But the existence of diamagnetism is unexpected because a repulsive force indicates a net dipole moment aligned opposite to the field. Diamagnetism results from the effects of the magnetic field on the orbital motions of the electrons. An electron orbiting an atom or molecule is effectively a current, and so there is a magnetic dipole moment associated with the orbital state, as well as the spin state, of the electron. The curious feature of these orbital dipole moments, however, is that the net dipole moment is oriented opposite to the external magnetic field.

Diamagnetism can be understood in a rough classical physics way by looking at the oversimplified picture of two atoms with electrons orbiting the nucleus in different directions (Figure 7.9). The orbital magnetic dipole moment is opposite for the two different orbital directions, and both directions of rotation are equally likely. With no magnetic field, the net magnetization is zero. The stability of the electron orbit is due to the balance between the inward electrical force and the outward centrifugal force due to the electron's velocity. When a magnetic field is added, the additional magnetic force on the electron is inward for one sense of orbital motion and outward for the other. If the velocities of the electrons adjust to rebalance the forces, one is sped up and the other slowed down, increasing the magnetic dipole moment aligned opposite to the field and decreasing the other. The net magnetization is then opposite to the field.

All materials have diamagnetic effects due to orbital electron motions that create a magnetization aligned opposite to the field, and some materials in addition have paramagnetic effects due to unpaired electron spins that create a magnetization aligned with the field. The net magnetization that results reflects the balance between diamagnetic and paramagnetic effects, and the classification of materials as diamagnetic or paramagnetic reflects the outcome of this balance. But both diamagnetism and paramagnetism are relatively weak effects, in that the magnetic forces on such materials even in a magnetic field as high as those used for imaging are still only about 1% of the force of gravity.

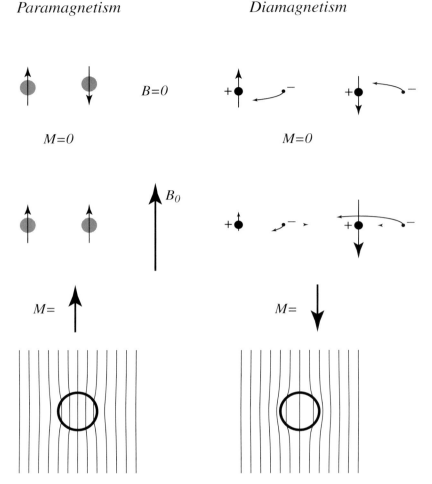

Figure 7.9. Paramagnetism and diamagnetism. Magnetic dipole moments (unpaired electrons and nuclei) align with the magnetic field to produce a magnetization aligned with B_0 (paramagnetism, left). The magnetic dipole moments due to the orbital motions of electrons are altered to produce a net magnetization aligned opposite to the field (diamagnetism, right). For diamagnetism, the diagrams suggest how the added force due to the magnetic field either adds to or subtracts from the centrifugal force on the electron, so that the electron velocity for stability increases or decreases depending on the direction of motion. The bottom row shows distortions of uniform magnetic field lines by a magnetized sphere.

A striking exception to this discussion of materials that interact weakly with a magnetic field is a ferromagnetic material, which can be strongly magnetized when placed in a magnetic field and can retain that magnetization when the field is removed. The very large magnetization induced in such materials corresponds to the coordinated alignment of many electron spins, although the magnetic interactions of the spins are not responsible for the coordination. In ferromagnetic materials such as iron, unpaired electrons are in a lower energy state when they are aligned with each other, for reasons related to the quantum nature of the spins. The unpaired electron spins of nearby atoms in a crystal of iron then tend to become aligned with each other, forming a small volume of material with a uniform orientation, called a *domain.* A large block of material consists of many domains, with a random direction of orientation within each domain. Each domain is still microscopic but nevertheless contains billions of atoms, and so the magnetic field associated with the aligned electrons is quite large. But in the absence of an external magnetic field, there is no net magnetization because of the random orientation of the domains. When the iron is placed in a magnetic field, the domains aligned with the field are energetically favored, and they begin to grow at the expense of the other domains. That is, the electrons in a neighboring domain switch their orientation to join the favored domains. The result is the creation of a very large magnetization, and even after the external field is turned off the rearranged domain structure tends to persist, leaving a permanent magnetization.

Ferromagnetic materials are always excluded from the vicinity of a magnetic resonance imaging system. Small fragments of ferromagnetic material can severely distort MR images. Even a sample as small as a staple can produce a large area of signal dropout in an image. More seriously, the inadvertent use of ferromagnetic tools in the vicinity of a large magnet is a severe safety risk. In the field of a 1.5-T magnet, the magnetic force on a 2-lb iron wrench is more than 50 lb, and the wrench will fly toward the scanner. Care should always be taken to check carefully any equipment brought into the MR scan room to ensure that no ferromagnetic components can become dangerous projectiles. In addition, subjects must be carefully screened to ensure that they have no ferromagnetic materials in their body, such as metal plates, old surgical clips, or even small metal fragments from sheet metal work. From here on we will focus only on materials that are weakly magnetized.

Magnetic Susceptibility

In addition to the magnetic forces discussed in the last section, a second effect of placing a sample of a material in a magnetic field is that the local magnetic field is distorted by the interaction of the internal dipole moments with the field. Each cubic millimeter of the material contains many magnetic dipole moments, and each of these dipoles creates its own dipole field. In a magnetic field, the dipole moments tend to align with the field if the material is paramagnetic, or opposite to the field if it is diamagnetic, and the sum of the moments of each of these dipoles is the net magnetization of the material. The net magnetization M is the equivalent dipole density in the material and so depends both on the intrinsic dipole density and on the degree of alignment of the dipoles. The creation of a net magnetization has two important effects for MR imaging. The first is that the part of M due to the alignment of nuclear dipoles is the magnetization that can be manipulated to generate the NMR signal. The second effect is that other dipole moments, such as unpaired electrons, contribute a much larger net magnetization, and this creates an additional, nonuniform magnetic field that adds to the main field B_0. For example, the effect on the total magnetic field of placing a sphere of diamagnetic or paramagnetic material in a uniform field is illustrated in the bottom row of Figure 7.9. In the absence of the sphere, the field lines are vertical and parallel. For a paramagnetic sphere the field lines are pulled in and concentrated within the sphere, and for the diamagnetic sphere the lines are pushed out from the sphere. These field inhomogeneities produce distortions and signal loss in MR images, but they also are the basis for functional imaging exploiting the BOLD effect or using injected contrast agents.

The degree to which a material becomes magnetized is measured by the *magnetic susceptibility*, χ, of the material: the local magnetization is $M = \chi B_0$. The magnetization M has the same dimensions as the magnetic field B_0, so χ is dimensionless. This can be a bit confusing because M is the equivalent density of magnetic dipoles, rather than a magnetic field, despite the fact that they have the same units. The magnetic fields produced in the neighborhood of a magnetized body are on the same order as M, but they also depend on the geometrical shape of the body. For most materials χ is on the order of a few parts per million, so the additional weak field that results from the alignment of intrinsic magnetic dipoles in matter is typically only a few parts per million of the main magnetic field B_0. The susceptibility χ may be positive (paramagnetic) or negative (diamagnetic), depending on whether the component of magnetization due to unpaired electrons or the component due to orbital motions is dominant. Exogenous contrast agents are paramagnetic.

It is important to maintain a clear distinction between the local magnetization of a magnetized body and the magnetic field created *by* that magnetized body. Whenever a body with a uniform composition is placed in a uniform magnetic field, it becomes uniformly magnetized. This means that in any small volume of the body, the partial alignment of the magnetic dipoles of the body is the same, so that they add up to a uniform magnetization M throughout. All this is independent of the shape of the body; it is a direct effect of the interaction of each of the dipoles with the magnetic field, leading to partial alignment. A collection of partially aligned dipoles, in turn, creates its own magnetic field through all of space, and this field adds to B_0. This additional field depends strongly on the geometry of the body.

However, if the local magnetization of a body depends on the partial alignment of the dipoles with the local field, and the local field is then altered by the additional field produced by the magnetized body, shouldn't this feed back on the local magnetization itself and alter it? The presence of the magnetized body does alter the local field, and indeed this does alter the local magnetization, but by a negligibly small amount. The field distortions in the human head are only about 1 ppm of B_0, so the variations in the local magnetization due to this additional field are only 1 ppm *of* 1 ppm, and so are negligibly small. For practical purposes then, we can assume that a body of arbitrary shape but uniform composition, when placed in a uniform magnetic field B_0, becomes uniformly magnetized with a dipole moment density $M = \chi B_0$.

The field distortions around a magnetized body depend on the shape of the body. Figure 7.10 shows pattern of field offsets around a uniformly magnetized sphere. For this simple spherical geometry field distortion is again a dipole field pattern. That is, adding up the contributions from each of the individual dipoles produces a field that is equivalent to one big dipole at the center of the sphere. However, this is only true for the perfect symmetry of a sphere; a body with a more

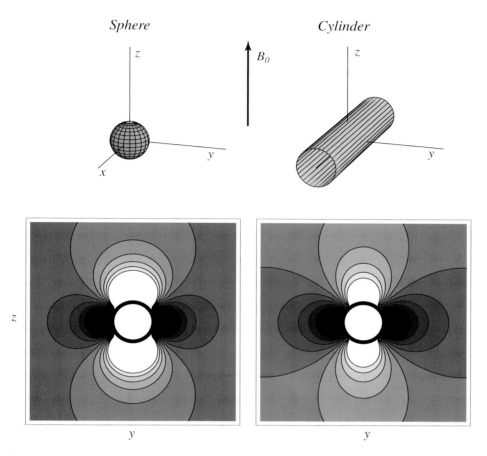

Figure 7.10. Magnetic field distortions around magnetized objects. Contour plots of the offset of the z-component of the field, B_z, in a plane cutting through a uniformly magnetized sphere (left) and cylinder (right). Both patterns have a dipolelike shape.

complex shape would produce a more complex field distortion. Another simple geometrical shape that is relevant for fMRI is a long cylinder oriented perpendicular to the magnetic field (Figure 7.10). The field distortion is qualitatively similar to the distortion around a sphere, although the radial dependence is different: the field offset falls off as $1/r^3$ for the sphere, but $1/r^2$ for the cylinder (r is the radial distance). At the surface of the cylinder, the maximum field offset is $\Delta B = 2\pi\Delta\chi B_0$, where $\Delta\chi$ is the susceptibility difference between the inside and the outside of the cylinder, and this maximum offset is independent of the radius of the cylinder. A magnetized cylinder is a useful model for thinking about magnetized blood vessels due to the presence of deoxyhemoglobin and the resulting BOLD effect.

In the preceding discussion we focused on the field distortions outside a magnetized body, but for most shapes the field inside is distorted as well. The sphere and the infinitely long cylinder are special cases in that they produce a uniform field offset inside. A short cylinder produces an external field intermediate between that of a sphere and a long cylinder, and the internal field is also distorted.

Field Distortions in the Head

The significance of these magnetic susceptibility effects is that whenever a body is placed in a uniform, external magnetic field B_0, the net field is distorted both outside and inside the body. This happens even if the body has a perfectly uniform composition and depends strongly on the shape of the body. Furthermore, if the body is heterogeneous, composed of materials with different magnetic susceptibilities, the field distortion is even worse. Figure 7.11 (shown earlier as Figure 5.10) shows the field distortion within a human head when placed in a uniform magnetic field. To a first approximation the head consists of three types of material: water, bone, and air. Field distortions are evident in the vicinity of interfaces between these materials. The large sinus cavities produce a local field distortion rather like a dipole field that extends through several centimeters of the brain, and also there is a broad field gradient in the superior/inferior direction due to the presence of the rest of the body. In general, the size of the field distortion in terms of the volume affected is comparable to the size of the heterogeneity. The largest field offsets are due to the air/water interface near the sinus cavities. Detailed modeling of the air spaces of the head predict field offsets of a few parts per million, in good agreement with what is measured (Li et al., 1995).

In MRI such field distortions within the body are a nuisance. A central assumption of MRI is that the magnetic field is uniform so that any field offsets measured when the field gradients are applied are entirely due to the location of the source of the signal, and not due to intrinsic field nonuniformity. Field distortions due to magnetic susceptibility variations between tissues thus lead to distortions in the MR images, and for some imaging techniques (e.g., EPI) these distortions can be severe. For this reason, MR scanners are equipped with additional coils called *shim coils,*

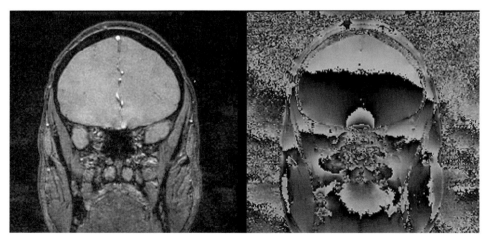

Figure 7.11. Magnetic field distortions in the head. A coronal gradient echo image, with the magnitude on the left and the phase on the right. The phase map shows magnetic field distortions due to the heterogeneity of the brain. Distortions include a dipolelike field near the sinus cavity and a superior/inferior gradient.

which can be used to flatten the magnetic field. This process is called shimming the magnetic field, and it is important to remember that this involves correcting for the intrinsic inhomogeneities of the human body as well as for nonuniformities of the magnet itself.

The macroscopic field distortions shown in Figure 7.11 are an unwanted byproduct of tissue heterogeneity. However, *microscopic* field distortions around small blood vessels are the basis for both contrast agent studies of blood volume and BOLD functional MRI. A contrast agent such as gadopentetate dimeglumine (Gd-DTPA) alters the susceptibility of the blood, creating field offsets in the space around the vessels (Villringer et al., 1988). At the peak of the passage of a bolus of Gd-DTPA through the vasculature, the susceptibility change of the blood is about 0.1 ppm (Boxerman et al., 1995), and if we model the vessels as long cylinders, this produces maximum field offsets of about 0.6 ppm. The BOLD effect is based on the fact that during brain activation the oxygen content of the venous blood is increased, which in turn alters the blood susceptibility relative to the surrounding tissue water. The susceptibility change due to increased oxygenation of the blood in the activated state is on the order of 0.01 ppm (Weisskoff and Kiihne, 1992), so the maximum field offsets are about 0.06 ppm. Because the susceptibility difference between the blood and the surrounding water is reduced when the blood is more oxygenated, the signal increases slightly. Magnetic susceptibility effects relevant to fMRI thus span nearly two orders of magnitude, from the large-scale heterogeneity of the brain that produces field variations of a few parts per million and image artifacts, to blood oxygenation-dependent microscopic susceptibility differences of a few hundredths of a part per million that reveal areas of functional activity.

REFERENCES

Alsop, D. C. and Detre, J. A. (1996) Reduced transit-time sensitivity in noninvasive magnetic resonance imaging of human cerebral blood flow. *J Cereb Blood Flow and Metab* **16,** 1236–1249.

Boxerman, J. L., Hamberg, L. M., Rosen, B. R. and Weisskoff, R. M. (1995) MR contrast due to intravascular magnetic susceptibility perturbations. *Magn. Reson. Med.* **34,** 555–566.

Feynman, R. P., Leighton, R. B. and Sands, M. (1965) *The Feynman Lectures on Physics.* Addison-Wesley: New York.

Frank, L. R., Wong, E. C. and Buxton, R. B. (1997) Slice profile effects in adiabatic inversion: Application to multislice perfusion imaging. *Magn. Reson. Med.* **38,** 558–564.

Grant, P. E., Vigneron, D. B. and Barkovich, A. J. (1998) High resolution imaging of the brain. *MRI Clinics of North America* **6,** 139–154.

Li, S., Williams, G. D., Frisk, T. A., Arnold, B. W. and Smith, M. B. (1995) A computer simulation of the static magnetic field distribution in the human head. *Magn. Reson. Med.* **34,** 268–275.

Purcell, E. M. (1965) *Electricity and Magnetism.* McGraw-Hill: New York.

Silver, M. S., Joseph, R. I. and Hoult, D. I. (1985) Selective spin inversion in nuclear magnetic resonance and coherent optics through an exact solution of the Bloch-Riccati equiation. *Phys. Rev. A* **31,** 2753–2755.

Villringer, A., Rosen, B. R., Belliveau, J. W., Ackerman, J. L., Lauffer, R. B., Buxton, R. B., Chao, Y.-S., Wedeen, V. J. and Brady, T. J. (1988) Dynamic imaging with lanthanide chelates in normal brain: contrast due to magnetic susceptibility effects. *Magn. Reson. Med.* **6,** 164–174.

Weisskoff, R. M. and Kiihne, S. (1992) MRI susceptometry: image–based measurement of absolute susceptibility of MR contrast agents and human blood. *Magn. Reson. Med.* **24,** 375–383.

8

Relaxation and Contrast in MRI

INTRODUCTION

The contrast between one tissue and another in a magnetic resonance (MR) image varies over a wide range depending just on the pulse sequence used for imaging. This dramatic soft-tissue contrast makes magnetic resonance imaging (MRI) sensitive to subtle differences in anatomy. In this chapter we will consider the basic factors that affect the MR signal and determine the contrast characteristics of an image. How this signal is mapped to produce an MR image is taken up in Chapter 10, but it is helpful to remember that an MR image is essentially a snapshot of the distribution of the MR signal, and we will illustrate some of the signal characteristics with images. The flexibility of MRI comes about largely because the MR signal depends on a number of tissue properties. The utility of MRI for clinical studies stems from the variability of the relaxation times between one tissue type and another and between healthy and diseased tissue. The important questions for clinical imaging then tend to focus around issues of static signal contrast, and pulse sequences for best emphasizing the tissue differences (Hendrick, Nelson, and Hendee, 1984). For functional imaging, however, physiological changes such as altered blood oxygenation have more subtle effects on the MR signal, and the goal is to detect dynamic changes in the signal over time.

In the following sections, the sources of contrast in an MR image are discussed in terms of how the intrinsic nuclear magnetic resonance (NMR) properties of the tissue, such as the relaxation times and the proton density, interact with different pulse sequence parameters to affect the signal intensity. We then examine the physical factors and conditions that determine these NMR properties.

THE SPIN ECHO SIGNAL

Spin Echoes

In a simple FID experiment, the generated signal decays away faster than it should due to T_2 decay alone because of magnetic field inhomogeneity. Spins sitting in different magnetic fields precess at different rates, and the resulting phase dispersion reduces the net signal. The apparent relaxation time T_2^* then is less than T_2. We can separate the decay of the net signal from a sample into two processes: the intrinsic decay of the local signal from a small, uniform region, which is governed by T_2, and the mutual cancellation of signals from different nearby locations due to phase dispersion caused by field inhomogeneities. The net decay is described by T_2^*, but it is sometimes useful to isolate the decay due to inhomogeneities from that due to T_2 (Hoppel et al., 1993). This additional decay due to inhomogeneities alone has been called T_2' decay. The assumed relationship between these three quantities is: $1/T_2^* = 1/T_2 + 1/T_2'$. The inverse of a relaxation time is a relaxation *rate constant,* and it is the rates that add to give the net relaxation effects. But it is important to remember that this relationship is really only qualitative. It would be a correct quantitative description if inhomogeneities always create a monoexponential decay, but that is rarely the case. Nevertheless, it is useful to think of signal decay in these terms.

As introduced in Chapter 4, signal loss due to field inhomogeneity can be reversed by applying a second radiofrequency (RF) pulse that causes the magnetization vectors to come back into phase and create an echo of the original free induction decay (FID) signal (a *spin echo*) at a time TE (the *echo time*) after the original excitation pulse. To review how this remarkable effect comes about, imagine two small magnetized regions sitting in slightly different magnetic fields. After a 90° excitation pulse the magnetization vectors are tipped into the transverse plane. As they begin to precess at slightly different frequencies, the phase difference between them grows larger. After waiting a time TE/2, a 180° RF pulse is applied along the *y*-axis in the rotating frame. The action of the 180° pulse is to flip the transverse plane like a pancake, reversing the *sign* of the phase of each magnetization vector. In other words, the phase φ_1 of the first magnetization is changed to $-\varphi_1$, and the phase φ_2 of the second group is changed to $-\varphi_2$. After the RF pulse, the phase of each magnetization continues to evolve, just as before, so that after another time delay TE/2 the first group again acquires an additional phase φ_1, and the second group again acquires an additional phase φ_2. But the net phase of each group is then zero, meaning that they are back in phase and add coherently to form a strong net signal (the echo) at time TE.

In fact, the echoing process is quite general, and any RF pulse will create an echo, although with flip angles other than 180°, the refocusing is not complete. In particular, repeated RF pulses generate a rich pattern of echoes, and we will consider this phenomenon in more detail later in the chapter. To understand the formation of echoes, it is helpful to examine how a 180° RF pulse rotating spin vectors around the same axis as the original 90° pulse (the *x*-axis of the rotating frame), also produces an echo. Figure 8.1 illustrates the formation of an echo by a 180° pulse by following the fate of four representative spin vectors. After a 90° pulse around *x* tips the spin vectors into the transverse plane, they each begin to precess at a different rate due to field inhomogeneity. In Figure 8.1, spin vector 1 has the highest offset of the precession frequency, vector 3 is on-resonance and so appears to be stationary in the rotating frame, and vectors 2 and 4 have plus and minus precession frequency offsets half as large as that for vector 1. After a time sufficient for vector 1 to accumulate a phase offset of 180° from vector 3, the vectors have spread evenly in the

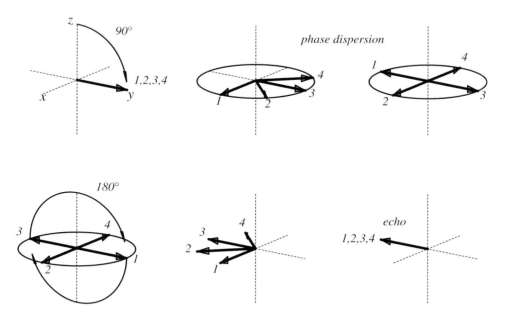

Figure 8.1. Formation of a spin echo. The separate fates of four representative spin vectors are depicted during a spin echo pulse sequence. After being tipped into the transverse plane by a 90° pulse around the *x*-axis in the rotating frame, the spins precess at different rates due to field inhomogeneities, spreading into a disk in the transverse plane (top). A 180° pulse around *x* flips the disk, and the continued precession of each spin causes an echo to form along the −*y*-axis.

transverse plane. The 180° RF pulse then flips this plane around the x-axis, reversing the positions of vectors 1 and 3 and leaving vectors 2 and 4 unchanged. Each vector then continues to precess, and after an equal elapsed time they are all in phase along the $-y$-axis, creating an echo. The distinction between this example and the first example is that the 180° pulse is applied along the x-axis rather than the y-axis. In the first example, the echo formed along the $+y$-axis, and in the second example (with the RF along x-axis) the echo formed along the $-y$-axis, but in both cases all of the spin vectors come back into phase to form a strong echo. In short, a 180° RF pulse applied along any axis will create a strong echo, but the orientation of this echo depends on the axis of the RF pulse.

Note that although a 180° pulse will correct for field inhomogeneities, it will *not* refocus true T_2 decay. The reason an echo forms is that the phase acquired during the interval before the 180° pulse is exactly the same as the phase acquired during the interval after the pulse. But the phase variations associated with T_2 decay are due to *fluctuating* fields, and the pattern of fluctuations is not repeated before and after the RF pulse. In short, a spin echo reverses the dephasing effects of static fields but not fluctuating fields. As a result, the echo signal intensity is weaker than the initial FID signal due to T_2 decay during the interval TE. After the echo the signal again decays because of T_2^* effects, but another 180° RF pulse will create another echo. This can be continued indefinitely, but each echo will be weaker than the last because of T_2 decay.

The basic spin echo (SE) pulse sequence can be summarized as

90° pulse – wait TE/2 – 180° pulse – wait TE/2 – measure

Typically, this pulse sequence is repeated at a regular interval TR called the *repetition time*. In a conventional MRI setting it is necessary to repeat the pulse sequence many times to collect all the data needed to reconstruct the image. The contrast between one tissue and another in the image will depend on the magnitude of the SE signal generated at each location.

SE Signal Intensity and Image Contrast

The mathematical expression for the SE signal is derived in Box 8. The signal is always proportional to the local proton density but also depends on the relaxation times. There are two pulse sequence parameters that are operator controlled: the repetition time TR and the echo time TE (Figure 8.2). These parameters control how strongly the local tissue relaxation times, T_1 and T_2, affect the signal. The echo time is the time when the spin echo occurs due to the refocusing effects of the 180° pulse and is typically the time when the MR signal is measured. By lengthening TE (i.e., waiting a longer time after the excitation pulse before applying the 180° refocusing pulse), there is more time for transverse (T_2) decay. The repetition time, on the other hand, controls how much longitudinal relaxation is allowed to happen before the magnetization is tipped over again when the pulse sequence is repeated. During the period TR, a sample with T_1 much shorter than TR will relax nearly completely, so that the longitudinal magnetization just before the next 90° pulse is large. But a sample with T_1 longer than TR will be only partly relaxed, and the

BOX 8. THE MR SIGNAL EQUATIONS

From the Bloch equations (Box 7), the expected signal intensity for any pulse sequence can be derived. And from such signal equations, expressing the dependence on M_0, T_1, T_2, and the pulse sequence parameters, the expected image contrast between tissues can be calculated. We can illustrate the procedure by deriving the signal intensity for the spin echo pulse sequence, a 90° RF pulse followed by a 180° pulse after a delay TE/2, and with the pulse sequence repeated after a repetition time TR. The pulse sequence can be described in a compact way as

$$90° - \text{wait TE/2} - 180° - \text{wait TE/2} - \text{measure} - \text{wait TR} - \text{TE}$$

Note that the repetition time, the interval between the initial 90° pulse and the next repeat of the 90° pulse is TR, the sum of each of the waiting intervals in this notation. If TR is not much longer than T_1, then the magnetization will not have fully recovered during the TR interval. After the pulse sequence is repeated a few times, a steady state will develop such that the magnetization just before each 90° RF pulse is the same, and the signal generated is then described as the steady-state signal for that pulse sequence. We wish to calculate this steady-state signal. If $M_z(0)$ is the longitudinal magnetization just before the 90° pulse, the initial magnitude of the *transverse* magnetization after the pulse will also be $M_z(0)$. The signal is measured at the echo time TE, and so the SE signal is simply $M_z(0)e^{-\text{TE}/T_2}$. The question then is: what is $M_z(0)$?

We can calculate the steady-state longitudinal magnetization by following through the pulse sequence, rotating the components of the magnetization as required by the RF pulses, incorporating relaxation in the intervals between RF pulses as dictated by the Bloch equations, and then applying the steady-state condition that the resulting magnetization at time TR must be the same as what we started with at time zero. Mathematically, the growth of z-magnetization can be described as an exponential decay of the *difference* between the current value of M_z and the equilibrium value M_0 so that if the z-magnetization starts at M_{z1} and relaxes for a time t, the final magnetization is

$$M_z = M_0 - (M_0 - M_{z1})\, e^{-t/T_1}$$

We can now apply this rule twice to calculate how the z-magnetization evolves. The progressive changes in the z-component of the magnetization are as follows. The 90° pulse tips $M_z(0)$ into the transverse plane, and the longitudinal component then begins to grow from zero, reaching a value of

$$M_z = M_0 - [M_0 - M_z(0)]\, e^{-\text{TE}/2T_1}$$

by time TE/2. The 180° pulse flips the regrown component from $+z$ to $-z$, and it then begins to regrow from this negative value. After relaxing for a time TR − TE/2, the longitudinal magnetization is back to the starting point, just before the 90° pulse, and so this magnetization is again $M_z(0)$ in the steady state. Applying the same relaxation rule for the period after the 180° pulse to the expression for M_z directly gives an expression for $M_z(0)$. The full SE signal intensity is then

$$S_{SE} = M_0 e^{-\text{TE}/T_2} \left(1 - 2e^{-(\text{TR}-\text{TE}/2)/T_1} + e^{-\text{TR}/T_1}\right) \qquad [\text{B8.1}]$$

(continued)

BOX 8, continued

Note that if TE is very short, the signal is approximately

$$S_{SE} \approx M_0 e^{-TE/T_2} (1 - e^{-TR/T_1})$$ [B8.2]

We can apply the same type of reasoning to other pulse sequences to derive appropriate expressions for the NMR signal. For the inversion recovery (IR) pulse sequence with a spin echo acquisition, the form of the pulse sequence is

180° – wait TI – 90° – wait TE/2 – 180° – wait TE/2 – measure – wait TR-TI-TE

The initial 180° pulse acts as a preparation pulse, modifying the longitudinal magnetization, and the transverse magnetization is not created until the 90° pulse is applied after the inversion time TI. The second 180° pulse creates a spin echo of this transverse magnetization. The resulting signal intensity is

$$S_{IR} = M_0 e^{-TE/T_2} (1 - 2e^{-TI/T_1} + 2e^{-(TR-TE/2)/T_1} - e^{-TR/T_1})$$ [B8.3]

And if TR $\gg T_1$, the IR signal is approximately

$$S_{IR} \approx M_0 e^{-TE/T_2} (1 - 2e^{-TI/T_1})$$ [B8.4]

The IR signal differs from the SE signal in two ways. First, the signal is more T_1-weighted because of the factor 2 in Equation [B8.4] compared with Equation [B8.2]. This expresses the fact that the IR signal is recovering over a range twice as large ($-M_0$ to M_0) as the range of the SE signal (0 to M_0). The second unique feature of the IR signal is that there is a null point when the longitudinal magnetization, relaxing from a negative value, passes through $M_z = 0$. A 90° pulse applied at this time will generate no signal because the longitudinal magnetization is zero. The null point occurs when TI $= T_1$ ln 2 $= 0.693 T_1$ so that the expression in parentheses in Equation [B8.4] is zero. This effect is used in imaging to suppress the signal from particular tissues. For example, fat has a short T_1, and so the fat signal is nulled when TI is about 150 ms. This is described as a *short TI inversion recovery (STIR) sequence.*

The preceding calculations of signal intensities are relatively simple because of an implicit assumption that TR $\gg T_2$ so that the transverse magnetization has completely decayed away before the pulse sequence is repeated. But for gradient echo pulse sequences this is often not true. The calculation of signal intensity is then quite a bit more complicated because all three components of the magnetization must be considered (Buxton et al., 1989; Gyngell, 1988). Another way of stating the complexity of this problem is that when TR is shorter than T_2, each RF pulse creates echoes of the previous transverse magnetization, and these echoes add to form the net signal. However, with a spoiled GRE pulse sequence the formation of these echoes is prevented (the echoes are spoiled), and for this case the signal can be calculated in the same manner as for the SE and IR signals (Buxton et al., 1987). The pulse sequence is then very simple:

α – wait TE – measure – wait TR – TE

The flip angle is now taken to be an arbitrary angle α, and the effect of this is that the longitudinal magnetization is not reduced to zero with each excitation pulse. Taking this into account, the resulting signal intensity is

$$S_{GRE} = M_0 e^{-TE/T_2^*} \sin \alpha \, \frac{1 - e^{-TR/T_1}}{1 - \cos \alpha \, e^{-TR/T_1}} \qquad \text{[B8.5]}$$

Note that the transverse decay now depends on T_2^*, rather than T_2, because there is no spin echo to refocus the effects of magnetic field inhomogeneity. This expression for the signal exhibits some interesting properties that differ from the SE and IR cases. When TR is long, the maximum signal is produced with a flip angle of 90°, as one would expect. But as TR becomes shorter, the flip angle that produces the maximum signal is reduced. This flip angle for maximum signal is called the Ernst angle α_E (Ernst and Anderson, 1966) and is given by

$$\cos \alpha_E = e^{-TR/T_1} \qquad \text{[B8.6]}$$

For example, with TR = 30 ms and T_1 = 1000 msec, the maximum signal is achieved with $\alpha_E = 25°$.

Furthermore, when α is smaller than the Ernst angle, the signal is relatively independent of the value of T_1. In the limit of small flip angle so that $\cos \alpha$ is close to one, Equation [B8.5] reduces to

$$S_{GRE} \approx M_0 e^{-TE/T_2^*} \sin \alpha \qquad \text{[B8.7]}$$

and the signal is independent of T_1. Thus, the flip angle is an important parameter for manipulating contrast in GRE images. With large flip angles the signal is strongly T_1-weighted, but with small flip angles the T_1-sensitivity is suppressed, and the signal is just density- and T_2^*-weighted.

longitudinal magnetization will be smaller. After the next 90° pulse this longitudinal magnetization becomes the transverse magnetization and generates a signal, so the short T_1 sample will produce a stronger signal.

The SE signal can be viewed as having some degree of proton density-weighting, T_1-weighting, and T_2-weighting in the sense that all these parameters contribute to the signal, and different tissues can be distinguished in an image based on how their differences in M_0, T_1, and T_2 modify the local signal intensity. The SE sequence is always proton-density-weighted because the equilibrium magnetization is proportional to the proton density, and the maximum signal that can be generated is proportional to M_0. But this maximum signal is only achieved when TR is much longer than T_1 so that the longitudinal magnetization fully recovers between repetitions, and when TE is much smaller than T_2 so that the signal decay during TE is negligible. For other pulse sequence parameters, there will be some degree of T_1-weighting and T_2-weighting in the local signal. The sensitivity of the signal to T_1 is controlled by TR, with longer TR decreasing the T_1-weighting of the signal, and the sensitivity to T_2 is controlled by TE, with shorter TE decreasing T_2-weighting.

It seems plausible that we could then maximize the contrast between two tissues by maximizing the sensitivity to both T_1 and T_2 differences. However, this turns out to be a bad idea. In the body, proton density, T_1 and T_2 are positively correlated, so that more watery tissues (e.g., cerebrospinal fluid) tend to have larger proton den-

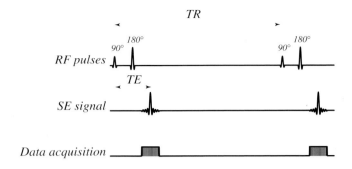

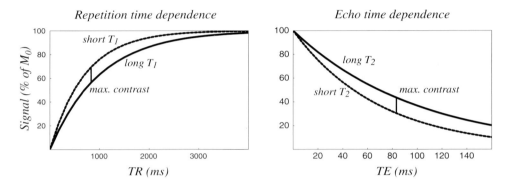

Figure 8.2. Spin echo signal. The SE pulse sequence is defined by two operator-controlled parameters, the repetition time TR and the echo time TE (top). The SE signal increases with longer TR in a way that depends on T_1 and decreases with increasing TE in a way that depends on T_2. Maximum T_1-weighted contrast between tissues occurs when TR is about equal to T_1, and maximum T_2-weighted contrast occurs when TE is about equal to T_2.

sity and longer T_1 and T_2, and this leads to conflicting contrast effects. T_1-weighting produces a stronger signal from tissues with short relaxation times, whereas T_2-weighting tends to produce a stronger signal from the tissues with long relaxation times (see Figure 8.2). If the signal is sensitive to both T_1 and T_2, these effects tend to cancel one another and produce poor tissue contrast. This means that if one wants to produce a signal with strong T_1-weighting, the sensitivity to T_2 must be suppressed. A T_1-weighted SE sequence thus uses short TR to increase T_1-weighting and short TE to minimize T_2-weighting. Similarly, a T_2-weighted SE sequence uses long TR to minimize T_1-weighting and long TE (approximately equal to T_2) to maximize T_2-weighting. Finally, a purely density-weighted sequence uses long TR to suppress T_1-weighting and short TE to suppress T_2-weighting.

The contrast characteristics of the SE pulse sequence applied to brain imaging are illustrated in Figure 8.3. The top row shows examples of T_1-weighted, density-weighted, and T_2-weighted images. The contrasts between gray matter (GM), white matter (WM), and cerebrospinal fluid (CSF) are radically different in the three images. White matter is brightest and CSF is darkest in the T_1-weighted image, and this pattern is reversed in the T_2-weighted image. In the so-called density-weighted

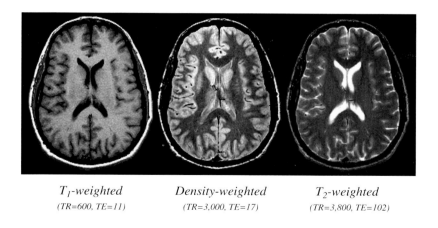

T_1-weighted
(TR=600, TE=11)

Density-weighted
(TR=3,000, TE=17)

T_2-weighted
(TR=3,800, TE=102)

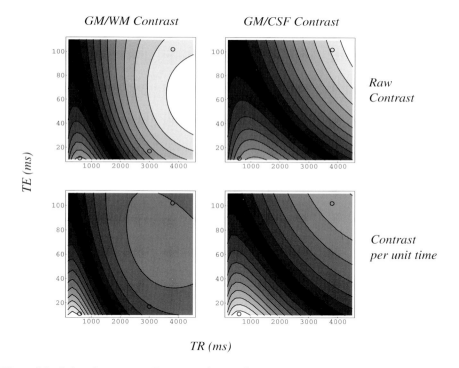

Figure 8.3. Spin echo contrast. Images at the top show examples of T_1-weighted, density-weighted, and T_2-weighted contrast (timing parameters given in milliseconds). Contour plots show contrast in the TR/TE plane for two tissue pairs: GM/WM (left) and GM/CSF (right). The first row shows raw signal difference between tissues, whereas the second row shows the contrast-to-noise ratio per unit time.

image, gray matter is brightest despite the fact that CSF has the highest proton density. The reason for this is that the T_1 of CSF is so long that for TR = 3 s the CSF signal is still substantially T_1-weighted. In comparing these images it is important to keep in mind that we have followed the common practice of adjusting the window and level of each image individually to best bring out the intrinsic tissue contrast. In

TABLE 8.1 Typical NMR Parameters in the Brain

Tissue	M_0 (arb. units)	T_1 (ms)	T_2 (ms)
Gray matter	85	950	95
White matter	80	700	80
CSF	100	2500	250

other words, the gray scale is different for each image so that even though it looks like the CSF is brighter on the T_2-weighted image than on the density-weighted image, the absolute signal is not. It is just that the CSF signal has decayed much less than GM or WM with long TE so that relative to these tissues it is much brighter.

To see in a more continuous way how the contrasts change when the pulse sequence parameters TR and TE are varied, we can calculate the contrast for a pair of tissues from the SE signal intensity equation in Box 8 and assumed values for the NMR parameters for particular tissues. These parameters are somewhat variable, but typical numbers are given in Table 8.1. The lower panels in Figure 8.3 show contour plots of the absolute value of the contrast between GM and WM (left) and between GM and CSF (right) in the TR/TE plane. The first row shows the raw contrast calculated for one repetition of the pulse sequence. For GM/WM contrast there are two islands of high contrast, corresponding to T_1-weighted and T_2-weighted images, with a diagonal trough of poor contrast running between them. For WM/CSF contrast there are also two islands, but slightly shifted. Both contrasts are maximized using a T_2-weighted sequence with a very long TR and a moderately long TE.

However, this comparison of the raw signal differences between tissues does not address a critical factor: the noise in the image. In most applications the ability to distinguish one tissue from another in an image depends not just on the raw contrast but rather on the contrast-to-noise ratio (CNR) (Hendrick et al., 1984; Wehrli et al., 1984). The image noise is independent of TR and TE, so for one repetition of the pulse sequence the noise will be about the same for any TR or TE. But the total time required for a pulse sequence to play out is TR, so a sequence with a short TR can be repeated several times and averaged in the same time it takes a long TR sequence to play out once, and averaging reduces the noise in proportion to the square root of the number of averages. For example, for the same total imaging time a sequence with TR = 500 ms can be repeated four times as many times as a sequence with TR = 2000 ms, so the noise is cut in half in the short TR sequence. A figure of merit for comparing different pulse sequences that takes this into account is the CNR per unit time, which is just proportional to the CNR divided by $\sqrt{TR}$. The bottom row of panels in Figure 8.3 shows the CNR per unit time for GM/WM contrast and GM/CSF contrast. In this example, both contrasts are largest for the T_1-weighted pulse sequence because the long TR required for a T_2-weighted sequence is inefficient. A substantial amount of clinical MR research is directed toward identifying optimal pulse sequence parameters for different applications, and other criteria in addition to CNR affect these decisions. For example, pathological tissue is more readily detected when it is brighter than normal tissue, and so because many types of lesion involve lengthening of the relaxation times, T_2-weighted images are often used. In practice, clinical imaging usually includes a mixture of T_1-weighted, T_2-weighted, and proton-density-weighted images.

The terminology of *density-weighted* and *T_1-weighted* is widely used but somewhat misleading, as we saw above in Figure 8.3. The MR signal is always proportional to the proton density, and so to be precise *all* signals are density-weighted. The important difference between the long TR signal and the short TR signal is that with long TR there is *only* density-weighting, whereas with short TR there is T_1-weighting as well. From Table 8.1, T_2-weighting and density-weighting are mutually supportive, in the sense that both tend to make the signal with long T_2 and high spin density larger. But with short TR the T_1-weighting is in direct conflict with density-weighting and T_2-weighting. For example, the proton density difference between GM and CSF would tend to make the CSF signal stronger, whereas the T_1 difference tends to make the GM signal stronger, and the trough in the contour plots reflects the region where these conflicting effects reduce the contrast. The terminology is also potentially misleading because a particular TR may be longer than T_1 for some tissues but comparable to T_1 for others. As noted earlier, with TR = 3 s, the T_1-sensitivity is suppressed for GM and WM but is strong for CSF. The descriptive terms T_1-weighted, T_2-weighted, and density-weighted are used frequently, but bear in mind that this terminology is imprecise.

Generalized Echoes

The process of spin echo formation was described earlier in terms of the action of a 180° RF pulse. In fact, the echoing process is much more general, and any RF pulse can create an echo of previous transverse magnetization. To see how this comes about, consider two 90° pulses applied in succession with a delay T between them, and assume that the RF pulse is applied along the x-direction in the rotating frame. The original demonstration of spin echoes used such 90° pulses, rather than 180° pulses (Hahn, 1950). The first RF pulse rotates the longitudinal magnetization from the z-axis to the y-axis in the rotating frame, where it begins to precess (Figure 8.4). During the period T the individual spin vectors precess at different rates due to field inhomogeneities. In the rotating frame precessing at the mean precession rate, the spin vectors will spread into a fan and eventually a disk covering the plane so that the net magnetization is reduced to zero. The second 90° pulse then rotates this disk around the x-axis, putting some of the magnetization along the z-axis, but preserving some of the magnetization in the transverse plane. To simplify the picture, the fates of four representative spin vectors are plotted in Figure 8.4, in a similar fashion to those in Figure 8.1. By the time of the second 90° pulse, these vectors have spread evenly in the transverse plane, lying along the $+x$-, $-x$-, $+y$-, and $-y$-axis. After the second 90° pulse, the x-axis vectors are unaffected, but the $+y$ vector is rotated to $-z$, and the $-y$ vector is rotated to the $+z$-axis. After a second evolution period T, each of the x-vectors will acquire the same phase offset as during the first T interval, $+90°$ for one and $-90°$ for the other. They are then back in phase along the $-y$-axis, creating a spin echo. But this spin echo is weaker than the echo created by a 180°

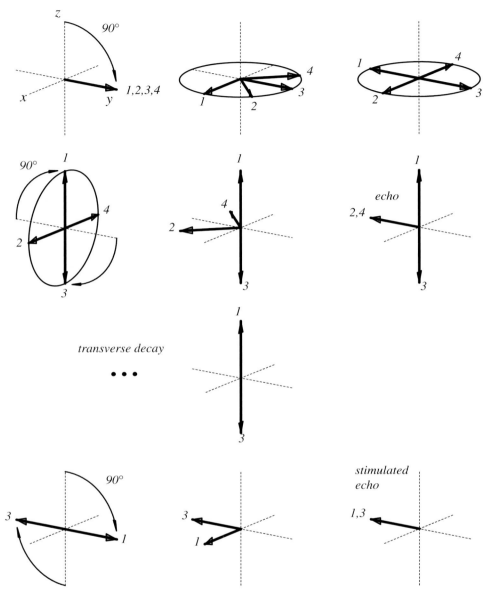

Figure 8.4. Formation of echoes with 90° pulses. The fate of four spin vectors is shown during application of three 90° pulses, presented as in Figure 8.1. The first 90° pulse tips the spin vectors into the transverse plane, where they precess at different rates and spread into a disk. The second 90° pulse tips the disk so that vectors 1 and 3 lie on the z-axis. Spin vectors 2 and 4 continue to precess and form an echo along the −y-axis. Over time the transverse components decay away with time constant T_2, but spin vectors 1 and 3 decay more slowly, with time constant T_1. A third 90° pulse tips these spin vectors back to the transverse plane, and resumed precession produces another echo, called a stimulated echo.

pulse because some of the original transverse magnetization is now stored along the z-axis and so does not contribute to the echo. In general, the smaller the flip angle of the refocusing pulse, the weaker the echo. Over time the transverse components decay away.

What happens to the magnetization that was parked along the z-axis? Over time it also will relax back toward equilibrium, but with a time constant T_1 instead of T_2. However, if instead it is tipped back down to the transverse plane before it has fully relaxed, another echo will be formed, called a *stimulated echo*. A third 90° pulse around x returns this magnetization to the transverse plane, putting the original $+y$ vector along $–y$, and the original $–y$ vector along $+y$. Now that these vectors are back in the transverse plane, they will begin to precess again at the same rate as before. After another interval T, the vector that had originally precessed 180° to end up on the $–y$-axis, will precess another 180° and return to the $–y$-axis, where it adds to the vector that stays along the $–y$-axis to form the stimulated echo. Like the direct spin echo that formed after the second RF pulse, the stimulated echo is weaker than the full echo of a 180° pulse because only a part of the transverse magnetization is refocused.

A series of RF pulses can thus generate both direct and stimulated echoes. An example that suggests just how complicated this can become is illustrated in Figure 8.5, which shows the echo pattern formed by an initial 90° pulse followed by two α-degree pulses. To emphasize that echo formation results simply from free precession, interrupted by occasional RF pulses, the curves in Figure 8.5 were calculated without including any relaxation effects. In these simulations, spin vectors with a random distribution of precession frequencies freely precess, and the net signal is the average y-component of the ensemble of spins. When $\alpha = 180°$, the situation is the standard SE pulse sequence: the initial pulse generates an FID, and each 180° pulse creates a full echo of the original transverse magnetization, for a total of two echoes. The first echo is along the $–y$-axis and so appears negative in the plot, and the second echo, being an echo of the first echo, is positive. In other words, with repeated 180° RF pulses along the x-axis, the successive echoes alternate sign.

However, if α is reduced to 135°, the echo pattern develops an interesting complexity. The original two echoes are reduced in amplitude, as we might expect, but in addition two new echoes appear, both with a negative sign. The weak echo occurring before the second of the original echoes is the stimulated echo described in Figure 8.4. The second new echo, occurring later than the original two echoes, is an echo of the original signal due to the initial 90° pulse refocused by the second α-pulse. As the flip angle is reduced, the original two echoes grow progressively weaker, with the second echo decreasing in amplitude more quickly than the first. The reason for this is that this second echo is really an echo of an echo, so if each echoing process is only partial, it will depend more strongly on the flip angle, and in this example it is not detectable if the flip angle is reduced to as low as 45°. In contrast, the stimulated echo increases as the flip angle is reduced, peaking at 90° but remaining as the strongest echo for lower flip angles. Finally, the fourth echo also increases in amplitude with decreasing flip angle, peaking at 90°. One can think of this echo (a bit loosely) as formed from spin vectors that were not completely refocused by the first

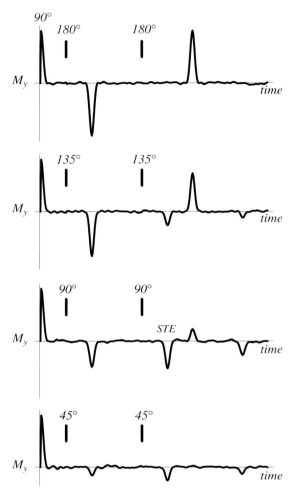

Figure 8.5. Echo patterns from three RF pulses. Each row shows the echoes formed by two successive α-degree pulses, with α = 180°, 135°, 90°, and 45° (top to bottom). Each time course begins with a 90° pulse and the resulting FID. The curves show a simulation of T_2^* losses and echo refocusing by plotting the average value of M_y for 2,000 spins, each precessing at its own constant rate, but with small random differences of the precession frequency among the spins. The top row shows the simple double echo pattern resulting from 180° pulses, but with smaller RF pulses more echoes appear, including a stimulated echo (STE).

RF pulse but are then refocused by the second RF pulse. This echo does not occur for a 180° pulse because all the spin vectors do refocus after the first RF pulse, so the second RF pulse only creates an echo of the echo.

This example illustrates that the echo pattern formed by a string of RF pulses can be quite complex. It also shows that a 180° pulse is in some sense an exception, in that the echo pattern is fairly simple. This can present practical problems in a multiecho pulse sequence because real 180° pulses are never perfect. In imaging applications the flip angle can vary through the thickness of the slice, so in reality we must deal with refocusing pulses with a range of flip angles. The resulting unwanted echoes can cause artifacts in the images if they are not carefully controlled.

Furthermore, the foregoing example was simplified by ignoring relaxation effects. By starting with a 90° pulse so that the longitudinal magnetization was reduced to zero and by neglecting any regrowth of that magnetization, the role of each RF pulse as a refocusing pulse was emphasized. But in reality each pulse (except for the special case of a perfect 180° pulse) would also produce new coherent transverse magnetization. This illustrates a basic feature of RF pulses that is important for understanding the fast gradient echo imaging sequences discussed later. Whenever a series of RF pulses is applied, each RF pulse does two things: it produces a new FID itself, but it also contributes to creating an echo of previous FIDs. Furthermore, if the RF pulses are equally spaced, the echoes occurring by different routes occur at the same time, such as a direct echo from the previous FID and a stimulated echo of the FID produced by the pulse two back. In fast imaging with short repetition times, these echoes can build up and strongly affect the measured signal, adding an interesting complexity to the signal measured with gradient echoes and short TR.

THE GRADIENT ECHO SIGNAL

Gradient Echoes

The simplest pulse sequence consists of a single RF pulse with arbitrary flip angle α applied repeatedly with a repetition time TR, and with the signal measured at a time TE after each RF pulse. The prototype of such a pulse sequence is FLASH (fast low-angle shot) (Haase et al., 1986). In an imaging setting such a pulse sequence is described as a gradient recalled echo (GRE) or simply a gradient echo (GE). The terminology refers to the fact that the gradient pulses used for imaging are usually constructed with an initial negative lobe so that a gradient echo forms at the center of data collection when the effects of the positive frequency encoding gradient just balance the effects of the initial gradient lobe. In other words, at the gradient echo the net effect of the gradients applied up to that time is zero. The term *gradient echo imaging* is somewhat unfortunate because it suggests that this method uses gradient echoes *instead* of RF echoes. There is indeed no 180° RF pulse in GRE imaging, but as described in the previous section on generalized echoes, a series of closely spaced RF pulses of any flip angle can also create echoes that affect the steady-state signal. Furthermore, gradient echoes are an integral part of both SE and GRE imaging. The distinction between the two is really just that GRE pulse sequences do not contain a 180° refocusing pulse. We will adopt this standard terminology even though we will not be considering the effects of imaging gradients until Chapter 10. For now we will simply explore the signal and contrast properties of the GRE pulse sequence. Even though there is no 180° refocusing pulse involved, and thus no explicit echo at the time when the signal is measured, we still refer to the data collection time as TE for consistency with the SE pulse sequence.

T_2* and Chemical Shift Effects

There are two important differences in the signal characteristics of the GRE and SE signals. The first is a direct result of the fact that there is no 180° refocusing pulse in a GRE pulse sequence. As a consequence, the dephasing effects of field inhomogeneities are not reversed, and so the signal decays exponentially with increasing TE with a decay constant T_2*, rather than T_2. Because the head itself is inhomogeneous, a GRE image with a long TE usually shows areas with reduced signal where the local T_2* is shortened in areas with inhomogeneous fields (Figure 8.6). This can be an asset in studies of brain iron (Wismer et al., 1988) or in studies of hemorrhage, where the evolution and breakdown of blood products leads to measurable variations in the GRE signal (Thulborn and Brady, 1989). But the sensitivity to field inhomogeneities also leads to artifactual signal dropouts due just to the nonuniformity of the head (e.g., near sinus cavities). Furthermore, the T_2* of an imaging voxel may depend on the size of the voxel because a larger voxel may contain a larger spread of precession frequencies causing the signal to decay more quickly (see the example in Figure 8.6). For this reason, the TE is usually kept short in GRE imaging, often as small as a few milliseconds.

An exception to this is fMRI based on the Blood Oxygenation Level Dependent (BOLD) effect, where the goal is to detect small local changes in T_2* due to microscopic field variations between the intravascular and extravascular spaces, and within the blood itself, arising from changes in blood oxygenation. For BOLD studies, TE is usually in the moderate range of 30–60 ms, as in the example in Figure 8.6. Thus, there is always an essential conflict involved in BOLD imaging due to T_2* effects. A somewhat long TE is required so that the signal will be sensitive to the T_2* changes produced by the BOLD effect, but this brings in added sensitivity to signal dropouts due to the nonuniformity of the head. For this reason, shimming the magnet to try to flatten out the broad field inhomogeneities is an important part of fMRI studies.

GRE imaging also exhibits a chemical shift effect because the resonant frequencies of the hydrogen nuclei in fat and water differ by about 3.5 ppm (Wehrli et al., 1987). Because there is no 180° RF pulse to refocus the phase differences that develop between the fat and water signals, the net signal from a voxel containing both fat and water shows oscillations in intensity with increasing TE as the fat and water signals come in and out of phase. Figure 8.6 shows an example of this chemical shift effect in a voxel in the scalp. Note that the troughs of the signal, when fat and water are out of phase, are sharper than the peaks, as illustrated in Figure 8.6 with both an experimental curve and a theoretical curve. At 1.5 T the cycle time for water to precess a full cycle relative to fat is only about 4.4 ms, and so this is the period of the oscillations in the signal decay curve. The interference of the fat and water signals can be used to estimate the fat content of tissues or partly to suppress the signal from tissues containing fat by choosing TE to be at a point where the fat and water signals are out of phase. For example, in MR angiography applications in which the goal is to achieve good contrast between blood and surrounding tissue, an out-of-phase TE of 2.2 or 6.6 ms is often used partly to suppress the tissue signal. In

Magnetic field mapping

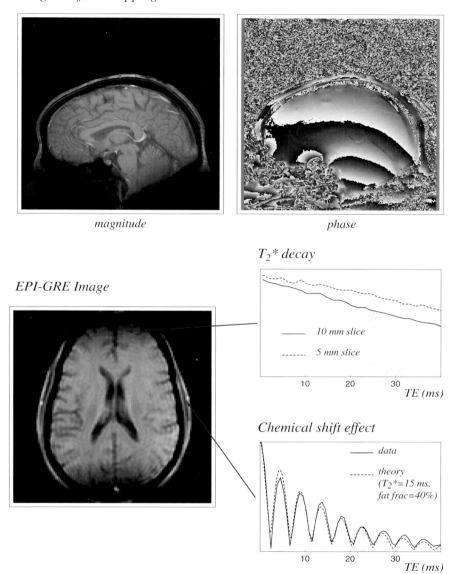

EPI-GRE Image

Figure 8.6. Echo time effects on the GRE signal. With no 180° RF refocusing pulse, the phase of the local GRE signal at the time of measurement (TE) is proportional to the local magnetic field offset, as illustrated by the magnitude and phase images shown in the top row. When the signals contributing to the net signal of an imaging voxel have different resonant frequencies, phase dispersion leads to signal loss (T_2* effect). And when the voxel contains both fat and water, the dependence of the signal on TE contains an oscillation as the fat and water signals come in and out of phase.

the healthy brain a fat signal is seen only in the scalp and skull marrow. The lipids that make up the myelin sheath of nerves are highly structured and so have a very short T_2 and are not observed in standard MRI.

Short TR Effects

The second important difference between the GRE and SE signals arises because the repetition times used with GRE pulse sequences are usually much shorter than those used with SE pulse sequences. The use of short TRs is made possible in part because there is no 180° RF pulse. The essential limitation on how short TR can be is set by government guidelines limiting RF exposure to the subject. Each time an RF pulse is applied, heat is deposited in the body. The amount of deposited energy is proportional to the square of the flip angle, so one repetition of an SE pulse sequence with a 90° and a 180° RF pulse deposits 45 times as much energy as one repetition of a GRE pulse sequence with a single 30° RF pulse. For this reason TR can be drastically shortened while keeping the rate of energy deposition (the *specific absorption rate,* SAR) below the guidelines. In practice, the TR for a GRE pulse sequence can be as short as 5 ms, and with a total imaging time as short as a few seconds, motion artifacts due to respiration can be significantly reduced by collecting the entire image during one breath-hold. Alternatively, three-dimensional volume acquisitions with high spatial resolution can be collected in a few minutes.

An essential useful feature of GRE pulse sequences is thus the ability to use very short repetition times. But before tackling the more complex problem of understanding the signal with short TR, we begin with the long TR case. When TR is much greater than T_2, so that any transverse magnetization generated by one of the RF pulses has decayed away by the time of the next pulse, the contrast characteristics are similar to those of the SE pulse sequence. If the flip angle α is 90°, all the longitudinal magnetization is flipped into the transverse plane. This is often described as a *saturation recovery pulse sequence,* and the 90° pulse is called a saturation pulse because it reduces the longitudinal magnetization to zero. If TR is much longer than T_1, the magnetization fully recovers between RF pulses, producing a proton-density-weighted signal such that CSF is brightest and WM is darkest. As TR is reduced, the signal becomes more T_1-weighted, just as it does with an SE pulse sequence. If TR were the only way to influence the degree of T_1-weighting, the contrast characteristics of the GRE and SE pulse sequences would be similar. But an additional parameter to vary in a GRE pulse sequence is the flip angle α.

Figure 8.7 (top) shows the effect on the contrast of reducing the flip angle α for short TR, when TR is shorter than T_1 but longer than T_2 (curves were calculated from the equation derived in Box 8). The plot shows signal curves for two tissues with the same proton density but with T_1s of 1,000 and 700 ms, calculated for TR = 4,000 and 500 ms. As expected, for long TR there is little T_1-weighting, and the signals of the two tissues are nearly equal for all flip angles. With shorter TR and a flip angle near 90°, the signal is strongly T_1-weighted as described earlier, with the tissue with a shorter T_1 creating a larger signal. But as α is reduced, the signal becomes less and less T_1-weighted until for small α it is essentially just density-weighted. For the calculated curves in Figure 8.7, the proton densities were assumed to be equal, so all the

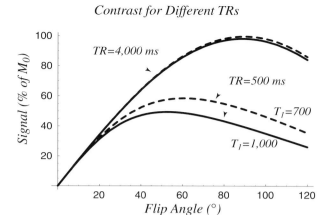

Contrast for Different TRs

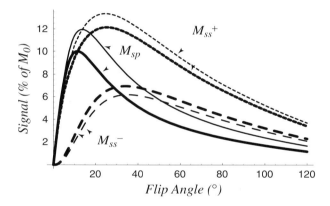

Contrast for Different GRE Signals

Figure 8.7. Effect of flip angle on GRE signals. Top: Curves are plotted for two tissues with a 30% difference in both relaxation times (solid line: $T_1 = 1,000$ ms and $T_2 = 100$ ms; dashed line: $T_1 = 700$ and $T_2 = 70$). T_1-weighting can be minimized with either a long TR or with a small flip angle. Bottom: Curves show the contrast between the same two tissues for very short TR (20 ms) for the three types of GRE signal (in each pair the bold lines are for the tissue with longer relaxation times).

signal curves are the same for small flip angles. That is, even though TR < T_1, so that there is little time for recovery of the longitudinal magnetization, the signal nevertheless can be made insensitive to T_1 by using a small flip angle (Buxton et al., 1987). The source of this useful effect is that tipping the magnetization by a small angle leaves most of the longitudinal magnetization intact near the equilibrium value, so T_1 relaxation makes a negligible change in the longitudinal component and the resulting signal is then insensitive to T_1. In short, the MR signal can be made insensitive to T_1 either by increasing TR or by decreasing the flip angle with short TR.

When TR >> T_2, the transverse magnetization decays away before the next RF pulse. As a result, the measured signal is entirely due to the FID generated by the most recent RF pulse. But when TR < T_2, this situation is changed in an interesting way. Each pulse still produces new transverse magnetization, but the transverse magnetization from previous RF pulses will not have decayed away completely. Different components of this previous transverse magnetization will have acquired different phases due to local field offsets (e.g., applied gradients or main field inhomogeneity) so that this old transverse magnetization may be incoherent. But if these field offsets are the same during each TR period, the RF pulses will create echoes of the previous transverse magnetization at multiples of TR. These echoes will add to the new transverse magnetization from the most recent RF pulse, creating a strong coherent signal immediately before and after each RF pulse (Figure 8.8). After a number of RF pulses are applied, the magnetization will approach a steady state in which the signal pattern is repeated in the same way during each TR

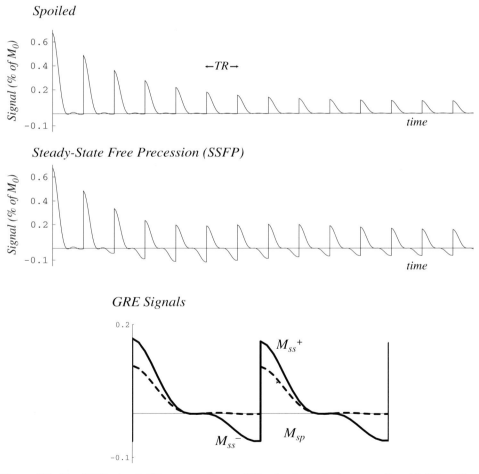

Figure 8.8. The GRE signal. When an α-degree RF pulse is applied repeatedly with TR < T_2, a steady state develops after several pulses. If the echoes are spoiled, a coherent magnetization (M_{sp}) is created after each RF pulse. If the echoes are not spoiled, a coherent magnetization forms both before (M_{ss}^-) and after (M_{ss}^+) each pulse. There are thus three distinct signals that could be measured with a GRE pulse sequence.

period. In this condition of *steady-state free precession (SSFP)* the coherent signal just after the RF pulse, M_{ss}^+, and the signal just before the RF pulse, M_{ss}^-, are both constant (Gyngell, 1988; Patz, 1989).

The coherent magnetization M_{ss}^- is the net result of the echoes of all the FIDs generated by the previous RF pulses. The next RF pulse then partly flips this coherent transverse magnetization and also adds to it a new FID signal to create the coherent magnetization M_{ss}^+. So for an SSFP pulse sequence such as this, there are two possible signals to measure, and both M_{ss}^+ and M_{ss}^- depend on the echoing process resulting from many closely spaced RF pulses. But in addition to these two signals, a third possible signal is the spoiled signal that results when the echoes are suppressed. The echoes occur because whatever phase precession occurs during one TR interval is exactly repeated in the next. The echo formation can be blocked by inserting random gradient pulses into each TR interval after data collection to produce a random additional precessional phase before the next RF pulse (*gradient spoiling*). Alternatively, the echoes can be spoiled by varying the flip axis of the RF pulse *(RF spoiling)*, which also adds a variable phase angle to the precession during each TR interval. With the echoes spoiled, there is no coherent magnetization before each RF pulse ($M_{ss}^- = 0$), and the signal just after the RF pulse, M_{sp}, consists only of the FID generated by that pulse with no echo component. Note that if the TR is very long so that the echoes are naturally attenuated by T_2 decay, the magnetization M_{ss}^+ is the same as the spoiled magnetization M_{sp}, and M_{ss}^- is zero.

For imaging with short TR, different GRE pulse sequences are used depending on which of the signals M_{ss}^+, M_{ss}^-, or M_{sp} is to be measured. Unfortunately, each manufacturer of MR imagers has given a different name to these pulse sequences, and this can lead to confusion. Each of these names is an acronym, but the full names generally do not make the matter any clearer. Although there are many variations of GRE pulse sequences, they can all be grouped according to which of these three signals is being measured. Some common GRE pulse sequence acronyms, and the associated signal being imaged, are

M_{sp}: FLASH, SPGR
M_{ss}^+: GRASS, FISP, FAST
M_{ss}^-: SSFP, PSIF, CE-FAST

Figure 8.7 (bottom) shows plots of the three signals M_{ss}^+, M_{ss}^-, and M_{sp} as a function of flip angle for a short TR for relaxation times similar to GM and WM. These curves illustrate several interesting properties of the GRE signal. For small flip angles the echoes are weak, and so M_{ss}^-, which consists solely of echoes, is weak. Also, M_{ss}^+ is similar to M_{sp}, again because the echoes are weak. But notice that what small contribution there is from echoes actually decreases the steady-state signal slightly compared to the spoiled signal. As the flip angle increases, the M_{ss}^- signal increases, and the contrast between two tissues is essentially T_2-weighted so that the tissue with the longer T_2, and thus the stronger echoes, is brighter. Both the M_{ss}^+ and the M_{sp} signals increase rapidly with increasing flip angle up to a critical angle called the Ernst angle (see Box 8). The Ernst angle α_E

is the flip angle that produces the maximum signal with a spoiled pulse sequence, and it is also the flip angle where the steady-state and spoiled signals cross. For flip angles greater than α_E, the steady-state signal M_{ss}^+ is larger than the spoiled signal M_{sp} because of the coherent addition of the echo signals. But notice that the contrast between two tissues often is greater for the spoiled signal, despite the fact that the signal itself is intrinsically weaker. This is another example of the conflict between T_1-weighted and T_2-weighted signals that we encountered when considering SE contrast. In this case, a long T_1 tends to reduce the magnitude of each FID because there is less longitudinal recovery during TR, but a long T_2 tends to increase the signal because the echoes are stronger. The result is reduced contrast between tissues with the steady-state signal.

The fact that a moderate flip angle (e.g., 30°) produces a larger spoiled signal than a 90° pulse may at first seem somewhat surprising. After all, a 90° pulse flips all the longitudinal magnetization into the transverse plane, whereas a 30° pulse flips only a fraction of it. And indeed, if only one RF pulse were applied, the 90° pulse *would* create a larger signal. But here we are interested in the *steady-state* signal that develops when many RF pulses are applied in succession. The signal still depends on how much of the longitudinal magnetization is flipped into the transverse plane, but it also depends on how large that longitudinal magnetization *is,* and that also depends on the flip angle. For a small flip angle the longitudinal magnetization is only slightly disturbed, whereas for a 90° flip angle it is destroyed completely, and so the longitudinal magnetization that regrows during TR will be quite small. Thus, for large flip angles the signal is a large part of a small magnetization, and for small flip angles it is a small part of a larger magnetization. The optimal balance that produces the largest signal is an intermediate flip angle, the Ernst angle, which depends on T_1.

SOURCES OF RELAXATION

Fluctuating Fields

In the earlier discussion of the physics of NMR in Chapter 7, the phenomenon of relaxation was attributed to the effects of fluctuating fields. These fluctuations determine the relaxation times T_1 and T_2, and in the previous sections we discussed how the spin echo and gradient echo signals depend on these tissue parameters. In particular, by manipulating pulse sequence parameters such as TR, TE, and the flip angle, the sensitivity of the MR signal to these relaxation times can be controlled. Pulse sequences can be optimized to detect subtle differences between one tissue and another, as in anatomical imaging, or changes over time, as in functional imaging. In this section we will focus on the physical origins of these relaxation times.

Our goal is to understand, at least in part, why the observed relaxation times are what they are. However, this is not a simple task, and despite the importance of relaxation effects for medical imaging, a full understanding of NMR relaxation in the body is still lacking. In the NMR literature a considerable body of work has developed around the theory of relaxation in NMR (Bloembergen, 1957; Bloembergen, Purcell, and Pound, 1948; Solomon, 1955). However, the sources of relaxation in biological systems is an active area of research, and in this section we will only brush the surface by introducing a few key concepts. A natural first question when thinking about T_1 and T_2 is: why are they so long? The most basic time constant associated with NMR is the period of the precessional motion. Yet, broadly speaking, the relaxation times are on the order of 1 s, nearly eight orders of magnitude longer than the precession period in a 1.5-T magnetic field. If this were not so, MRI would be extremely difficult. Frequency encoding depends on reliably measuring frequency differences on the order of 1 ppm. This is only possible if the signal oscillates millions of times before it decays to undetectable levels. Two related questions are: why is T_1 longer than T_2? And, why do the relaxation times differ from one tissue to another? If the relaxation times of all tissues were the same, the contrast in MR images would be due just to differences in proton density, which varies over a much more limited range than the relaxation times. The sensitivity of MRI for detecting subtle pathological anatomy or functional activation would be greatly reduced.

To address these questions, we can examine the physical sources of relaxation. Relaxation results from the effects of fluctuating magnetic fields, and the ultimate source of fluctuating fields is the random thermal motions of the molecules. Each water molecule is in constant motion, colliding with other molecules, rotating, vibrating, and tumbling randomly. The basic conceptual model for understanding the effects of such fluctuations is the random walk. We will use it both to understand how fluctuating fields lead to phase dispersion and signal loss through relaxation, and also in the next chapter to understand how the MR signal is affected by random motions of molecules through spatially varying magnetic fields. As a water molecule tumbles, each hydrogen nucleus feels a fluctuating magnetic field. In a pure water sample, the primary source of this fluctuating field is the dipole field of the other hydrogen nucleus in the same water molecule. As the molecule rotates to a new position, the relative orientation of the two nuclei changes, and because the dipole field produced by the proton has a strong directional dependence, the magnetic field felt by a nucleus fluctuates randomly.

To illustrate how these field fluctuations lead to relaxation, we can look at how T_2 decay arises. Suppose that we examine a sample of pure water after applying a $90°$ RF pulse that generates a coherent transverse magnetization. We can picture this magnetization as being due to a set of identical dipoles, starting out in alignment and precessing together in phase. However, in addition to the primary magnetic field B_0, each dipole also feels a fluctuating field due to the magnetic moments of other nuclei. The z-component of this field adds to (or subtracts from) B_0 and so briefly alters the precession rate. Then for each nucleus, the full precessional motion is a combination of a uniform precession due to B_0, plus a weaker, jerky precession added in. It is easiest to think about this by imagining that we are in a rotating frame of reference rotating at the average precession rate $\omega_0 = \gamma B_0$. Then the additional precessional motions appear as a slow, irregular fanning out of the dipole vectors because the pattern of random fields felt by each dipole is different. We can describe this phase dispersion by plotting the distribution of the phase angle φ for the set of dipoles, as in Figure 8.9. Because the net phase angle is the accumulation of many small random steps, we expect that this distribution will be Gaussian. We can call the

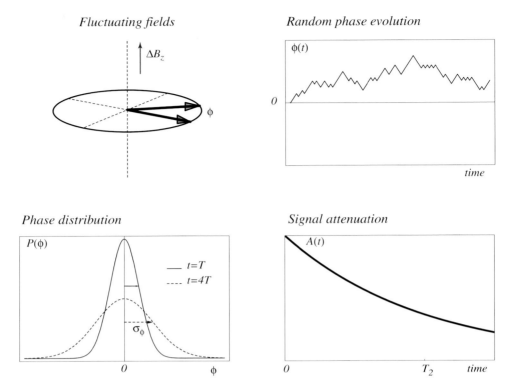

Fluctuating fields

Random phase evolution

Phase distribution

Signal attenuation

Figure 8.9. Effect of fluctuating magnetic fields on the net signal. Each spin feels a randomly fluctuating component of B_z, producing a random phase angle φ, which grows over time in a random walk fashion (top row). For a collection of spins, each undergoing an independent random walk, the width of the phase distribution grows in proportion to the square root of time, which creates an attenuation of the signal that is exponential in time (bottom row).

standard deviation of the phase distribution $\sigma_\varphi(t)$, and over time σ_φ will grow as the phase dispersion increases. The net signal is then the sum of many dipole vectors with this distribution of phases, and due to the phase dispersion the net signal is attenuated from the value it would have if all the spin vectors added coherently. We can calculate an expression for this attenuation factor A by integrating $\cos\varphi$ over a Gaussian distribution of phases, which gives

$$A(t) = e^{-\sigma_\varphi^2/2} \qquad [8.1]$$

The time dependence of the signal decay then depends on how $\sigma_\varphi(t)$ increases with time.

To understand the time dependence of the phase dispersion, we can simplify the physics with a random walk model. Imagine that the water molecule stays in one position for a time τ, called the *correlation time*, and then randomly rotates to a new position. During each interval τ, a nucleus feels a constant magnetic field B added to the main field B_0. During the first τ interval the magnitude of the random field is B_1, during the second interval it is B_2, and so on. Then during each interval the dipole acquires a phase offset $\varphi_n = \gamma B_n \tau$, where γ is the gyromagnetic ratio, and the net phase offset after a total time t is the sum of all of these random phase offsets. Because each phase increment is directly proportional to B_n, the net phase is proportional to the sum of all the B values. To calculate this sum, we can further simplify the physics and assume that each value of B_n has the same magnitude B_{av}, but the sign switches randomly between positive and negative. (This may sound like a gross oversimplification, but in fact it is identical to letting the field take on a range of values if B_{av}^2 is the average squared magnitude.) The pattern of fluctuating fields can then be viewed as a random walk with step size B_{av}. After N steps the sum of the B values will be different for each nucleus, and the standard deviation of the accumulated phase will be proportional to the standard deviation of the sum of the B_n. For a random walk the standard deviation of the sum of the B_n is $B_{av} \sqrt{N}$. We can relate the number of steps and the total time by $N = t/\tau$, and putting all these arguments together the variance of the phase is

$$\sigma_\phi^2(t) = \gamma^2 B_{av}^2 \tau t \qquad [8.2]$$

The key result of this equation is that the phase dispersion grows with the square root of time (or the variance grows in proportion to time). When Equation [8.2] is substituted into Equation [8.1], the attenuation factor $A(t)$ is a monoexponential decay, and we can identify the decay constant as

$$\frac{1}{T_2} = \frac{1}{2} \gamma^2 B_{av}^2 \tau \qquad [8.3]$$

Although this is only a rough and somewhat simplified calculation, it nevertheless illustrates the factors that give rise to T_2. The transverse relaxation rate ($1/T_2$) increases whenever the magnitude of the fluctuating fields or the correlation time increases. For a hydrogen nucleus in a sample of pure water, the primary source of fluctuating magnetic fields is the dipole moment of the other hydrogen nucleus in the water molecule. In a more complex biological fluid, the relaxation of hydrogen spins also is influenced by additional fluctuating dipole fields due to other nuclei and to unpaired electrons. Furthermore, in this simple argument, we only considered the slow fluctuations of the magnetic field. With a rapidly varying field, there are also fluctuations at the Larmor frequency that contribute to relaxation, and these fluctuations are critical for understanding T_1 relaxation.

The Difference Between Longitudinal and Transverse Relaxation

As previously noted, in a pure water sample T_1 and T_2 are similar and long. Why is T_1 so much longer than T_2 in the body? To understand the difference between the two, we need to consider the magnitude of the fluctuating fields at different frequencies. In the previous arguments we only considered the average of the fluctuating fields over time, and this is essentially just the field fluctuations at zero frequency. The key difference between T_1 and T_2 relaxation is that T_2 depends on these zero-frequency fluctuations, but T_1 does not. To produce T_1 relaxation, the fluctuations must occur at the Larmor frequency. To see this, consider what is required to cause transverse and longitudinal relaxation. Fluctuations in B_z cause T_2 relaxation, as already described because they produce added random precession around the z-axis. But precession around the z-axis does not alter the z-component of the magnetization and so does not contribute to T_1 relaxation. To change the z-component, the fluctuating field must act like an excitation RF pulse, producing a slight tipping of the magnetization. But just as with the RF pulses applied in the NMR experiment, this requires a magnetic field along the x- or y-axis fluctuating at the Larmor frequency. Then in the rotating frame, the fluctuating field looks like a nonzero average field in the transverse plane, and the magnetization will precess slightly around this field, changing the z-component. Fluctuations at the Larmor frequency also affect T_2, and so the fundamental reason why T_1 is longer than T_2 is that transverse relaxation is promoted by both fluctuations at zero frequency and at the Larmor frequency, while longitudinal relaxation is unaffected by the zero-frequency fluctuations.

In our earlier simplified analysis of T_2, we effectively only considered the zero-frequency fluctuations. A more complete theory, even for simple dipole-dipole inter-actions, must include contributions at the Larmor frequency and also at twice the Larmor frequency. Nevertheless, Equation [8.3] captures the essential dependence of relaxation on the magnitude and correlation time of the fluctuating fields. And by comparing the intensity of the fluctuations at zero frequency and at the Larmor frequency, we can see in a rough way why T_1 and T_2 are different.

A useful way to characterize the frequency spectrum of the fluctuations is in terms of the correlation time τ. Figure 8.10 suggests how the energy in different frequency components for the same magnitude of fluctuating fields changes with different values of τ. The spectrum is relatively flat up to frequencies around $1/\tau$ and then falls off rather sharply. The amplitude of the initial plateau decreases as τ becomes shorter and the energy of the fluctuations is spread over a wider range of frequencies. From this plot we can get a rough idea of how the relaxation times vary by assuming that $1/T_2$ is proportional to the amplitude of the spectrum at zero frequency, and $1/T_1$ is proportional to the amplitude at the Larmor frequency. For very long τ, the amplitude at zero frequency is large, so T_2 is short. But the Larmor frequency is past the roll-off frequency of the spectrum, so fluctuations are ineffective in promoting longitudinal relaxation and T_1 is long. As τ decreases, the amplitude at zero frequency steadily decreases, lengthening T_2. On the other hand, the amplitude at the Larmor frequency increases, so T_1 becomes shorter. However, there is a minimum of T_1 when $1/\tau$ is about equal to the Larmor frequency. For shorter τ, the amplitude at the Larmor frequency begins to decline again, lengthening T_1. If $1/\tau$ is much larger than the Larmor frequency, both T_1 and T_2 are long. The fact that the two relaxation times are comparable in a room temperature sample of pure water indicates that the correlation time is very short. The fact that T_1 is about 10 times longer than T_2 in the body indicates that the more complex composition of tissue, with slowly tumbling macromolecules and biological structures, produces fluctuating fields with longer correlation times so that T_2 is affected more than T_1.

Considerations of the frequency spectrum of the fluctuating fields also help to explain how the relaxation times change with different magnetic field strengths B_0. Changing B_0 changes the Larmor frequency and so shifts the point on the frequency spectrum that controls T_1 relaxation. Because the amplitude of the fluctuating fields

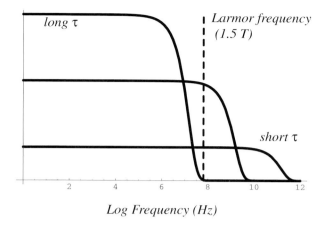

Log Frequency (Hz)

Figure 8.10. Sources of relaxation. Schematic plots of the frequency spectrum of fluctuating fields suggest how the amplitudes at different frequencies depend on the correlation time τ of the fluctuations. For shorter τ the energy of the fluctuations is spread over a wider frequency range, and the amplitude at zero frequency is reduced. Roughly speaking, $1/T_2$ is proportional to the amplitude at zero frequency, and $1/T_1$ is proportional to the amplitude at the Larmor frequency. Fluctuations with a long τ promote transverse relaxation, making T_2 short, but have little effect on T_1.

tends to decrease at higher frequencies, the T_1 at higher magnetic fields tends to increase. On the other hand, the T_2 is primarily determined by the fluctuations at zero frequency and so is relatively independent of field strength. For example, in going from 1.5 to 4 T, the T_1 of gray matter increases from about 1,000 ms to about 1,250 ms (Barfuss et al., 1988; Breger et al., 1989).

In short, the tissue relaxation times are determined by the magnitude and correlation times of the local fluctuating magnetic fields, and these in turn depend on the local environment of the water molecules. In general, for a more structured environment the correlation times are long so field fluctuations are concentrated in the low frequencies, and the result is that T_2 is shorter than T_1. In the brain, for example, the more structured environments of gray matter and white matter have shorter relaxation times than the more fluid CSF. Lesions in the brain of various kinds tend to have longer relaxation times. In very highly organized structures, such as bone or the myelin sheath around nerves, the correlation times are quite long. These longer correlation times drastically shorten T_2 and lengthen T_1. For example, bone mineral contains calcium phosphate compounds, which potentially can be imaged with ^{31}P-NMR (Ackerman, Raleigh, and Glimcher, 1992). But the challenge for imaging is that the T_2 may be as short as a few hundred microseconds, whereas the T_1 may be as long as 60 s!

Contrast Agents

In clinical MRI studies, contrast agents are often used to enhance the contrast between different tissues by altering the local relaxation times. These agents affect the magnitude and correlation times of the fluctuating fields, and the basics of how these agents work can be understood from the preceding arguments. The most commonly used contrast agents are gadolinium (Gd) compounds (Young et al., 1981; Yuh et al., 1992). There are different forms, but each is essentially a gadolinium atom attached to a chelating agent, such as DTPA, which binds the agent in a nontoxic form. Gadolinium alters the relaxation time because it contains unpaired electrons, and the water molecules can approach near enough for the magnetic moment of the electrons to have an effect on the relaxation of the protons. The magnetic field produced by an electron is 3 orders of magnitude stronger than the field of the proton, so the magnitude of the fluctuating fields is greatly increased. The correlation time is short, so gadolinium affects both T_1 and T_2. In fact, the change in the two relaxation rates is the same, but because the initial transverse relaxation rate is typically 10 times larger than the longitudinal relaxation rate, the fractional change in T_1 is much larger than the change in T_2. For example, if the initial transverse relaxation rate is 10 s^{-1} (T_2 = 100 ms), and the longitudinal relaxation rate is 1 s^{-1} (T_2 = 1,000 ms), and if Gd produces a change of 1 s^{-1} in each of the relaxation rates, then this will be a 50% change in T_1 (1,000 to 500 ms) but only a 10% change in T_2 (100 to about 90 ms). For this reason, agents such as this are described as T_1-agents.

A second class of contrast agents effectively reduces T_2 more than T_1 by producing large spatial variations in the magnetic field. These agents possess a large magnetic moment, and if they remain in the blood, they alter the blood magnetic susceptibility relative to the surrounding tissue, creating field gradients through the tissue. This has a direct effect on T_2* because the heterogeneity of the field leads to signal decay due just to the static field offsets. However, T_2 itself is also affected because diffusion of the water molecules leads to random displacements of the dipoles, and as they move through the inhomogeneous field, they precess at different rates and phase dispersion develops. Technically speaking, this is a diffusion effect due to the heterogeneity of the tissue, rather than a true alteration of T_2, but for classification purposes we can describe this as a T_2 effect because it produces large signal changes on a T_2-weighted image. Such diffusion effects will be taken up in Chapter 9.

The primary agent in clinical use that behaves in this fashion is in fact Gd-DTPA (Villringer et al., 1988). That is, in addition to its relaxivity effect, which primarily alters the local T_1, gadolinium also creates a susceptibility effect when it is confined to the vasculature, and this affects T_2 and T_2*. The effects of gadolinium on the signal intensity thus can be rather complex. Imagine that a bolus of Gd-DTPA is injected in a patient, and a series of rapid images of the brain is acquired. In the healthy portions of the brain, the blood brain barrier prevents the gadolinium from leaving the vasculature. As the bolus passes through the blood volume, the T_2* and to a lesser extent the T_2 are reduced, and the signal intensity thus drops transiently as the bolus passes. This is the basis for using Gd-DTPA to measure blood volume because the dip is accentuated when the cerebral blood volume is larger (this is discussed more fully in Chapter 14). But now consider what happens if there is a brain tumor with a leaky blood brain barrier. The gadolinium then enters the tissue and reduces the local T_1, which increases the signal from the tumor in a T_1-weighted image. This enhancement of tumors is the primary diagnostic use of gadolinium.

Other agents lack the relaxivity effects of gadolinium but possess a similar large magnetic moment and so produce only the T_2^* and T_2 effects. For example, dysprosium (Dys) has a larger magnetic moment than gadolinium, and Dys-DTPA produces a larger change in transverse relaxation without a change in T_1 (Villringer et al., 1988). Other compounds exploit the magnetic properties of iron (Chambon et al., 1993; Kent et al., 1990; Majumdar, Zoghbi, and Gore, 1988). Superparamagnetic particles carry a large magnetic moment and so strongly affect transverse relaxation. Finally, a natural physiological agent is deoxyhemoglobin. Deoxyhemoglobin is paramagnetic, but oxyhemoglobin is diamagnetic. As a result, if the concentration of deoxyhemoglobin changes, the susceptibility of the blood changes, and this produces weak field gradients through the tissue. As introduced in Chapter 6, this effect is the basis for most of the fMRI studies done today to map patterns of brain activation because blood oxygenation changes with activation. The susceptibility differences produced naturally by deoxyhemoglobin alterations during activation are about an order of magnitude smaller than those due to a typical bolus of gadolinium. As a result, the extravascular signal change is only a few percent.

REFERENCES

Ackerman, J. L., Raleigh, D. P., and Glimcher, M. J. (1992) Phosphorous-31 magnetic resonance imaging of hydroxyapatite: A model for bone imaging. *Magn. Reson. Med.* **25,** 1–11.

Barfuss, H., Fischer, A., Hentschel, D., Ladebeck, R., and Vetter, J. (1988) Whole-body MR imaging and spectroscopy with a 4 T system. *Radiology* **169,** 811–16.

Bloembergen, N. (1957) Proton relaxation times in paramagnetic solutions. *J. Chem. Phys.* **27,** 572.

Bloembergen, N., Purcell, E. M., and Pound, R. V. (1948) Relaxation effects in nuclear magnetic resonance absorption. *Phys. Rev.* **73,** 679.

Breger, R. K., Rimm, A. A., Fischer, M. E. T_1 and T_2 measurements on a 1.5 T commercial imager. *Radiology* **71,** 273–6.

Buxton, R. B., Edelman, R. R., Rosen, B. R., Wismer, G. L., and Brady, T. J. (1987) Contrast in rapid MR imaging: T_1- and T_2-weighted imaging. *J. Comput. Assist. Tomogr.* **11,** 7–16.

Buxton, R. B., Fisel, C. R., Chien, D., and Brady, T. J. (1989) Signal intensity in fast NMR imaging with short repetition times. *J. Magn. Reson.* **83,** 576–85.

Chambon, C., Clement, O., Blanche, A. L., Schouman-Claeys, E., and Frija, G. (1993) Superparamagnetic iron oxides as positive MR contrast agents: In vitro and in vivo evidence. *Magn. Reson. Imag.* **11,** 509–19.

Ernst, R. R., and Anderson, W. A. (1966) *Rev. Sci. Instrum.* **37,** 93.

Gyngell, M. L. (1988) The application of steady-state free precession in rapid 2DFT NMR imaging. *Magn. Reson. Imag.* **6,** 415–19.

Haase, A., Frahm, J., Matthaei, D., Haenicke, W., and Ferboldt, K.-D. (1986) Flash imaging: Rapid NMR imaging using low flip-angle pulses. *J. Magn. Reson.* **67,** 258–66.

Hahn, E. L. (1950) Spin echoes. *Phys. Rev.* **80,** 580–93.

Hendrick, R. E., Nelson, T. R., and Hendee, W. R. (1984) Optimizing tissue differentiation in magnetic resonance imaging. *Magn. Reson. Imag.* **2,** 193–204.

Hoppel, B. E., Weisskoff, R. M., Thulborn, K. R., Moore, J. B., Kwong, K. K., and Rosen, B. R. (1993) Measurement of regional blood oxygenation and cerebral hemodynamics. *Magn. Reson. Med.* **30,** 715–23.

Kent, T., Quast, M., Kaplan, B., Lifsey, R. S., and Eisenberg, H. M. (1990) Assessment of a superparamagnetic iron oxide (AMI-25) as a brain contrast agent. *Magn. Reson. Med.* **13,** 434–43.

Majumdar, S., Zoghbi, S. S., and Gore, J. C. (1988) Regional differences in rat brain displayed by fast MRI with superparamagnetic contrast agents. *Magn. Reson. Imag.* **6,** 611–15.

Patz, S. (1989) Steady-state free precession: An overview of basic concepts and applications. *Adv. Magn. Reson. Imag.* **1,** 73–102.

Solomon, I. (1955) Relaxation processes in a system of two spins. *Phys. Rev.* **99,** 559.

Thulborn, K. R., and Brady, T. J. (1989) Iron in magnetic resonance imaging of cerebral hemorrhage. *Magn. Reson. Quart.* **5,** 23–38.

Villringer, A., Rosen, B. R., Belliveau, J. W., Ackerman, J. L., Lauffer, R. B., Buxton, R. B., Chao, Y.-S., Wedeen, V. J., and Brady, T. J. (1988) Dynamic imaging with lanthanide chelates in normal brain: Contrast due to magnetic susceptibility effects. *Magn. Reson. Med.* **6,** 164–74.

Wehrli, F. W., MacFall, J. R., Glover, G. H., Grigsby, N., Haughton, V., and Johanson, J. (1984) The dependence of nuclear magnetic resonance (NMR) image contrast on intrinsic and pulse sequence timing parameters. *J. Magn. Reson. Imag.* **2,** 3–16.

Wehrli, F. W., Perkins, T. G., Shimakawa, A., and Roberts, F. (1987) Chemical sift induced amplitude modulations in images obtained with gradient refocusing. *Magn. Reson. Imag.* **5,** 157–8.

Wismer, G. L., Buxton, R. B., Rosen, B. R., Fisel, C. R., Oot, R. F., Brady, T. J., and Davis, K. R. (1988) Susceptibility induced MR line broadening: applications to brain iron mapping. *J. Comput. Assist. Tomogr.* **12,** 259–65.

Young, I., Clarke, G., Bailes, D., Pennock, J., Doyle, F., and Bydder, G. (1981) Enhancement of relaxation rate with paramagnetic contrast agents in NMR imaging. *J. Comput. Assist. Tomogr.* **5,** 543–7.

Yuh, W., Engelken, J., Muhonen, M., Mayr, N., Fisher, D., and Ehrhardt, J. (1992) Experience with high-dose gadolinium MR imaging in the evaluation of brain metastases. *AJNR* **13,** 335–45.

9

Diffusion and the MR Signal

Introduction
Diffusion Imaging
    The Nature of Diffusion
    Diffusion in a Linear Field Gradient
    Techniques for Diffusion Imaging
    Multicompartment Diffusion
    Diffusion Imaging in Stroke
Anisotropic Diffusion
    Restricted Diffusion
    Anisotropic Diffusion
    The Diffusion Tensor
    Measuring the Trace of the Diffusion Tensor
    Mapping White Matter Fiber Tracts
    Beyond the Diffusion Tensor
Diffusion Effects in fMRI
    Diffusion Around Field Perturbations
    Motional Narrowing

    BOX 9: THE PHYSICS OF DIFFUSION

INTRODUCTION

Water molecules in the body are in constant motion. In Chapter 8, we considered how these thermal motions lead to random rotations of the water molecule, producing fluctuations of the local magnetic field felt by the hydrogen nucleus. These fluctuating fields lead to relaxation; in particular, the low-frequency fields reduce T_2 without affecting T_1. But in addition to random rotations of the molecule, thermal motions also produce random displacements, the process of *diffusion*. In a nonuniform magnetic field, as a spin moves randomly to another position, there are corresponding random changes in its precession rate, and thus an additional dephasing of the spins and greater signal loss. This additional signal decay due to diffusion through inhomogeneous fields is exploited in three ways in magnetic resonance imaging (MRI). First, by applying a strong linear field gradient and measuring the additional signal attenuation, the local diffusion coefficient D can be measured. This is the basis of diffusion imaging, and one of the primary applications of diffusion imaging is in early assessment of injury due to stroke (Baird and Warach, 1998). Conventional MRI does not reveal the affected area in stroke until several hours after the event, when T_2 changes become apparent. But the apparent diffusion coefficient is reduced very early in the development of a stroke, and maps of altered D in the acute phase correlate well with the T_2 maps of the affected area made several hours later.

Second, the ability to measure the local diffusion coefficient provides a potentially powerful tool for mapping the connections between brain regions (Conturo et al., 1999). In white matter, the diffusion of water is *anisotropic,* with D about ten times larger along the fibers than across the fibers. Mapping the diffusion anisotropy thus provides a way to map white matter fiber tracts. As these methods mature, they will provide a new structural approach to the investigation of the functional organization of the brain that will complement functional magnetic resonance imaging (MRI) studies of dynamic patterns of activation.

Finally, the third way in which diffusion effects enter MRI is that injected contrast agents such as Gd-DTPA, or intrinsic agents such as deoxyhemoglobin, create microscopic field perturbations around the small blood vessels, and the presence of the agent can be measured by measuring the change in T_2^* or T_2. If the water molecules did not diffuse, such microscopic, static field offsets would affect only T_2^*, and not T_2. But with diffusion the spins move in a random way through these field perturbations, and so the effects are not fully refocused with a spin-echo experiment. Spin echo fMRI methods based on these diffusion effects are potentially more accurate in localizing the site of neuronal activity than the more commonly used GRE fMRI techniques (Lee et al., 1999).

DIFFUSION IMAGING

The Nature of Diffusion

Water is a highly dynamic medium, with water molecules continuously tumbling and colliding with one another and with other molecules. With each collision, a water molecule is both rotated to a new angle, and deflected to a new position. These effects are random, in the sense that the small deflection or rotation in one collision is unrelated to the effects of the last collision. Both of these effects are important in understanding the NMR signal. As a molecule rotates, the relative orientation of a hydrogen nucleus in the magnetic field produced by the other hydrogen nucleus in the molecule changes, and so each nucleus feels a randomly fluctuating magnetic field. These fluctuations lead to relaxation, as described in Chapter 8. The fact that each molecule also undergoes random displacements of position means that a group of molecules, which are initially close together, will

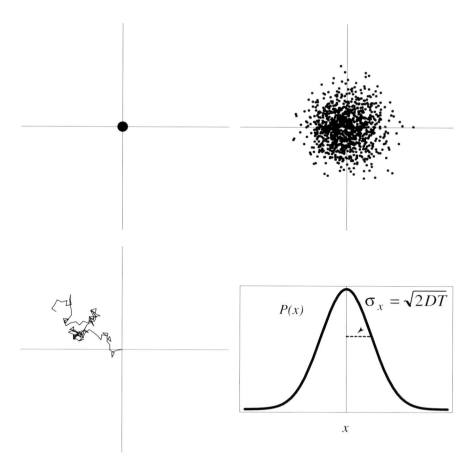

Figure 9.1. Diffusion. Water molecules that start from the same location (upper left) over time spread out (upper right), like a drop of ink in a clear fluid. Each molecule undergoes a random walk (lower left) in which each step is in a random direction. The mean displacement of many molecules that start at the same location is zero, but the standard deviation of the spread of their positions increases in proportion to the square root of DT, where D is the diffusion coefficient and T is the elapsed time (lower right).

eventually disperse like a drop of ink in water (Figure 9.1). This self-diffusion of water produces only small displacements of the spins, but these displacements are nevertheless measurable with NMR.

The essential nature of diffusion is that a group of molecules that start at the same location will spread out over time. Each molecule suffers a series of random displacements so that after a time T the spread of positions along a spatial axis x has a variance of

$$\sigma_x^2 = 2DT \tag{9.1}$$

where D is the diffusion coefficient, a constant characteristic of the medium. (Box 9 contains a more complete derivation of this equation.) In other words, during the

BOX 9. THE PHYSICS OF DIFFUSION

The effects of diffusion can be understood with a simple random walk model, such that in each time interval τ a molecule moves a distance s in a random direction. This view of diffusion as a random walk may seem to have little to do with the classical concept of diffusion as a flux of particles down a concentration gradient as described by Fick's law:

$$J = -D \frac{dC}{dx} \tag{B9.1}$$

where J is the particle flux (number of particles passing through a unit area per second), dC/dx is the gradient of the particle concentration, and D is the diffusion coefficient. Based on this equation, it is sometimes said that diffusion is "driven" by a concentration gradient. This seems inconsistent with the random walk model in which each step is random regardless of the concentration. However, Equation [B9.1] is the natural result of random motions: there is a net flux from high to low concentrations simply because more particles start out from the region of high concentration.

To relate the parameters of a random walk (s and τ) to D, consider a one-dimensional random walk and the net flux past a particular point x. The local density of particles along the line is $C(x)$. Additionally, for one time step, we need only look at the particles within a distance s of x to calculate the flux because these are the only particles that can cross x in one step. Let $C_L = C(x - s/2)$ be the mean concentration on the left and $C_R = C_L + s\, dC/dx$ is then the mean concentration on the right of x. In a time interval τ (one step), on average half of the particles within a distance s to the left of x will move to the right past x, so the number of particles crossing x from the left is $sC_L/2$, giving a positive flux (particles per unit time) of $J^+ = sC_L/2\tau$. Similarly, half of the particles within a distance s to the right will move left to form a negative flux $J^- = sC_R/2\tau$. The net flux $J = J^+ - J^-$ is then

$$J = -\frac{s^2}{2\tau} \frac{dC}{dx} \tag{B9.2}$$

The classical diffusion coefficient D thus is related to the parameters of a random walk as

$$D = \frac{s^2}{2\tau} \tag{B9.3}$$

For a one-dimensional random walk of N steps, the mean final displacement is zero because each step is equally likely to be to the left or the right. But the variance of the final positions is $\sigma^2 = Ns^2$. That is, the width of the spread of final positions grows in proportion to the square root of the number of steps. Noting that the total time T is simply the number of steps N times the step interval τ of the random walk, we can complete the connection between the classical diffusion coefficient D and the random walk:

$$\sigma^2 = 2DT \tag{B9.4}$$

Diffusion imaging is built around the effects of diffusion through a linear field gradient. A basic diffusion pulse sequence is shown in Figure 9.2. After a 90° excitation pulse, a strong gradient pulse is applied with amplitude G and duration δt. At a time T after the beginning of the first pulse, a second pulse is applied with equal amplitude but opposite sign. If the spins did not diffuse, the second pulse would exactly balance the effects of the first pulse, creating a gradient echo. The net effect would be as if the gradient pulses were not applied at all. (If the experiment is done as a spin echo, with a 180° refocusing pulse between the two gradient pulses, then the second gradient pulse also should be positive to balance the first pulse.) But with diffusion, each spin is likely to be in a different location when the second pulse is applied than it was when the first pulse was applied. The result is that the effects of the two gradient pulses will not balance, leaving each spin with a small random phase offset that depends on how far it moved between the two pulses. The net signal is then reduced because of these random phase offsets.

To quantify this diffusion effect on the MR signal, we can simplify the experiment so that δt is very short. Then we do not have to worry about how diffusion during the gradient pulse affects the signal. Instead, we can focus just on how far a spin has moved between the first pulse and the second. That is, we can consider that the effect of each gradient pulse is to mark the current position of a spin by its phase. A spin at position x will acquire a phase $\varphi = \gamma G x \delta t$ during the first gradient pulse, and the second gradient pulse will add a phase $-\varphi$ if the spin does not move, unwinding the effect of the first pulse. But if the spin has moved a net final distance x_f by diffusion during the interval T, then the net effect of the two gradient pulses will be a phase offset $\Delta\varphi = \gamma G x_f \delta t$. We know that the distribution of x_f is Gaussian with a variance given by Equation [B9.4], so the distribution of phase offsets is then also Gaussian with a variance σ_φ^2 proportional to the variance of the displacements:

$$\sigma_\varphi^2 = 2(\gamma G \delta t)^2 \, DT \qquad [B9.5]$$

As noted in Chapter 8, a Gaussian distribution of phases produces an exponential attenuation of the signal. The result is that the additional attenuation due to diffusion can be written as

$$A(D) = e^{-bD} \qquad [B9.6]$$

where the factor b incorporates all the amplitude and timing parameters of the gradient pulses. From the preceding argument, b would be $(\gamma G \delta t)^2 T$. A more careful analysis, taking account of the diffusion effects during the application of the gradient pulse, yields (Stejskal and Tanner, 1965)

$$b = (\gamma G \delta t)^2 \, (T - \delta t/3) \qquad [B9.7]$$

By measuring the MR signal with no gradient pulses and by comparing that with the signal for a reasonably large b, the attenuation due to diffusion can be calculated. From the measured attenuation, the diffusion coefficient can be calculated. By incorporating such diffusion weighting into an imaging pulse sequence, the local value of D can be mapped.

time interval T, any particular molecule moves a distance on the order of σ_x, but it is equally likely to move in either direction. Furthermore, the typical displacement of a particle grows only as the square root of time. This is fundamentally different from motion at a constant velocity, where displacement is proportional to time. For example, compare the average displacement of a water molecule diffusing with a diffusion coefficient $D = 10^{-5}$ cm^2/s (a typical number for brain) and a water molecule being carried along in the blood of a capillary with a speed of 1 mm/s. In 2 ms each will move about 2 μm, but while the time for the flowing molecule to move 20 μm is only 20 ms, the time for the diffusing molecule to move the same distance is 200 ms. Diffusion is thus reasonably efficient for moving molecules short distances, but it is highly inefficient for transport over large distances. It is a remarkable fact that such small displacements as these (tens of micrometers) can have a measurable effect on the magnetic resonance (MR) signal.

Diffusion in a Linear Field Gradient

Diffusion imaging is built around the effects of diffusion through a linear field gradient (see Box 9). The MR signal is made sensitive to diffusion by adding a pair of strong bipolar gradient pulses to the pulse sequence (Figure 9.2) (Stejskal and

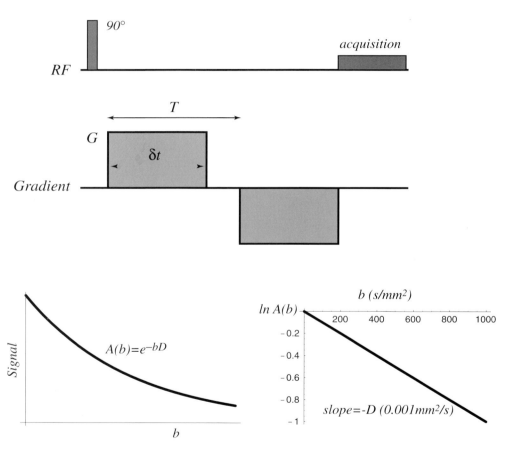

Figure 9.2. Measuring the diffusion coefficient with NMR. The NMR signal is made sensitive to diffusion by applying a bipolar gradient pulse between signal excitation and signal detection (top). If spins were stationary, the additional position-dependent precessional phase acquired during the first gradient pulse would be precisely unwound by the second gradient pulse, and there would be no effect on the net measured signal. With diffusion, the random displacements of water molecules between the two gradient pulses produce random phase offsets and signal attenuation. The attenuation is exponential in the term bD, where b is an experimental parameter that depends on the gradient strength and duration, and D is the local diffusion coefficient (bottom).

Tanner, 1965). The two gradient pulses are balanced so that their net effect would be zero for a spin that does not move, but each spin that moves during the interval between pulses acquires a phase offset proportional to how far it has moved. The result is a phase dispersion that is proportional to the dispersion of positions, producing an attenuation of the net signal by a factor that depends on the diffusion coefficient D (LeBihan, 1991):

$$A(D) = e^{-bD} \tag{9.2}$$

The b-factor depends only on the amplitude and timing parameters of the applied gradient pulses (see Box 9). The local tissue diffusion coefficient D can be calculated by measuring the signal with no gradients applied ($b = 0$) and again with a large value of b. The ratio of the two signals is the attenuation factor $A(D)$. Note that in these two measurements the echo time TE must be kept the same, so that the effects of T_2 decay are identical. In practice, there are two ways of displaying diffusion-sensitive images (Figure 9.3). The first is to calculate pixel by pixel the diffusion coefficient D and then to create an image of D. Such an image is usually called an ADC map (short for *apparent diffusion coefficient*), and in these images the tissues with the largest D are brightest. An alternative is to display the diffusion-weighted image itself (i.e., the image made with a large b-value), and in such an image the tissues with the largest D tend to be the darkest because they suffer the most attenuation. Note, however, that a diffusion-weighted image will have other contrast characteristics as well (e.g., some degree of T_2-weighting) and so is not a pure reflection of diffusion effects, in contrast to an ADC map.

A typical value of D in the brain is 0.001 mm^2/s. To measure D, b must be sufficiently large to produce a measurable attenuation. For example, a b-value of 1,000 s/mm^2 would attenuate the signal by a factor of e, but $b = 100$ s/mm^2 would only attenuate it by 10%. The b-factor depends on both the gradient strength and dura-

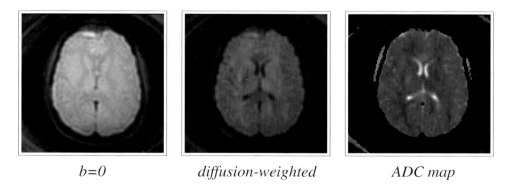

b=0	*diffusion-weighted*	*ADC map*

Figure 9.3. Diffusion-weighted imaging. An image without diffusion-weighting ($b = 0$) from a healthy human brain is shown on the left. When bipolar gradients are added to the imaging pulse sequence, each local signal is diffusion-weighted (middle). Cerebrospinal fluid (CSF), with the largest apparent diffusion coefficient (ADC), is the most attenuated. From these two images made with different b-values, a map of the ADC can be calculated on a voxel-by-voxel basis (right). Images were made with a spiral acquisition. (Data courtesy of L. Frank.)

tion, and so in principle a large value of b can be created with weak gradients if they are on for a long enough time. But the time during which diffusion can act is limited by T_2, the lifetime of the signal, so strong gradients are essential for creating large values of b. Example numbers for an MRI system are a gradient amplitude of 20 mT/m, with each pulse lasting 27 ms and a diffusion time between the start of the first pulse and the start of the second pulse of 57 ms (i.e., two 27-ms pulses with a 30-ms gap between them), which produces $b = 1000$ s/mm^2 (Shimony et al., 1999). Note that it takes a substantial amount of time to play out the gradient pulses to achieve sufficient diffusion sensitivity. For this example, the TE was 121 ms.

The basic procedure for calculating D is to measure the signals with a range of b-values, including $b = 0$. The attenuation factor A is calculated by dividing the signal for a particular b by the signal with $b = 0$, and then a plot of the natural logarithm of the attenuation ($\ln A$) vs. b yields a straight line with a slope of $-D$ (Figure 9.2). The minimum data required are just two measurements, one with $b = 0$ and one with b sufficiently large to produce a measurable attenuation. For a two-point measurement, the optimum choice of b to maximize the signal-to-noise ratio (SNR) is a value of $1/D$, where D is the diffusion coefficient of the tissue being measured.

Techniques for Diffusion Imaging

Diffusion sensitivity can be added to any imaging pulse sequence by inserting a bipolar gradient pulse after the excitation pulse and before the signal readout. For example, the gradient pulses shown in Figure 9.2 could be directly inserted into a gradient recalled echo (GRE) pulse sequence. Note that the axis of the diffusion-sensitizing gradient is arbitrary and can be adjusted by the experimenter. For a spin echo (SE) pulse sequence, the two gradient pulses are usually put on opposite sides of the 180° radio frequency (RF) refocusing pulse. In this case, the two gradient pulses have the same sign, such that if there were no motion, the 180° pulse would create a full echo of the signal. That is, the local phase change induced by the first gradient pulse would be reversed by the 180° pulse, and the second gradient pulse would then unwind the local phase offset.

One of the limitations of diffusion imaging is the need to have long echo times in order to apply the diffusion-sensitizing gradient pulses. In other words, the *diffusion time*, the time available for spins to diffuse apart, is limited by TE and so ultimately is limited by the T_2 of the tissue. This makes it very difficult to study tissues with short T_2 and small D. Stimulated echo techniques offer a way to solve this problem (Merboldt, Hanicke, and Frahm, 1985; Tanner, 1970). Stimulated echoes (STE) were introduced in Chapter 8. The simplest STE pulse sequence for diffusion imaging uses three sequential 90° RF pulses, with gradient pulses after the first and third. Then the first gradient pulse produces a transverse magnetization, and the gradient pulse changes the local phase in proportion to the spins' location. The second 90° pulse tips a part of the transverse magnetization back onto the longitudinal axis, and the part remaining in the transverse plane decays away with time constant T_2. But the components parked along the longitudinal axis decay much more slowly with a time constant T_1. The third 90° pulse then returns this magnetization to the transverse plane, and the second gradient pulse then refocuses the signal to create the stimulated echo. The power of the STE method is that the diffusion time, the time between the second and third 90° pulses, can be made quite long because the magnetization decays only with T_1.

Finally, diffusion imaging also can be done using GRE steady-state free precession (SSFP) pulse sequences (LeBihan, 1988). As described in Chapter 8, SSFP occurs in a string of closely spaced RF pulses when TR < T_2, so that a steady-state signal forms both before and after each pulse. Each of these signals has a strong contribution of echoes, with each RF pulse forming a partial echo of the signals generated by the previous RF pulses. In particular, the signal that forms just before each RF pulse (M^-_{ss} in the notation of Chapter 8) is composed entirely of echoes. These echoes are a combination of direct spin echoes and stimulated echoes, and so the SSFP signal is strongly sensitive to diffusion when diffusion-weighting gradients are added (Buxton, 1993). In fact, for the same b-value, the SSFP sequence is much more sensitive to diffusion than either the straight SE or STE pulse sequences, and this sensitivity is improved with smaller flip angles that maximize the STE component of the echoes. However, quantitation of D is not straightforward with an SSFP pulse sequence because the dependence of the attenuation on D is more complicated than Equation [9.2] and involves the local relaxation times as well.

In practice, diffusion imaging in the living human brain suffers from several potential artifacts. The purpose of adding the bipolar gradient pulses is to sensitize the MR signal to the small motions due to diffusion. However, this also makes the signal sensitive to other motions, such as blood flow in vessels and brain pulsations due to arterial pressure waves. The potential sensitivity of diffusion measurements to blood flow led to one of the earliest approaches to measuring perfusion with MRI, the intravoxel incoherent motion (IVIM) method (LeBihan et al., 1988). This method has been superceded by newer approaches, described in Chapters 13–15, but the IVIM technique was an important milestone in the development of MRI. Because of the very high motion-sensitivity of a diffusion-weighted image, brain motions due to arterial pulsations can severely degrade the images. Often diffusion imaging is done with the TR gated to the cardiac cycle to minimize the effects of motions due to arterial pulsatility. Single-shot echo planar imaging (EPI) avoids these motion artifacts, although EPI images can be distorted when using strong gradient pulses due to eddy current effects (Haselgrove and Moore, 1996; Jezzard, Barnett, and Pierpaoli, 1998).

Multicompartment Diffusion

The linear decrease in ln A with increasing b (Equation [9.2] and Figure 9.2) describes the diffusion behavior of a simple substance such as pure water. Brain tissues, however, are complex structures, and this leads to a rich variety of diffusion effects that alter this basic picture. The first effect is the heterogeneity of the tissue, such that, in any volume of tissue that we might sample in an imaging experiment (e.g., an image voxel of a few cubic millimeters), we are likely to be looking at multiple pools of water. For example, in the brain two diffusing components have been identified, with D differing by about a factor of 5 between the two components (Niendorf et al., 1996). (These components may be intracellular and extracellular water, but there are still some uncertainties in the interpretation of the data.) What type of diffusion decay curve would we expect to measure for such a two-compartment system? The answer depends on two factors: (1) the rate of exchange of water between the two compartments, and (2) the range of b-values used. If a typical water molecule moves back and forth between the two compartments multiple times during the experiment, the system is described as being in the *fast exchange* regime. In this case, all the water molecules have similar histories, in the sense that each one spends about the same amount of time in each compartment. As a result, the system behaves like a uniform system with a diffusion coefficient equal to the volume-weighted average of the diffusion coefficients of the two compartments:

$$D_{av} = v_a D_a + v_b D_b \qquad\qquad [9.3]$$

where v_a and v_b are the volume fractions of the two compartments (e.g., 0.2 for the extracellular space and 0.8 for the intracellular space), and D_a and D_b are the respective diffusion coefficients. In this fast exchange limit, the diffusion attenuation curve is linear with a slope equal to $-D_{av}$.

But if the exchange of water is slow so that the two compartments are effectively isolated during the experiment, the attenuation takes on a biexponential form (Figure 9.4):

$$A = v_a e^{-b D_a} + v_b e^{-b D_b} \qquad\qquad [9.4]$$

For small b, this biexponential curve is well approximated by a single exponential with $D = D_{av}$, and so initially the slope of $\ln A$ is just $-D_{av}$. But for larger b, this approximation breaks down, and the compartment with the larger D is more attenuated and so contributes less to the signal. The result is that the slope of $\ln A$ approaches a value corresponding to the smaller D, so there is an upward curvature of the diffusion attenuation curve (see Figure 9.4). In short, this curve deviates from a straight line when two conditions are satisfied: (1) there are multiple

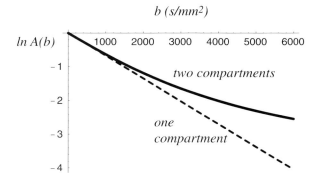

Figure 9.4. Diffusion in more complex systems. With multiple compartments of diffusing water, the diffusion attenuation curve depends on how rapidly the water molecules exchange between compartments. With rapid exchange, the system behaves like a single compartment, and the decay curve is a single exponential. With slow exchange, the decay curve is similar to the single compartment decay curve for low b-values, but for higher b-values the curve bends upward as the signal from the compartment with the higher D is more attenuated.

isolated or slowly exchanging water compartments with different Ds, and (2) large b-values are used. To probe multicompartment diffusion in a tissue, one must make measurements with many b-values to characterize this curvature. Or, put another way, with a two-point measurement of D in a multicompartment, slow-exchange system the value measured will vary depending on what b-value is used. The measured value will lie somewhere between the true average, D_{av}, and the smaller of the two Ds. By using a small b-value, one can ensure that the measured value is close to the true average, but the cost of such a measurement is reduced SNR.

Diffusion Imaging in Stroke

One of the primary applications of diffusion imaging in clinical studies is in the early assessment of stroke (Baird and Warach, 1998). A stroke begins with a sudden interruption of blood flow to a region of the brain, starting a cascade of destructive events that ultimately leads to ischemic injury and infarction. The therapeutic window for delivering drugs to break up the embolus and restore flow before irreversible damage has occurred is the first few hours after onset (Brott et al., 1992). In the acute stages of stroke, conventional MRI, such as T_1-weighted, T_2-weighted, or density-weighted images, and computed tomography (CT) all appear normal. These conventional techniques show the area of the stroke only several hours after the event. However, diffusion-weighted imaging shows a drop in the ADC within minutes of the interruption of blood flow (Kucharczyk et al., 1991). In human studies, the size of the lesion measured acutely with diffusion-weighted imaging (DWI) correlated strongly with the neurologic deficit assessed 24 h after the stroke onset (Tong et al., 1998). Other disorders such as status epilepticus (Zhong et al., 1993) and spreading depression (Takano et al., 1996) also exhibit early changes in the ADC value. For this reason, diffusion imaging is widely used clinically for the early assessment of stroke and other disorders and is also a standard technique for animal studies investigating the pathophysiological changes involved in stroke.

The reason for the abrupt decrease of the ADC in stroke is not fully understood. It is generally thought that the diffusion coefficient of water in the intracellular space is less than that of water in the extracellular space. An early proposal attributes the change in the ADC to cytotoxic edema, with a water shift from the extracellular to the intracellular space that changes the average ADC (Benveniste, Hedlund, and Johnson, 1992; Moseley et al., 1990). Other investigators have argued, on the basis of an observed biexponential behavior, that a simple averaging of diffusion coefficients is not adequate to understand the ADC changes fully (Niendorf et al., 1996). An alternative theory is that the intracellular swelling increases the tortuosity of the diffusion paths in the extracellular space, decreasing the extracellular ADC (Niendorf and Norris, 1994). Other data indicate that the diffusion coefficient is reduced in both the intracellular and extracellular compartments, possibly because of a reduction in cytoplasmic motions (Duong et al., 1998). All these mechanisms may play a role in reducing the ADC, but a quantitative understanding of the phenomenon is lacking.

ANISOTROPIC DIFFUSION

Restricted Diffusion

There is another effect, common in measurements of D in biological tissues, that also produces an upward curvature of the diffusion attenuation curve similar to Figure 9.4. In biological structures, the motion of water molecules is restricted by natural barriers such as cell membranes and large protein molecules, an effect called *restricted diffusion* (Cooper et al., 1974). In contrast to the multicompartment effects described earlier, this effect depends on precisely *how b* is changed to generate the attenuation curve. There are two distinct ways in which we could alter b. The first is to step through multiple gradient strengths while keeping the timing fixed. The second is to keep the gradient pulses at a fixed amplitude but to vary the diffusion time T between the pulses. If we generated diffusion attenuation curves with both schemes, a tissue exhibiting restricted diffusion would show a normal linear curve when the diffusion time is constant, but an upward bending curve similar to Figure 9.4 if T is varied, suggesting that D appears to be smaller when T is long. For comparison, if the upward curvature were due to multicompartment diffusion, the two curves would look the same regardless of how b was varied.

The cause of this restricted diffusion effect is the heterogeneous structure of tissue. With large macromolecules and numerous membranes and other barriers, water is not freely diffusing. Imagine water molecules compartmentalized in a small box with impermeable walls. For short diffusion times, the water molecules do not move far, and most of them do not reach the edge of the box, so the barriers have little effect on how far a molecule diffuses. But for longer diffusion times, more molecules reach the walls of the box and are bounced back rather than diffusing past. The result is that the spread of displacements is not as large as it would be if the water were freely diffusing, and so the diffusion coefficient appears to be smaller with longer diffusion times.

From these arguments we can expect that the diffusion coefficient will vary between tissues, depending on the structure of the tissues. Furthermore, in addition to being heterogeneous, tissues are often *anisotropic*. That is, there are oriented structures, such as nerve fibers in white matter, and this raises the interesting possibility that diffusion within a tissue also depends on direction.

Anisotropic Diffusion

Figure 9.5 shows diffusion-weighted images in a healthy brain. In the two images, the diffusion-sensitizing gradients were perpendicular to each other. For many tissues, the attenuation is about the same, indicating that the diffusion is reasonably isotropic. But for white matter, the diffusion attenuation depends strongly on the orientation. This diffusion anisotropy can be both a problem and a useful tool. For stroke studies, where the goal is to identify regions with low D, the natural anisotropy of white matter can produce false identifications of affected areas. But the anisotropy also makes possible mapping of the orientation of the fiber tracts.

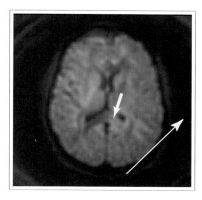 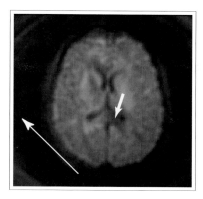

Figure 9.5. Anisotropic diffusion. In some tissues, the magnitude of the signal reduction with dif-fusion weighting depends on the orientation of the diffusion-sensitizing gradient (anisotropic diffusion). This is pronounced in white matter, with the diffusion coefficient along the fiber direction as much as ten times larger than that for the perpendicular direction. Note the dramatic change (fat arrows) when the gradient direction (thin arrows) is changed by 90°. (Data courtesy of L. Frank.)

The question, then, is how to measure anisotropic diffusion. Naively, we might imagine that measurements of D along three perpendicular axes (e.g., x, y, and z) would completely describe the diffusion at a point in the brain. But diffusion is sub-tler than this, and three measurements are not sufficient to characterize diffusion fully. In fact, six measurements are required, each along a different axis. To see why this is so, it is helpful to simplify the problem to just two dimensions, x and y, and imagine that diffusion takes place only in these two dimensions. For this 2D case, three measurements are required to characterize diffusion (instead of two). To illus-trate this, imagine that we are measuring a sample of white matter in which the fibers are oriented along an axis at an angle θ to the x-direction (Figure 9.6). We will call this axis x', and the perpendicular axis y'. These are the natural axes of symme-try of the diffusion process, called the *principal axes*. The diffusion coefficient along the fibers (x') is D_1, and perpendicular to the fibers (y') it is D_2, a smaller value. Now suppose that we measure D with a gradient oriented along the x-axis. What value of D will we measure? Both D_1 and D_2 should contribute because both diffusion along the fibers and perpendicular to the fibers contributes to the displacement of spins along the gradient direction (x).

We can think of any one molecule as undergoing two random and independent displacements, one along x' and one along y', and the projection of each of these onto the x-axis is the contribution to the net displacement of that molecule along x. The displacements along x due to diffusion along x' are characterized by a standard deviation $\sigma_1 = (2D_1T)^{1/2} \cos\theta$, and the displacements along the x-direction due to diffusion along y' have a standard deviation $\sigma_2 = (2D_2T)^{1/2} \sin\theta$. These two dis-placements are both random with zero mean, and so the net standard deviation when two independent random variables are added together is given by $\sigma^2 = \sigma^2_1 + \sigma^2_2$. From Equation [9.1], this variance is equivalent to an effective diffusion coeffi-cient D_x of

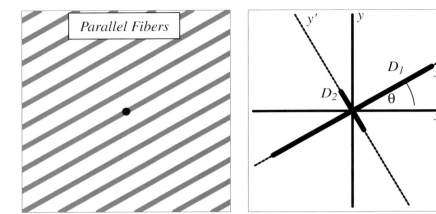

Figure 9.6. Diffusion in white matter fiber tracts. In a system with parallel fibers, the diffusion along the fibers is greater than diffusion perpendicular to the fibers ($D_1 > D_2$). In this example, the fibers are oriented at an unknown angle θ with respect to the x- and y-axes of the imager coordinate system. The coordinates aligned with the fibers, x' and y', are the principal axes. To characterize local diffusion for this 2D example, three measurements of diffusion along different axes are required because there are three quantities to be measured (D_1, D_2, and θ).

$$D_x = D_1 \cos^2 \theta + D_2 \sin^2 \theta \qquad [9.5]$$

Thus, the effective D will lie between D_1 and D_2 and depends on the angle θ that defines the orientation of the fibers. Equation [9.5] also demonstrates a somewhat surprising property of these diffusion measurements. Suppose that D is measured along two arbitrary but perpendicular axes. For example, in addition to the D measured along x, we also measure D along y. Taking the projections of displacements along x' and y' onto the y-axis, the measured D is

$$D_y = D_1 \sin^2 \theta + D_2 \cos^2 \theta \qquad [9.6]$$

If we add these two measurements together, we find $D_x + D_y = D_1 + D_2$ (because $\sin^2 \theta + \cos^2 \theta = 1$ for any θ). That is, regardless of the orientation of the fibers, the sum of the Ds measured along orthogonal axes is always the same. This fact is very useful for measuring an average diffusion coefficient, averaged over different directions to remove anisotropy effects. In mathematical terms, the sum of the Ds along orthogonal directions is the *trace* of the *diffusion tensor* (we will return to this mathematical formalism in the next section).

We can generalize the previous arguments with an expression for D measured along an arbitrary axis at an angle φ to the x-axis:

$$D(\varphi) = D_1 \cos^2 (\theta - \varphi) + D_2 \sin^2 (\theta - \varphi) \qquad [9.7]$$

Then $\varphi = 0$ corresponds to the diffusion coefficient measured with a gradient along the x-axis, and $\varphi = 90°$ corresponds to the D measured with a gradient along the y-axis. We can illustrate this angular dependence by plotting a curve such that the distance from the origin to the curve along an axis at angle φ is proportional to the

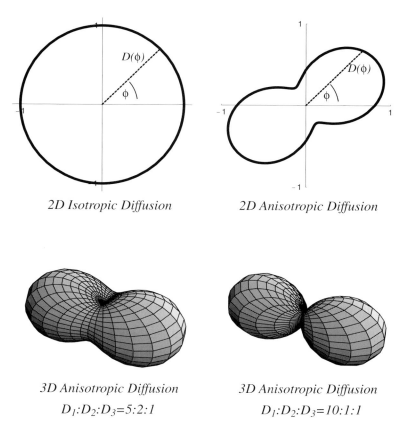

2D Isotropic Diffusion   2D Anisotropic Diffusion

3D Anisotropic Diffusion   3D Anisotropic Diffusion
$D_1:D_2:D_3=5:2:1$ $D_1:D_2:D_3=10:1:1$

Figure 9.7. Anisotropic diffusion. In anisotropic diffusion, the measured value of D is different for different directions. We can visualize this by plotting a curve (in two dimensions) such that the distance to the curve along an angle φ is proportional to the value of D that would be measured along that direction. For isotropic diffusion, this curve is a circle (upper left), but for anisotropic diffusion, it takes on a dumbbell shape (upper right). In three dimensions, the equivalent curve is a peanut-shaped surface (lower plots).

value of D along that axis, as in Figure 9.7. For isotropic diffusion with $D_1 = D_2$ the curve is a circle, but when D_1 and D_2 are distinctly different it takes on more of a dumbbell (or peanut) shape.

From these arguments, we can see why three measurements of D along different axes are necessary to characterize 2D diffusion. There are three unknown quantities $(\theta, D_1,$ and $D_2)$ that must be determined, so at least three different measurements of diffusion will be required. If only two measurements are made, for example along x and y, the two measured points will be consistent with many diffusion curves, as illustrated in Figure 9.8. An additional measurement (e.g., at an angle of 45°) is necessary to identify the correct curve. Note that a diffusion curve such as this characterizes diffusion measurements made at one point in the brain. With imaging, many spatial points can be measured at the same time, and each imaging voxel will have its own diffusion curve that must be calculated from the image data.

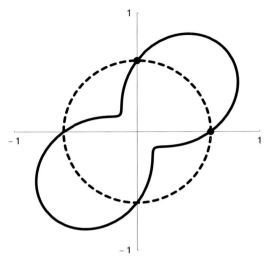

Figure 9.8. Ambiguities of diffusion measurements. In two dimensions, measurements of D along two axes (indicated by dots) are consistent with a family of different diffusion curves (in this case an isotropic diffusion curve and a highly anisotropic diffusion curve). An additional measurement of diffusion along an axis at 45° would resolve the ambiguity.

The same ideas apply to 3D anisotropic diffusion. The diffusion properties at one point in the tissue can be described by three diffusion coefficients (D_1, D_2, and D_3) along three perpendicular (but unknown) principal axes, as illustrated in Figure 9.7. If we now measure diffusion along an arbitrary direction, the projections of each of the independent distributions of displacements along each of the principal axes will add to form the net displacement along the gradient axis, and the net variance is the sum of each of the projected variances (Hsu and Mori, 1995). The measured D is then

$$D = D_1 \cos^2 \theta_1 + D_2 \cos^2 \theta_2 + D_3 \cos^2 \theta_3 \qquad [9.8]$$

where each θ_i is the angle between the ith principal axis and the measured axis. For the general case of 3D anisotropic diffusion, the measured diffusion along an arbitrary axis depends on six quantities: three diffusion coefficients along the principal axes and three angles that specify how these principal axes are oriented with respect to the measurement axis. The 3D curve of D as a function of orientation then looks like the peanut in Figure 9.7.

In practice, the calculation of the local diffusion characteristics does not use Equation [9.6] or [9.8] directly. Instead, the calculations are framed in terms of the diffusion tensor, which is mathematically equivalent. But before turning to the diffusion tensor formalism, we should clarify a subtle point that is often misleading in the literature. In most papers on diffusion tensor imaging, the geometrical shape of the diffusion tensor is described as an ellipse, and yet the fundamental geometry we have described is distinctly different from an ellipse (e.g., Figure 9.7). The diffusion curves in Figure 9.7 describe the variance of the displacements of the water molecules along an arbitrary axis, and by Equation [9.1] this variance is interpreted as an effective diffusion coefficient along a particular axis. However, this is not the same as the spatial distribution of *final positions* of diffusing particles. That is, if the diffusion process leads to independent displacements along three principal axes, the distribution of final positions *is* elliptical, and the widths of the distribution along each of the principal axes is proportional to the square root of the principal diffusivity along that axis. But the diffusion tensor describes the variance of the *total* distribution along one direction, not just those points that happen to end up lying along that particular axis. In other words, what the diffusion tensor tells us is the variance of the *projection* of the final positions of all the particles onto a particular axis. So if we imagine projecting that elliptical distribution onto axes at different angles and then calculating the variance of each projection, the resulting curve of D looks like our dumbbell-shaped curve. In short, it is reasonable to think of anisotropic diffusion producing an elliptical spread of particle positions, but it is important to remember that the quantity we measure, $D(\varphi)$, has a more complex shape.

The Diffusion Tensor

In mathematical terms, the added complexity of anisotropic diffusion is that D must be considered to be a tensor, rather than a scalar. That is, instead of being characterized by a single number, it is described by a 3×3 matrix of numbers. In a diffusion imaging experiment, the diffusion coefficient is measured along a particular axis, which we can indicate by a unit vector $\boldsymbol{u}$. For example, if the diffusion-sensitizing gradient pulses are applied along the x-axis, $\boldsymbol{u} = \{1,0,0\}$, or if the measurement axis is at an angle θ to the x-axis and in the x-y plane, $\boldsymbol{u} = \{\cos\theta, \sin\theta, 0\}$, then the measured value of D along any axis $\boldsymbol{u}$ is given by (Hsu and Mori, 1995):

$$D = (u_x\, u_y\, u_y) \begin{pmatrix} D_{xx} & D_{xy} & D_{xz} \\ D_{yx} & D_{yy} & D_{yz} \\ D_{zx} & D_{zy} & D_{zz} \end{pmatrix} \begin{pmatrix} u_x \\ u_y \\ u_z \end{pmatrix} \qquad [9.9]$$

With a more compact notation, we can use the symbol $\boldsymbol{D}$ to distinguish the diffusion matrix from a particular value of the diffusion coefficient and the superscript T to indicate the transpose and write

$$D = \boldsymbol{u}^T \boldsymbol{D}\, \boldsymbol{u} \qquad [9.10]$$

The diffusion tensor is symmetric, with $D_{ik} = D_{ki}$, so there are six unknown quantities: the elements down the diagonal, and the three elements in one corner. Measuring all six components is described as measuring the full diffusion tensor. The values of these tensor components depend on the coordinate system used (i.e., measurements are done in the coordinate system defined by the imager gradients). In one special coordinate system, called the principal axes, the diffusion tensor is diagonal (all the off-diagonal components are zero), and the three values along the diagonal are called the *principal diffusivities*. The diffusion tensor in this principal axis coordinate system then has the form

$$\boldsymbol{D}_{pa} = \begin{pmatrix} D_1 & 0 & 0 \\ 0 & D_2 & 0 \\ 0 & 0 & D_3 \end{pmatrix} \qquad [9.11]$$

where D_1, D_2, and D_3 are the principal diffusivities. The diffusion tensor in any other coordinate system is directly related to the principal axis form of the tensor and the rotation matrix R that converts coordinates in the principal axis system into the coordinate frame in which the measurements are performed (i.e., the coordinate system defined by the imager gradients) such that

$$D = RD_{pa}R^{-1} \qquad\qquad [9.12]$$

where R^{-1} is the matrix inverse of R. In practice, this procedure is done in reverse. The diffusion tensor is measured in a particular coordinate system, and one must then find the coordinate transformation that produces a diagonal matrix and thus identifies the principal axes. In other words, the six measured components of the diffusion tensor are used to calculate the three rotation angles that define the transformation to the principal axes system and the three principal diffusivities. These computations are equivalent to solving for the six unknown quantities in Equation [9.8]. Calculations are done pixel by pixel in an imaging experiment.

In practice, these calculations are done with a generalized version of Equation [9.2], in which the diffusion sensitivity of the pulse sequence is characterized by a matrix b_{ik} (called the b-matrix) instead of a single scalar b (Mattiello, Basser, and Bihan, 1997). Then in the expression for the decay of the signal, bD is replaced by a sum of terms in which each b_{ik} is multiplied by the corresponding term D_{ik} in the diffusion tensor. The accuracy of the diffusion tensor measurements can be improved by including in the b-matrix the diffusion effects of the imaging gradients themselves in addition to the gradients applied specifically for diffusion weighting.

A common approach to measuring D is to acquire one image with $b = 0$ and six images with b about equal to 1,000 s/mm^2 but with the gradient pulses applied along six different directions. Figure 9.9 shows an example data set collected and processed according to the recommendations of Basser and Pierpaoli (1998). From these data, the local value of each of the six independent values of the diffusion tensor are calculated for each voxel. Two useful combinations of these tensor components are the *trace* and the *relative anisotropy (RA) index*. The trace is simply the average D_{av} of the principal diffusivities and represents the isotropic part of the diffusion tensor. The relative anisotropy index is a measure of the ratio of the magnitudes of the anisotropic and isotropic parts of the diffusion tensor (Basser and Pierpaoli, 1998). If the three principal diffusivities are D_1, D_2, and D_3, then the relative anisotropy RA is

$$RA = \frac{\sqrt{[(D_1 - D_{av})^2 + (D_2 - D_{av})^2 + (D_3 - D_{av})^2]/3}}{D_{av}} \qquad [9.13]$$

In the case where the diffusion is known to be cylindrically symmetric, only four diffusion-weighted images instead of six are required (Conturo et al., 1996; Hsu and Mori, 1995). For example, diffusion in a nerve fiber would be higher along the fiber, but all directions perpendicular to the fiber axis should be equivalent. In this case, two of the unknowns are eliminated because two of the principal axes have the same diffusivities, and the orientation of the principal axes is described by just two angles.

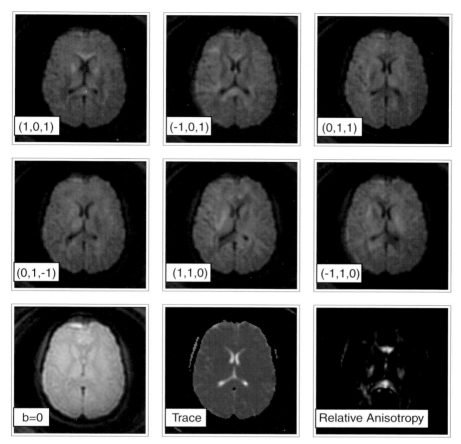

Figure 9.9. Diffusion tensor imaging. To measure the full 3D diffusion tensor, a total of seven images are required, six measured with a large *b*-value with the gradient along different axes (top two rows) and one with *b* = 0. Labels indicate the *(x, y, z)* direction of the gradient. From these data, the six elements of the diffusion tensor are calculated, and maps of the local values of these elements can be displayed as an image. The trace is the isotropic part of the diffusion tensor, the average of the three principal diffusivities. The relative anisotropy index is a measure of how different the three principal diffusivities are from one another. (Data courtesy of L. Frank.)

Because the diffusion tensor is described by six numbers, it can be awkward to display the full diffusion information contained in a data set in which **D** is measured at each point in the brain. Several measures of anisotropy have been proposed as a way of collapsing the information of the full diffusion tensor into a single number that could then be presented as a map (Conturo et al., 1996; Pierpaoli and Basser, 1996; Shrager and Basser, 1998). All these measures essentially describe how different the three principal diffusivities are from one another.

Measuring the Trace of the Diffusion Tensor

The sum of the three components along the diagonal of the matrix is the trace of the diffusion tensor, and the trace is the same regardless of the coordinate system used to represent the tensor. In particular, in the principal axis coordinate system, the trace is the sum of the principal diffusivities. And because the trace is independent of the coordinate system used to measure D, it can be calculated from just three measurements of D along any set of orthogonal axes. That is, measuring D along the x-, y-, and z-directions will yield the same sum regardless of the orientation of the principal axes. This is a very useful way to derive an isotropic, average diffusion coefficient.

The trace can be measured with a single pulse sequence by successively applying bipolar gradient pulses along separate axes. For example, for the simple 2D case discussed in the previous section, we could apply a pair of bipolar x-gradient pulses followed by a pair of y-gradient pulses, as shown in Figure 9.10. The first pair will attenuate the signal by a factor e^{-bD_x}, and the second pair will further attenuate the signal by a factor e^{-bD_y}. The logarithm of the net attenuation is then $-b(D_x + D_y)$, giving a direct measurement of the trace. In measuring the trace, it is tempting to save time and apply the two pairs of gradient pulses at the same time, as in the bot-

Measuring the trace of the diffusion tensor

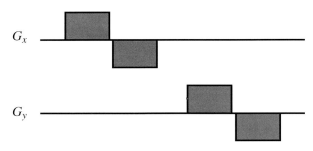

Measuring diffusion along a diagonal axis

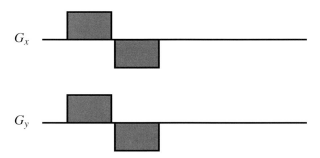

Figure 9.10. Measuring the trace of the diffusion tensor. The trace of the diffusion tensor is the sum of the diagonal elements (the principal diffusivities) and reflects the average diffusion coefficient in an anisotropic medium. The plots illustrate gradient patterns for 2D diffusion imaging. Sequential bipolar gradients along different axes (top) produce a net signal attenuation that depends on the trace. However, applying the same gradient pulses simultaneously (bottom) is not sensitive to the trace but instead is sensitive to diffusion along a single axis at an angle of 45° to x and y.

tom of Figure 9.10. Intuitively, it seems that this ought to produce the same amount of diffusion attenuation, but in fact the measured D with such a pulse sequence is not simply $D_x + D_y$. When two equal gradient pulses are applied simultaneously along two orthogonal axes, this creates a gradient along an axis at 45° to the other two. This pulse sequence is, thus, sensitive to one set of net displacements along this diagonal axis, whereas the original pulse sequence is sensitive to two separate, sequential sets of displacements along x and y.

The reason the two measurements are different is that with anisotropic diffusion the displacements along x and y during the same time interval are not statistically independent of each other. If there were no correlation between the random displacements Δx and Δy, then the aligned gradient scheme sensitive to one set of displacements would work because the separate attenuations produced by the x and y gradients are independent processes. But the problem is that, in general, the displacements along x and y are correlated. We can calculate this correlation for our 2D example with principal axes x' and y', with x' tilted at an angle θ with respect to the x-axis (as in Figure 9.6). The displacements along the principal axes, $\Delta x'$ and $\Delta y'$, are uncorrelated, but the measured displacements Δx and Δy have contributions from both:

$$\Delta x = \Delta x' \cos \theta - \Delta y' \sin \theta$$

$$\Delta y = \Delta x' \sin \theta + \Delta y' \cos \theta \qquad [9.14]$$

Each $\Delta x'$ is drawn from a distribution with standard deviation σ_1, and each $\Delta y'$ is drawn from a distribution with standard deviation σ_2. With this in mind, we can examine the correlation between Δx and Δy by calculating the expected value of the product $\Delta x \Delta y$:

$$\Delta x \Delta y = (\Delta y'^2 - \Delta x'^2) \sin \theta \cos \theta + \Delta x' \Delta y' (\cos^2 \theta - \sin^2 \theta)$$

$$\langle \Delta x \Delta y \rangle = (\sigma^2_2 - \sigma^2_1) \sin \theta \cos \theta \qquad [9.14]$$

The term in $\Delta x' \Delta y'$ is zero on average because these variables are truly uncorrelated, but the remaining terms produce a nonzero average unless either $\sigma_1 = \sigma_2$, or the angle θ is zero or a multiple of 90°. In other words, displacements along x and y are correlated unless the diffusion is isotropic or our measurement axes happen to line up with the principal axes. To avoid the effect of these correlations, a measurement of the trace must look at separate displacements along orthogonal axes, such as the sequential measurement in the top of Figure 9.10. This pattern of gradients works but is not the most time-efficient, and cleverer sets of gradient pulses have been designed to pack the gradients in tightly while avoiding correlations in the measured displacements (Chun, Ulug, and Zijt, 1998; Wong, Cox, and Song, 1995).

Mapping White Matter Fiber Tracts

One of the most promising applications of diffusion tensor imaging (DTI) in basic studies of the brain is mapping white matter fiber tracts. In regions of oriented fibers, the local diffusion is anisotropic, with a larger diffusion coefficient along the fiber direction than perpendicular to it. Measurements in monkeys found that in structures with a regular, parallel arrangement of fibers the average value of D along the fibers was nearly a factor of ten times larger than the D measured perpendicular to the fibers (Pierpaoli and Basser, 1996). Local fiber orientation can be mapped by measuring the full diffusion tensor and identifying the first principal axis, the one with the largest D.

In a recent study, Conturo and co-workers used this technique to map the connections between different brain regions by drawing trajectories based on the local first principal axis (Conturo et al., 1999). The diffusion tensor was measured with 2.5-mm isotropic resolution using single-shot EPI. Trajectories were calculated from many initial seed points by moving in small steps in the direction of the local fiber orientation. Connections between two regions were then visualized by displaying all the trajectories passing through both regions.

This technique is new, and issues of error propagation, particularly with lower resolution images, need further investigation. Nevertheless, mapping fiber tracts with DTI represents an exciting approach to investigating connectivity in the brain, and this anatomical approach is nicely complementary to the functional approach of fMRI.

Beyond the Diffusion Tensor

A critical problem in mapping fiber tracts with DTI is that the local geometry is not always the simple one of parallel fibers. An imaging voxel may contain several sets of overlapping fibers, and the interpretation of diffusion tensor measurements then becomes more complicated. To understand this problem, we need to ask two questions: (1) what is the diffusion tensor when there are multiple fiber orientations, and (2) what does MR imaging show in this case?

As an example, suppose that a voxel contains equal proportions of two sets of parallel fibers oriented at an angle of 90° to each other. In each set, the value of D along the fibers is D_1 and perpendicular to the fibers it is D_2. We will compare diffusion in this mixed system with the case of isotropic diffusion with the average diffusion coefficient, $D = (D_1 + D_2)/2$, and for simplicity we treat this example as two-dimensional diffusion. The crossed fiber arrangement is highly symmetric, but the diffusion characteristics are nevertheless quite distinct from the case of isotropic diffusion. Figure 9.11 illustrates the diffusion pattern that would be found in each of these two examples: isotropic diffusion leads to a spherical spread of displacements, and the crossed fibers produce a cross-shaped diffusion pattern. However, despite the fact that the diffusion patterns are distinct, the diffusion tensors are identical. That is, if we were to measure the diffusion coefficient along any axis, the measured D would be constant for both systems. To see this, suppose we calculate D along an axis at an angle φ to the first principal axis of one set of fibers, which means that it is also at an angle φ to the *second* principal axis of the other set of fibers. The net variance of displacements along the axis is then

$$D(\varphi) = \frac{1}{2} (D_1 \cos^2 \varphi + D_2 \sin^2 \varphi) + \frac{1}{2} (D_1 \sin^2 \varphi + D_2 \cos^2 \varphi)$$

$$= \frac{D_1 + D_2}{2} \qquad\qquad [9.16]$$

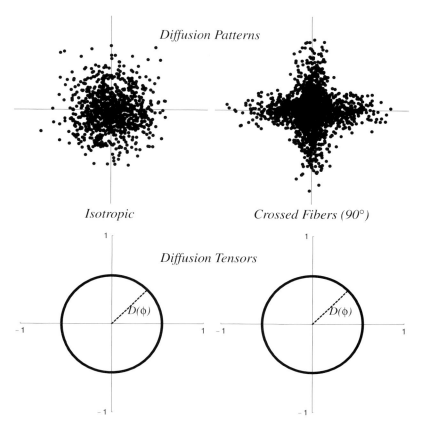

Figure 9.11. Ambiguities of the diffusion tensor. Isotropic diffusion (top left) and crossed-fiber anisotropic diffusion (top left) create different patterns of diffusion, yet the diffusion tensors are identical. The diffusion tensor (bottom) describes the diffusion coefficient $D(\varphi)$ along different directions at an angle φ, and $D(\varphi)$ is proportional to the variance of the projection of the distribution shown at the top onto the axis at angle φ. For both examples, these projections are symmetric.

In other words, no matter which axis is chosen, the displacements along the principal axes of both sets of fibers combine to produce the same net variance. Because D is proportional to that variance, D is the same in all directions, and the diffusion tensor of the crossed fibers is identical to the diffusion tensor for isotropic diffusion.

This example shows that the diffusion tensor does not fully describe the diffusion characteristics of a medium. It *does* describe the net variance of displacements along any direction, but different diffusion patterns can create the same net variance. This brings us to the question of precisely what is measured in MR diffusion imaging. If MRI is only sensitive to the mean squared displacement along an axis, then diffusion imaging data is fully described by the diffusion tensor. If this were the case, the example shown in Figure 9.11 would be an insurmountable problem: the symmetric crossed fibers would be indistinguishable from isotropic diffusion. Fortunately, however, recent work shows that MR measurements are potentially sensitive to aspects of diffusion beyond what is described by the conventional diffusion tensor (Tuch et al., 1999).

In fact, we have already encountered this aspect of diffusion imaging in the earlier context of multicompartment diffusion. If two compartments with different diffusion coefficients are both present within an imaging voxel, then for small values of b the apparent diffusion coefficient is the true average of the Ds for the two compartments. But for larger values of b, the decay becomes biexponential (as in Equation [9.4]). The key result of this effect is that the MR signal attenuation does not depend just on the net variance of the displacements but instead depends on the *separate* variances in the two compartments. This effect carries directly over to DTI. With large b-values, the MR signal is no longer sensitive just to the net variance of displacements, which is what the diffusion tensor describes, but depends on the separate variances of the different compartments. For example, if the voxel contains equal fractions of two identical sets of fibers at right angles to each other, the signal attenuation measured with diffusion sensitivity b along an axis at an angle φ is

$$A(\varphi) = \frac{1}{2} e^{-b \, (D_1 \cos^2 \varphi + D_2 \sin^2 \varphi)} + \frac{1}{2} e^{-b \, (D_1 \sin^2 \varphi + D_2 \cos^2 \varphi)} \qquad [9.17]$$

For small b-values, this expression is equivalent to Equation [9.16], and the diffusion attenuation is sensitive only to the average D. However, with large b-values, the nonlinear form of Equation [9.17] becomes important.

Figure 9.12 illustrates this effect for 2D diffusion by plotting the MR signal attenuation as a function of angle, $A(\varphi)$, for the example of crossed fibers. (These plots are analogous to the plots of $D(\varphi)$: the distance to the curve is proportional to A, the ratio of the signal measured with b greater than zero to the signal with b = 0.) For small b, the diffusion tensor does approximately describe the diffusion effects, and the attenuation pattern is essentially isotropic. However, as b is increased, the shape of $A(\varphi)$ begins to change, and with very large values of b (e.g., 3,000 s/mm^2) $A(\varphi)$ reveals the true diffusion pattern. However, the interpretation of $A(\varphi)$ involves some subtleties. Figure 9.13 shows the diffusion pattern when the proportions of the two sets of crossed fibers are not equal. In this example, 70% of the voxel volume is occupied by fibers running left/right, so the cross-shaped diffusion pattern is elongated in this direction. However, the corresponding plot of $A(\varphi)$ is elongated along the vertical axis. The reason for this is that this direction is dominated by the short axis of the left/right fibers, and so this direction shows the least attenuation (i.e., A is largest). In short, $A(\varphi)$ is sensitive to the more complex diffusion pattern of crossed fibers, but the pattern must be interpreted carefully to identify the dominate fiber direction.

In their original implementation of this idea, Tuch and co-workers measured A along 126 different directions and used this data to plot the diffusion surface for each point in the brain (Tuch et al., 1999). Moving beyond the diffusion tensor description of diffusion is thus a potentially powerful approach for resolving ambiguities due to crossed fibers and for fully exploiting the diffusion sensitivity of MRI. This approach is still in its infancy, but it holds great promise for future developments.

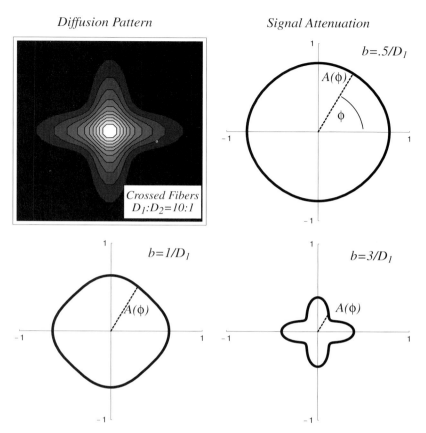

Figure 9.12. Angular dependence of MR signal attenuation. For the 2D example of crossed fibers, the diffusion pattern has the shape of a blurred cross (top left). The other plots show the attenuation of the MR signal measured with different values of b as a function of the angle φ of the diffusion encoding axis. For weak values of b, the shape of $A(\varphi)$ is governed by the diffusion tensor, and so $A(\varphi)$ is reasonably symmetric. For larger values of b, the pattern of $A(\varphi)$ begins to reveal the true diffusion pattern.

DIFFUSION EFFECTS IN fMRI

Diffusion Around Field Perturbations

The preceding sections dealt with the effects on the MR signal of diffusion in a linear magnetic field gradient. Random motions lead to a degree of signal attenuation that is directly related to the strength of the gradient and the local diffusion coefficient. In diffusion imaging, the field gradient is applied by the experimenter and so is controllable in magnitude and orientation. But there are a number of important situations in which the field variations are intrinsic to the tissue, and these local field variations are generally nonlinear. These might arise due to the intrinsic heterogeneity of the tissue or to the presence of contrast agents. The primary effect of this sort related to fMRI occurs when the susceptibility of the blood differs from

Diffusion Pattern   *Signal Attenuation*

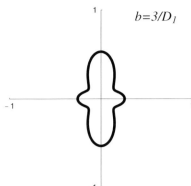

Figure 9.13. MR signal attenuation with unequal proportions of crossed fibers. The interpretation of the angular dependence of the signal attenuation $A(\varphi)$ shown in Figure 9.12 involves some subtleties. When the proportions of the two sets of fibers are not equal, the asymmetry of the diffusion pattern (left) is opposite to the asymmetry of $A(\varphi)$.

the surrounding tissue space, either because of an intrinsic change in deoxyhemoglobin or because of the presence of a contrast agent (Fisel et al., 1991; Hardy and Henkleman, 1991; Majumdar and Gore, 1988; Ogawa et al., 1993; Weisskoff et al., 1994; Yablonsky and Haacke, 1994). Field gradients then develop around the vessels, and as the water molecules diffuse around the vessels they move through different magnetic fields. This physical picture is more complex than the simple case of diffusion in a linear field gradient discussed earlier and is better described as diffusion through field perturbations. Because of the complexity of this process, the discussion is necessarily more qualitative than that mentioned earlier.

The physical picture of this process is that the blood vessels are scattered randomly throughout the medium, with each one creating a local field distortion in its vicinity (Figure 9.14). Without diffusion, spins near a vessel would precess at a different rate than spins far away. For a simple gradient recalled echo (GRE) pulse sequence, this would produce a shortening of T_2^* because the spins would dephase more quickly. But for an SE pulse sequence, the 180° RF pulse refocuses the effects of field offsets so that the signals from the near and far spins come back into phase and create the spin echo. Without diffusion, the SE signal would be unaffected by the presence of field perturbations.

With diffusion, though, both the SE and the GRE signals are affected. However, the nature of the diffusion effect is quite different from the effects in a linear gradient, and, in fact, the effects on SE and GRE signals can even be in opposite directions. It is helpful to describe these effects as an effective change in the transverse relaxation rate. Normal T_2 decay is a simple exponential with a decay rate $R_2 = 1/T_2$, and for a GRE experiment the decay rate is $R_2^* = 1/T_2^*$. We can keep this form and describe the additional signal attenuation due to the field perturbations by the term ΔR_2. So for a decay time t, the additional attenuation is

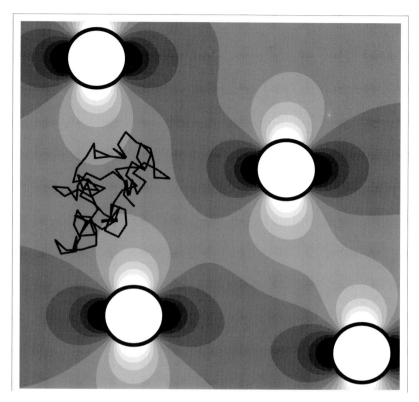

Figure 9.14. Diffusion around magnetized capillaries. Small blood vessels containing paramagnetic contrast agent or deoxyhemoglobin create dipolelike magnetic field distortions in their vicinity, shown as a contour plot of the field. A diffusing water molecule undergoes a random walk (jagged line), carrying the precessing nuclei through different magnetic fields. The random phase changes due to the varying field lead to attenuation of the net signal.

$$A_{SE}(t) = e^{-\Delta R_2 t}$$
$$A_{GRE}(t) = e^{-\Delta R_2^* t} \hspace{6cm} [9.17]$$

The changes in the relaxation rates (ΔR_2 and ΔR_2^*) capture the effects of the field perturbations, and it is these changes that we want to understand. Characterizing these effects in this manner is useful, even if the additional attenuation is not strictly monoexponential. In this case, the changes would be functions of time (i.e., functions of the echo time). For example, for spin echo measurements in a linear field gradient, we can use the results from Box 9, where the decay is of the form e^{-bD}. For a continuous gradient, both the diffusion time T and the duration of the pulse δt are proportional to t, so $b \propto t^3$. Then in the form of Equation [9.16], we would write this as $\Delta R_2 \propto t^2$. Because ΔR_2 usually does depend on time, we can simplify things by looking at a fixed time corresponding to a typical echo time (e.g., TE = 40 ms), and then see how ΔR_2 and ΔR_2^* depend on D.

Describing the attenuation in terms of relaxation rates also ties in directly with the line width measured in spectroscopy. Because of the decay of the signal, the proton spectral line from a sample is not infinitely thin. The faster the signal decays, the broader the spectral line will be. The frequency width of the line is directly proportional to R_2 or R_2^*, depending on the type of experiment. So, for example, the effect of field perturbations in a SE experiment can be described in three equivalent ways: (1) an additive change in the transverse relaxation rate, ΔR_2, (2) a decrease in the signal measured at a particular time TE, or (3) a broadening of the spectral line. All three descriptions are used in the literature.

Motional Narrowing

Suppose now that we perform a thought experiment in which we start with a fixed collection of field perturbations (e.g., a network of magnetized capillaries) and vary the diffusion coefficient, beginning with no diffusion ($D = 0$) and then increasing D, repeating our SE and GRE experiments as we go. Each experiment is done with the same fixed TE, so true T_2 effects are the same, and variations in the signals are then due to ΔR_2 and ΔR_2^*. Figure 9.15 shows the effects of changing D by plotting the change in the relaxation rates and the resulting signal attenuation as functions of D. The attenuation plots show just the additional attenuation due to ΔR_2 and ΔR_2^* so that $A = 1$ corresponds to the signal that would be measured without field perturbations. Starting with $D = 0$ on the left side of the plots, there is substantial additional attenuation of the signal in the GRE experiment and no signal loss in the SE experiment because the spin echo refocuses the effects of the field perturbations. From the preceding discussion of diffusion in linear field gradients, we might naively expect that as D increases we will have more signal loss (increased ΔR_2), and initially we do see the SE signal decrease. However, the GRE signal *increases* with increasing D (i.e., ΔR_2^* *decreases*). As we continue to increase D, the GRE signal continues to increase, but the SE signal exhibits a more complex behavior. As D increases, the SE signal first decreases but then begins to plateau, and finally, when D is large enough, the SE signal begins to increase. In this regime, the SE and GE signals are nearly the same.

The effect that leads to this behavior is called *motional narrowing*, referring to the narrowing of the spectral line (reduction of ΔR_2^* or ΔR_2) when D is large. It occurs when the typical distance moved by a spin due to diffusion during the experiment is much larger than the size of the local field perturbation so that each spin samples a range of field offsets. The key physical difference between diffusion through an array of magnetized cylinders and diffusion in a linear field gradient is that with the cylinders the range of fields a spin can experience is limited. The field offset is maximum at the surface of the cylinder and diminishes with increasing distance. But in a linear field gradient, the farther a spin moves, the larger the field offset, and spins that tend to diffuse in different directions will acquire large phase differences. If the cylinders are small enough (or the diffusion coefficient is high enough), it is possible for a spin to diffuse past many cylinders and thus sample the full range of field distortions. If all the diffusing spins also sample all the field variations, the net phase acquired by each is about the same, corresponding to precession in the average field. With relatively little phase dispersion present, the signal is only slightly decreased. If D increases (or the cylinder diameter decreases), the averaging will be even more effective and there will be less attenuation.

Transverse Relaxation Rates

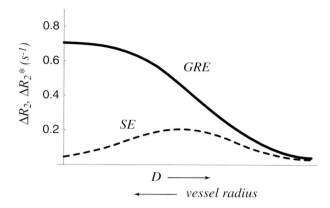

Signal Attenuation

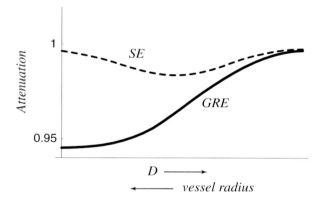

Figure 9.15. Effects of diffusion through random fields on the MR signal. Diffusion through random field perturbations due to magnetized blood vessels produces changes in the transverse relaxation rates ΔR_2 and ΔR^*_2 (top) and results in signal attenuation (bottom). The effect of diffusion depends on how the typical diffusion distance compares with the vessel radius, so these curves can be viewed as showing the effects of increased diffusion coefficient D moving to the right or increased vessel radius moving to the left. The maximum spin echo (SE) attenuation occurs at approximately the capillary radius, and the maximum gradient echo (GRE) effect occurs for the largest vessels.

This argument addresses the question of why ΔR_2^* for the GRE experiment steadily decreases as D increases. But ΔR_2 for the SE experiment exhibits a more complicated pattern, initially increasing as D increases, but after reaching a peak it then decreases again. We can think of this peak in ΔR_2 as a cross-over point for two processes affecting the SE signal. The intrinsic signal that could potentially be recovered by the 180° RF pulse is the GRE signal decrease, and we have already seen how the GRE signal loss improves with increasing D due to motional narrowing. But in addition, the ability of the spin echo to refocus the remaining phase offsets *decreases* with increasing D. This decrease is due to the fact that when spins are moving through variable fields the pattern of field fluctuations felt before the 180° pulse will have increasingly less relation to the fields felt after the 180° pulse as D increases. The result is that the spin echo is less effective in refocusing the phase offsets. In other words, the SE signal is not attenuated at either extreme of D values. When D is small, the field offsets are refocused by the 180° pulse. When D is large, there is little spread in the phase offsets because each spin samples all the field offsets, so there is no need for refocusing. It is only when the motional narrowing effect is not complete, but D is large enough to disrupt the refocusing effect, that the SE signal is attenuated. This peak of the SE attenuation occurs when the distance moved by diffusion during the experiment is about the same size as the spatial scale of the field perturbations (i.e., neither much larger nor much smaller).

This specificity of the SE diffusion effect is potentially useful in localizing signal changes in the microvasculature from those due to larger vessels. In the preceding arguments, we imagined changing D for a fixed set of magnetized blood vessels. But the same arguments apply when considering one value of diffusion but a range of vessel sizes (Kennan, Zhong, and Gore, 1994). For any magnetized blood vessel, the spatial scale of the magnetic field perturbations is on the scale of the vessel diameter. Then for a fixed diffusion coefficient, the effects around large vessels would correspond to the left side of the plots in Figure 9.15, and decreasing vessel size corresponds to moving right on the plots. During the course of the experiment, a water molecule will move a distance Δx on the order of $\Delta x^2 = 2DTE$, and for TE = 40 ms and D = 1 $\mu m^2/s$, this is about 9 μm. This distance is close to the diameter of a capillary (5–8 μm), and so we would expect that an SE experiment would only show an appreciable attenuation due to magnetized vessels of capillary size, whereas a GRE experiment would be more sensitive to larger vessels (Lee et al., 1999). We will return to this difference in the discussion of the BOLD effect in Chapter 16.

REFERENCES

Baird, A. E., and Warach, S. (1998) Magnetic resonance imaging of acute stroke. *J. Cereb. Blood Flow Metabol.* **18,** 583–609.

Basser, P. J., and Pierpaoli, C. (1998) A simplified method to measure the diffusion tensor from seven MR images. *Magn. Reson. Med.* **39,** 928–34.

Benveniste, H., Hedlund, L. W., and Johnson, G. A. (1992) Mechanism of detection of acute cerebral ischemia in rats by diffusion-weighted magnetic resonance microscopy. *Stroke* **23,** 746–54.

Brott, T. G., Haley, E. C., Levy, D. E., Barsan, W., Broderick, J., Sheppard, G. L., Spilker, J., Kongable, G. L., Massey, S., and Reed, R. (1992) Urgent therapy for stroke I: Pilot study of tissue plasminogen activator administered within 90 minutes. *Stroke* **23,** 632–40.

Buxton, R. B. (1993) The diffusion sensitivity of fast steady-state free precession imaging. *Magn. Reson. Med.* **29,** 235–43.

Chun, T., Ulug, A. M., and Zijl, P. C. M. v. (1998) Single-shot diffusion-weighted trace imaging on a clinical scanner. *Magn. Reson. Med.* **40,** 622–8.

Conturo, T. E., Lori, N. F., Cull, T. S., Akbudak, E., Snyder, A. Z., Shimony, J. S., McKinstry, R. C., Burton, H., and Raichle, M. E. (1999) Tracking neuronal fiber pathways in the living human brain. *Proc. Natl. Acad. Sci. USA* **96,** 10422–7.

Conturo, T. E., McKinstry, R. C., Akbudak, E., and Robinson, B. H. (1996) Encoding of anisotropic diffusion with tetrahedral gradients: a general mathematical diffusion formalism and experimental results. *Magn. Reson. Med.* **35,** 399–412.

Cooper, R. L., Chang, D. B., Young, A. C., Martin, C. J., and Ancker-Johnson, B. (1974) Restricted diffusion in biophysical systems. *Biophys. J.* **14,** 161–77.

Duong, T. Q., Ackerman, J. J. H., Ying, H. S., and Neil, J. J. (1998) Evaluation of extra- and intracellular apparent diffusion in normal and globally ischemic rat brain via 19F NMR. *Magn. Reson. Med.* **40,** 1–13.

Fisel, C. R., Ackerman, J. L., Buxton, R. B., Garrido, L., Belliveau, J. W., Rosen, B. R., and Brady, T. J. (1991) MR contrast due to microscopically heterogeneous magnetic susceptibility: Numerical simulations and applications to cerebral physiology. *Magn. Reson. Med.* **17,** 336–47.

Hardy, P. A., and Henkleman, R. M. (1991) On the transverse relaxation rate enhancement induced by diffusion of spins through inhomogeneous fields. *Magn. Reson. Med.* **17,** 348–56.

Haselgrove, J. C., and Moore, J. R. (1996) Correction for distortion of echo-planar images used to calculate the apparent diffusion coefficient. *Magn. Reson. Med.* **36,** 960–4.

Hsu, E. W., and Mori, S. (1995) Analytical expressions for the NMR apparent diffusion coefficients in an anisotropic system and a simplified method for determining fiber orientation. *Magn. Reson. Med.* **34,** 194–200.

Jezzard, P., Barnett, A. S., and Pierpaoli, C. (1998) Characterization of and correction for eddy current artifacts in echo planar diffusion imaging. *Magn. Reson. Med.* **39,** 801–12.

Kennan, R. P., Zhong, J., and Gore, J. C. (1994) Intravascular susceptibility contrast mechanisms in tissues. *Magn. Reson. Med.* **31,** 9–21.

Kucharczyk, J., Mintorovitch, J., Asgari, H. S., and Moseley, M. (1991) Diffusion/perfusion MR imaging of acute cerebral ischemia. *Magn. Reson. Med.* **19,** 311–15.

LeBihan, D. (1988) Intravoxel incoherent motion imaging using steady-state free precession. *Magn. Reson. Med.* **7,** 346–51.

LeBihan, D. (1991) Molecular diffusion nuclear magnetic resonance imaging. *Magn. Reson. Quart.* **7,** 1–30.

LeBihan, D., Breton, E., Lallemand, D., Aubin, M.-L., Vignaud, J., and Laval-Jeantet, M. (1988) Separation of diffusion and perfusion in intravoxel incoherent motion MR imaging. *Radiology* **168,** 497–505.

Lee, S. P., Silva, A. C., Ugurbil, K., and Kim, S. G. (1999) Diffusion-weighted spin-echo fMRI at 9.4 T: microvascular/tissue contribution to BOLD signal changes. *Magn. Reson. Med.* **42,** 919–28.

Majumdar, S., and Gore, J. C. (1988) Studies of diffusion in random fields produced by variations in susceptibility. *J. Magn. Reson.* **78,** 41–55.

Mattiello, J., Basser, P. J., and Bihan, D. L. (1997) The b matrix in diffusion tensor echo-planar imaging. *Magn. Reson. Med.* **37,** 292–300.

Merboldt, K. D., Hanicke, W., and Frahm, J. (1985) Self-diffusion NMR imaging using stimulated echoes. *J. Magn. Reson.* **64,** 479–86.

Moseley, M. E., Cohen, Y., Mintorovich, J., Chileuitt, L., Shimizu, H., Kucharczyk, J., Wendland, M. F., and Weinstein, P. R. (1990) Early detection of regional cerebral ischemia in cats: comparison of diffusion- and T2-weighted MRI and spectroscopy. *Magn. Reson. Med.* **14,** 330–46.

Niendorf, T., Dijkhuizen, R. M., Norris, D. G., Campagne, M. v. L., and Nicolay, K. (1996) Biexponential diffusion attenuation in various states of brain tissue: Implications for diffusion-weighted imaging. *Magn. Reson. Med.* **36,** 847–57.

Norris, D. G., Niendorf, T., and Leibfritz, D. (1994) Healthy and infarcted brain tissues studied at short diffusion times: the origins of apparent restriction and the reduction in apparent diffusion coefficient. *NMR Biomed.* **7,** 304–10.

Ogawa, S., Menon, R. S., Tank, D. W., Kim, S.-G., Merkle, H., Ellerman, J. M., and Ugurbil, K. (1993) Functional brain mapping by blood oxygenation level–dependent contrast magnetic resonance imaging: A comparison of signal characteristics with a biophysical model. *Biophys. J.* **64,** 803–12.

Pierpaoli, C., and Basser, P. J. (1996) Toward a quantitative assessment of diffusion anisotropy. *Magn. Reson. Med.* **36,** 893–906.

Shimony, J. S., McKinstry, R. C., Akbudak, E., Aronovitz, J. A., Snyder, A. Z., Lori, N. F., Cull, T. S., and Conturo, T. E. (1999) Quantitative diffusion-tensor anisotropy brain MR imaging: Normative human data and anatomic analysis. *Radiology* **212,** 770–84.

Shrager, R. I., and Basser, P. J. (1998) Anisotropically weighted MRI. *Magn. Reson. Med.* **40,** 160–5.

Stejskal, E. O., and Tanner, J. E. (1965) Spin-diffusion measurements: spin echoes in the presence of a time-dependent field gradient. *J. Chem. Phys.* **42,** 288–92.

Takano, K., Latour, L. L., Formato, J. E., Carano, R. A. D., Helmer, K. G., Hasegawa, Y., Sotak, C. H., and Fisher, M. (1996) The role of spreading depression in focal ischemia evaluated by diffusion mapping. *Ann. Neurol.* **39,** 308–18.

Tanner, J. E. (1970) Use of stimulated echo in NMR diffusion studies. *J. Chem. Phys.* **52,** 2523–6.

Tong, D. C., Yenari, M. A., Albers, G. W., O'Brien, M., Marks, M. P., and Moseley, M. E. (1998) Correlation of perfusion- and diffusion-weighted MRI with NIHSS score in acute (<6.5 hour) ischemic stroke. *Neurology* **50,** 864–70.

Tuch, D. S., Weisskoff, R. M., Belliveau, J. W., and Wedeen, V. J. (1999) High angular resolution diffusion imaging of the human brain. In: *Seventh Meeting of the International Society for Magnetic Resonance in Medicine,* pp. 321: Philadelphia.

Weisskoff, R. M., Zuo, C. S., Boxerman, J. L., and Rosen, B. R. (1994) Microscopic susceptibility variation and transverse relaxation: Theory and experiment. *Magn. Reson. Med.* **31,** 601–10.

Wong, E. C., Cox, R. W., and Song, A. W. (1995) Optimized isotropic diffusion weighting. *Magn. Reson. Med.* **34,** 139–43.

Yablonsky, D. A., and Haacke, E. M. (1994) Theory of NMR signal behavior in magnetically inhomogenous tissues: The static dephasing regime. *Magn. Reson. Med.* **32,** 749–63.

Zhong, J., Petroff, O. A. C., Prichard, J. W., and Gore, J. C. (1993) Changes in water diffusion and relaxation properties of rat cerebrum during status epilepticus. *Magn. Reson. Med.* **30,** 241–6.

IIB

Magnetic Resonance Imaging

10

Mapping the MR Signal

INTRODUCTION

There are many techniques for producing a magnetic resonance (MR) image, and new ones are continuously being developed as the technology improves and the range of applications grows. The variety of techniques available is in part an illustration of the intrinsic flexibility of magnetic resonance imaging (MRI). The MR signal can be manipulated in many ways: radio frequency (RF) pulses as excitation pulses tip magnetization from the longitudinal axis to the transverse plane to generate a detectable MR signal and as refocusing pulses create echoes of previous signals; gradient pulses eliminate unwanted signals when used as spoilers and, in their most important role, serve to encode information about the spatial distribution of the signal for imaging. By manipulating the RF and gradient pulses, many pulse sequences can be constructed.

The large variety of available pulse sequences for imaging also reflects the variety of goals of imaging in different applications. In most clinical imaging applications, the goal is to be able to identify pathological anatomy, and this requires a combination of sufficient spatial resolution to resolve small structures and sufficient signal contrast between pathological and healthy tissue to make the identification. Because the MR signal depends on several properties of the tissue, and the influence of these properties can be manipulated by adjusting the timing parameters of the pulse sequence, MR images can be produced with strong signal contrast between healthy and diseased tissue. For example, in Chapter 4, MRI was introduced with an illustration (Figure 4.1) of the range of tissue contrast that results simply from manipulating the repetition time (TR) and the echo time (TE) of a spin-echo pulse sequence.

In other applications, the speed of imaging is critically important to be able to follow a dynamic process or simply to minimize artifacts due to subject motion. On modern scanners, an image can be acquired in as little as 30 ms, and images can be collected continuously at rates exceeding 10 images/s. Figure 10.1 shows an image collected with an echo planar imaging (EPI) pulse sequence in only 60 ms. In morphometric mapping to measure the volumes of brain structures with high precision, spatial resolution rather than imaging speed is the primary concern. With volume imaging, the resolved volume element *(voxel)* can be smaller than one cubic millimeter, although the time required to collect such high-resolution images of the whole brain is 5–10 min. Figure 10.1 also shows one slice from a magnetization prepared rapid acquisition gradient echo (MP-RAGE) volume acquisition with a voxel volume of 1 mm^3, requiring 6 min to acquire a full 140-slice data set covering the head. For comparison, the EPI image of the same slice in Figure 10.1 has a voxel volume of 45 mm^3.

An ideal imaging technique would have rapid acquisition of data to provide good temporal resolution, high spatial resolution to be able to resolve fine details of anatomy, and a high signal-to-noise ratio (SNR) to distinguish tissues of interest by differences in the MR signal they generate. But these goals directly conflict with one

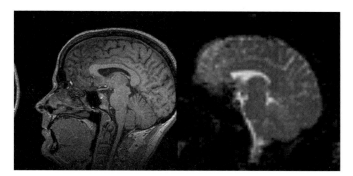

Figure 10.1. Spatial and temporal resolution in MRI. On the left is a high-spatial-resolution image collected with an MP-RAGE pulse sequence in about 6 min, with a voxel volume of 1 mm^3. On the right is a rapid, but low spatial resolution, image collected with an EPI pulse sequence in about 60 ms, with a voxel volume of 45 mm^3.

another. As spatial resolution is improved, the smaller image voxel generates a weaker signal relative to the noise. A very-high-resolution image, with voxel volumes much less than 1 mm^3, could be acquired with standard equipment, but the SNR would be so degraded that the anatomical information would be lost. In addition, as the voxel size decreases, the total number of voxels in the image increases, requiring a longer imaging time to collect the necessary information. In some applications, the goal of achieving a particular tissue contrast also requires a long imaging time. For example, with conventional imaging, T_2-weighted contrast requires a long repetition time, and thus a long total imaging time. With newer techniques for fast imaging there is much more flexibility in dealing with the trade-offs of image contrast and imaging time, but the essential conflicts involved in simultaneously achieving high SNR, high spatial resolution, and high temporal resolution still remain. The different imaging pulse sequences reflect different approaches to balancing these conflicting goals.

The central concept in understanding how MRI works is the idea of k-space, the spatial Fourier transform (FT) of the image. The FT of the image, rather than the image itself, is directly measured in MRI. Different imaging techniques are distinguished by two features: how they sample k-space to collect sufficient data to reconstruct an image of the transverse magnetization at one time point and what the magnitude of the local magnetization *is* at that time point. The k-space sampling determines the basic parameters of the image, such as field-of-view, spatial resolution, and speed of acquisition. But the second feature, the magnitude of the local MR signal, determines whether an image will show useful contrast between one tissue and another. The two features of imaging, how k-space is sampled and the nature of the local signal, can be considered independently. In Chapter 8, the focus was on the signal itself, and this chapter focuses on how an image of that signal distribution is created.

A brief word about the naming of pulse sequences is in order. Sometimes the naming is based on the nature of the signal (e.g., spin echo, SE), sometimes it is based on the acquisition technique (e.g., echo planar imaging, EPI), and sometimes it is both to specify precisely the imaging (e.g., SE-EPI). Acronyms are ubiquitous in MRI, and the sheer number of named pulse sequences is often daunting to the novice trying to get a handle on how MRI works. Sometimes the acronyms are helpfully descriptive, but usually they simply serve to distinguish one pulse sequence from another, and this author, at least, can rarely remember exactly what the acronyms stand for. To add to the confusion, the same pulse sequence sometimes has different names depending on the manufacturer of the scanner (e.g., GRASS, FISP, and FAST). The goal of this chapter is to clarify the basic principles on which MRI is based rather than to provide a comprehensive survey of existing imaging techniques. Nevertheless, a number of imaging pulse sequences are described along the way.

BASICS OF IMAGING

Magnetic Field Gradients

MRI exploits the physical fact that the resonant frequency is directly proportional to the magnetic field. By altering the magnetic field in a controlled way so that it varies linearly along a particular axis, the resonant frequency also will vary linearly with position along that axis. Such a linearly varying field is called a *gradient field* and is produced by additional coils in the scanner. An MR imager is equipped with three orthogonal sets of gradient coils so that a field gradient can be produced along any axis. Because these gradient fields usually are turned on for only a few milliseconds at a time, they are referred to as *pulsed gradients.*

Compared to the main magnetic field B_0, the field variations produced by the gradients are small. Typical gradient strengths used for imaging are a few milliTesla per meter (mT/m), and conventional MR imagers usually have maximum strengths of 10–30 mT/m. At maximum strength, the magnetic field variation across a 30-cm object is 3 mT with a 10-mT/m gradient, only 0.2% of a typical B_0 of 1.5 T. For the following discussion of spatial encoding, it is convenient to express field gradients in units of the resonant frequency change they produce per centimeter (Hz/cm): 10 mT/m = 4,258 Hz/cm for protons.

Slice Selection

In most applications, the first step in image acquisition is the application of a slice-selective RF pulse that tips over the magnetization in only a particular desired slice. To do this, the RF pulse is shaped so that it contains only a relatively narrow band of frequencies centered on a particular frequency ω_0. While the RF pulse is applied, a magnetic field gradient along the slice-selection axis *(z)* is applied, so that the resonant frequency at the center of the desired slice is ω_0. (We will call the slice-selection axis *z,* but the actual orientation is arbitrary.) In the presence of the field gradient, the resonant frequency varies with position along the *z*-axis, so the RF pulse is on-resonance for only a small range of *z*. Then only those spins within a narrow range centered on the desired slice are excited by the RF pulse. The process of slice selection was described in more detail in Chapter 7.

The process of slice selection produces a precessing transverse magnetization at each point of the selected plane. The rest of this chapter deals with how we make an image of the spatial distribution of that magnetization. An MR image is essentially a snapshot of the local amplitude of the transverse magnetization at a particular time point. The central task of MRI then is to encode information about the *x*- and *y*-positions of each signal in such a way that an image of the signal distribution in the *x-y* plane can be reconstructed. A remarkable aspect of MRI is that this spatial information is encoded into the signal itself.

Gradient Echoes

A central concept in MRI is the process of formation of a gradient echo. If a gradient pulse is applied after an RF excitation pulse, spins at different positions along the gradient axis will precess at different rates. The effect of the gradient pulse is thus to produce a large dispersion of phase angles, which grows while the gradient is on, and the net signal is severely reduced *(spoiled)*. In Figure 10.2 this is illustrated by drawing curves of the phase differences over time of spins with different *x*-positions. Initially the spins are in-phase, but when the gradient is turned on, they begin to dephase, and once the gradient is turned off, the phase dispersion remains but no

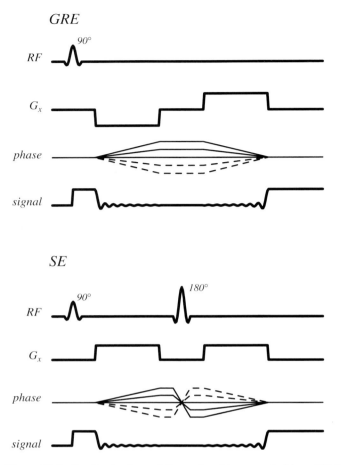

Figure 10.2. Gradient echoes. After a signal is generated by a 90° RF pulse, a gradient pulse will cause spins at different positions to precess at different rates, producing phase variations and a reduction of the net signal (spoiling). A second gradient pulse with opposite sign (or the same sign if a 180° RF refocusing pulse is applied first) will refocus the phase offsets, creating a gradient echo when the areas under the two gradient pulses are matched.

longer grows. However, if an opposite gradient pulse is then applied for the same duration, each spin will acquire a phase angle opposite to the phase it acquired during the first pulse. The phase dispersion diminishes until all the spins are back in-phase, and all spins add coherently to produce a strong signal called a *gradient recalled echo (GRE)*, or just a gradient echo. If a 180° RF pulse is placed between the two gradient pulses, the two gradients must have the same sign for a gradient echo to occur. The 180° RF pulse will reverse the phase of each spin group, and the second gradient pulse will then bring them back into phase (Figure 10.2).

ID Imaging

The simplest MR measurement is the generation of a free induction decay (FID), described in previous chapters. A 90° RF pulse tips over the longitudinal magnetization to generate a signal, and the signal decays over time with a time constant T_2^*. The simple FID pulse sequence, when used for imaging, is called a GRE pulse sequence. This terminology, although in standard use, can be confusing. Gradient echoes are an important part of the imaging process, but they are involved in every type of imaging, not just imaging an FID signal. The situation is further confused because sometimes a distinction is drawn between an SE pulse sequence and a GRE pulse sequence based on the type of echoing process involved: RF echoes for the SE, and gradient echoes for the GRE. But gradient echoes are ubiquitous in imaging; both SE and GRE imaging use gradient echoes. The difference between these two pulse sequences is that SE *also* includes an RF refocusing pulse to generate a spin echo, but GRE does not. The convention is that a pulse sequence, which does not explicitly contain a 180° refocusing pulse, is called a GRE pulse sequence.

Taking just this simple GRE pulse sequence, how can we separate and map the signals from different locations? Imaging is done by exploiting the basic relationship of nuclear magnetic resonance (NMR), that the local precession frequency is proportional to the local magnetic field, and so can be manipulated by applying gradient fields. When a gradient field is turned on, the total signal is spread out over a range of frequencies, and the precession frequency then varies linearly with position along the gradient direction. This basic picture of frequency encoding was introduced qualitatively in Chapter 5, and the following is a more quantitative development in terms of the Fourier transform and the important concept of k-space.

To begin with, consider the simple example of an object with a rectangular profile, as illustrated in Figure 10.3. We can think of this as a one-dimensional (1D) image $I(x)$, with $I(x)$ representing the density of transverse magnetization at x. That is, the net signal produced by spins located within a small range dx centered on x is $I(x)dx$. By the Fourier transform theorem, any function of position x can also be

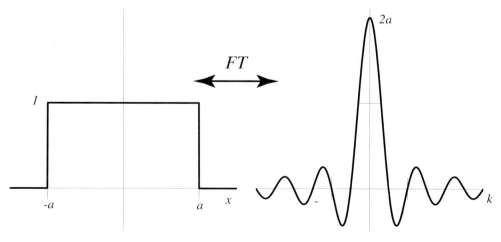

Figure 10.3. The Fourier transform. Any function of position, such as a profile through an image $I(x)$ (left), can also be described as a function of spatial frequencies $S(k)$ (right) where k is the inverse of the spatial wavelength. The functions $I(x)$ and $S(k)$ are related by the Fourier transform so that, given one representation, the other can be calculated.

expressed as a sum of sine and cosine waves of different wavelengths and amplitudes that spread across all of x. The different spatial frequencies of these waves are denoted by k, the inverse of the wavelength, so that small k-values correspond to low spatial frequencies and long wavelengths. Then, the profile $I(x)$ can be expressed as $S(k)$, where $S(k)$ is the amplitude of the wave with spatial frequency k. The two representations $I(x)$ and $S(k)$ are equivalent, in the sense that both carry the same information about the profile, just expressed in a different way. The importance of this k-space representation for imaging is that $S(k)$ is what is actually measured, and $I(x)$ is reconstructed from the raw data by calculating the Fourier transform.

The mathematical relationship between these two representations given by the Fourier transform is (Bracewell, 1965)

$$S(k) = \int_{-\infty}^{\infty} I(x)e^{i2\pi xk}dx \qquad [10.1a]$$

$$I(x) = \int_{-\infty}^{\infty} S(k)e^{-i2\pi xk}dk \qquad [10.1b]$$

The simplicity of the form of Equation [10.1] is in part due to the use of complex numbers. The FT could also be written in terms of real sines and cosines, but in a more cumbersome way. Furthermore, the complex notation is convenient for describing the MR signal produced by a precessing magnetization vector. The precessing transverse magnetization can be expressed as a complex number whose magnitude is the amplitude of the transverse magnetization and whose phase is the precessional phase angle. Mathematically, the magnetization is written as $Me^{i\theta}$, where M is the magnitude of the vector and θ is the phase angle in the transverse plane (Figure 10.4). Alternatively, an equivalent representation is the projection of the vector onto two perpendicular axes in the transverse plane, with the two projections treated as the real and imaginary parts of a complex number. If the two axes are labeled r and i for the real and imaginary components, then the complex magnetization is written as M_r+iM_i, where i is the square root of -1. Both components are, of course, real physical quantities, and the term "imaginary" just means that it is the term multiplied by i. With this in mind, we can treat $I(x)$, representing both the magnitude and phase of the local magnetization, as a complex number at each position x.

Figure 10.4 shows magnitude/phase and real/imaginary representations for a rectangular distribution of magnetization magnitude with a phase that varies linearly with x and so wraps around each time phase increases by 360°. A snapshot of the distribution of transverse magnetization along x can be represented in complex form as $M(x) = \rho(x)e^{i\theta(x)}$, where $\rho(x)$ is the density of magnetization along x, and $\theta(x)$ is the local phase angle at x. In general, both ρ and θ are also functions of time: ρ typically decreases due to relaxation, and θ steadily increases due to precession. But for now we are only interested in mapping the distributions of ρ and θ at one particular time, a snapshot of the distributions. The measured MR signal is the net signal from the entire object, which is calculated by integrating over the profile $M(x)$. The signal contributed from a small region between x and $x + dx$ is $M(x)dx$, so the net signal S is

$$S = \int_{-\infty}^{\infty} M(x)dx \qquad [10.2]$$

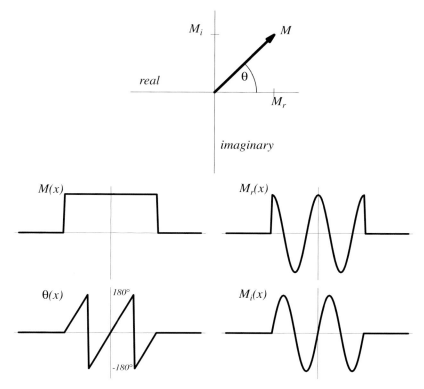

Figure 10.4. Complex numbers. In MR applications, it is useful to describe the local magnetization and the Fourier transform in terms of complex numbers. In the FT, the representations $I(x)$ and $S(k)$ each consist of two numbers, which can be taken as the magnitude and phase (left) or the real and imaginary parts (right) of a complex number. In this example, the magnitude profile $M(x)$ is rectangular, and the phase varies linearly across the object. Physically, the magnitude of $M(x)$ is the net magnitude of the local precessing magnetization vector at x, and the phase is the phase angle of this vector at the center of data acquisition.

All we can measure is this net MR signal from the object. Imaging is accomplished by turning on a gradient field and measuring the evolution of this net signal for a short time centered on our snapshot time. A gradient field has no effect on the center of the field of view ($x = 0$) but causes the total field to vary linearly with x, adding to B_0 for positive x and subtracting from B_0 for negative x. The magnitude G of the gradient is conveniently expressed in units of hertz per centimeter so that the resonant frequency offset of spins at position x is Gx. After precessing for a time t in this gradient field, the magnetization of a spin at position x will acquire an additional phase $\theta = 2\pi Gxt$. Because we are expressing the magnetization as a complex number consisting of a magnitude and a phase, the mathematical equivalent of adding a phase twist θ is a multiplication by $e^{i\theta}$. The gradient field thus modifies the local phase of the magnetization in a position-dependent way, and the net signal at time t becomes

$$S(t) = \int_{-\infty}^{\infty} M(x)e^{i2\pi Gxt}\mathrm{dx} \qquad\qquad [10.3]$$

But if we identify $k = Gt$, this is precisely the form of the Fourier transform in Equation [10.1]. That is, while the gradient is on, the net signal over time traces out the spatial FT of the object so that $S(t)$ is a direct measure of $S(k)$. After $S(t)$ has been measured, the image $I(x)$ can be reconstructed by applying the inverse FT to the data.

This remarkable relationship lies at the heart of all of MRI and provides a powerful way of thinking about different ways of doing imaging (Twieg, 1983). But there are some subtleties involved. First of all, we described this imaging procedure as taking a snapshot of the distribution of transverse magnetization at one time point, yet it takes some time to collect the data. There must be sufficient time for phase evolution under the influence of the gradient field to measure $S(k)$. But during this data acquisition period, the intrinsic transverse magnetization (i.e., the transverse magnetization without the effects of the gradient) is not constant. The phase angle continues to increase by precession, and the amplitude decreases by relaxation. Precession at the primary resonant frequency due to B_0 is not a problem; the receiver accounts for this known precession. But if the intrinsic resonant frequency is altered from the nominal value, by chemical shift or field inhomogeneities, the result will be artifacts in the image. The essential assumption of imaging is that, prior to turning on the gradient, all spins precess at precisely the same frequency. They are not necessarily in-phase with one another, but these phase offsets are assumed to be constant. The result when this ideal assumption does not hold is that spins with intrinsic resonant frequency offsets are mapped to the wrong location. These off-resonance effects, and the decay of the signal by relaxation during data acquisition, are sources of artifacts in imaging.

In short, MRI is built on an idealization that, during the data acquisition period, the intrinsic local MR signals are constant in amplitude and oscillating at frequency f_0 so that any changes observed in the net signal are due entirely to the effects of the applied gradient. That is, the evolution of the signal over time is interpreted as being a result of the distribution of magnetization in space interacting with the applied gradient, and not as an intrinsic change in the local signal. Because this idealization is never true, artifacts will result, and the magnitude of the artifacts will increase as the duration of data acquisition increases. In conventional MRI, the data acquisition window is relatively short (about 8 ms), and these artifacts do not seriously degrade the image. But with fast imaging techniques, the data acquisition window typically is much longer (up to 100 ms); consequently, these artifacts are more of a problem. Artifacts are discussed in more detail in Chapter 11.

The expression for the Fourier transform involves another somewhat subtle feature. Note that Equation [10.1b], the expression for the inverse FT used to reconstruct the image from the measured data, requires adding up the contributions from both positive and negative values of k. A negative spatial frequency may seem like a strange concept, but mathematically it is perfectly straightforward. The sign of k simply describes whether the phase increases or decreases with increasing x. The necessity of measuring negative as well as positive spatial frequencies makes the data acquisition slightly more complicated. In the simplest approach, a gradient is turned on and maintained at a constant value, and data are collected during this read-out gradient. But remembering that $k = Gt$, this only measures the positive spatial frequencies, and to measure the negative ks requires that either G or t must be negative. The negative frequencies could be measured by repeating the experiment and reversing the sign of the gradient, but this would then require two shots to measure the data from one profile. Instead, both positive and negative ks can be measured by creating a *gradient echo* at the center of the data acquisition window (Figure 10.5). Prior to applying the read-out gradient, a gradient pulse with opposite sign and half the duration is applied, sometimes called a *compensation* pulse. The physical effect of this is to wind up the local phase with the compensation pulse prior to applying the read-out gradient so that during the first half of data acquisition the phases unwind, with the effect of the compensation pulse neatly canceled at the center of the data acquisition window, creating a gradient echo when all spins are back in phase. In the second half of data acquisition, the local phases continue to increase. The mathematical effect of this is that the first half of the data acquisition samples the negative k-values, and the second half samples the positive k-values. Effectively, the zero of time, corresponding to $k = 0$ when all the spins are back in phase, has been moved from the beginning of the read-out window to the middle. If we think of MRI as a snapshot of the distribution of transverse magnetization at a particular time point, that time point is the time when the $k = 0$ sample is measured.

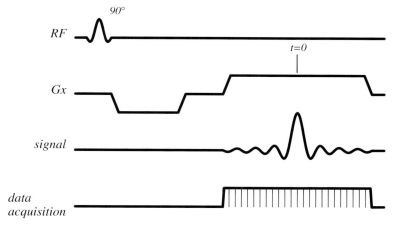

Figure 10.5. Frequency encoding. Pulse sequence diagram illustrating frequency encoding of position along the x-axis. By applying a field gradient along x during data acquisition, the signals from different positions along x are spread over different frequencies, with a one-to-one correspondence between position and temporal frequency. The measured quantity is the net signal over time, $S(t)$. The distribution of temporal frequencies is just the FT of this signal, which is then directly proportional to $I(x)$. In other words, the signal $S(t)$ directly maps out the spatial FT of the object, $S(k)$, with the correspondence between time (t) and spatial frequency (k) given by $k = Gxt$. Both positive and negative spatial frequencies are measured by preceeding the data acquisition with a negative gradient pulse so that the point where all spins are in-phase, corresponding to $t = 0$ (and thus $k = 0$) is moved to the center of the data acquisition window.

2D Imaging

The gradient echo is the basic tool of MRI. During data acquisition, the total signal maps out k-space, the spatial FT of the distribution of transverse magnetization at one instant of time. The time of this snapshot is when the data sample corresponding to $k = 0$ is measured. But everything mentioned to this point describes 1D imaging. Frequency encoding alone measures a 1D projection of a two-dimensional (2D) image onto the x-axis. That is, all the signals with a given x-coordinate, regardless of their y-position, contribute to the net signal corresponding to position x. How do we sort out the y distribution of the signals to make a 2D image? There are several ways, but the most common is to use phase encoding for the second dimension (Edelstein et al., 1980; Kumar, Welti, and Ernst, 1975). In fact, phase encoding is accomplishing the same thing as frequency encoding, but in a more discrete way.

To see how phase encoding works, it is helpful to examine how frequency encoding works in more detail. From the preceding discussion about the correspondence between temporal frequency and position during the read-out gradient, one might conclude that the key feature is the precession rate when a data sample is measured. But this is not quite right; the key feature is the accumulated phase differences between spins at the time of each sample. Imagine breaking the read-out gradient used in frequency encoding into a series of short pulses, with a data sample between each pulse (Figure 10.6). The resulting data are identical to the original data meas-

Frequency Encoding

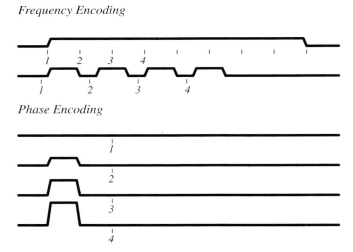

Phase Encoding

Figure 10.6. Equivalence of frequency encoding and phase encoding. Frequency encoding employs a constant gradient, but a series of short gradient pulses interleaved with data samples would produce identical measurements at times 1, 2, 3, and so on (top) because each sample measures the cumulative effects of all the previous gradient pulses. In phase encoding (bottom), the signal is measured after a single gradient pulse, and the magnitude of the gradient pulse is increased with each new excitation. The phase twists produced by a gradient pulse depend only on the area under the gradient pulse, so the numbered samples would be identical to those measured with frequency encoding. The primary difference is that with frequency encoding the samples are measured rapidly after one excitation pulse, whereas with phase encoding they are measured one at a time with separate excitations.

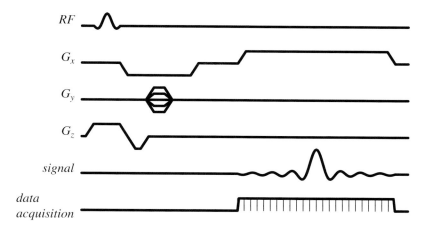

Figure 10.7. Gradient echo imaging pulse sequence. Each line shows the time sequence for different events. The pulse sequence begins with slice selection along the z-axis, followed by phase encoding along y and frequency encoding along x. The phase encoding gradient is incremented each time the pulse sequence is repeated, and each repetition measures one line in k-space. After sufficient repetitions (e.g., 128 or 256), the image is calculated as the FT of the k-space matrix.

ured with the continuous gradient; relative phase changes between spins at different locations grow only when the gradients are on because the spins precess at the same rate in the gaps. So inserting the gaps has no effect on the cumulative phase offsets produced at the time of each of the data samples, and indeed a sample could be collected at any time within the gap. In other words, it is not necessary that a gradient is on when a data sample is measured because the signal depends on the cumulative phase changes produced by previous gradient pulses, which remain locked in after the gradient is turned off. From the point of view of sampling in k-space, the sampling point moves when the gradient pulses are on and then pauses during the gaps. Each of these data samples simply records the cumulative effects of all the previous gradient pulses, and the net effect of a string of gradient pulses is identical to that of a single gradient pulse with the same amplitude and total duration. But the phase effects of a gradient pulse are the same for any gradient pulse that has the same *area* (the product of the gradient amplitude and duration) because the phase produced at a point is proportional to Gt. The same sampling in k-space could then be done one point at a time by applying gradient pulses of different amplitude followed by a data sample, as shown in Figure 10.6, and this process is called phase encoding. In short, the identical data samples measured in frequency encoding could be measured with phase encoding by repeating the pulse sequence to generate a new MR signal, applying a single gradient pulse whose amplitude is incremented each time the pulse sequence is repeated, and measuring one data sample for each generated MR signal.

Two-dimensional imaging is done by frequency encoding the x-axis and phase encoding the y-axis, and it is a remarkable fact that these two processes do not interfere with one another. Figure 10.7 shows the full pulse sequence diagram for a simple imaging sequence. Slice selection is done by applying a frequency-selective RF pulse in conjunction with a gradient in z. The selected z-plane is then mapped by frequency encoding and phase encoding, with the pulse sequence repeated for each new phase-encoding step. From the Fourier transform view, the measured data traces out the 2D FT of the image in a 2D k-space (k_x, k_y). Each time the pulse sequence is repeated, one line in k_x at a fixed k_y is measured with a gradient echo in x. Each phase-encoding pulse in y moves the k-space sampling to a new line at a new value of k_y. The data collection fills in a block of samples in k-space, and then the image is reconstructed by applying the FT to the data.

At first glance, phase encoding seems very inefficient compared to frequency encoding. With frequency encoding, for each RF excitation pulse to generate a signal, the full distribution in one direction is collected; however, with phase encoding, only one sample is collected for each RF pulse. Why can't we simply rotate the readout gradient and use frequency encoding again along the y-axis? This would yield a projection of the image onto the y-axis. But projections of an image onto two axes are not sufficient data to reconstruct the image. Projections onto many axes, with only a small angle of rotation between them, are required. This method is called *projection reconstruction* (PR) and is analogous to the technique used in x-ray computed tomography (CT) and positron emission tomography (PET). The first MR images were made with a projection reconstruction technique (Lauterbur, 1973). This technique is still in use for specialized applications, but most MRI now uses some form of phase encoding.

Mapping *k*-Space

With the preceding ideas, we can now formalize the idea of k-space and how it relates to the local magnetization. Any image is a distribution of intensities in the x-y plane, represented by $I(x,y)$. In MRI, the physical quantity imaged is the local transverse magnetization. Consequently, at each point (x,y), there are, in fact, two numbers needed to specify the local signal: the magnitude of the local magnetization vector and its phase angle. The local magnetization is precessing, so the phase angle is constantly changing, but we can think of an MR image as a snapshot of the transverse magnetization at one instant of time. Then the local phase angle may differ from one location to the next if, for example, the main magnetic field is different at the two locations so that the magnetization vectors precess at different rates. This is a useful way to map the magnetic field distribution in the head by simply imaging the relative phase angle distribution, as illustrated in Figure 10.8. Note that the map of phase angle shows abrupt transitions between white and black, which simply result from the fact that the phase is cyclic, so that moving from 359° to 0° is a smooth phase change, but the number describing the phase jumps. One can think of the bands of black and white as contour levels of phase, marking 360° phase changes.

With this in mind, we can treat $I(x,y)$, representing both the magnitude and phase of the local magnetization, as a complex number at each point of the x-y plane. Any distribution $I(x,y)$ can also be described as a function of spatial frequencies, $S(k_x, k_y)$, in a k-space with axes (k_x, k_y) (Figure 10.9). At each point in k-space, there is also a complex number, with a magnitude and a phase, and this number

Magnitude   *Phase*

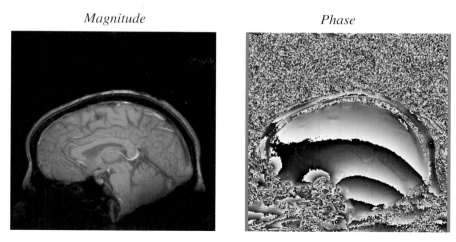

Figure 10.8. Magnitude and phase images. An MR image reflects the local transverse magnetization at the center of data acquisition (when the $k = 0$ data sample is measured). The local magnetization is described by a magnitude (left) and a phase angle (right). Magnetic field variations across the brain create different precession rates, resulting in different phase angles at the time of imaging with a GRE pulse sequence (an SE pulse sequence refocuses these phase offsets). The sharp transitions of the phase image are an artifact of the display due to the cyclic nature of phase, but they effectively serve as contour lines of the magnetic field distribution.

Image   *k-space*

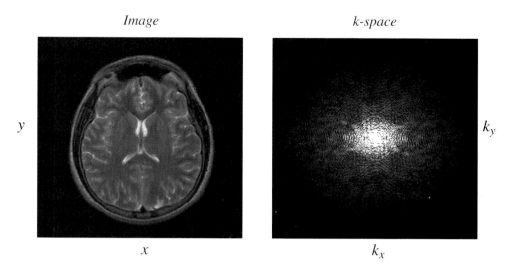

Figure 10.9. Image space and k-space. Any MR image can be equivalently represented as a matrix of intensities $I(x,y)$ or a matrix of spatial frequency amplitudes $S(k_x,k_y)$. The central portion of k-space describes the low-spatial-frequency components, and the outer edges describe the high frequencies, which determine image resolution. (Only the magnitude images are shown, and there is a corresponding phase map in each space.)

Image   *k-space*

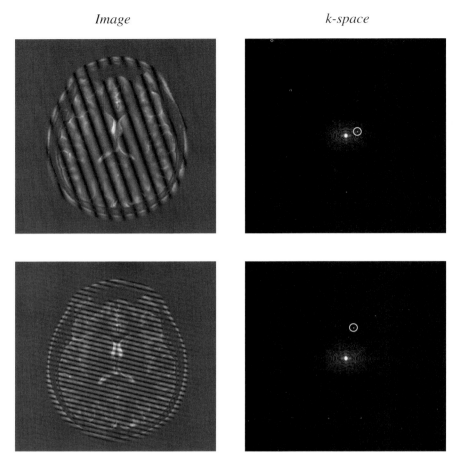

Figure 10.10. Effect on the image of individual *k*-space values. Each point in *k*-space represents a sine wave pattern across the image plane (illustrated for the two circled points), and the *k*-space amplitude is the amplitude of that wave in the image. The wavelength gets shorter moving away from the center of *k*-space, and the angle of the point in *k*-space determines the angle of the wave pattern in image space.

describes the amplitude and phase of a simple sine wave extending across the entire image plane, as illustrated in Figure 10.10. Each value of k is associated with a distinct wave, with the wavelength equal to the inverse of the magnitude of k, and the direction given by the location of the point in the k_x-k_y plane. Thus, small values of k correspond to long wavelengths, and large values of k correspond to short wavelengths. The amplitude $S(k_x,k_y)$ at each point in k-space describes the amplitude of the wave with spatial frequencies (k_x,k_y), and the phase describes how that wave pattern is shifted in the x-y plane. Figures 10.9 and 10.10 illustrate the basic relationships between image space and k-space. The low spatial frequencies usually have the largest amplitude and so contribute most to the image intensity, but the high spatial frequencies provide spatial resolution in the image. Given either distribution, $I(x,y)$

or $S(k_x, k_y)$, the other can be calculated with the Fourier transform, using the 2D form of Equation 10.1.

The power of thinking about imaging from the perspective of k-space is that k-space is actually measured in the imaging process, and image reconstruction just requires applying the FT to the raw data. The relationship at the heart of MRI is that by applying magnetic field gradients, the net MR signal from the entire slice is itself a direct measure of k-space. During data acquisition, as the local phase changes induced by the gradient field continue to evolve, the net signal sweeps out a trajectory in k-space. Each measured sample of the net signal is then a measured sample in k-space, and the task of imaging is to measure sufficient samples in k-space to allow reconstruction of an image.

Earlier, k-space sampling was introduced by discussing frequency encoding and gradient echoes, and we can now look at this as a k-space trajectory controlled by the applied gradients. Each time a gradient echo is acquired, a line through k-space is measured. For an x-gradient echo, the first sample starts at a large $-k_x$ value, moves through $k_x = 0$ at the peak of the gradient echo, and continues on to large $+k_x$ values at the end of data sampling. The phase-encoding steps in y prior to each sampled gradient echo serve to bump the sampling trajectory to a new k_y line in k-space. Then by stepping through many phase-encoding steps in y, and for each step acquiring a gradient echo with a frequency encoding gradient turned on in x, k-space is measured one line at a time with a raster scanning type of trajectory. This is the basic sampling pattern in conventional MRI.

We can generalize this by defining $\boldsymbol{k}(t)$ as a vector in k-space defining the location that is being sampled at time t. Then if $\boldsymbol{G}(t)$ is the total field gradient vector applied at time t, including both x and y gradient components, the general expression for $\boldsymbol{k}(t)$ is

$$\boldsymbol{k}(t) = \int_0^t \boldsymbol{G}(t)dt \qquad\qquad [10.4]$$

The sampled point in k-space at time t depends on the full history of the gradients that have been applied after the transverse magnetization was created at $t = 0$. When the gradients along each axis are balanced (at the time of a gradient echo), the $\boldsymbol{k} = 0$ point is sampled. In this equation, $\boldsymbol{G}$ is expressed in hertz per centimeter. The more familiar units for a magnetic field, Gauss or Tesla, are converted to an equivalent precession frequency by multiplying by the gyromagnetic ratio. This conversion of units emphasizes that the important role of a magnetic field gradient is to create a gradient of resonant frequency, so it is natural to express a field strength in terms of the resonant frequency it produces.

This is the basic imaging equation for MRI. At each time point t, the net signal from the entire slice measures the amplitude and phase at the point in k-space described by $\boldsymbol{k}(t)$. A prescribed pulse sequence defines how the gradients are applied and so defines $\boldsymbol{G}(t)$ and the trajectory through k-space. This equation is defined in two dimensions but is equally valid in three dimensions. The intensity at each point in a volume of space can be described by $I(x,y,z)$ and in the corresponding k-space, $S(k_x, k_y, k_z)$. Field gradients along all three spatial axes can be prescribed to create a three-dimensional (3D) trajectory in k-space.

PROPERTIES OF MR IMAGES

Image Field of View

Basic properties of the MR image, such as the field-of-view (FOV) and resolution, are determined by how k-space is sampled in the image acquisition process. To see how this comes about, we begin with the FOV, the spatial extent of the image from one edge to the opposite edge. In photography, the FOV is determined by a lens that restricts light entering the aperture so that only light rays originating within a narrow cone reach the film to produce the image. Light originating from outside the FOV is not a problem because it never reaches the film plane. But in MRI, there is no lens to restrict which signals reach the detector coil. A small surface coil is only sensitive to a small volume of tissue in its vicinity and so acts somewhat to restrict the FOV. But uniform imaging of the brain requires a head coil that is sensitive to signals generated anywhere within the head. The FOV of an MR image is not determined by the geometry of the detector coil but, instead, by how k-space is sampled. Specifically, the FOV is determined by the spacing Δk of measured samples in k-space.

To see how the k-space sampling interval determines the FOV, consider frequency encoding along the x-direction and the phase changes that develop between one measured sample of the signal and the next. Due to the gradient, spins at different x-positions precess at different rates and acquire a phase offset proportional to $G\Delta t$, where Δt is the time between data samples. Figure 10.11 shows several combinations of gradient strengths and sampling rates on the left, and a plot of the phase difference acquired between one sample and the next as a function of position is on the right. The slope of this phase vs. x curve depends just on the area under the gradient between two successive samples, so the slope is twice as great in the top set of curves as it is in the bottom set. As we move away from the center toward positive x, the phase difference grows until it reaches 180°; then, it drops to −180° and continues to increase from there. Because of this cycling of the phase angle, there is a characteristic separation distance that produces a 360° phase difference between two points. This distance is the FOV. The cycling of the phase means that the signal from any position x will be exactly in-phase with the signal from x + FOV, x + 2FOV, and so on. During the interval before the next sample of the net signal, the local signal at x + FOV will again acquire a 360° phase offset relative to the signal at x, and so on for all the measured samples. But a 360° phase change is indistinguishable from a 0° phase change; consequently, throughout the data acquisition, the signal at x + FOV behaves precisely like the signal from x, so the two signals are indistinguishable in the data. The result is that the signal from x + FOV (and x + 2FOV, etc.) is mapped to the same location as the signal from x in the reconstructed image. The effect in the image is *wraparound,* in which the signal arising outside the FOV on one side appears to be added in to the signal from the other side. In signal processing, this phenomenon is called *aliasing.* The MP-RAGE image in Figure 10.1 shows an example of wraparound, with the back of the head appearing in front of the nose.

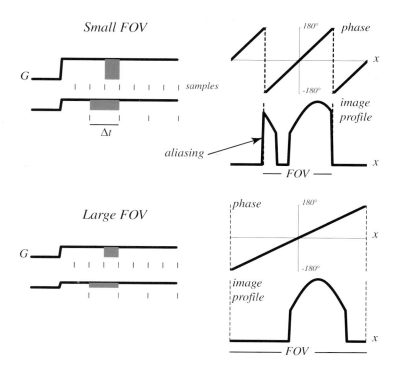

Figure 10.11. Image field-of-view. The FOV of an image is set by the area under the frequency-encoding gradient between one data sample and the next, and this area is simply the sampling interval in k-space: $\Delta k = G\,\Delta t$. The top plot on the left shows two combinations of gradient strength and sampling time that produce the same small FOV, and the bottom plot shows two combinations that produce a larger FOV. The phase offset acquired between one time sample and the next is plotted as a function of position on the right. Two positions that acquire phase offsets between time samples, which differ by 360°, are indistinguishable in the data and so are mapped to the same image point. This creates a wraparound of signals outside the FOV to the other side of the image. The FOV can be increased by decreasing either G or Δt.

The FOV is inversely proportional to the area $G\Delta t$ under the gradient during the interval between samples (the shaded areas in Figure 10.11). To enlarge the FOV, the gradient area must be decreased. This can be done either by decreasing the gradient strength or the sampling interval Δt, as shown in Figure 10.11. Returning to the k-space view and Equation 10.4, this area is just the sampling interval Δk in k-space. The wavelength corresponding to Δk is the FOV, and because k is reciprocally related to wavelength, the FOV increases as Δk is reduced. The same argument applies to all directions in k-space. An image with a rectangular FOV can be acquired by sampling with different intervals Δk_x and Δk_y. For example, an image in which FOV_x is half of FOV_y would be created if Δk_x is twice Δk_y.

In short, the FOV is determined by the sampling interval in k-space. If the object being imaged extends farther than the FOV, the parts outside the FOV are wrapped around to the other side.

Image Resolution

The spatial resolution of an image determines how well two signals can be distinguished when they originate close together in space and, in MRI, resolution is determined by the largest values of k that are sampled. Consider again frequency encoding along the x-axis. To distinguish between the signal arising at x and the signal from a short distance away Δx, there must be some data sample collected where the signals from x and $x + \Delta x$ have a significantly different phase. At the center of the gradient echo, these two signals are in-phase; as time continues, their relative phase will change due to the effect of the gradient. But because these two points are close together, the field difference between the two points due to the gradient is small, and so the phase evolution is slow. The maximum relative phase difference will occur in the last measured data sample, where the cumulative effect of the gradient is maximum. The resolution is defined as the distance Δx such that, for two signals separated by Δx, the phase difference in the last data sample is $180°$.

In k-space, the last data sample is a measurement at the highest sampled value of k_x, which we can call k_{max}. High spatial resolution requires sampling out to large values of k_{max}, as illustrated in Figure 10.12. Note that the wavelength associated with k_{max} is not Δx but rather $2\Delta x$ because two points separated by a distance Δx differ in phase by $180°$, not $360°$. For example, for a resolution of 1 mm, k_{max} must be 5 cycles/cm. As k_{max} increases, Δx becomes smaller, and resolution improves. As with the FOV, the spatial resolution need not be the same in all directions. If k_{max} in the k_y-direction is smaller than k_{max} in the k_x-direction, the resolution in the y-direction

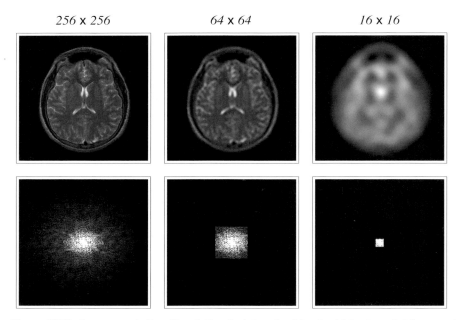

Figure 10.12. Image resolution. Resolution is determined by the highest spatial frequencies that are measured, the outer points in k-space. The image is progressively blurred (top) as the extent of sampling in k-space is reduced (bottom).

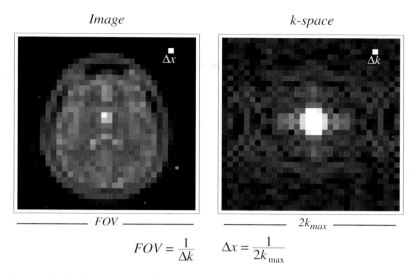

$$FOV = \frac{1}{\Delta k} \qquad \Delta x = \frac{1}{2k_{max}}$$

Figure 10.13. The symmetry between image space and k-space. The resolution in one domain is inversely proportional to the FOV in the other domain, and vice versa.

will be worse. That is, a rectangular sampling pattern in k-space will create an image with different spatial resolution in x and y. This relationship is symmetrical with that for FOV. There, a rectangular array in image space was associated with different separations in k-space, which is just the k-space "resolution." In general, the Fourier transform relationship is completely symmetrical: the resolution in one domain is determined by the FOV in the other domain (Figure 10.13).

In summary, MRI consists of sampling in k-space. The spacing of the samples determines the image field-of-view (FOV = $1/\Delta k$), and the largest k sampled determines the resolution ($\Delta x = 1/(2k_{max})$). Because both $-k$ and $+k$ locations are sampled, the total number of data samples along one axis in k-space is $N = 2k_{max}/\Delta k$ = FOV/Δx. In other words, for N measured samples in k-space, equally spaced along a line, the image FOV is divided into N resolution elements.

Pixels, Voxels, and Resolution Elements

When an image is reconstructed from the k-space data, it is presented as a matrix of signal values. Each point in this matrix is called a pixel (from "picture element"), and on a display screen each pixel is shown as a small square with uniform intensity. Because the imaging process collects data from a certain slice thickness, there is a volume associated with each pixel, called a voxel (loosely from "volume element"). In practice, from an $N \times N$ matrix of measured signal values in k-space, an $N \times N$ matrix of image intensities is reconstructed using an algorithm called the fast Fourier transform (FFT), which dramatically speeds up the calculation of the FT (Brigham, 1974). For the FFT, it is most convenient to work with matrices whose dimensions are a power of two, so it is common to deal with matrices with dimensions of 64×64, 256×256, and so on. The availability of the FFT has had a huge impact on many areas of technology, and it is difficult to overestimate its impor-tance. If the FFT did not exist, it is hard to imagine that MRI could have developed into the powerful tool it is today.

Because the FFT naturally converts an $N \times N$ matrix of points in k-space into an $N \times N$ matrix of points in image space, the image pixel size typically is the same as the resolution element. But it is important to note that there is nothing fundamental about this, and that in some applications it may be useful to reconstruct the image with the pixel size smaller than the true resolution element. In other words, it is tempting to think that because the FFT algorithm takes the $N \times N$ k-space data and calculates a specific grid of $N \times N$ points in the image plane, there is something spe-cial about those particular points, and that our imaging process has somehow pro-duced measured samples of the image intensity at those particular pixel locations. But in fact, each measured point in k-space describes a continuous wave covering *every* point in the image plane, so the data can be used to calculate the intensity at any point, not just the pixel centers that naturally emerge from the FFT. The sim-plest way to reconstruct the image with reduced pixel size is to place the measured, $N \times N$ k-space matrix in the center of a larger matrix, such as $4N \times 4N$, put zeroes in all of the locations where data were not measured (called *zero-padding*), and apply the FFT to produce a $4N \times 4N$ matrix of pixels in the image plane (Figure 10.14 illus-trates this with a low resolution 32×32 image). The spacing of samples in the k-space matrix has not changed, so the FOV of the larger image matrix is the same. Similarly, the true spatial resolution set by the sampling of k-space also has not changed, but now that resolution size is four pixels instead of one in the recon-structed image.

The effect of finite spatial resolution is to produce an image that is a blurred ver-sion of the true distribution of intensities. The process of zero-padding the data to

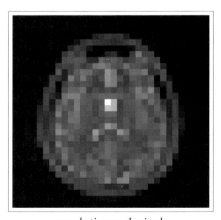
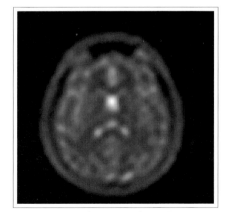

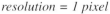
resolution = 1 pixel   *resolution = 4 pixels*

Figure 10.14. Pixels and resolution elements. The pixel size in an image display is often matched to the resolution (left), but the "tiled" look is entirely artifactual. When the same image is displayed with a smaller pixel size (right), the intrinsic blurring due to finite resolution is better visualized.

create a smaller pixel size does not add any information to that contained in the measured data; it simply makes the blurring associated with the true resolution easier to see. The nature of this blurring is described more fully in the next section. For now, it is important simply to note that any MR image, although based on only a finite amount of k-space data, can be reconstructed with any number of pixels that is desired. The imaging process creates a continuous, blurred image of the true distribution, and the pixel size is simply a choice of how to sample that blurred image for display. A pixel size that is matched to the true resolution can at times be a poor representation of the data, in the sense that the image described by the k-space data is nothing like a patchwork of square tiles. That is, the sharp jumps in intensity at the borders of pixels are entirely an artifact of the display; the MRI process creates a smoothed version of the true distribution rather than a sampled version. A good rule of thumb is that, if the individual pixels of the display are readily apparent to the eye, the pixel size should be reduced.

The Point Spread Function

Spatial resolution in the image was defined earlier in terms of the k-space sampling done in acquiring the image data. But how, precisely, does the blurring in the reconstructed image depend on the k-space sampling? Consider imaging a single, small point source, and imagine reconstructing an image with the pixel size much smaller than the true resolution Δx so the blurring can be easily seen. Ideally, we would find only a single pixel lit up, no matter how small we make the pixels in the reconstruction, because that is the true distribution. But instead, what we find is that the point source is spread out over many pixels in the image, and the shape that describes this is called, logically enough, the point spread function *(PSF)*.

To see how the PSF comes about, it is helpful to use an important property of the Fourier transform called the convolution theorem (Bracewell, 1965). The most familiar example of the mathematical process of convolution is smoothing. A function $f(x)$ can be smoothed in x by replacing the value at each location x with an average of the values in the vicinity of x. The set of weights used for constructing the average can be described by a function $w(x)$, such that $f(x)$ is smoothed with $w(x)$ by sliding w along the x-axis until it is centered on a point x, multiplying the two functions together, integrating to calculate the average, and then sliding $w(x)$ to a new location in x and repeating the calculation. Then if $h(x)$ is the resulting smoothed function, we write $h(x) = w(x)*f(x)$; $h(x)$ is the *convolution* of $w(x)$ and $f(x)$. The convolution theorem says that the Fourier transform of the convolution of two functions is the product of the FTs of the two functions: $H(k) = W(k)F(k)$. This is often a useful way to calculate convolutions, but for our purposes here it provides a powerful way of thinking about how processes in k-space, where MR data is measured, translate into effects on the reconstructed image.

To begin with, consider again the sampling in k-space during data acquisition. An ideal, true image of a continuous distribution of magnetization would specify an intensity value for every point in the plane, and the k-space representation of this distribution would similarly be continuous and extend to infinitely large values of k (top row of Figure 10.15). We can then look at the imaging process and the sampling in k-

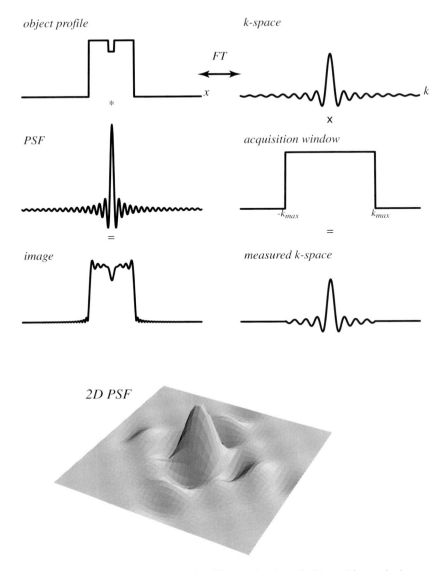

Figure 10.15. The point spread function. The production of a blurred image is shown as equivalent operations in the image domain (left column) and in k-space (right column). The limited extent of sampling in k-space is described by multiplying the full k-space distribution by a windowing function that cuts out the high spatial frequencies. The resulting image is the convolution of the true image with the Fourier transform of the windowing function, PSF(x). The full 2D version of the PSF is shown at the bottom.

space as modifying this true k-space distribution to create a k-space representation of a different image, but one that approximates the ideal image. There are two modifications in k-space: a discrete sampling with a spacing Δk and a windowing due to the finite extent of sampling, described by k_{max}. The discrete sampling leads to the wrap-around problem: Δk defines the field-of-view, and if the extent of the object is larger than the FOV, the signal wraps around. But as long as the FOV is sufficiently large to avoid wraparound, a regularly sampled k-space, with samples extending out to infinite values of k, would still represent the full resolution of the ideal image. Then the fact that k-space is only measured out to a maximum of k_{max}, instead of infinite k, is equivalent to multiplying the full k-space distribution by a rectangular windowing function that has the value one between $-k_{max}$ and $+k_{max}$, and zero everywhere else (middle row of Figure 10.15). Because windowing (multiplication) in one domain is equivalent to convolution in the other domain, multiplying the k-space distribution by this rectangular window is equivalent to convolving the true image with the FT of the windowing function. That is, the resulting reconstructed image is a smoothed version of the true image (bottom row of Figure 10.15), and the point spread function that describes the smoothing is the FT of the windowing function.

The resulting PSF, the FT of a rectangular window in k-space with an amplitude of one and a width of $2k_{max}$, is

$$PSF(x) = \frac{\sin(2\pi k_{max}x)}{\pi x} \qquad [10.5]$$

This form is called a *sinc* function, and Figure 10.3 shows the shape of this function (with $a = 2k_{max}$). It takes on both positive and negative values, with oscillating lobes that diminish in intensity moving away from the center. Sampling farther out in k-space reduces the width of the PSF, while preserving the same shape. The central value is $2k_{max}$, and the net area under $PSF(x)$ is one. The first zero-crossing occurs at $\Delta x = 1/2k_{max}$, the resolution of the image, and subsequent zero-crossings occur at integer multiples of Δx. The resulting image is then a convolution of the true image with $PSF(x)$.) That is, the intensity at each point is a weighted average of the true intensities in the vicinity of the point, with the weighting factors defined by $PSF(x)$. This is equivalent to replacing the intensity of each point in the true image with a spread-out version of that intensity given by $PSF(x)$, and then adding up each of these blurred points to produce the final image. In other words, $PSF(x)$ describes not just how a point is spread out but also how much the signal at different locations contributes to the reconstructed signal at one point. For example, the net signal measured at $x = 0$ comes mostly from signals arising between $-\Delta x$ and $+\Delta x$, which add coherently. But there are also negative signal contributions from $-1.5\Delta x$ and $+1.5\Delta x$. Finally, for display of this continuous, blurred version of the true image, samples are selected at discrete points defined by the pixel size. If the pixel is chosen to match the resolution so that the separation between pixels is Δx, then for each pixel all the other pixel locations fall on the zero-crossings of the $PSF(x)$. This has important consequences for the statistical correlations of the noise in the reconstructed pixels and is considered in more detail in later sections.

A More General Definition of Resolution

The imaging process itself produces a blurred version of the image, but in practice the image sometimes is further smoothed during reconstruction or in postprocessing. In smoothing, the image is convolved with a smoothing function, so this is equivalent to multiplying by another window in k-space, as illustrated in Figure

PSF due to acquisition   *acquisition window*

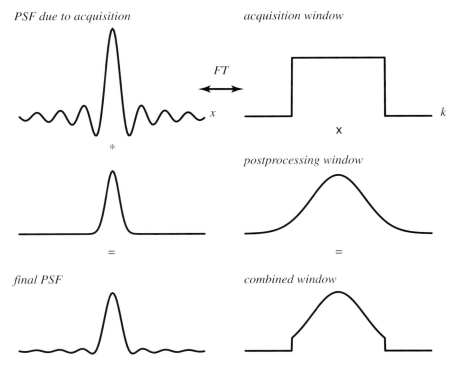

Figure 10.16. Effect of image smoothing on the PSF. The PSF is modified by additional image smoothing in postprocessing, illustrated here with a Gaussian smoothing. Convolving the image with a Gaussian is equivalent to multiplying the k-space acquisition window by a Gaussian (the FT of a Gaussian is another Gaussian) to create a combined windowing function. The final PSF is the FT of the combined window.

10.16. The rectangular block of data is multiplied by a function that is one at the center but rolls off smoothly in the vicinity of k_{max}. Again, the PSF is simply the FT of the windowing function, but because the sharp edges of the intrinsic rectangular window produced by the k-space sampling have been smoothed off, the sidelobes of the PSF are greatly reduced. The cost of this, however, is that the central lobe of the PSF is reduced and broadened, so the resolution is somewhat coarser because the high spatial frequencies are attenuated.

By altering the windowing function (i.e., filtering the k-space data), the shape of the PSF is altered, so the question of how to define the spatial resolution becomes a more subtle question. A full description of the blurring of the image depends on the full shape of the PSF, but we would like to be able to characterize the resolution by a single number in a meaningful way. A useful approach is to think about the intensity distribution in the reconstructed image of a point source. Imagine imaging a ID distribution of magnetization density $M(x)$ in which all the spins contributing to the signal are tightly clustered around the position $x = 0$. If the total magnetization of these spins is m, and they are confined within an interval δx, then the magnetization density is $M(0) = m/\delta x$. We can then imagine making δx smaller until it is much less than any resolution distance Δx we will consider, so that $M(x)$ is very large at $x = 0$ (approaching infinity as δx approaches zero) and zero everywhere else.

The imaging process then produces a smoothed version of $M(x)$, the magnetization density. For a resolution Δx, the net signal m from the point source is effectively spread out over the range Δx, and so the signal density in the image is $I(0) = m/\Delta x$ in the pixel containing the point source. As the resolution distance increases, the same net signal is further diluted in a larger Δx, and so the image intensity is reduced. This brings up a somewhat subtle point: it is tempting to think of the image intensity at a point in an MR image as the total signal arising from the voxel, but this is not really correct. Instead, the image intensity is the apparent *density* of magnetization, averaged over that voxel. In our example, the net signal m in the voxel at $x = 0$ is constant no matter how the imaging is done, but because $I(0)$ represents magnetization *density*, the pixel intensity will depend on the resolution. Multiplying the image intensity by the resolution will convert each density measurement into a measurement of the total signal from the voxel, which for a single image just rescales all the intensity numbers. Thus, for considering just one resolution, $I(x)$ can be taken as a measure of the net signal from each voxel. But when comparing images with different resolutions, it is important to remember that $I(x)$ is really apparent magnetization density.

The result of the foregoing argument is that the image intensity in a pixel containing a point source is inversely proportional to the resolution. We can now reverse this argument and use it to *define* the resolution for any shape of the PSF. If the effect of an altered PSF is to cut the image intensity of a point source in half, then the characteristic resolution distance has doubled. But we can also relate the image intensity of a point source directly to the central value of the PSF. The true image, with a point source of net signal m at $x = 0$, is convolved with PSF(x) to produce $I(x)$. Because $M(x)$ is a point source, the image value at $x = 0$ is simply mPSF(0). That is, PSF(x) describes the contribution of $M(x)$ to the net signal at $x = 0$, and since all the spins *are* at $x = 0$, the total contribution to $I(0)$ is m weighted with PSF(0). So if $I(0) = m/\Delta x$ from the original argument, and $I(0) = m$PSF(0) from the viewpoint of the point spread function, the central value of the PSF function is directly related to the resolution: PSF(0) $= 1/\Delta x$.

To summarize, the effect of filtering in k-space on resolution can be characterized in a quantitative way by how the filtering affects the image intensity of a point source, and this is described by the magnitude of the central value of the PSF. We can take this one step farther and ask how the peak value of the PSF is related to the shape of the window in k-space. A basic property of the Fourier transform is that, in either domain, the central value is equal to the integral of the function in the other domain. So, the area under the window function, A_w, is the central value of the PSF. For example, the image acquisition effectively multiplies the k-space distribution of the true image by a window that has an amplitude of one and a width of $2k_{max}$. The area under the window is then $A_w = 2k_{max}$, and so the resolution is $\Delta x = 1/A_w = 1/2k_{max}$, in agreement with our original definition of resolution.

If another windowing function is applied to the data, such as a smoothing in postprocessing, the resolution changes in proportion to the change in area, A_w. Specifically, the ratio of the area under the new windowing function to the original area is the same as the ratio of the old resolution to the new resolution. For example, if the area under the window is reduced by a factor of two, the characteristic resolution distance is increased by a factor of two. This definition of the resolution can be

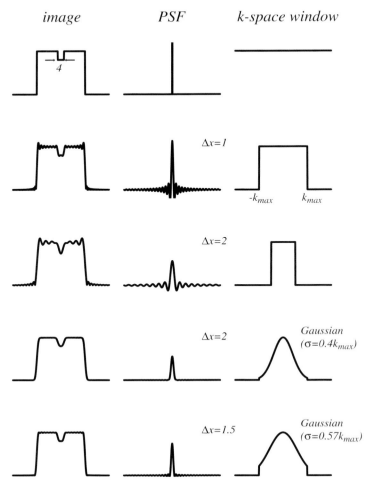

Figure 10.17. Effect of smoothing on image resolution. Examples of the effects of different combined windowing functions (right column) on the PSF (middle column) and the resulting image (left column) of an ideal image profile. The ideal image profile (top) is a rectangle with a 4-mm-wide intensity depression in the middle. Other rows show a high-resolution acquisition with no postprocessing, a low-resolution acquisition with no postprocessing, and examples of the high-resolution acquisition with two degrees of Gaussian smoothing. The resolution Δx, as defined by the reduction in signal of a point source, is the reciprocal of the area under the combined windowing function. The sharp edges of the acquisition window create significant ripples in the PSF and in the resulting image, and the Gaussian smoothing damps them out.

stated in another way, as the width of an equivalent rectangle that has the same area as the actual PSF and the same amplitude of the central point. Because the area under the PSF is one, the equivalent width must be the reciprocal of PSF(0). For the PSF given by Equation [10.5], the equivalent width is the distance from the center to the first zero-crossing (i.e., half the full width of the central lobe).

Figure 10.17 illustrates this principle with different window functions. The top row shows the true profile through the object, represented by a full *k*-space distribution. The object is a rectangle 32-mm wide, with a small area of reduced intensity in the middle that is 4-mm wide. The second row shows the image that results when the acquisition covers k-space out to $k_{max} = 5$ cm^{-1}, giving a resolution of 1 mm. Note that the sidelobes of the PSF create a ringing pattern in the image near the edges (discussed in the next section). The next three rows show examples of postprocessing windows to smooth the data. The third row uses a narrower rectangular window, whereas the fourth and fifth rows show the effect of Gaussian smoothing. In each case, the resolution is defined by the amplitude of PSF(0), but clearly the resolution itself does not fully describe the effect on the reconstructed image, as can be seen by comparing the third and fourth rows. Both have a resolution of 2 mm, but the sidelobes of the PSF and the ringing in the image are suppressed by the Gaussian smoothing. We will return to the question of image smoothing in the context of noise reduction in Chapter 11. But first we consider the source of the ringing artifact in more detail.

Gibbs Artifact

The filtering described previously to reduce the sidelobes of the point spread function illustrates a fundamental property of the Fourier transform: a sharp edge in one domain requires many components to represent it accurately in the other domain. In the filtering example, a sharp boundary to the sampling in k-space produces an extended PSF with many sidelobes in image space. When this PSF is convolved with a sharp edge in image space, such as the edge of the brain, the resulting image of that edge is both blurred and shows a "ringing" pattern that looks like small waves emanating from the edge into the brain (Figure 10.18). Mathematically, this pattern simply results from the lobes of the PSF. But another way of describing the problem is that a sharp edge requires an infinite range of spatial frequencies, and with the finite k-space sampling the highest frequencies are not measured.

We can then look at the process of building up a sharp edge by successively adding the spatial frequencies up to a given cut-off frequency (Figure 10.19). As more spatial frequencies are added, the resulting curve approaches closer to the sharp step function, with the slope of the blurred edge continuously increasing toward a vertical line. But there is a fascinating way in which the resulting shape still differs from a clean step function. The wavelength of the ripples on both sides of the edge decreases as more frequencies are added in, but the *amplitude* of the ripples stays the same. Specifically, the overshoot at the top and the undershoot at the bottom are always about 9% of the amplitude of the step. This curious effect of the FT was studied by the physicist Willard Gibbs around the turn of the century and is usually called Gibbs phenomenon (Bracewell, 1965). The ringing artifact near sharp edges in an MR image is usually referred to as a Gibbs artifact, or *truncation* artifact, because it results from the truncation of sampling in k-space.

To look more closely at how the Gibbs artifact comes about, consider a nonideal step in which the transition from one intensity level to another is described by a linear change over a distance δx. Such an edge is described by spatial frequencies up to about $1/\delta x$. If the cut-off of k-space sampling is much smaller than this frequency,

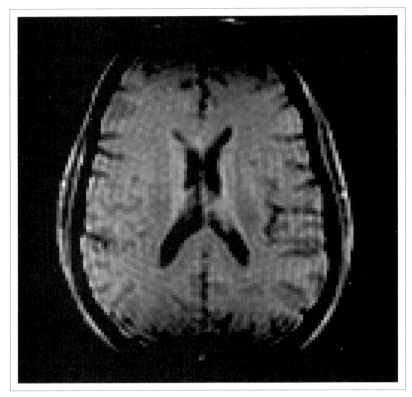

Figure 10.18. Gibbs artifact (or truncation artifact). The ringing pattern illustrated in this brain image occurs because of the ripples of the PSF in low-resolution images.

there will be a Gibbs artifact due to the missing spatial frequencies. But if the k-space sampling extends out far enough to include $k = 1/\delta x$, the edge is reproduced with reasonable fidelity. For a true step function, the required values of k extend to infinity. In practice, edges of tissues in an MR image are not perfectly sharp. The finite thickness of the imaged slice generally leads to some slight angling of tissue boundaries, so the transition is broadened. As a result, Gibbs artifact can usually be eliminated, or reduced to an acceptable level, by increasing spatial resolution. But for dynamic imaging, such as EPI for BOLD fMRI studies, the spatial resolution is coarse, and Gibbs artifact can be quite pronounced.

An interesting variation of the Gibbs artifact occurs when imaging a thin band embedded in a background with a different intensity. When the width of the band is large, the Gibbs artifact appears at both edges, but the center is reasonably flat. But when the width begins to approach the intrinsic resolution, the Gibbs artifacts from the two sides begin to overlap. When the width is four resolution elements, the ripples reinforce each other, creating a striking thin dark line down the middle of the band. This artifact can give a pronounced, but false, impression of a tri-laminar structure. Such an artifact is sometimes seen in imaging of the spinal cord and articular cartilage (Frank et al., 1997).

image   k-space

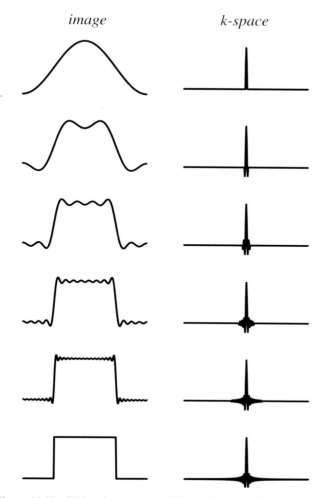

Figure 10.19. Gibbs phenomenon. Effect of representing a sharp edge (bottom row) with a finite range of k-space values. Because a sharp edge requires an infinite range of frequencies for an accurate description, any finite set of k-space samples creates ripples. Remarkably, the magnitude of the overshoot at the edge does not decrease with more samples, although the wavelength of the ripples becomes shorter.

REFERENCES

Bracewell, R. N. (1965) *The Fourier Transform and Its Applications.* McGraw-Hill: New York.

Brigham, E. O. (1974) *The Fast Fourier Transform.* Prentice-Hall: Englewood Cliffs, NJ.

Edelstein, W. A., Hutchison, J. M. S., Johnson, G., and Redpath, T. (1980) Spin warp NMR imaging and applications to human whole body imaging. *Phys. Med. Biol.* **25,** 751–6.

Frank, L. R., Brossman, J., Buxton, R. B., and Resnick, D. (1997) MR imaging truncation artifacts can create a false laminar appearance in cartilage. *AJR* **168,** 547–54.

Kumar, A., Welti, D., and Ernst, R. (1975) NMR Fourier zeugmatography. *J. Magn. Reson.* **18,** 69–83.

Lauterbur, P. C. (1973) Image formation by induced local interactions: Examples employing nuclear magnetic resonance. *Nature* **242,** 190–1.

Twieg, D. B. (1983) The *k*-trajectory formulation of the NMR imaging process with applications in analysis and synthesis of imaging methods. *Medical Physics* **10,** 610–21.

11

MRI Techniques

INTRODUCTION

Chapters 7–9 described the enormous flexibility of the MR signal, how it depends on several tissue properties such as relaxation times and diffusion, and how it can be manipulated to emphasize these different properties by adjusting pulse sequence parameters. The sensitivity to the relaxation times is controlled by adjusting timing parameters such as the repetition time TR or the echo time TE, and the magnetic resonance (MR) signal becomes sensitive to the self-diffusion of water by adding additional field gradient pulses. Chapter 10 described how images are made by using gradient fields and exploiting the fact that the nuclear magnetic resonance (NMR) precession frequency is directly proportional to the local magnetic field. The central idea of magnetic resonance imaging (MRI) is that the application of field gradients makes the net signal over time trace out a trajectory in k-space, the spatial Fourier transform (FT) of the distribution of the MR signal. The image is reconstructed by applying the FT to the measured data. Because the gradients are under very flexible control, many trajectories through k-space are possible.

In this chapter we bring together these ideas from the previous chapters to describe several techniques for imaging in terms of how they produce useful contrast and how they scan through k-space. This review is selective, focusing on techniques that illustrate basic concepts of imaging or that are commonly used for functional magnetic resonance imaging (fMRI). Most fMRI work is done with single-shot echo planar imaging (EPI), so this technique is presented in more detail.

A central idea running throughout MRI is that the signal is a transient phenomenon: it does not exist until we start the experiment, and it quickly decays away. When we make an image of that signal, we can think of it as a snapshot of the signal at a particular time. This is necessarily an approximation because the imaging process requires some time for the signal to evolve under the influence of the imaging gradients and trace out a trajectory in k-space. However, the contrast in an image is primarily determined by the magnitude of the MR signal when the sampling trajectory measures the $k = 0$ sample. This is the sample that directly reflects the raw signal, and all the other samples serve to encode the spatial distribution of the signal. So we can think of an MR image as a snapshot of the transient distribution of magnetization at the time the $k = 0$ sample is measured.

As described in earlier chapters, two broad classes of imaging techniques are spin echo (SE) and gradient echo (GRE). An SE technique includes a 180° radio frequency (RF) refocusing pulse that corrects for signal loss due to magnetic field inhomogeneities. After an excitation pulse, the SE signal decays exponentially with a time constant T_2, and for a GRE pulse sequence the signal decays through a combination of T_2 and local field inhomogeneity effects, described as T_2^* decay. For an echo time TE, the SE signal is attenuated by a factor e^{-TE/T_2}, and the attenuation of the GRE signal is attenuated by a factor e^{-TE/T_2^*}. Whenever we refer to the echo time of an imaging pulse sequence, we mean the time when the $k = 0$ sample is measured. In fact, T_2^* decay is a rather complicated process, depending on intrinsic properties of the tissue, chemical shift, and even the voxel size of the image. These complications will be considered in Chapter 12, and for now we can assume that the GRE signal simply decays exponentially with time constant T_2^* and consider the basic pulse sequences for SE and GRE imaging.

CONVENTIONAL IMAGING TECHNIQUES

Spin Echo and Asymmetric SE Acquisitions

A helpful graphical tool in understanding how imaging pulse sequences work is the pulse sequence diagram, showing how RF and gradient pulses are played out over time (e.g., Figure 11.1). A pulse sequence diagram shows a separate time line for each of the different events that occur. This includes lines for RF pulses, gradient pulses along each of the three spatial axes, and a data sampling line indicating when samples are measured. The full pulse sequence diagram for a conventional two-dimensional (2D) SE pulse sequence is shown in Figure 11.1. During the application of the 90° and 180° RF pulses, a slice-selective gradient is applied along the z-axis. After the 90° excitation pulse, the phase-encoding gradient in y is applied, and the

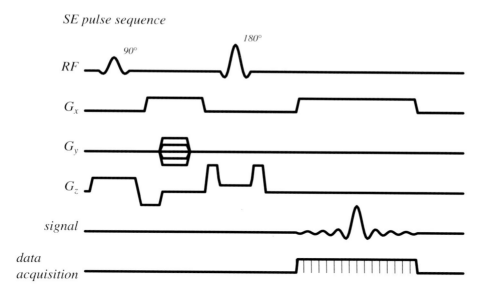

Figure 11.1. Pulse sequence diagram for a SE image acquisition. Each line shows how one component of the pulse sequence plays out over time. The RF pulses excite a signal, and the spatial information is encoded with slice selection along z, frequency encoding along x, and phase encoding along y.

stepped pattern in the diagram indicates that the amplitude of this gradient is incremented each time the pulse sequence is repeated. The data acquisition is centered on the spin echo and is collected with a read-out gradient turned on in the x-direction. The sampling trajectory in k-space is then a raster pattern, with one line in k_x measured after each excitation pulse.

In addition to these primary gradient pulses for slice selection along z, phase encoding along y, and frequency encoding along x, there are a few other gradient pulses shown in Figure 11.1 that are necessary to make high-quality images. After the slice-selection pulse in z, a shorter, negative z-gradient pulse is applied. The purpose of this z-compensation gradient is to refocus phase dispersion created by the slice-selection gradient. The slice-selective RF pulse takes some time to play out, typically 3 ms or more, so as the transverse magnetization begins to form during this excitation pulse, it also precesses at the frequency set by the slice-selection gradient. The spins at different z-positions within the selected slice will begin to get out of phase with one another, and if this phase dispersion through the slice thickness is not corrected, the image signal will be severely reduced. The negative z-gradient pulse performs the refocusing, effectively creating a gradient echo with spins at all z-levels back in phase at the end of the z-gradient pulse. For the gradient pulse during the slice-selective 180° RF pulse, the phase dispersion effects of the gradient are naturally balanced because of the symmetrical placement of the gradient pulse around the 180° pulse. In other words, whatever phase changes are produced by the first half of the gradient pulse are reversed by the 180° pulse, and the second half of the gradient pulse then cancels these phase changes.

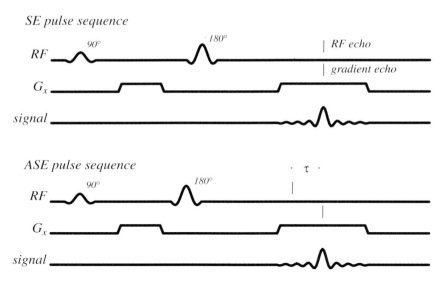

Figure 11.2. Asymmetric SE pulse sequence. In an SE imaging sequence, there are two echoing processes at work: an RF echo due to the 180° RF pulse and a gradient echo due to the read-out gradient pulses. In a standard SE, these two echoes occur at the same time (upper diagram). However, if the 180° pulse is shifted by a time $\tau/2$, the time of the RF echo is shifted by a time τ relative to the gradient echo (lower diagram). The time of the gradient echo marks the time when the $k = 0$ sample is measured, so this is the time that determines contrast in the image. Because the RF echo is displaced in this asymmetric (ASE) pulse sequence, the local phase evolves due to field inhomogeneities for a time τ, giving the ASE sequence a greater sensitivity to microscopic magnetic susceptibility effects.

Prior to the positive read-out gradient pulse along x, a negative x-gradient pulse, called the x-compensation pulse, is applied. As described in Chapter 10, this gradient pulse combination produces a gradient echo at the center of the data acquisition window so that Fourier components corresponding to both positive and negative values of k can be measured. The center of each line in k-space ($k_x = 0$) is sampled at the time of the gradient echo, and so this defines the time of our snapshot of the distribution of transverse magnetization. There are thus two echoing processes occurring during data collection in an SE pulse sequence: the gradient echo produced by the x-gradient pulses and the RF echo produced by the 180° pulse. In a standard SE sequence, these two echoes are aligned so that they occur at the same time. In this way, any dephasing of the spins due to field inhomogeneities is refocused when the center of k-space is measured, so the resulting image intensities depend only on T_2 decay, and not on T_2^*.

However, it is not necessary that the two echoes be aligned. In an asymmetric spin echo (ASE) pulse sequence, the relative timings of the gradient and RF pulses are offset so that the spin echo is shifted by a time τ from the center of acquisition, the time when the $k_x = 0$ sample is measured (Figure 11.2). As a result, the imaged signal is partly dephased due to effects of inhomogeneities. By making repeated measurements and varying τ but holding TE fixed, one could plot out a signal decay curve $S(\tau)$ (Hoppel et al., 1993). However, the time constant for decay of this curve is neither T_2 nor T_2^*. The decay with increasing τ has no T_2 component because TE is fixed, and signal decay results just from the dephasing effects of field inhomogeneities. To describe this additional decay in an ASE sequence in a semiquantitative way, we need to introduce an additional decay time, T_2':

$$\frac{1}{T_2'} = \frac{1}{T_2^*} - \frac{1}{T_2} \qquad\qquad\qquad [11.1]$$

In other words, $1/T_2'$ describes the part of the full unrefocused relaxation rate described by T_2^*, which is due only to field inhomogeneities, and not to T_2 decay itself. The reason this is a semiquantitative relation is that the effects of field inhomogeneities often do not produce a pure monoexponential decay. Nevertheless, this relation is useful in thinking about the different signal characteristics of SE, ASE and GRE pulse sequences. In short, the SE signal decays with increasing TE by T_2 effects alone, the GRE signal decays with TE by T_2 and field inhomogeneity effects, and the ASE signal decays with τ by the field inhomogeneity effects alone.

The ASE pulse sequence was originally introduced as a way of separating the fat and water signals in an image (Buxton et al., 1986; Dixon, 1984). Roughly speaking, the protons in lipids precess at a rate 3.5 ppm different from those of water. In fact, there are a number of lipid proton resonances corresponding to different chemical forms of hydrogen, and there is even a resonance near that of water. But the average effect can be approximated as though it were a single resonance shifted from water. In an SE acquisition, these chemical shift effects are refocused so that the fat and water signals are back in phase. (However, the fat signal is displaced in the image because of the resonant frequency shift, as discussed in Chapter 12.) With an ASE sequence, the fat and water signals precess relative to each other at a rate determined by the resonant frequency shift. At 1.5 T, fat and water complete a full 360° relative phase rotation every 4.4 ms. Then for a voxel containing both fat and water, the ASE signal will oscillate as τ is increased: when $\tau = 2.2$ ms, the two signals are out of phase, and so subtract from each other, but at $\tau = 4.4$ ms, they add coherently again. A GRE sequence also shows this oscillation but is superimposed on an overall decay due to T_2 (e.g., see Figure 8.6).

In fMRI studies based on the Blood Oxygenation Level Dependent (BOLD) effect, the goal is to measure small changes in the MR signal produced by microscopic field inhomogeneities due to the presence of deoxyhemoglobin. The SE pulse sequence is the least sensitive to these effects. In fact, if the spins generating the MR signal were perfectly static, the spin echo would perfectly refocus the phase changes produced by these field offsets, and the SE signal would be insensitive to the BOLD effect. The reason that the SE sequence is sensitive to the BOLD effect at all is that the spins move around due to diffusion, wandering through regions of variable field and accumulating phase offsets that are not completely refocused by the spin echo (see Chapter 9). The GRE sequence is the most sensitive to the BOLD effect because the phase offsets due to field inhomogeneities grow during the full TE. The ASE sequence is intermediate in sensitivity between SE and GRE, and because the time for field offset effects to accumulate depends on τ, rather than TE, there is somewhat more flexibility in tuning the sensitivity of the pulse sequence.

Gradient Echo Acquisitions

The diagrams for three different types of GRE imaging pulse sequences are shown in Figure 11.3. The defining characteristic of a GRE pulse sequence is the absence of a 180° RF refocusing pulse. A gradient echo is still required at the center of data acquisition (TE), so the sign of the initial *x*-compensation gradient is

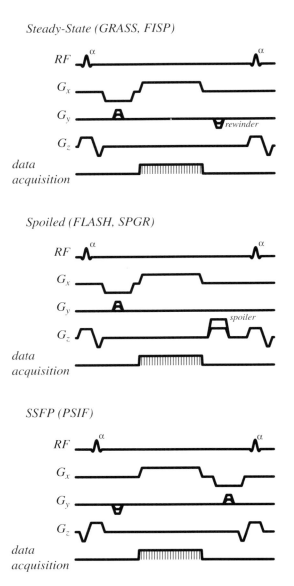

Figure 11.3. Three types of GRE imaging. In GRE imaging with short TR, each RF pulse generates both a new FID and echoes of previous FIDs. With a steady-state sequence (top), both the new FID and the echoes contribute to the signal; with a spoiled sequence (middle), the echo component is destroyed; and with a steady-state free precession (SSFP) sequence (bottom), only the echoes contribute to the signal.

reversed from the SE sequence. Other than this change, the rest of the pulse sequence is similar to the standard SE sequence, and the sampling trajectory in k-space is the same: one line in k_x is measured for each RF excitation pulse. But a critical practical difference between the conventional SE and GRE acquisitions is that the repetition time TR can be made much shorter with a GRE sequence (Wehrli, 1990). The limiting factor on the TR of the SE sequence is the rate of deposition of RF energy in the subject. The RF energy increases with the square of the flip angle, so a 90°–180° combination in an SE sequence deposits 45 times as much energy as a single 30° RF pulse! So with a GRE sequence with a reduced flip angle, the TR can be reduced to a very short time (<10 ms) without exceeding regulations on RF heating of the subject. With a TR of 20 ms, acquisition of an image with 128 phase encode steps requires only about 2.5 s. The prototype GRE fast imaging sequence is called FLASH (fast low-angle shot) (Haase et al., 1986), but many variations have now been developed.

In Chapter 8, the characteristics of the MR signal when TR is shorter than T_2 were discussed. With very short TR, there is a general echoing process such that each RF pulse both creates a new free induction decay (FID) and generates echoes of the previous FIDs. When this process reaches a steady state, the net signal after each RF pulse contains two components: the FID from the most recent RF pulse plus echoes of the previous FIDs. The magnitudes of both components depend strongly on the flip angle as well as TR. Furthermore, the contributions of these two components to the imaged signal can be manipulated by applying appropriate spoiler pulses. There are then three types of signal that one could choose to image with a short-TR GRE sequence: both components, the FID component alone, or the echo component alone. The first diagram in Figure 11.3 shows the pulse sequence for imaging the FID and echo components together, the net steady-state signal. This pulse sequence is usually called GRASS (gradient recalled acquisition in the steady-state) or FISP (fast imaging with steady-state precession), depending on the manufacturer of the MR imager. The key element for preserving the echo component is a rewinder gradient pulse along the y-axis that reverses each of the phase-encoding gradients before the next RF pulse. For the echoes to form, the phase evolution during each of the TR periods must be the same. An unbalanced phase-encoding gradient pulse that varied with each TR would act as a spoiler, destroying the echoes.

The second diagram in Figure 11.3 shows a spoiled-GRE sequence designed to image only the FID component of the signal. By inserting a spoiler gradient pulse on the z-axis after the data collection and by varying the strength of the pulse with each repetition of the pulse sequence, the echoes do not form because the net phase accumulation in different TR periods is randomized. The FID component is generated before the spoiler pulse is applied, and so is not affected. On current scanners, the spoiling is often done by varying the RF pulse so that the magnetization is tipped onto a different axis with each TR. The flip angle stays the same, so the magnitude of the transverse magnetization is the same. However, by varying the axis of rotation, the phase in the transverse plane is altered with each phase encode step, preventing the echoes from forming. In its current form, FLASH is a spoiled sequence, and this pulse sequence is also called SPGR (spoiled GRASS). Note that leaving the phase-encoding gradient unbalanced would also produce some spoiling, but in a nonuniform way. Near $y = 0$ in the image, the phase-encoding gradient has little effect on the local precession, so the spoiling would be ineffective in this part of the image.

Finally, to image only the echoes, the odd-looking pulse sequence at the bottom of the figure is used. Note that the pattern of gradient pulses looks like a time-reversed version of the GRASS sequence. The reason for this is that we do not want the FID from the most recent RF pulse to contribute to the signal, but we do want the echoes of all the previous FIDs to contribute. So the gradients after the RF pulse are left unbalanced, to spoil the FID component, but after the next RF pulse the same gradients are applied again to create an echo during the data collection window. This pulse sequence usually is called SSFP (steady-state free precession) or PSIF (FISP spelled backwards).

Another way of looking at these different GRE signals is to consider that the steady state that forms when a long string of RF pulses is applied produces a coherent magnetization M^- just before each RF pulse and M^+ just after each RF pulse. Then a data collection window between two RF pulses could potentially contain contributions from both M^- and M^+. Whether these signals contribute depends on whether the gradient pulses are balanced during the interval between the time when the coherent signals form and when the center of data acquisition is measured. This is the data sample corresponding to $k = 0$, and so for a signal to contribute to the image the net area under the x- and z-gradients must be zero at this time. For example, in the steady-state GRASS sequence, the gradients between M^+ and the center of data acquisition sum to zero, but those between M^- and the $k = 0$ sample do not. The result is that only the M^+ signal contributes. Similarly, in the echo-only SSFP sequence, the gradients between the center of data acquisition and M^-, but not M^+, are balanced.

The contrast between tissues in these three types of imaging was discussed in Chapter 8. In brief, for small flip angles, the steady-state GRE signal and the spoiled GRE signal are both primarily density-weighted, and there is little difference between the two because the echo component is weak with small flip angles. For larger flip angles, the steady-state GRE signal is much larger than the spoiled GRE signal because the echo component is larger, but contrast between tissues is better with the spoiled signal. The reason for this is that the spoiled signal is strongly T_1-weighted, whereas the steady-state signal also contains T_2-weighting due to the echoes, and this tends to conflict with the T_1-contrast. As T_1 and T_2 become longer, the FID component decreases, but the echo component increases, so the net steady-state signal has poor contrast.

In SSFP, the echo-only signal is strongly T_2-weighted. To emphasize this, the pulse sequence is often described as one in which TE is longer than TR. The rationale for this is that the FID generated by an RF pulse will not contribute to the measured signal until the next TR interval when it returns as an echo. For example, if TR is 30 ms and the data acquisition is at the center of the TR interval, then the TE would be called 45 ms because that is the time interval between the echo and the FID from two RF pulses back, the most recent FID that contributes to the echo. But unfortunately, this terminology can be misleading. The echo signal that is imaged contains contributions from the echoes of *all* previous FIDs (except the most recent one) in addition, and each of these echoes has a different echo time. Furthermore, if one is concerned about the effects of field inhomogeneities, the relevant time for T_2^* effects to develop is not the stated TE, but rather the time interval between the center of data collection and the next RF pulse (15 ms in this example).

Echo-Shifted Pulse Sequences

Conventional gradient echo pulse sequences are useful in many applications because fast acquisitions are possible with short TR. However, for applications such as fMRI and bolus tracking of a contrast agent, there is a basic conflict between the need for a short TR to provide high temporal resolution for dynamic imaging and a reasonably long TE to make the image sensitive to magnetic susceptibility effects. As noted earlier, the echo time in an SSFP sequence is often described as being longer than TR, but this is not true for T_2^* effects. Echo-shifted (ES) sequences were introduced as a way to truly produce an echo time for phase evolution that is longer than the TR (Chung and Duerk, 1999; Duyn et al., 1994; Liu et al., 1993b; Moonen et al., 1992).

The basic idea of an echo-shifted pulse sequence is that additional gradient pulses are added so that the transverse component produced by an RF pulse is dephased during the read-out period right after it is generated, but rephased during the read-out in the next TR period. Figure 11.4 illustrates this idea with a stripped-

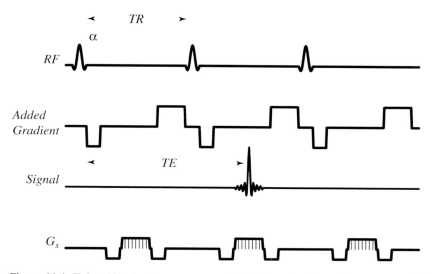

Figure 11.4. Echo-shifted pulse sequences. In fMRI applications of conventional GRE imaging, there is a conflict between the need for a short TR to provide high temporal resolution and the need for a sufficiently long TE to provide sensitivity to magnetic susceptibility (T_2^*) effects. Echo shifting makes possible a TE longer than TR by adding additional gradient pulses so that the signal generated from one RF pulse is dephased during the read-out period in that TR frame but refocused in the next TR read-out period.

down pulse sequence showing just the gradient pulses used to shift the echo and the read-out gradient. The other imaging gradients have been left out for simplicity, and the read-out gradient simply shows when data acquisition occurs. The echo-shifting effect is due entirely to the additional gradient pulses. The FID generated by the first RF pulse is quickly spoiled by the first gradient pulse, so it does not contribute to the signal in the first read-out window. However, as this magnetization continues to precess in the transverse plane, the subsequent gradient pulses create a gradient echo at the time of the second read-out window. That is, between the initial RF pulse and the second read-out window, the gradient pulses are balanced so that the net area under the gradients is zero. For all subsequent read-out windows, the net area is nonzero, so the signal generated by the first RF appears only in the next TR period. The TE in this example is then equal to 1.5 TR.

The preceding argument ignored the effect of the second RF pulse on the transverse magnetization. We simply imagined the transverse magnetization to carry through subsequent RF pulses and focused just on the effects of the gradient pulses. But each RF pulse does have an effect on the transverse magnetization. Imagine an imaging voxel containing spins precessing at the same rate. In the absence of any gradient pulses, these spins would remain coherent as they precess, generating a strong signal. When a strong gradient pulse is applied, spins at different locations within the voxel along the gradient axis precess at different rates; and if the gradient is strong enough, these spin vectors will fan out into a disk in the transverse plane. The next RF pulse will tip this disk, reducing the amplitude of the vectors that remain in the transverse plane. For example, if the RF pulse rotates the disk around x by an angle α, then the y-component of each spin vector is reduced by a factor $\cos \alpha$. When the spin vectors are refocused by the next gradient pulse, the amplitude of the net vector will be reduced. However, if the flip angle of the RF pulse is small, this reduction in amplitude is relatively minor. And, most importantly, the phase of the refocused vector corresponds to precession for the full time between the first RF pulse and the second read-out window. In other words, the second RF pulse slightly reduces the amplitude of the echo but does not affect the phase. Because of this, the effective echo time TE for the development of magnetic susceptibility effects is longer than TR.

Variations on this idea have been used to develop pulse sequences in which the echo can be shifted by any number of TR periods (Liu et al., 1993b). The echo-shifted technique has been adapted for fMRI studies in a version called PRESTO (principles of echo shifting with a train of observations) (Duyn et al., 1994; Liu et al., 1993a) and also applied to bolus tracking studies of contrast agent dynamics (Moonen et al., 1994).

Volume Imaging

Volume acquisitions require trajectories that cover a three-dimensional (3D) k-space. Any 2D imaging trajectory can, of course, be used to acquire images of a volume by acquiring separate images of the individual planes that make up the volume. In multislice acquisitions, the data for multiple slices can be acquired in an interleaved fashion to improve the time efficiency. However, true 3D volume acquisitions in which the scanning trajectory moves throughout a 3D k-space are possible. The most important difference between 2D and 3D approaches to measuring a volume of data is the signal-to-noise ratio (SNR). With the 2D approach, signal is collected from a particular voxel only when the slice containing that voxel is excited. The acquisition of data from other slices does nothing to improve the SNR of that voxel. In contrast, with a 3D acquisition, each measured signal contains contributions from every voxel in the volume, and so each contributes to the SNR of that voxel. The SNR in an image is discussed more fully in Chapter 12, but for now the important point is that 3D acquisitions offer an SNR advantage over 2D acquisitions, and this SNR can be traded against resolution to acquire high-resolution images with very small voxels.

The most commonly used trajectory in 3D imaging is a rectilinear scanning with a gradient echo along x, with phase-encoding pulses along y and z to move the scanning line to a new k_y and k_z position. A popular pulse sequence for acquiring high-resolution anatomical images is SPGR, which provides good T_1-weighted contrast between white matter and gray matter and so is useful for segmenting brain images into tissue types. With this type of acquisition, the typical scanning trajectory is to cover a k_x-k_y plane at one value of k_z and then to move to a new plane at a new k_z. With each excitation RF pulse, one line in k_x is acquired at fixed k_y and k_z. From this k-space data, the images are usually reconstructed and stored as a set of 2D images in (x, y) corresponding to different z-locations. If the data were acquired with the same resolution along each axis (isotropic voxels), the 3D block can be resliced in any orientation to create a new set of slices. In doing this, the voxels that make up the image are often treated as small blocks that are rearranged to form new slices, but it is important to remember the earlier discussion in Chapter 10 of the point spread function (PSF). With this type of acquisition, the PSF is a sinc function along each axis (see Figure 10.15).

Another popular pulse sequence for acquiring high-resolution structural images is magnetization prepared rapid gradient echo (MP-RAGE) (Mugler and Brookeman, 1990). In MP-RAGE, the trajectory in k-space is again a rectilinear sampling, but RF inversion pulses are added periodically to improve the T_1-weighted contrast. After each sampling of a plane at fixed k_z, an inversion pulse is added, so the longitudinal magnetization then follows an inversion recovery (IR) curve during acquisition. The excitation pulses use small flip angles that do not strongly disturb the longitudinal magnetization. As a result, during the acquisition of one plane in k_x-k_y, the signal is slowly varying due to the relaxation of the longitudinal component as the k-space sampling proceeds. The primary effect of the inversion pulses is to improve contrast by sampling the center of k-space at the part of the inversion recovery curve that is most sensitive to T_1. But a secondary effect is that the changing intrinsic signal affects the measured net signal and so affects the sampling in k-space. Such relaxation effects create an additional blurring in the image and are discussed in more detail later in the chapter. Despite the complexities introduced by imaging a signal that varies during image acquisition, the MP-RAGE pulse sequence produces high-resolution images with superior contrast between gray matter and white matter.

Exploiting Symmetries of k-Space

In the preceding discussion of conventional SE and GRE imaging, the importance of reducing TR in speeding up data acquisition was emphasized. With these conventional techniques, the basic k-space sampling trajectory is unchanged: one line of k-space is sampled following each RF excitation pulse, and with GRE imaging, this is simply done faster with a shorter TR. But a more general approach to performing fast imaging is to consider different k-space trajectories, and in particular to develop trajectories that collect more than one k-line for each RF pulse. But before considering some of these ultrafast techniques, there are ways to decrease acquisition time even with a conventional trajectory by exploiting some symmetries of k-space.

In conventional imaging, one line of k-space is collected each time a signal is excited. For a total of N lines of data, the total imaging time is N TR. One approach to reducing the data acquisition time is a *partial k-space* acquisition, which exploits a symmetry of k-space that sometimes occurs (Feinberg et al., 1986; Haacke, Mitchell, and Lee, 1990). If the intrinsic distribution of transverse magnetization is all in-phase, as for example at the peak of a spin echo, then the negative half of k-space is redundant. The value at $-k$ is the same as that at $+k$, but with opposite phase, so it is only necessary to measure half of k-space. The division of k-space into two parts can be either along k_x or k_y. When only a part of the full k_x range is measured, it is described as a *partial echo* acquisition. By reducing the x-compensation gradient, the time TE of the gradient echo, where the $k_x = 0$ sample is measured, is moved closer to the beginning of data sampling. When only half of the k_y range is sampled, it is referred to as a *half-NEX* or *half-Fourier* acquisition, where NEX is a common abbreviation for the number of excitations used for each phase-encoding step (i.e., the number of averages). Because the signal from each excitation is used to collect two lines in k-space, one measured directly and the other inferred from the first, the number of excitations per line in k-space is only $1/2$.

But with a pure gradient echo acquisition, with no refocusing spin echo, the spins in different locations continue to precess at different rates due to field inhomogeneities. Nevertheless, the phase variations across the image plane are often relatively smooth, and the central points in k-space can be used effectively to reconstruct a low-resolution image of the phase distribution and to use this image to correct the full data. To do this, some data must also be collected in the second half of k-space, but often collecting 60 or 70% of the total k-space data is sufficient. The cost of partial k-space acquisition is a reduced SNR because fewer measurements go into the reconstructed image (Hurst et al., 1992). But there are advantages as well. A half-NEX acquisition reduces the total imaging time by a factor of 2. A partial echo acquisition does not shorten the imaging time because the same number of phase-encoding steps are collected, but it does make possible a shorter echo time (TE), which can improve the SNR. Short TE is especially important in angiography applications, where the motion of the flowing spins through the applied gradient fields leads to a rapid phase dispersion and a resulting loss in signal.

FAST IMAGING TECHNIQUES

k-Space Sampling Trajectories for Fast Imaging

Partial *k*-space acquisitions can reduce the minimum imaging time by up to a factor of 2. Much larger reductions can be realized by acquiring more than one line in *k*-space from each excited signal, and there are now a number of ways of doing this (Figure 11.5). In fast spin echo (FSE, also called turbo SE, TSE), multiple 180° pulses are used to create a train of echoes, and each echo is phase encoded differently to measure a different line in *k*-space (Atlas, Hackney, and Listerud, 1993). For example, an echo train of 8 echoes will reduce the minimum imaging time by a factor of 8. This makes it possible to acquire T_2-weighted images, which require a long TR, in less than 1 minute. By increasing the number of spin echoes, a low-resolution image can be acquired in a single-shot mode by

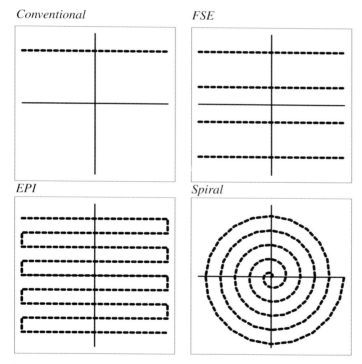

Figure 11.5. *k*-space sampling trajectories. In conventional MRI one line in *k*-space is measured with each excited signal (upper left). Each time the pulse sequence is repeated the phase-encoding gradient shifts the sampling to a new line in *k*-space. In fast spin echo imaging (upper right), multiple echoes are generated for each excited signal, and each echo is separately phase encoded to measure several lines in *k*-space with each shot. In echo planar imaging, the gradients are rapidly switched so that with a single shot the *k*-space trajectory scans back and forth across the full range of *k*-space required for an image. Spiral trajectories use sinusoidally varying gradients to create a trajectory that spirals out from the center. EPI and spiral trajectories can be used in either single-shot mode for the highest temporal resolution or in a multishot mode for higher spatial resolution.

acquiring 64 echoes of one excited signal, a technique called RARE (Rapid Acquisition with Relaxation Enhancement) (Hennig and Friedburg, 1988; Hennig, Nauerth, and Friedburg, 1986). The RARE technique was the original version of a pulse sequence that used multiple spin echoes to encode different lines in k-space, and FSE is essentially a multishot version of RARE. A newer version of this technique is HASTE (half-Fourier acquisition with a single-shot turbo spin echo), which combines the idea of multiple spin echoes with a half-Fourier acquisition, to take advantage of the symmetry of k-space to produce single-shot images (Kiefer, Grassner, and Hausmann, 1994).

In EPI, a rapid series of gradient echoes is generated to cover k-space in a back and forth scanning pattern (Schmitt, Stehling, and Turner, 1998b). In single-shot EPI, a block of k-space equivalent to a low-resolution image can be measured from one excitation pulse. To improve spatial resolution, multishot EPI can be used to cover more of k-space. GRASE (gradient and spin echo) combines spin echo and gradient echo acquisition by generating a series of spin echoes and then generating several gradient echoes under the envelope of each spin echo, with each gradient echo measuring a new line in k-space (Feinberg and Oshio, 1992). This pulse sequence is less sensitive to $T_2{*}$ effects than a standard EPI acquisition.

The scanning trajectories for the foregoing pulse sequences are essentially a raster scanning type. Each gradient echo samples one straight line across k-space, a new phase-encoding pulse moves the sampling to a new line, and a new straight line is sampled. But many scanning patterns are possible. By turning on gradients in x and y simultaneously, but varying the proportions, a radial pattern of sampling is produced. Each line passes through the center of k-space, but at a different angle. This technique is called projection reconstruction (PR) imaging (Glover and Lee, 1995) and is analogous to x-ray computed tomography (CT). With PR imaging, it is possible to collect each ray one half at a time, using two excitation pulses with sampling starting in the center of k-space. Each sampled line is then a ray starting out from zero. This is not very fast imaging, but it makes possible an extremely short TE because the center of k-space is sampled right after the excitation pulse. Such pulse sequences are useful when there are very short T_2 or $T_2{*}$ components in the signal, which would be gone by the time of more standard image acquisitions. PR pulse sequences are not available on standard imagers but are used in specialized research applications.

A promising strategy is spiral imaging, in which the sampling trajectory spirals out from the center of k-space. This can be done in a single-shot fashion, or higher resolution images can be acquired with multiple spirals. Spiral imaging efficiently uses the available gradient strength because the k-space trajectory is smoothly varying, and it is relatively insensitive to motion (Glover and Lee, 1995; Noll, 1995). Spiral imaging is not widely available on MR imagers, but a few institutions are using spiral imaging for fMRI studies with great success (Cohen et al., 1994; Engel et al., 1994; Gabrieli et al., 1997; Noll et al., 1995). Another novel approach to fast imaging is burst imaging, described in Box 11, which is much quieter than other imaging techniques but suffers from a poor signal-to-noise ratio.

BOX 11. QUIET IMAGING WITH BURST TECHNIQUES

One of the most surprising features of MRI when one is first exposed to a scanner is the loud acoustic noise associated with the image acquisition. The gradient coils used for imaging carry large currents and are sitting in a large magnetic field, and so are subject to large forces. When the current is pulsed in the coil, a sharp pulsed force is applied, and the acoustic noise is due to the flexing of the coils under this force. The gradient coil thus acts like a large loudspeaker system. This can be a significant complicating factor in fMRI experiments. With EPI, the sound can reach levels of 130 dB, with the energy centered on the fundamental switching frequency of the EPI acquisition (about 1000 Hz) (Savoy et al., 1999). This poses problems for any auditory fMRI study and makes studies of sleep very difficult.

The acoustic noise is directly related to the fast gradient switching that makes possible fast imaging with EPI. A single read-out period during an EPI acquisition is on the order of 1 ms long, so the read-out gradient is switched from a large negative amplitude to a large positive amplitude roughly every millisecond during acquisition. This rapid switching drives the sampling trajectory in k-space. With a constant gradient, the sampling trajectory is a straight line in k-space, and so to scan back and forth and cover a plane in k-space the trajectory must bend. But bending the trajectory requires switched gradients, so the loud acoustic noise is tightly connected to the ability to do single-shot imaging. And indeed, from this argument, it is difficult to see how the acoustic noise could be eliminated. Both the amplitude of the sound and the fundamental frequency can be reduced by using weaker gradients and slower rise times, which then extends the image acquisition time. But even though such an approach can reduce the noise, it cannot eliminate it. Remarkably, however, there is a pulse sequence that is virtually silent and acquires an image in less than 50 ms. The technique is called burst imaging (Hennig and Hodapp, 1993; Jakob et al., 1998; Lowe and Wysong, 1993), and it has recently been applied to fMRI studies of sleep (Jakob et al., 1998; Lovblad et al., 1999).

A simple pulse sequence for burst imaging is shown in Figure 11.6. A series of RF pulses with low flip angle α is applied in the presence of a constant x-gradient. A 180° RF pulse is then applied, and afterwards the same x-gradient is turned on again as a read-out gradient. During this read-out, the FIDs produced by each of the original α-RF pulses create a string of echoes. Each of these echoes is a frequency-encoded signal and, in the absence of any other gradient, would simply scan across the same line in k-space. By turning on a y-gradient as well during the read-out period, each successive echo is shifted to a different line in k-space. Each scanned line is at an angle because the y-gradient is also on during acquisition, but this tipped k-space sampling nevertheless covers the plane.

Burst imaging thus produces a rapid image with hardly any gradient switching. The reason it is able to do this is that, unlike EPI, burst imaging does not generate one signal and then use that signal to map a continuous trajectory through k-space. Instead, burst generates many signals and then moves each one on a straight line through k-space. For example, consider the signal generated by the first α-pulse. The remainder of the first x-gradient pulse moves this signal far out in k_x, way past the maximum of the image. The

(continued)

BOX 11, continued

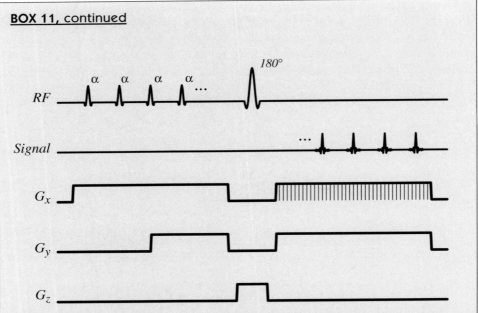

Figure 11.6. Burst imaging. Burst imaging is a nearly silent imaging technique because it elim-
inates the rapid gradient switching used in techniques such as EPI. A series of small flip angle
RF pulses is applied in the presence of a constant gradient G_x. A slice-selective 180° pulse is
then applied. With the same x-gradient turned on again, a series of echoes forms from each of
the signals excited by the original string of RF pulses. Each of these echoes samples a single
line in k-space. By collecting the data with a gradient in y also turned on, each line is effectively phase encoded differently. (The k-space trajectory is actually parallel lines but tipped at
an angle because of the constant G_y.) Although burst imaging is virtually silent and very rapid,
it suffers from a much lower SNR compared with EPI.

second x-gradient then reverses the trajectory, moving back toward $k = 0$. When the y-
gradient is turned on, the trajectory tips up slightly, and it is then this straight but slightly
angled line that passes through the region of k-space that will be used for imaging. But
this trajectory is never turned around to make another pass through. Instead, the next
line is measured with the second generated signal, and so on.

Burst imaging can thus be viewed as a technique that generates a number of signals,
and each one provides a single line through k-space. However, this description brings out
the problem with burst imaging: the signal-to-noise ratio is poor. We can think of the initial local longitudinal magnetization as the available signal we have for imaging. With an
EPI acquisition with a 90° RF pulse, all this signal is generated at once and then moved
through k-space to generate the image. But with burst imaging, this signal is broken into
many small parts, with each one moved through k-space on a single line. For a rapid
acquisition such as this, there is no time for any significant longitudinal relaxation, so the
flip angle α must be small so that the longitudinal magnetization is not completely
destroyed. Each generated signal is then smaller than the full available signal by at least
a factor of $\sin \alpha$ (after each α-pulse the longitudinal magnetization is slightly reduced, so
after the first pulse the generated transverse magnetization is even less). Then for any

line in k-space, the amplitude of the signal used for mapping is much less with burst than with EPI, so the SNR is correspondingly much less.

The signal loss of a full burst sequence compared to EPI is complicated to calculate because each of the α-pulses has some effect on the transverse magnetization created by the previous pulses. Careful optimization of the phase of each of the RF pulses is necessary to minimize the effects of these interactions (Zha and Lowe, 1995). For now we can ignore these complications to try to estimate the highest SNR that could be achieved with this approach even if there were no interactions. Specifically, suppose that each RF pulse generates an MR signal that is then unaffected by subsequent RF pulses, and further suppose that relaxation is negligible during the experiment. Then the amplitude of the signal produced with each pulse directly measures the intrinsic signal amplitude when scanning through k-space. For EPI, this intrinsic signal is equal to the full longitudinal magnetization because EPI uses a 90° pulse to put all the available magnetization into the transverse plane. But for burst imaging, this signal is reduced by a factor $\sin \alpha$, so the key question is: how large can α be? The problem is that each α-pulse reduces the longitudinal magnetization, so the signal generated by the next pulse is weaker. This is undesirable for scanning through k-space because the idealization of imaging is that the intrinsic signal is constant, so that any changes in the net signal are the result of the spatial distribution of the signal interacting with the imaging gradients. In other words, a variable intrinsic signal while scanning through k-space leads to distortions and blurring in the image.

We can imagine dealing with this variable signal problem by using progressively larger flip angles in the RF pulse train so that each generates the same magnitude of transverse magnetization. If this string of RF pulses is optimized to use all the available longitudinal magnetization for imaging, then the final RF pulse should be 90° to bring the last bit of magnetization fully into the transverse plane. This optimization of the RF flip angles is not standard in burst imaging, but it is a fruitful way to think about how burst imaging could be optimized for SNR. So the key question is: how do we design a string of N equally spaced RF pulses so that the full longitudinal magnetization M is broken into N equal transverse magnetization components M_T, leaving no longitudinal magnetization at the end? This would divide up the available signal evenly among the individual lines of k-space, and the SNR of burst relative to EPI then is M_T/M. Naively, we might expect that if the longitudinal magnetization is divided into N transverse components, the intrinsic burst signal would be M/N. However, this is not right, and it turns out that a longitudinal magnetization M can produce N transverse components each with amplitude $M/\sqrt{N}$. Clearly, magnetization is not conserved when going from longitudinal to transverse! The SNR of burst thus is reduced from that of EPI by a factor of $\sqrt{N}$. Because N is the number of lines measured in k-space, N also is the number of resolved voxels along the y-axis. In other words, as the resolution of the image improves, the SNR of burst becomes even worse compared to EPI. Even for a low-resolution image matrix of 64 voxels, the SNR of EPI is eight times better. The cost of silent imaging is thus a very large hit in SNR.

To see how this factor of $\sqrt{N}$ comes about, we start by imagining that we have a string of optimized RF pulses with flip angle $\alpha_1, \alpha_2, ..., \alpha_N$, each of which produces the same

(continued)

BOX 11, continued

(but unknown) transverse magnetization M_T. The full longitudinal magnetization M is consumed in this process, so the last pulse must put all the remaining longitudinal magnetization into the transverse plane ($\alpha_N = 90°$). The first RF pulse produces a transverse magnetization $M_T = M \sin \alpha_1$, so the ratio of the SNRs of burst compared with EPI is $\sin \alpha_1$. To calculate the optimal flip angles, imagine that we are looking somewhere in the middle of the pulse train. Let the remaining longitudinal magnetization just before the nth RF pulse be M_n. After the nth pulse, the transverse magnetization is $M_T = M_n \sin \alpha_n$, and the remaining longitudinal magnetization is $M_n \cos \alpha_n$. After the next RF pulse, this remaining longitudinal component is tipped over to create a transverse component $M_T = M_n \cos \alpha_n \sin \alpha_n+1$. Equating these two expressions for M_T, the relationship between subsequent flip angles is

$$\sin(\alpha_{n+1}) = \tan(\alpha_n)$$

$$\frac{1}{\sin^2(\alpha_{n+1})} = \frac{1}{\sin^2(\alpha_n)} - 1 \qquad [B11.1]$$

where the second form shows the simple relation in terms of the sine of each flip angle. We can now calculate the string of flip angles by starting with the last, which we know must be $\alpha_n = 90°$. Moving toward the beginning of the train, $1/\sin^2 \alpha_n$ is simply one plus the value for α_n+1. So, the initial flip angle that produces the maximum attainable SNR of burst compared with EPI is

$$\sin(\alpha_1) = \frac{1}{\sqrt{N}} \qquad [B11.2]$$

Consequently, although burst imaging has a number of unique and interesting features, it is not optimal for general fMRI studies because of its intrinsically low SNR. Nevertheless, it is a promising approach for sleep studies or other studies that are incompatible with the loud sounds of EPI.

Echo Planar Imaging

The previous section suggests the diversity and flexibility of pulse sequences for MRI. Virtually every type of imaging has been used in some form of functional MRI experiment. But the most common imaging technique for fMRI at 1.5 T is single-shot EPI, and so it is worth looking more closely at how EPI works. The idea of echo planar imaging was proposed early in the history of magnetic resonance imaging (Mansfield, 1977), but it is only in the last few years that this technique has become widely available. A comprehensive history and survey of current applications of EPI can be found in Schmitt et al. (1998b). Figure 11.7 shows a simplified pulse sequence diagram for a single-shot (EPI) pulse sequence. Because of the rapid gradient reversals, it is not possible to show the full diagram, and the small boxed region is repeated $N/2$ times, where N is the total number of lines measured in k-space. Not shown in this diagram is the preparation module to saturate fat that is almost always

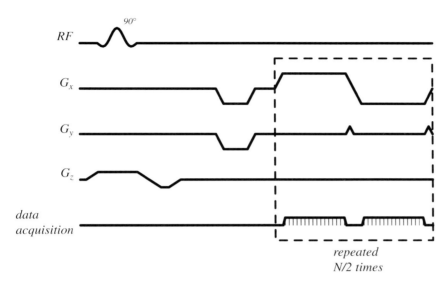

Figure 11.7. Echo planar imaging. The pulse sequence diagram shows the rapidly switched gradient pulses used for a back and forth scanning of k-space. The read-out gradient (x) alternates between positive and negative values, creating a gradient echo at the center of each read-out window. During a constant gradient, the scanning trajectory in k-space is a straight line in k_x, with the sign of G_x determining whether the trajectory moves to the left or the right. The small y-gradient pulses (blips) shift the k-space sampling to a new k_y line, so the full trajectory is as shown in Figure 11.5.

used in EPI. The initial negative gradient pulses in x and y move the location of k-space sampling to $-k_{max}$ on both the k_x- and k_y-axes. After that, the repeated gradient echo module produces a back and forth scanning of k-space. The small phase encoding pulses along y are called *blips*.

EPI requires strong gradients and rapid switching capabilities. A central problem in doing single-shot imaging is that the data acquisition window is limited by T_2^*. If it is much longer than T_2^*, the intrinsic signal will have significantly decayed during data acquisition. The corresponding k-space samples will then be reduced because of the intrinsic decay. Since the later samples are often the larger k samples describing the high spatial frequencies, this amounts to an additional blurring of the image. Such effects are considered in more detail in Chapter 12, but for now the essential problem is that the acquisition window is limited by T_2^* effects to about 100 ms to sample a block of k-space sufficient to reconstruct an image.

From Equation [10.4], the trajectory through k-space depends on the temporal pattern of the applied gradient fields. Under the influence of the gradients, the evolving net signal is a direct measure of the k-space distribution of the image. Choosing a desired field-of-view (FOV) and resolution for the image defines a grid of points in k-space that must be sampled. The total imaging time required then depends on how quickly the sampling point can be moved over the grid in k-space, and this depends on two properties of the gradient coils used for imaging: the maximum gradient strength and how fast the gradient can be changed (Figure 11.8). The

EPI gradient waveform   *k-space trajectory*

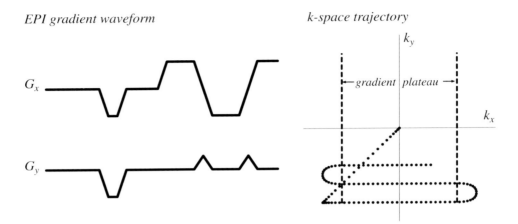

Figure 11.8. The EPI k-space trajectory. The correspondence between the timing of gradient pulses (left) and the k-space trajectory is illustrated for part of an EPI pulse sequence. The dots in k-space show the location of the sampling point at equal time steps to give a sense of the varying speed of the trajectory through k-space. The initial gradient pulses in x and y move the sampling to the left and down, and then the oscillating gradient G_x creates the back and forth motion while the periodic blips in G_y move the sampling to a new k_y-line. The part of the trajectory corresponding to the plateaus of G_x are indicated on the right. Note that, during the ramps, the trajectory extends to larger values of k_x, and these data can also be used if corrections are applied for the different speeds of the k-space trajectory.

gradient amplitude is usually expressed in units of milliTesla per meter (mT/m) or Gauss per centimeter (G/cm, with 1 G/cm = 10 mT/m), and the maximum gradient strength on current MR imagers is typically in the range of 20–30 mT/m. To put the gradient strength in perspective, consider again frequency encoding in which samples from $-k_{max}$ to $+k_{max}$ are acquired during a gradient echo. With stronger gradients, this k-space line can be sampled more quickly, so a natural measure of the maximum gradient strength is the minimum time required to scan over a specified range of k_x. A convenient range is $-k_{max}$ to $+k_{max}$, for the k_{max} needed to achieve a resolution of 1 mm. With a gradient strength of 25 mT/m, the time required to scan one line in k-space equivalent to a resolution of 1 mm is about 1 ms. For increased gradient strength, this number is decreased in proportion; for higher spatial resolution, this time is increased in proportion to the improvement of the resolution.

The second factor that affects the speed of scanning is how fast the gradient can be reversed so that the direction of sampling in k-space can be reversed. There are two common ways of expressing this: the slew rate, which describes the maximum rate of change of the field gradient, usually expressed in Tesla per meter per second (T/m-s), and the rise time, which describes the time required to increase the gradient amplitude from zero to its positive maximum value. Typical numbers for a 1.5-T scanner are a slew rate of 80–120 T/m-s and a rise time of 200–300 µs. These parameters are, of course, related: the maximum gradient strength divided by the rise time is the slew rate. The rise time directly measures how much time must be spent in changing the direction of sampling in k-space. One can think of sampling in k-space as analogous to a car racing along a winding track with sharp turns. The time to complete the circuit depends on both how fast the car moves on the straightaway (governed by the gradient strength) but also on how fast the car can corner (determined by the gradient rise time).

To see more specifically how gradient strength and rise times affect EPI data collection, we can consider the primary gradient waveform used in EPI, the basic oscillating pattern used to collect successive gradient echoes sampling a line in k_x. Between gradient echoes, phase-encoding blips in y are applied to shift the k-space sampling to a new k_y line. Ideally, the oscillation of the x-gradient would be a square wave, but the gradient rise times limit the possible shapes to more rounded forms (Figure 11.8). For example, if the plateau duration is 1 ms and the rise time is 0.3 ms, a total of 1.6 ms is required for each gradient echo. For an image matrix size of N resolution elements, N gradient echoes are required for a full k-space acquisition, giving a total data collection time of 102 ms for a 64×64 matrix.

In the earlier discussion of sampling in k-space, the sampling was done during application of a constant read-out gradient. But because the rise times are typically fairly long, waiting for the gradient to reach the plateau means that data are collected during only a fraction of the time (about 62% in the previous example). This waiting wastes some of the gradient power that is available. One way to think about this is to note that the resolution in x is inversely proportional to the area of the gradient pulse. In the previous example, the area under the full trapezoidal gradient is 30% more than the area under the plateau portion alone. Instead of collecting data only on the gradient plateau, the signal also can be sampled on the ramps to achieve better spatial resolution with the same gradient waveforms. The problem then is that the samples are not uniformly spaced along k_x (Figure 11.8). During the ramps, the sampling point moves more slowly through k-space because the gradient is weaker, so for evenly spaced samples in time, the samples in k-space are bunched together during the ramps. Before applying the FFT to reconstruct the image, the unevenly spaced k-space samples must be interpolated onto an evenly spaced grid. This can slow down the reconstruction time because of the additional computations required. Alternatively, the sampling in time can be adjusted to match the trajectory through k-space, with a longer interval between the samples during the ramps so that the measured samples in k-space are evenly spaced. This scheme requires a longer setup time because the appropriate sampling intervals must be calculated before the sequence is run, but the reconstruction is then faster.

Safety Issues

In conventional MRI, safety concerns related to pulse sequences generally focus on heating the body by the applied RF pulses (Shellock and Kanal, 1996). Each RF pulse deposits energy in the body, and the rate of energy deposition measured in watts per kilogram of tissue is called the specific absorption rate (SAR). The U.S. Food and Drug Administration provides guidelines for the maximum SAR, and calculations of SAR are usually done in the pulse sequence code so that the operator is informed if the RF heating of the prescribed sequence is excessive. The limits on SAR are most critical for fast SE acquisitions, which use many 180° refocusing pulses. The energy of an RF pulse depends on the square of the amplitude of the electromagnetic field, so when the flip angle is changed by altering the strength of the RF field with the duration held constant, the SAR depends on the square of the flip angle. Reduced flip angle GRE acquisitions thus deposit much less energy than SE acquisitions. Ultrafast imaging with EPI acquisitions use fewer RF pulses and so are not significantly limited by SAR guidelines.

In fast imaging with EPI, there are two safety concerns related to the fast gradient switching necessary to scan rapidly through k-space. The first is the very loud acoustic noise associated with fast gradient switching. Magnetic fields exert forces on currents, so when a current is pulsed through the gradient coil, the force flexes the coil and produces a sharp tapping sound. In fact, the gradient coil acts much like a loudspeaker, and the sound level can be as high as 130 dB (Savoy, Ravicz, and Gollub, 1999). For this reason, subjects must always wear ear protection such as ear plugs or close-fitting headphones.

The second safety concern with EPI is nerve stimulation due to the rapid gradient switching, which depends on the gradient strength and the slew rate (Schmitt, Irnich, and Fischer, 1998a). Nerve stimulation can occur when the rate of change of the local magnetic field (dB/dt) exceeds a threshold value (Reilly, 1989). Note that it is not the amplitude of the magnetic field, but rather its rate of change, that causes the problem. A large but constant magnetic field has little effect on the human body, but a changing field induces currents in the body in the same way that a precessing magnetization induces currents in a detector coil. When the current in a gradient coil is reversed, and the gradient strength is ramped quickly between its maximum negative and positive values, the rate of change of the local magnetic field can be quite large.

The value of dB/dt depends on the slew rate and gradient strength, but it also depends on location within the coil. At the center, the coil produces no additional field, so there is nothing to change. The largest field changes are at the ends of the coil, at the maximum distance along the gradient direction.

For imaging applications, only the z-component of the magnetic field matters, and when we refer to a gradient field, we mean the gradient of the z-component. But for considerations of dB/dt, we must also consider the fields perpendicular to z created by the coil. All magnetic field lines must form closed loops, so the field lines running through the coil bend around at the ends of the coil. For example, a transverse y-gradient coil creates a strong field near the ends of the coil running in the y-direction, perpendicular to the main field. When the gradient is pulsed, this perpendicular field creates a large dB/dt. Furthermore, nerve stimulation depends on the electric field created by the changing magnetic field. If we imagine a loop of wire near the end of the coil, the current induced in the loop is proportional to the rate of change of the flux of the magnetic field through the loop and so is proportional to the size of the loop. Thinking of the body as a current loop, the larger the cross section of the body exposed to the changing magnetic field, the larger the induced currents will be. The largest cross section is in the coronal plane. Because the y-gradient produces a magnetic flux change through this plane, the y-gradient is the most sensitive for generating nerve stimulation. For this reason, the y-gradient is generally not used for frequency encoding in EPI (e.g., a sagittal image with frequency encoding in the anterior/posterior direction).

Different governments and agencies have set different regulations on the maximum rate of change of the magnetic field, but generally values of dB/dt below 6 T/m are considered a level of no concern (see Schmitt et al., 1998a, for a review of current guidelines). Note that this limit does not directly limit the slew rate because a shorter coil can operate with a larger slew rate while keeping the maximum dB/dt below threshold (Wong, Bande Hini, and Hyde, 1992). The imaging speed of acquisition techniques such as EPI currently is limited by these concerns about physiological effects rather than hardware performance.

REFERENCES

Atlas, S. W., Hackney, D. B., and Listerud, J. (1993) Fast spin-echo imaging of the brain and spine. *Magn. Reson. Quart.* **9,** 61–83.

Buxton, R. B., Wismer, G. L., Brady, T. J., and Rosen, B. R. (1986) Quantitative proton chemical-shift imaging. *Magn. Reson. Med.* **3,** 881–900.

Chung, Y. C., and Duerk, J. L. (1999) Signal formation in echo shifted sequences. *Magn. Reson. Med.* **42,** 864–75.

Cohen, J. D., Forman, S. D., Braver, T. S., Casey, B. J., Servan-Schreiber, D., and Noll, D. C. (1994) Activation of the prefrontal cortex in a non-spatial working memory task with functional MRI. *Human Brain Mapping* **1,** 293–304.

Dixon, W. T. (1984) Simple proton spectroscopic imaging. *Radiology* **153,** 189–94.

Duyn, J. H., Mattay, V. S., Sexton, R. H., Sobering, G. S., Barrios, F. A., Liu, G., Frank, J. A., Weinberger, D., and Moonen, C. T. W. (1994) 3-Dimensional functional imaging of human brain using echo-shifted FLASH MRI. *Magn. Reson. Med.* **32,** 150–5.

Engel, S. A., Rumelhart, D. E., Wandell, B. A., Lee, A. T., Glover, G. H., Chichilnisky, E.-J., and Shadlen, M. N. (1994) fMRI of human visual cortex. *Nature* **369, 370 [erratum],** 525, 106 [erratum].

Feinberg, D. A., Hale, J. D., Watts, J. C., Kaufman, L., and Mark, A. (1986) Halving MR imaging time by conjugation: Demonstration at 3.5 kG. *Radiology* **161,** 527–31.

Feinberg, D. A., and Oshio, K. (1992) Gradient-echo shifting in fast MRI techniques (GRASE) for correction of field inhomogeneity errors and chemical shift (communication). *J. Magn. Reson.* **97,** 177–83.

Gabrieli, J. D., Brewer, J. B., Desmond, J. E., and Glover, G. H. (1997) Separate neural bases of two fundamental memory processes in the human medial temporal lobe. *Science* **276,** 264–6.

Glover, G. H., and Lee, A. T. (1995) Motion artifacts in fMRI: Comparison of 2DFT with PR and spiral scan methods. *Magn. Reson. Med.* **33,** 624–35.

Haacke, E. M., Mitchell, J., and Lee, D. (1990) Improved contrast using half-Fourier imaging: Application to spin-echo and angiographic imaging. *Magn. Reson Imag.* **8,** 79–90.

Haase, A., Frahm, J., Matthaei, D., Haenicke, W., and Ferboldt, K.-D. (1986) Flash imaging: Rapid NMR imaging using low flip-angle pulses. *J. Magn. Reson.* **67,** 258–66.

Hennig, J., and Friedburg, H. (1988) Clinical applications and methodological developments of the RARE technique. *Magn. Reson. Imag.* **6,** 391–5.

Hennig, J., and Hodapp, M. (1993) Burst imaging. *MAGMA* **1,** 39–48.

Hennig, J., Nauerth, A., and Friedburg, H. (1986) RARE imaging: A fast imaging method for clinical MR. *Magn. Reson. Med.* **3,** 823–33.

Hoppel, B. E., Weisskoff, R. M., Thulborn, K. R., Moore, J. B., Kwong, K. K., and Rosen, B. R. (1993) Measurement of regional blood oxygenation and cerebral hemodynamics. *Magn. Reson. Med.* **30,** 715–23.

Hurst, G. C., Hua, J., Simonetti, O. P., and Duerk, J. L. (1992) Signal-to-noise, resolution and bias function analysis of asymmetric sampling with zero-padded magnitude FT reconstruction. *Magn. Reson. Med.* **27,** 247–69.

Jakob, P. M., Schlaug, G., Griswold, M., Lovblad, K. O., Thomas, R., Ives, J. R., Matheson, J. K., and Edelman, R. R. (1998) Functional burst imaging. *Magn. Reson. Med.* **40,** 614–21.

Kiefer, B., Grassner, J., and Hausmann, R. (1994) Image acquisition in a second with half-Fourier acquisition single shot turbo spin echo. *J. Magn. Reson. Imag.* **4(P),** 86.

Liu, G., Sobering, G., Duyn, J., and Moonen, C. T. W. (1993a) A functional MRI technique combining principles of echo shifting with a train of observations (PRESTO). *Magn. Reson. Med.* **30,** 764.

Liu, G., Sobering, G., Olson, A. W., Gelderen, P. v., and Moonen, C. T. (1993b) Fast echo-shifted gradient-recalled MRI: Combining a short repetition time with variable T2* weighting. *Magn. Reson. Med.* **30,** 68–75.

Lovblad, K.-O., Thomas, R., Jakob, P. M., Scammell, T., Bassetti, C., Griswold, M., Ives, J., Matheson, J., Edelman, R. R., and Warach, S. (1999) Silent functional magnetic resonance imaging demonstrates focal activation in rapid eye movement sleep. *Neurology* **53,** 2193–5.

Lowe, I. J., and Wysong, R. E. (1993) DANTE ultrafast imaging sequence (DUFIS). *J. Magn. Reson.* **101,** 106–9.

Mansfield, P. (1977) Multi-planar image formation using NMR spin echoes. *J. Phys.* **C10,** L55–8.

Moonen, C. T., Liu, G., Gelderen, P. v., and Sobering, G. (1992) A fast gradient-recalled MRI technique with increased sensitivity to dynamic susceptibility effects. *Magn. Reson. Med.* **26,** 184–9.

Moonen, C. T. W., Barrios, F. A., Zigun, J. R., Gillen, J., Liu, G., Sobering, G., Sexton, R., Woo, J., Frank, J., and Weinberger, D. R. (1994) Functional brain MR imaging based on bolus tracking with a fast T2*-sensitized gradient echo method. *Magn. Reson. Imag.* **12,** 379–85.

Mugler, J. P., and Brookeman, J. R. (1990) Three dimensional magnetization prepared rapid gradient echo imaging (3D MP-RAGE). *Magn. Reson. Med.* **15,** 152–7.

Noll, D. C. (1995) Methodologic considerations for spiral k-space functional MRI. *Int. J. Imag. Syst. Tech.* **6,** 175–83.

Noll, D. C., Cohen, J. D., Meyer, C. H., and Schneider, W. (1995) Spiral k-space MR imaging of cortical activation. *J. Magn. Reson. Imag.* **5,** 49–56.

Reilly, J. (1989) Peripheral nerve stimulation by induced electric currents: Exposure to time varying magnetic fields. *Med. Biol. Eng. Comput.* **27,** 101–10.

Savoy, R. L., Ravicz, M. E., and Gollub, R. (1999) The psychophysiological laboratory in the magnet: Stimulus delivery, response recording, and safety. In: *Functional MRI,* pp. 347–65. Eds. C. T. W. Moonen and P. A. Bandettini. Springer: Berlin.

Schmitt, F., Irnich, W., and Fischer, H. (1998a) Physiological side effects of fast gradient switching. In: *Echo Planar Imaging: Theory, Technique and Application,* pp. 201–52. Eds. F. Schmitt, M. K. Stehling, and R. Turner. Springer: Berlin.

Schmitt, F., Stehling, M. K., and Turner, R. (1998b) *Echo Planar Imaging: Theory, Technique and Application.* Springer: Berlin.

Shellock, F. G., and Kanal, E. (1996) Bioeffects and safety of MR procedures. In: *Clinical Magnetic Resonance Imaging*, pp. 391–434. Eds. R. R. Edelman, J. R. Hesselink, and M. B. Zlatkin. Saunders: Philadelphia.

Wehrli, F. W. (1990) Fast-acan magnetic resonance: principles and applications. *Magn. Reson. Quart.* **6,** 165–236.

Wong, E. C., Bandettini, P. A., and Hyde, J. S. (1992) Echo-planar imaging of the human brain using a three axis local gradient coil. In: *Eleventh Annual Meeting, Society of Magnetic Resonance in Medicine,* p. 105: Berlin.

Zha, L., and Lowe, I. J. (1995) Optimized ultra-fast imaging sequence (OUFIS). *Magn. Reson. Med.* **33,** 377–95.

12

Noise and Artifacts in Magnetic Resonance Images

Image Noise
>   Image Signal-to-Noise Ratio
>   The Noise Distribution Depends on SNR
>   Spatial Smoothing to Improve SNR
>   Spatial Correlations in the Noise
>
>   BOX 12: SPATIAL SMOOTHING AND IMAGE NOISE

Image Distortions and Artifacts
> $N/2$ Ghosts in EPI
> T_2* Effects on Image Quality
>   Image Distortion Due to Off-Resonance Effects
>   Motion Artifacts
>   Physiological Noise

IMAGE NOISE

Image Signal-to-Noise Ratio

Chapter 10 described how the local magnetic resonance (MR) signal is mapped with magnetic resonance imaging (MRI). However, noise enters the imaging process in addition to the desired MR signal, so the signal-to-noise ratio (SNR) is a critical factor that determines whether an MR image is useful (Hoult and Richards, 1979; Macovski, 1996; Parker and Gullberg, 1990). The signal itself depends on the magnitude of the current created in a detector coil by the local precessing magnetization in the body. The noise comes from all other sources that produce stray currents in the detector coil, such as fluctuating magnetic fields arising from random ionic currents in the body and thermal fluctuations in the detector coil itself.

The nature of the noise in MR images is critical for the interpretation of functional magnetic resonance imaging (fMRI) data. The signal changes associated with blood oxygenation changes are weak, and the central question that must be addressed when interpreting fMRI data is whether an observed change is real, in the sense of being due to brain activation, or whether it is a random fluctuation due to the noise in the images. This remains a difficult problem in fMRI because the noise has several sources and is not well characterized. Noise is a general term that describes any process that causes the measured signal to fluctuate when the intrinsic NMR signal is stable. In MRI, there are two primary sources of noise: thermal noise and physiological noise. We will begin with the thermal noise because it is better understood and take up physiological noise at the end of the chapter. In many applications, the thermal noise is the primary source of noise, but in dynamic imaging the dominant source of noise often is physiological.

The SNR depends strongly on the radio frequency (RF) coil used for signal detection. A small surface coil near the source of the signal picks up less stray noise from the rest of the body, and for focal studies, such as fMRI experiments measuring activation in the visual cortex, the SNR can be improved by using a well-placed small surface coil for RF detection. The limitation of small coils, however, is that they provide only limited coverage of the brain. The trade-off between small coils for better SNR and large coils for better coverage can be overcome by using multiple small coils in a phased array system (Grant, Vigneron, and Barkovich, 1998). This requires a scanner hardware configuration with multiple receiver channels to accommodate the multiple coils. The result is the SNR of a small coil but with more extended coverage, although the sensitivity pattern of a phased array system is not as uniform as the pattern of a larger head coil optimized for uniformity.

Once the hardware has been optimized to provide the most sensitive detection of the MR signal, the SNR in an image still depends strongly on the pulse sequence used to acquire the data. Three factors affect this pulse-sequence-dependent SNR. The first is the intrinsic magnitude of the generated transverse magnetization M at the time of data acquisition. The flexibility of MR as an imaging modality comes from the ease with which we can manipulate M so that its magnitude reflects different properties of the tissue, as described in Chapters 7–9. Density-weighted, T_1-weighted, and T_2-weighted images all are commonly used, and M is manipulated to reflect these weightings by adjusting pulse sequence parameters such as the repetition time TR and the echo time TE. The maximum value of M is M_0, the local equilibrium magnetization. With higher magnetic field strengths (B_0), M_0 increases because of the greater alignment of spins with the field. Because M_0 sets the scale for the magnitude of M, the SNR improves with increasing B_0, and this is a primary motivation for the development of high field MRI systems.

The second factor that affects the SNR is the voxel volume, ΔV. When more spins contribute to the local signal, we would naturally expect the SNR to be larger. But from the discussion of the point spread function (PSF) of the image in Chapter 10, the voxel volume may appear to be a somewhat slippery concept. Intuitively, we would like to be able to look at one point in the reconstructed image and interpret the intensity there as an average of the signals over a small volume ΔV. In general, however, the reconstructed signal at a point has contributions from the entire image plane, defined by the PSF, although the reconstructed intensity is certainly dominated by the nearby signals. The definition of voxel volume is thus somewhat approximate, describing the volume that contributes most of the signal to the intensity at a point in the image. A useful definition of voxel volume is to treat it as a rectangular block with dimensions on each side equal to the corresponding resolution on each axis, giving a volume ΔV. In the same fashion, we earlier defined the resolution along an axis as the equivalent width of a rectangular PSF with the same central value as the actual PSF. For the standard sinc-shaped PSF due to a rectangular window in k-space (Equation [10.5]), the resolution is the distance from the center to the first zero-crossing. The voxel volume is then the product of these resolution dimensions along each of the three spatial axes. This view, although only a rough approximation, is useful for manipulating data, such as reslicing a 3D block of data to construct a new plane. But it is important to remember that a rectangular block is only a crude picture of the resolution of an MR image. The true resolved volume has a more complicated appearance described by the PSF in each of the directions.

Finally, the third factor that affects the SNR of a voxel is the total time spent collecting data from that voxel. The total time, T, depends on the length of the data acquisition window, the number of repetitions of the acquisition required to sample k-space, and the number of averages performed for each of the sampled points in k-space. Specifically, if the pulse sequence is repeated n times in collecting data for the image, and the acquisition time on each repetition is T_{acq}, then $T = nT_{acq}$. The SNR is then

$$\text{SNR} \propto M\,\Delta V\,\sqrt{T} \qquad\qquad [12.1]$$

This expression is written as a proportionality because the absolute number depends on the coil configuration used. Equation [12.1] is useful for describing how changes in the pulse sequence will affect SNR for the same coil setup. The SNR is directly proportional to the intrinsic signal M and the volume of tissue contributing to each voxel, ΔV, both of which are intuitively clear. The SNR is also proportional to the square root of the time spent collecting data, a dependence that is familiar from averaging data, in which the SNR increases with the square root of the number of averages.

It may seem surprising that the expression for SNR is as simple as this. Imaging pulse sequences use different gradient strengths and data sampling rates, and yet these parameters do not enter directly into the expression for SNR. In fact, these parameters are important, and one can look at SNR from the point of view of the bandwidth associated with each voxel. For example, using a stronger frequency-encoding gradient produces a larger spread of frequencies across the field-of-view (FOV) and so associates each voxel with a larger bandwidth (Figure 12.1). Noise enters uniformly at all frequencies, with a net amplitude proportional to the square root of the bandwidth, and so the larger bandwidth means that more noise enters each voxel. But to produce the same voxel size in the image (i.e., the same sampling in k-space), the signal during the stronger read-out gradient would have to be sampled more rapidly because the relative phases of signals at different locations would be evolving more rapidly, and the total data collection time would be reduced. This is why we can represent the SNR just in terms of the total time spent collecting data. All the manipulations of the gradients and sampling rates that modify the band-

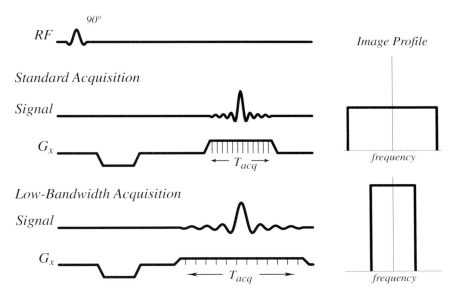

Figure 12.1. Changing the image acquisition time. The diagrams show two forms of the read-out gradient pulses used for frequency encoding that measure the same points in k-space (left). In the low-bandwidth version, the gradient amplitude is reduced, and the time between samples is increased so that the area under the gradient between samples is held constant. With a weaker gradient, the signal from the object being imaged is spread over a narrower range of frequencies (right). Because noise enters the data uniformly at all frequencies, the SNR is improved with the low-bandwidth sequence.

width per voxel, for the same image resolution, simply translate into a change in the data acquisition time. A pulse sequence that uses a longer read-out time with a reduced gradient amplitude to improve SNR is often called a low-bandwidth sequence.

Equation [12.1] explains some features of MRI that are not immediately obvious. An important practical question is whether averaging the k-space samples for an image with a small FOV gives a better SNR than collecting more k-space samples to image a larger FOV. Consider two images of the same plane, made with the same resolution. In the first image, the FOV is 20 cm measured with 128 phase-encoding steps, and each phase-encoding step is measured twice to improve the SNR. In the second image, the FOV is 40 cm measured with 256 different phase-encoding steps, with each step measured only once. Then the total time required to collect each image is the same (both acquisitions collect a total of 256 phase-encoding steps), and the resolution is the same. In the second image, the head appears smaller in the frame because the FOV is larger, but it is a 256 matrix compared to the 128 matrix of the first image. The central 128 matrix from the second image is then identical to the first image in imaging time, FOV, and resolution. Which image has the higher SNR? Naively, it seems that in the second image the extra work done by the additional phase-encoding steps was to provide an extensive view of the empty space around the head, data that seems irrelevant to the central image of the brain. The first image seems somehow more tightly focused on imaging the head, and so it seems plausible that averaging this more critical data should provide a better SNR. But in fact, the SNR is identical in the two images, as shown by Equation [12.1]. The voxel volume is the same, and the total time spent collecting the data is the same. In short, using different phase-encoding steps instead of repeating a more limited set for the same resolution exacts no cost in SNR and yet provides an image of a larger FOV.

The Noise Distribution Depends on SNR

In MRI each measured signal intensity during data acquisition corresponds to a sample in k-space, as described in Chapter 10. Our goal now is to understand how random noise in the measured k-space samples produces noise in the reconstructed image intensities. Each k-space sample can be thought of as a complex number with a real and an imaginary component, and independent noise is added to each component. To clarify the nature of the noise in a concrete way, consider a simple one-dimensional (1D) imaging experiment in which 128 samples are measured in k-space, with the data reconstructed as a 512-point 1D image. Furthermore, suppose that the intensity profile being imaged is perfectly flat in the middle and somewhat rounded at the edges so that the Gibbs artifact is not important, as illustrated in Figure 12.2. The ideal, noiseless image is shown as a dashed line, and an image with noise is shown as a solid line. Subtracting the two gives an image of just the noise

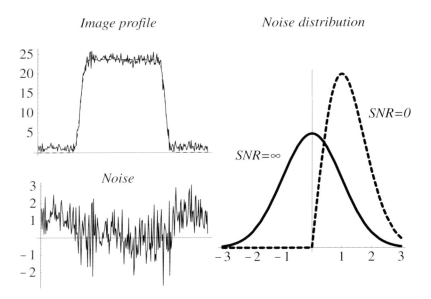

Figure 12.2. Noise in MR images. Noise added to the measured k-space samples is transformed into noise in the reconstructed images. A 1D profile of a magnitude image illustrates how the noise appears different in regions of high SNR (top left) and in the background air space with no intrinsic signal (bottom left). For normal Gaussian noise in the k-space data, the noise in a magnitude image is approximately Gaussian for high SNR but distinctly non-Gaussian when the SNR is low (right).

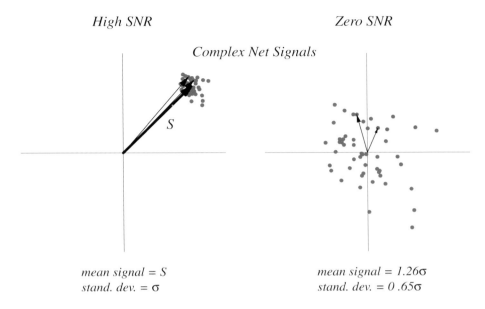

High SNR   *Zero SNR*

Complex Net Signals

S

mean signal = S   mean signal = 1.26σ
stand. dev. = σ   stand. dev. = 0 .65σ

Figure 12.3. Noise in magnitude images. The full net signal reconstructed in each pixel is a complex number, and noise in the measured *k*-space samples adds independently to each of the complex components (the variability of the measured vector due to noise is shown as gray dots). In a magnitude image, the pixel intensity is the magnitude of this complex number. For high SNR, only the noise component along the intrinsic signal vector contributes, so the image noise has a mean of zero and a standard deviation σ. However, when there is no intrinsic signal, as in the air space around the head, the mean of the noise is 1.26σ instead of zero (because there are no negative magnitudes) and the standard deviation is 0.65σ (see distributions in Figure 12.2).

component, amplified in Figure 12.2 to make it clearer. The first effect to notice is that the noise looks different outside the object than it does inside. Inside, the noise has a mean of zero, and the distribution of values around zero has a standard Gaussian shape. But outside the object, the noise distribution is distinctly non-Gaussian, and the mean is not zero.

This peculiar behavior is due to the fact that we have reconstructed a *magnitude* image. When the image is reconstructed with the Fourier transform (FT), the noise signals in each component of the *k*-space signal are transformed into noise in the real and imaginary components of the image. The net signal in a reconstructed voxel is then the sum of the intrinsic MR signal and the complex noise signal, and we can think of this as adding two vectors in the complex plane (Figure 12.3). When the SNR is large, a small random noise vector is added to a large signal vector. In this case, only the component of the noise along the direction of the intrinsic signal vector contributes significantly to changing the magnitude of the net vector, and the fluctuations of any one component of the noise are normally distributed with a mean of zero. As a result, the distribution of measured magnitudes is centered on the intrinsic magnitude and normally distributed. But when the SNR is zero, there is no intrinsic signal, just a small randomly oriented noise vector in the complex plane. In the magnitude image, the measured pixel value will be the length of this random vector. But the distribution of the lengths of a random vector in a plane is very different from a Gaussian. The magnitude can never have a negative amplitude, and the probability that the net vector will have a length near zero is small. If the standard deviation with high SNR is σ, then in the background of the image, where there is no intrinsic signal, the mean is 1.26σ and the standard deviation is 0.65σ.

In short, the noise distribution in the image is Gaussian only when the SNR is high. In practice, for an SNR > 10, the assumption of a Gaussian distribution is a reasonable approximation, although it is good to remember that, strictly speaking, this is only true for infinite SNR. This also illustrates that one must be careful when estimating the amplitude of the noise from measurements in the background air space of the image. The mean of the background is not zero, but this does not mean that an offset has been added to every point in the image; when the SNR is high, there is no offset of the mean. Furthermore, either the background mean or standard deviation can be used to estimate the noise in an image, since both are proportional to σ, but the measured values must be appropriately scaled as described above to measure the σ appropriate for the high SNR parts of the image.

Spatial Smoothing to Improve SNR

In most imaging applications, the raw signal-to-noise ratio is sufficiently high that the alterations of the noise distribution associated with working with a magnitude image are negligible, and we can assume a normal distribution for the noise. The raw SNR is given by Equation [12.1] and depends on the image voxel size and the time spent collecting data from that voxel. In fMRI applications, the goal is to be able to identify small changes in the signal, so to improve the SNR of each voxel measurement, the images are often further smoothed in postprocessing. In Chapter 10, the effect of smoothing in postprocessing on spatial resolution was considered. Smoothing with a function $w(x)$ is equivalent to multiplying the k-space distribution by a windowing function $W(k)$, the Fourier transform of $w(x)$. Smoothing worsens the spatial resolution, and the resolution distance is increased in proportion to the reduction in area under $W(k)$ compared with the original rectangular sampling window in k-space (see Figure 10.17). Then, for example, a rectangular sampling window extending out to only $k_{max}/2$, or a Gaussian window with $\sigma = 0.404\ k_{max}$, both reduce the area under the windowing function by a factor of 2, and so double the resolution distance. Both of these smoothings should improve the SNR at a point as well, but by how much?

To answer this question, we need to separate the effects of smoothing on the intrinsic signal itself and on the noise. The effect of smoothing on the intrinsic signal depends on the size and uniformity of the object. So for now we will restrict the question just to the noise component: what is the effect of smoothing on the random noise component added to the signal in a pixel? And to further simplify matters, we will continue to consider 1D imaging. Based on our intuitive understanding of averaging, we might naively expect that the noise should be reduced by the square root of the increase in the resolution distance. But the behavior of the noise turns out to be somewhat subtle (see Box 11). The improvement in the noise amplitude does not depend

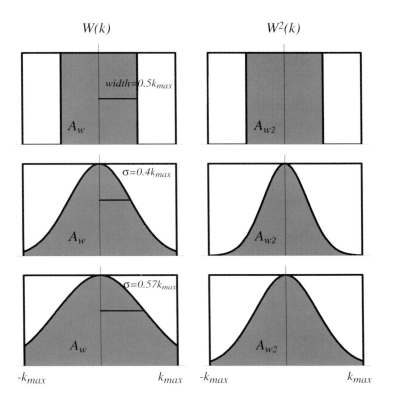

$W(k)$ $W^2(k)$

$$resolution\ distance\ =\ 1/A_w$$

$$noise\ correlation\ distance\ =\ 1/A_{w2}$$

$$SNR\ =\ SNR_0\sqrt{A_{w2}}$$

Figure 12.4. Effect of image smoothing on resolution, noise correlations, and SNR. Smoothing an image is equivalent to multiplying the k-space data by a windowing function $W(k)$. In these examples, the original window due to k-space sampling is shown as a rectangle with amplitude one extending from $-k_{max}$ to k_{max}. With smoothing, the change in the resolution distance is determined by A_w, the fractional area under $W(k)$ compared with the area of the original rectangular sampling window. However, the noise correlation distance and the SNR depend on A_{w2}, the fractional area under $W^2(k)$. For a rectangular window, $A_w = A_{w2}$ (top row), but for a Gaussian window (or any window other than a rectangle), the two are different. The Gaussian window that increases the resolution distance by a factor of 2 (middle) is narrower than the Gaussian window that increases the correlation distance by a factor of 2 (bottom).

on the area under $W(k)$, which governs how the resolution changes with smoothing, but rather on the area under $W^2(k)$ (Figure 12.4). For rectangular windows, this distinction does not matter because the amplitude of the rectangle is one: the square of the window function then is the same as the function itself. So, if the image is smoothed by multiplying k-space by a narrower rectangle (i.e., by simply deleting the samples corresponding to high spatial frequencies), the SNR improves by the square root of the increase in the resolution distance, in agreement with our naive intuition, that doubling the resolution distance decreases the noise by $\sqrt{2} \cong 1.41$.

Multiplying k-space with a rectangular window is equivalent to smoothing the image with a sinc function (Equation [10.5]). But smoothing with any other function will affect the noise differently. For example, a Gaussian window has a value of one at the center of k-space, but less than one at all other points (Figure 12.4). That is, this window modifies the amplitudes in k-space, rather than eliminating some of them entirely as with the rectangular window. The curve $W^2(k)$ is then narrower than $W(k)$. For the Gaussian with $\sigma = 0.404k_{max}$, the area under $W(k)$ is reduced by a factor of 2, but the area under $W^2(k)$ is reduced by a factor of about 2.8. Thus, the resolution distance is increased by a factor of 2, but the SNR is increased by $\sqrt{2.8} \cong$ 1.67. The differential effect of smoothing on resolution and noise comes about because the postprocessing smoothing changes the shape of the point spread function. If the new PSF were the same shape as the original (i.e., if the new window is a narrower rectangle), the noise change would be inversely proportional to the square root of the resolution change. But the Gaussian window alters the shape as well as broadening the PSF, and the result is that the benefit of improved SNR is greater than one might naively expect given the cost in loss of resolution.

These considerations of the effects of smoothing on resolution and noise bring us to an important issue. Spatial smoothing occurs in the imaging process itself due to the finite range of k-space sampling, but it can also be applied in postprocessing. If the goal is to maximize the SNR for a given spatial resolution, what is the most efficient way to collect and process the data? Consider three strategies for producing a 1D image with a given resolution in a fixed data acquisition time: (1) acquire an image with resolution twice as good as needed, and then smooth the image with a sinc function to increase the resolution distance by a factor of 2; (2) acquire the same image, but smooth with a Gaussian to achieve the same resolution distance; or (3) acquire an image with the desired resolution, and since this only takes half as long as the first two, acquire it again, average to reduce the noise, and do no postprocessing. These three strategies produce images with the same resolution in the same total data acquisition time, but which has the best SNR? To begin with, let the raw SNR in the images acquired with better resolution than is needed be SNR_0, and we can then see how each strategy improves it. For strategy 3, there is no smoothing in postprocessing, but the raw voxel size is larger by a factor of 2, so by Equation [12.1], $SNR_3 = 2\, SNR_0$. For strategy 1, smoothing with a sinc function to increase the resolution distance by a factor of 2 increases SNR by $\sqrt{2}$, so $SNR_1 = 1.41\, SNR_0$. In fact, smoothing with a sinc function is equivalent to throwing away the outer k-space samples (windowing with a narrower rectangle), so the final k-space sampling locations are identical to those acquired with strategy 3. But whatever time was spent collecting those large k samples was wasted, and so strategy 3 is more efficient. Finally, strategy 2 produces $SNR_2 = 1.67\, SNR_0$, as discussed earlier, and so is intermediate between the other two strategies.

In short, collecting data sufficient to produce a high-resolution image, and then smoothing it to the desired coarser resolution, is an inefficient way to improve SNR. It is better to collect only the data required for the desired resolution, and then to use the extra time to average that data. This seems to contradict the argument made earlier concerning acquisition of extra k-space data to increase the FOV. There we argued that, for constant resolution, acquiring extra points in k-space to reconstruct an image with a larger FOV produced the same SNR as an image with a smaller FOV that was averaged for the same total time. The argument was that in both cases the total acquisition time T in Equation [12.1] was the same. But here we are arguing the opposite for acquiring extra k-space samples to reconstruct an image with better spatial resolution, that the SNR of the smoothed image is degraded compared to what it could have been by focusing only on the desired k-space samples.

The root of this apparent paradox is whether the extra k-space samples are higher or lower than the desired k_{max}. The extra samples that increase the FOV are between the original samples, and so for all these samples, $k < k_{max}$. The samples that improve resolution beyond what is desired are all high spatial frequencies with $k > k_{max}$. All k-space samples with $k < k_{max}$ contribute to the SNR, whereas samples with $k > k_{max}$ are wasted. One way to think about this is to imagine that we are imaging a single small cube with the dimensions of the desired voxel (i.e., $1/(2k_{max})$) and to examine the amplitude of each of the measured samples of the signal by considering the sine wave pattern across that cube corresponding to different values of k. For low values of k, the wavelength is longer than the voxel dimension, so all the signals within the voxel add approximately coherently, and the signal is strong. The image reconstruction process then adds up each of these signals, so each contributes to the SNR in a way equivalent to simple averaging. But for high values of k, corresponding to wavelengths smaller than the voxel dimension, there is substantial phase variation within the voxel, and so the net signal is greatly reduced. If we imagine averaging these signals with the others, they do not improve the SNR. They add very little of the intrinsic signal and yet contribute noise to the average.

So, in general, spatial smoothing in postprocessing is a poor strategy for improving SNR. Nevertheless, it is often done for practical reasons. For example, the available pulse sequences on the MR scanner may not allow complete control over these parameters. Also, in the preceding example comparing a Gaussian smoothed high-resolution image with an acquired and averaged low-resolution image, the final resolution distance is the same, but the images are not identical because the point spread functions have a different shape. The Gaussian smoothed image shows much less of a Gibbs artifact (see Figure 10.17). Furthermore, a Gaussian smoothed image may be easier to work with when considering the statistical correlations of noise in the image. For example, in fMRI, to improve the sensitivity for detecting small signal changes, clustering algorithms that look for several nearby pixels activated together are sometimes used. The rationale for this is that the probability of several adjacent pixels all showing spurious activations due to noise is much more unlikely than a single pixel showing the same magnitude of random signal change (Lange, 1996; Poline et al., 1997). But to interpret the significance of clusters of activated pixels, it is necessary to understand how the noise is correlated between one pixel and another. The statistical analysis of Gaussian random fields is well developed, so Gaussian smoothing will put the images closer to a more convenient form (Friston, 1996). But it is important to remember that choosing such a strategy, of significant smoothing in postprocessing, makes a sacrifice in the SNR that could be attained by optimizing the image acquisition instead.

Spatial Correlations in the Noise

The preceding arguments considered the noise that appears in one pixel of the reconstructed image. That is, if we repeated the 1D experiment in Figure 12.2 many times, looking at the noise values at one pixel, we would find SNR-dependent distributions like those shown. In particular, if we look just at the high SNR plateau, the noise is normally distributed. However, we can reconstruct the image with as many pixels as we like, and clearly the noise in two adjacent pixels cannot be entirely independent. Intuitively, we would expect that N samples in k-space, each with an independent noise contribution, could lead to no more than N independent noise signals in the image. In an image reconstructed with the pixel size smaller than the intrinsic resolution, there will be correlations of the noise in nearby pixels. The practical effect of noise correlations becomes clear when we try to average the data on the plateau. For example, for two independent measurements of the same intrinsic signal, we expect the noise samples to add incoherently, so the net increase in the noise component is only $\sqrt{2}$, whereas the intrinsic signal doubles. The SNR then improves by $\sqrt{2}$. But if the noise samples are correlated, they add more coherently, and the improvement in SNR is not as great. In the extreme case of perfectly correlated noise, there is no improvement with averaging at all.

To be specific, suppose that our goal is to measure the average value of the signal on the plateau in Figure 12.2 by averaging all the pixel values covering a distance range R in the image. Assume that there are M pixels in this range and that the average signal-to-noise ratio in a pixel is SNR_0. If the noise in each of the pixels is independent, then the SNR of the average will improve by $SNR_{av} = \sqrt{M}\, SNR_0$. For correlated noise, we can use this relation to define an effective number of independent points, M_{eff}, such that the actual improvement in SNR with averaging is by a factor $\sqrt{M_{eff}}$. We can then use this to define an effective correlation distance, $x_{corr} = R/M_{eff}$. With this definition, averaging pixels over a range R improves the SNR in proportion to $1/\sqrt{x}_{corr}$.

In the raw acquired MR image, the correlation length is equal to the resolution length. If the image is reconstructed with the number of pixels equal to the number of samples in k-space, the separation between adjacent pixel centers is one resolution element, and the noise in each pixel is independent. Averaging over M pixels will then improve the SNR by a factor of $\sqrt{M}$. If the image is then smoothed in post-processing by applying a windowing function $W(k)$ in k-space, then both the resolution distance Δx and the correlation distance x_{corr} increase. However, just as we found earlier for the change in resolution and SNR, the increase in these two distances is not the same (see Box 12 and Figure 12.4). The resolution distance depends on the area under $W(k)$, but the correlation distance depends on the area under $W^2(k)$. That is, the correlation distance and the SNR both depend on the area under the *square* of the window function. If $W^2(k)$ decreases the area by a factor of 2, then the correlation distance increases by a factor of 2, and the SNR in one pixel increases by $\sqrt{2}$.

The fact that changes in the correlation distance and the SNR improvement with smoothing should be closely connected makes intuitive sense: more averaging both

BOX 12. SPATIAL SMOOTHING AND IMAGE NOISE

The noise in MR images is a critical concern in fMRI experiments where the signal-to-noise ratio is often the limiting factor in detecting brain activation. For this reason, the images are often smoothed, which improves the SNR but also introduces correlations in the noise of nearby pixels. There are two practical effects of the noise correlations. First, adding up the signals of nearby voxels, as is done in a region of interest (ROI) calculation, does not improve the SNR as much as it would if the noise in each voxel were independent. And second, the likelihood of clusters of nearby pixels showing false activation due to noise is greater than it would be if the pixel noise were independent. To understand how spatial smoothing of the images affects the SNR and the noise correlations in a quantitative way, we can examine a simplified case of 1D imaging.

Consider a 1D imaging experiment in which we measure N points in k-space covering the range $-k_{max}$ to $+k_{max}$. We assume that the object we are imaging has a strong signal of its own so that the noise inside the object will have a Gaussian distribution. In other words, we can think of imaging the object with a rectangular profile shown in Figure 12.2, and we will only look at noise on the plateau. We can further simplify the problem by assuming that the local precessing magnetization at each point in the object is in-phase so that the image is entirely real. In this way, we can focus just on the real part of the Fourier transform in calculating the image from the k-space samples. Then for each point in k-space, there are two measured numbers, the real and imaginary parts of the measured signal, and to each of these components a random noise signal is added. (We need to consider both the real and imaginary parts of the k-space measurement because both will contribute to the real part of the image.) For the sample at k_j, we will call the noise signal in the real component n_j and the noise in the imaginary component m_j, with all of the n_j and m_j independent of each other and normally distributed with a mean of zero and a standard deviation of σ. Finally, after data collection, the raw data is postprocessed by multiplying by a windowing function $W(k)$, and we will use W_j to indicate the value of $W(k)$ at sample j.

The first question then is: how do these noise samples in k-space translate into the noise in a particular pixel? The Fourier transform is linear; so the FT of the noise component is simply added to the FT of the object itself. And since we have simplified matters by assuming that the object is real, then we are only interested in the real part of the transform given in Equation [10.1]. But this equation is represented as a continuous transformation, and what we have are discrete samples in k-space. There is a standard mathematical transform, called the discrete Fourier transform, that converts one string of sampled numbers into another string of discrete numbers with the same length, and this is the calculation actually performed by the FFT. But for now we want something between the continuous FT and the discrete FT to emphasize the fact that a limited set of samples in k-space provides an estimate of the image intensity at *every* point x, and not just at a set of discrete samples. So, for this argument, we will approximate the integral as a sum but allow x to take on any arbitrary value.

From the basic equation for the Fourier transform (Equation [10.1]), the real part of the noise signal in the reconstructed image has two contributions: the real part of the

(continued)

BOX 12, continued

noise in the sample at k_j weighted with a cosine function and the imaginary part weighted with a sine function. Because we have only measured k-space between $-k_{max}$ and $+k_{max}$, the limits of the integral in Equation [10.1] are replaced with these values. The integral can then be approximated by a sum over the measured samples, with a spacing $\Delta k = 2k_{max}/N$ between samples, as

$$I_n(\mathrm{x}) = \Delta k \sum_{j=N/2+1}^{N/2} W_j n_j \cos{(2\pi j \, \Delta k \, x)} + \Delta k \sum_{j=N/2+1}^{N/2} W_j n_j \sin{(2\pi j \, \Delta k \, x)} \qquad [\text{B12.1}]$$

where $I_n(x)$ is the noise signal at position x in the reconstructed image. The variance of the image noise in a pixel can then be calculated from the expected value of this noise signal squared. Because the noise values n_j and m_j are independent, the expected value of any product of different ns and ms is zero, and the expected value of n^2_j and m^2_j is σ^2. Then the variance of the noise in an image is

$$\sigma_x^2 = \langle I_n^2(x) \rangle = \Delta k \sum_{j=N/2+1}^{N/2} W^2_j \left[\cos^2{(2\pi j \, \Delta k \, x)} + \sin^2{(2\pi j \, \Delta k \, x)} \right] \qquad [\text{B12.2}]$$

But the term in brackets is always one. Furthermore, we can identify in this expression the area under the square of the windowing function,

$$A_{w^2} = \int_{-\infty}^{\infty} W^2\,(k)\,dk = \Delta k \sum_{j=N/2+1}^{N/2} W^2_j \qquad [\text{B12.3}]$$

That is, A_{w^2} is the area under the net window squared, where the net window is a combination of a rectangular window from $-k_{max}$ to $+k_{max}$ multiplied by some other smoothing window (such as a Gaussian). Then the noise variance in the image is simply

$$\sigma^2_x = \sigma^2 \, \Delta k \, A_{w^2} \qquad [\text{B12.4}]$$

It is helpful to consider the dimensions of the terms in Equation [B12.4]. An image intensity $I(x)$ is a measure of signal density; so its dimensions for this 1D example are signal/length, and the noise σ_x should have the same dimensions. The intrinsic noise σ has signal dimensions, and Δk has dimensions of 1/length. The area under the window $W(k)$ is proportional to k and so also has dimensions of 1/length; consequently, the dimensions of σ_x are correct for a signal density. We can emphasize the role of spatial dimensions by substituting the intrinsic resolution set by the k-space sampling, $\Delta x_0 = 1/(2k_{max}) = 1/N\,\Delta\,k$, and the distance associated with the area under the window, $x_{corr} = 1/A_{w^2}$. Then the noise can be expressed as

$$\sigma^2_x = \frac{\sigma^2}{N \, \Delta x_0 \, x_{corr}} \qquad [\text{B12.5}]$$

The inverse of A_{w^2} is called x_{corr} because it turns out that this is the characteristic separation in x between noise signals that are uncorrelated (discussed in more detail later). If the windowing function is simply a rectangle between $-k_{max}$ and $+k_{max}$ (i.e., if no further smoothing is done), then $x_{corr} = 1/(2k_{max}) = \Delta x_0$, but for any other window $x_{corr} > \Delta\,x_0$. (We are only concerned with windows that are one at the center; more peculiar windows, such as an edge enhancement filter that suppresses the samples near $k = 0$ fall outside of this framework because they produce a point spread function that does not have a unit area.)

To see why x_{corr} is the characteristic correlation distance of the noise, consider what happens when we average the signals of many pixels together. Specifically, suppose that we image an object with a rectangular profile and, to begin with, perform no smoothing in postprocessing and reconstruct the image with the pixel size equal to the resolution, Δx_0. Then the resulting noise signals in the N pixels are all statistically independent (uncorrelated). (One can demonstrate this by using the expression for $I(x)$ in Equation [B12.1] to calculate the correlation of two noise signals separated by a distance δx explicitly and to show that the correlation is zero when $\delta x = \Delta x_0$.) We can now average together the signals from M contiguous pixels on the plateau of the image profile. The intrinsic signal is the same for all pixels, so averaging will not change it. But we expect the average noise signal to be reduced, and because the noise is independent in each pixel, σ_x should be reduced by a factor $\sqrt{M}$. Now suppose that we first smooth the data and then perform the same calculation, averaging the values for M pixels on the plateau. If we are averaging pixels over a much larger range than the characteristic width of the smoothing function, the fact that we have smoothed the data first should not affect the variance of the final average. Before smoothing, x_{corr} is equal to Δx_0, so the smoothing will reduce σ_x by a factor of $\sqrt{x_{corr}/\Delta x_0}$ by Equation [B12.5], and the subsequent averaging will further reduce σ_x by a factor of $\sqrt{M_{eff}}$. We have introduced M_{eff} here to describe the fact that if the noise signals being averaged are partially correlated by the smoothing, then we would expect there to be less of a reduction in σ_x on subsequent averaging. But the final average should come out the same with either approach (i.e., smoothing first and then averaging should not make much difference as long as x_{corr} is still much smaller than $M \Delta x_0$, the range we are averaging over). So the net reduction in σ_x should be the same, which implies that $M_{eff}/M = \Delta x_0/x_{corr}$. In other words, if we average over a range R of x in the image containing M pixels (i.e., $M = R/\Delta x_0$), the actual number of statistically independent points is $M_{eff} = R/x_{corr}$, and so x_{corr} is the typical noise correlation distance in the image.

This argument is meant to demonstrate the practical significance of the length x_{corr}. In fact, the full noise correlations between pixels must be described by a full correlation function. But it is often useful to have a practical definition of the correlation distance. The argument used here is similar to the argument used in Chapter 10 to define resolution, which also requires a full function (the point spread function) to define fully the contributions from different spatial locations to the signal measured at a point. In analyzing the effects of smoothing, two length scales naturally emerge: $1/A_w$ and $1/A_{w2}$. We have shown how $1/A_w$ can be interpreted as a characteristic resolution distance, in terms of how the signal of a point source changes with smoothing. In a similar fashion, we argued that $1/A_{w2}$ can be interpreted as a characteristic noise correlation distance in terms of the degree of improvement of SNR to be expected from averaging signals from different pixels.

It is interesting that smoothing the image has different effects on resolution and noise correlation. To summarize the arguments here and in the main text, we can think of three characteristic distances in the image: (1) the intrinsic resolution Δx_0, set by the initial

(continued)

BOX 12, continued

acquisition in k-space; (2) the final resolution Δx after smoothing with a windowing function $W(k)$; and (3) the noise correlation distance x_{corr} resulting from applying $W(k)$. These three distances are

$$\Delta x_0 = \frac{1}{2 k_{max}}$$

$$\Delta x = \frac{1}{A_w}$$ [B12.6]

$$x_{corr} = \frac{1}{A_{w2}}$$

where A_w is the area under $W(k)$ and A_{w2} is the area under $W^2(k)$. If no postprocessing is done, these three distances are the same, and if $W(k)$ is rectangular in shape, these three distances change by the same amount. But if, for example, k-space is multiplied by a Gaussian window with $\sigma_w = 0.57\, k_{max}$, then $\Delta x \cong 1.5\, \Delta x_0$, and $x_{corr} \cong 2\, \Delta x_0$. From the preceding arguments, the reduction in image noise follows the change in correlation length rather than the change in resolution, so SNR is improved by $\sqrt{2}$ in this example. The changes in the three lengths are different because smoothing with any function $W(k)$ other than a rectangle changes the shape of the point spread function.

improves SNR and increases spatial correlations in a direct way. Consider again the earlier example of smoothing with a sinc or a Gaussian function to increase the resolution distance by a factor of 2. Smoothing with a Gaussian gave a greater increase in SNR but would also produce a correspondingly greater increase in the correlation distance. For any smoothing function, the improvement in SNR is the square root of the increase in the correlation distance.

IMAGE DISTORTIONS AND ARTIFACTS

N/2 Ghosts in EPI

One of the most common image artifacts encountered in fMRI studies with EPI are faint ghost images shifted by half an image (Figure 12.5). Specifically, the ghost appears as an image of the head shifted in the phase-encoded direction by $N/2$ pixels, where N is the number of resolved voxels along this axis (we will refer to the phase-encoded axis as y even if it is not the vertical axis of the image). The half of the ghost shifted out of the image frame is wrapped around to the other side of the image. This artifact illustrates a useful way of thinking about how artifacts arise in MRI; we will use this way of thinking throughout this chapter. To understand the artifact, we examine how the sampling in k-space has been affected. For the EPI ghost, the problem arises from the way the lines in k-space are sampled. With EPI, the k-space trajectory is a back and forth motion, with the k-space sampling moving

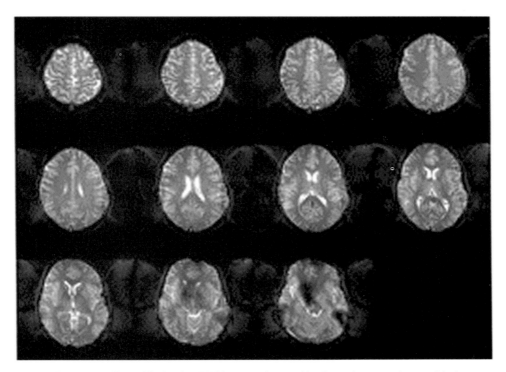

Figure 12.5. EPI artifacts. Single-shot EPI images of several brain sections are shown with the gray-scale window set to reveal the weak ghosts in the background. Any systematic effect that causes alternate lines in k-space to differ produces $N/2$ ghosts, an image of the brain shifted by half an image frame and wrapped around the other side. The inferior images also show signal dropouts due to magnetic susceptibility variations and a resulting shortening of T_2^*. (Data courtesy of E. Wong.)

to the left for one line and back to the right for the next line. This alternation in scanning direction can lead to a systematic difference between the odd and even lines in k-space. For example, if the gradients are not precisely balanced, the gradient echo can be displaced from the center of data acquisition in each read-out period. Furthermore, if the gradient echo occurs earlier when the odd k_y-space lines are collected, it will occur later when the even lines are collected. Alternating lines in k_y then are consistently different.

We can think about this periodic modulation of the k-space samples by imagining the full data to consist of a true set of k-space samples that accurately reflect the true image plus another set that consists of the true k-space values multiplied by another function $A(k)$. That is, the first set are the correct values, and the second set is the error set that will produce an artifact in the image. The Fourier transform used to reconstruct the image is linear, so the image is the sum of the separate images of these two sets of k-space samples. The true set of samples produces the correct image, but added to this is the artifactual image. Then we can look at the formation of the artifact just as we earlier looked at smoothing (convolution) in the image domain as a multiplication by a windowing function $W(k)$. The resulting artifactual image is the convolution of the true image with the FT of $A(k)$.

For the case of the $N/2$ ghosts, the effect of multiplying by $A(k)$ is to produce a modulation in k_y that alternates with each line. We can see the general form of the FT of $A(k)$ just from the nature of the k-space description and the symmetry of the FT. If we were to reverse domains, and instead look at a periodic modulation of the image domain, we know that a pattern repeating with every other line in the image is in fact the highest spatial frequency component in the image, and it is described by a single point at the maximum value of k_y in the k-space domain. Then because the FT is symmetric, the FT of a pattern that alternates with each line in k_y is a single point at the maximum value of y (i.e., at the edge of the image). And the convolution of the true image with a spike (a δ function) at the edge of the image simply moves the image to be centered on the spike. In other words, the artifactual ghost image is shifted by half of the image frame.

Note that this type of ghost could arise from any effect that causes alternate sampled lines in k-space to vary. The structure of the artifact is directly related to the periodicity in k-space. In the following, we examine a number of sources of artifacts in terms of how they affect the k-space data.

T_2^* Effects on Image Quality

Turning back now to the intrinsic SNR due to image acquisition itself, Equation [12.1] suggests that the raw SNR can be improved by lengthening the data acquisition time, T_{acq}. Consider again the prototype measurement of a gradient echo to sample one line in k-space, as illustrated in Figure 12.1. The data acquisition window can be lengthened, while maintaining the same spatial resolution and FOV, by reducing the gradient strength and sampling the signal more slowly in time. The relative phase changes induced by the weaker gradient evolve more slowly, so the total time needed to sample the same points in k-space is increased. Halving the read-out gradient and the data sampling rate and doubling the acquisition window would yield the same sampling in k-space, but with SNR improved by $\sqrt{2}$ due to the longer acquisition time. By the SNR argument alone, using even weaker gradients and longer acquisition times would continue to improve the image SNR. But two other effects become important as the data acquisition window is increased: relaxation effects and off-resonance effects.

As the data acquisition time is increased, we begin to come into direct conflict with one of the basic assumptions of MRI, that the MR image is a snapshot of the distribution of transverse magnetization at one instant of time. This cannot be perfectly true because some time is required to allow the applied field gradients to induce local phase changes, which creates the sampling in k-space. To be more precise, the basic premise of MRI is that the intrinsic local magnetization has a constant amplitude during data acquisition so that the measured signal changes are all due to the controlled interference of these signals induced by the gradients, and not due to changes in the intrinsic signals themselves. This is a good approximation if the acquisition time is much less than T_2^*, the apparent transverse relaxation rate for a voxel. But as the acquisition time is increased, relaxation effects can cause a signal change unrelated to the effects of the gradient pulses. Because the signal measured over time is interpreted as samples in k-space, relaxation effects alter the k-space data. In this way, they act like a natural filter, analogous to the applied filter for smoothing discussed earlier. Relaxation effects thus alter the windowing function in k-space and so modify the point spread function. In the extreme case of using a data acquisition window much longer than T_2^*, the PSF is dominated by T_2^* effects rather than the applied gradients. Although large values of k_{max} are measured, if the intrinsic signal has decayed away by the time these samples are measured, the associated amplitude in k-space is near zero. The high spatial frequencies are then suppressed, and the image is blurred. For this reason, T_2^* sets a practical upper limit for the data acquisition time.

The blurring effect of T_2^* signal loss during data acquisition is, in fact, somewhat subtle. In most acquisitions, the k-space trajectory moves from $-k_{max}$ to $+k_{max}$, with the $k = 0$ sample measured in the center of the acquisition window. The high positive k-values are attenuated relative to the intrinsic signal at the time of the $k = 0$ sample due to T_2^* decay. But the samples for negative k-values are enhanced relative to the $k = 0$ sample, in the sense that the intrinsic signal has not decayed as much when these samples are measured. The added windowing function in k-space due to T_2^* decay thus is not symmetric around the $k = 0$ sample. This effect is illustrated in Figure 12.6. In effect, the amplified negative large k-values partly offset the diminished positive large k-values so that the blurring for $T_{acq} = T_2^*$ is not very significant. For $T_{acq} = 3T_2^*$, the point spread function is more severely distorted.

The apparent transverse relaxation rate is a somewhat ill-defined number. The true, intrinsic T_2 is the natural decay time for transverse magnetization, and although it depends on the type of tissue, it does not depend on the size of the imaging voxel. But T_2^* includes both intrinsic relaxation and the effects due to field inhomogeneity, and the latter effects can depend on the voxel size. For example, magnetic susceptibility differences between tissues can produce broad field gradients running through the head. A larger voxel lying in this intrinsic field gradient will include a wider range of frequencies; consequently, the spins contributing to the net signal from the voxel will get out of phase with one another more rapidly, producing a shorter T_2^*. This effect can be seen in the lower images in Figure 12.5 showing transverse cuts through the brain near the sinus cavity. The susceptibility difference between the sinus (air) and the brain (water) produces broad field gradients. The magnitude of signal dropouts depends on the slice thickness, the orientation of the frequency and phase-encoding gradients (Figure 12.7). With thick slices, there is substantial signal dropout due to short T_2^*. With thinner slices, T_2^* is longer, and signal dropout is less of a problem. For gradient echo (GRE) acquisitions, signal dropouts are more severe than with spin echo (SE) acquisitions because the SE refocuses the phase dispersion due to field offsets. An asymmetric spin echo (ASE) is intermediate between an SE and a GRE acquisition. Note that the SE acquisition can also contain strong signal fluctuations independent of the T_2^* effects due to image distortions (discussed later).

The problem of signal dropouts with thicker slices illustrates the complicated effect of voxel size on the SNR. From Equation [12.1], the SNR is directly proportional to the voxel volume, so an increase in the voxel size should increase SNR. However, the effective T_2^* of a voxel tends to decrease with increasing voxel size as

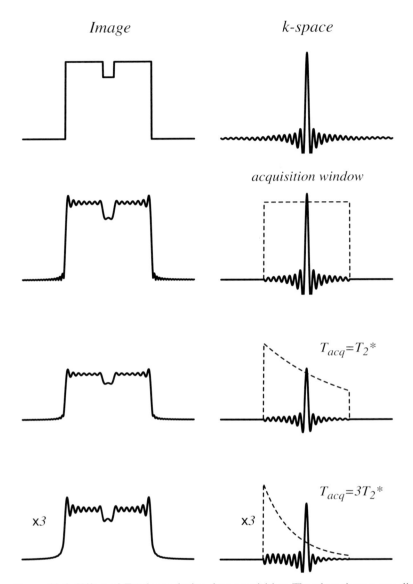

Figure 12.6. Effect of T_2^* decay during data acquisition. The plots show a one dimensional image space (left) and the corresponding k-space (right). The true shape of the imaged object is described by an infinite range of k-space (first row), so the finite rectangular acquisition window introduces some ringing (Gibbs artifact) in the reconstructed image (second row). If the intrinsic signal decreases during acquisition by T_2^* decay, the effect on the image is equivalent to smoothing with an asymmetric window in k-space. With the acquisition time T_{acq} equal to T_2^* (third row), there is little additional effect on the image except for the overall reduction of the amplitude by a factor e^{-TE/T_2^*}, where TE is the time of the center of acquisition when the $k = 0$ sample is measured. For $T_{acq} = 3T_2^*$, the distortion of the resulting image is more severe (fourth row).

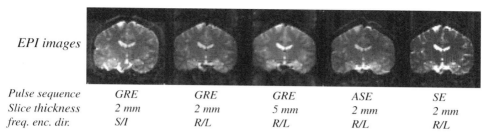

EPI images					
Pulse sequence	*GRE*	*GRE*	*GRE*	*ASE*	*SE*
Slice thickness	*2 mm*	*2 mm*	*5 mm*	*2 mm*	*2 mm*
freq. enc. dir.	*S/I*	*R/L*	*R/L*	*R/L*	*R/L*

Figure 12.7. Signal dropouts in EPI. In regions of susceptibility variation, short T_2^* can produce signal dropouts, as in the areas near the sinus cavities and the temporal lobes. Examples are shown for gradient echo, asymmetric spin echo, and spin echo acquisitions. The severity of the dropouts depends on slice thickness and the orientation of the frequency-encoding gradient. (Data courtesy of E. Wong.)

spins with a wider range of precession frequencies are included in the net signal. For example, if the field varies linearly across the voxel, the range of field offsets would double if the voxel size doubled. The shorter T_2^* with larger voxels tends to decrease the SNR. Because of this conflict, the optimal voxel size for maximizing SNR depends on the part of the brain under examination.

Relaxation effects thus have two separate, though related, effects on the reconstructed image: the local signal mapped to each point is attenuated due to T_2^* decay, but in addition the larger k-space samples are attenuated by signal decay during data acquisition, leading to blurring in the image. These two effects are somewhat separable: signal dropout depends primarily on the echo time TE when the $k = 0$ sample is measured, whereas the additional blurring due to T_2^* depends on the length of the data acquisition time T_{acq}. For example, if the shortest T_2^* is around 30 ms, then an image made with a 10-ms acquisition window centered on TE = 100 ms will show signal reductions due to T_2^* decay, but minimal blurring due to T_2^*. But when the data acquisition time is longer than the T_2^* values of the tissues, as it often is in echo planar imaging (EPI), the local T_2^* affects the local spatial resolution as well. One can visualize the full effect of this by imagining breaking up the full image plane into multiple image planes segregated on the basis of local T_2^*. For example, as a first approximation, we can imagine a slice through the brain to consist of three separate images of cerebrospinal fluid (CSF), gray matter, and white matter, each characterized by a different T_2^*, and the full image is the sum of these three images. We could then further subdivide the image based on variations in T_2^* within a tissue type, such as gray matter or white matter near the sinus cavities with reduced T_2^*. Then we can look at the effect of T_2^* on each of these subimages separately. In each case, the relaxation effects modify the k-space samples and so alter the PSF. Then the imaging process produces a convolution of each of the subimages with its appropriate, T_2^*-dependent PSF, and the net reconstructed image is then the sum of the individually blurred subimages. In general, short local T_2^* will reduce the later measured samples in k-space, and because these are large k samples for most k-space sampling trajectories, this produces additional blurring of the image. In areas where T_2^* is very short, the signal may drop out completely. The result is that the net reconstructed image is blurred in a nonuniform way, with the most blurring in the regions with short T_2^*, and with signal dropouts in regions with very short T_2^*.

Image Distortions Due to Off-Resonance Effects

As the data acquisition time is increased, off-resonance effects, in addition to T_2^* effects, become important. Like the T_2^* effects described in the previous section, these artifacts can be viewed as arising because a basic premise of MRI is violated. In this case, the assumption is that all spins precess at the same rate in the absence of the applied gradients. Then any relative phase changes that develop during data acquisition are due entirely to the effects of the gradient fields and so are directly related to the location of the signals. Any intrinsic resonant frequency offset thus leads to errors in localizing the signal.

The primary example of a resonance offset in the body is the 3.5-ppm resonant frequency difference of fat and water protons. This is a chemical shift effect, resulting from the partial shielding of the nucleus by electronic molecular orbitals, so that when placed in the same magnetic field B_0, the hydrogen nuclei in lipids feel a slightly different magnetic field and so precess at a slightly different rate than do the hydrogen nuclei in water. Although the frequency difference is only a few parts per million, this is sufficient to produce large errors in the localization of fat relative to water. In brain imaging, there is usually no detectable fat signal from the brain itself. Although myelin consists of lipids, the highly structured environment of the myelin creates a very short T_2 for the lipid protons, so any signal generated in an imaging experiment has decayed away by the time the imaging data are measured. So, in imaging of the head, the measurable fat signal arises from the skull marrow and the scalp.

The artifact that results can be understood by again considering the basic gradient echo measurement of one line in k-space (Figure 12.1). Position along the axis of the gradient is frequency encoded, so any intrinsic frequency offset will appear as a location offset. The image of fat is thus shifted along the frequency-encoded axis relative to water. In a conventional image, the shift typically is about two resolution elements because the frequency offset between fat and water is about twice the bandwidth per resolution element. This chemical shift artifact can be reduced by increasing the bandwidth per resolution element sufficiently so that the shift is less than the resolution, but this hurts the SNR. In practice, for conventional clinical imaging, the radiologist simply learns to recognize the chemical shift artifact and, in some cases, even to make use of it. The appearance of the artifact tends to highlight the boundaries between fatty tissues and tissues composed mostly of water. At a fat/water boundary, this can appear as a dark edge, if the fatty tissue is moved away from the water, or as a bright edge, if the fat signal from one tissue is moved on top of the water signal from the adjacent tissue so that the fat and water signals add.

However, in EPI off-resonance artifacts are much more of a problem. In EPI, successive lines in k-space are sampled in the k_x-direction with successive gradient echoes, with a phase-encoding pulse along the y-direction inserted between the gradient echoes to shift the sampling to a new value of k_y. The gradient amplitude for the x-gradient echoes is usually quite large, so the displacement of fat along the *x*-direction is much less than the resolution and so is not apparent. Instead, there is a large shift of fat along the phase-encoded *y*-direction. The nature of off-resonance effects in EPI at first glance seems puzzling. The off-resonance of fat in a conventional image is a small displacement of the image of fat along the frequency encoded direction, but in EPI the effect is a large displacement of fat along the phase-encoded direction. To understand how this comes about, we need to look at off-resonance effects in a slightly different way.

In conventional MRI, the intrinsic MR signal is created fresh for each phase-encoding step. Spins that are off-resonance acquire additional phase offsets as time evolves, but this unwanted phase evolution is reset before each new phase-encoding step because a fresh signal is generated with each new excitation pulse. There is no phase evolution across phase-encoding steps; whatever phase offsets are present when the signal is measured after the first phase-encoding step are the same for all the steps. And a constant phase offset simply appears in the phase of the reconstructed image and has no effect on the magnitude image. Conventional phase encoding thus is insensitive to errors due to off-resonance effects, and the chemical shift artifact appears as a pure shift in the frequency-encoded direction alone. But in single-shot EPI, all *k*-space is sampled after one intrinsic MR signal is generated. The phase offsets due to off-resonance effects are not reset before each phase-encoding pulse, and because the phase-encoding blips are spread throughout the data acquisition period, there is time for substantial unwanted phase offsets to accumulate. Think of the blipped phase encoding done in EPI as equivalent to frequency encoding using a very weak gradient during the entire acquisition time with widely spaced samples. That is, the series of sharp gradient pulses, with a data sample after each pulse, is equivalent to a continuous gradient with the same integrated area between samples as the blipped gradient. Because the equivalent gradient is so weak, the bandwidth per resolution element is small, and the shift of the fat image along *y* is many resolution elements.

The magnitude of the off-resonance effect can be characterized in terms of how much time is required to scan completely through one axis in *k*-space. In EPI, for example, a single pass through the k_x direction might require about 1 ms, whereas a full pass through k_y might take about 60 ms (the full data acquisition time T_{acq}). Now consider the signals from two positions separated by one resolution element in *x*. In moving from the $k_x = 0$ sample to the $k_x = k_{max}$ sample, the gradient-induced relative phase between these two signals is 180°, so after a full pass along k_x from $-k_{max}$ to $+k_{max}$, the induced phase offset is 360°. We can use this to calibrate the off-resonance effect, relating the observed shift in the image to the amount of artifactual phase evolution due to off-resonance precession. The fat is shifted by one resolution element for each 360° of phase evolution during the time required to sample from $-k_{max}$ to $+k_{max}$, and the same argument applies to both the frequency-encoded and the phase-encoded directions. For fat at 1.5 T, the 3.5-ppm frequency offset is about 220 Hz. Then, during a 1-ms scan through k_x, the additional phase evolution is only 0.22 cycles (79°), and so the displacement in the image is only 0.22 resolution elements along *x*. But if a full scan from $-k_{max}$ to $+k_{max}$ in *y* requires 60 ms, the extra phase accumulation of the fat signal is 13.2 cycles, and so the fat image

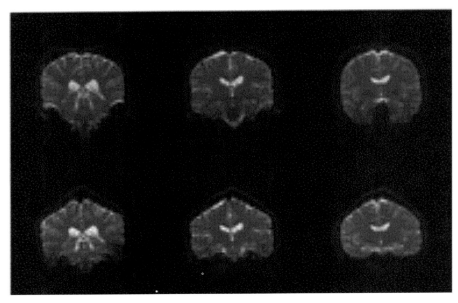

Figure 12.8. Off-resonance distortions in EPI. Coronal single-shot EPI images for three slices (columns) are shown. The phase-encoding gradient is vertical, but reversed in direction in row 2 compared with row 1 (compare with rows 3 and 4 of Figure 12.9). Note the vertical shift of the temporal lobes and the distortion of the top of the head. (Data courtesy of E. Wong.)

is shifted about 13 resolution elements in y. For an image with only 64 total resolution elements across the FOV, this is a substantial shift.

This discussion has focused on the chemical shift artifact due to fat and water, but the arguments also apply to other sources of off-resonance precession, such as field inhomogeneities due to magnetic susceptibility differences. Unlike chemical shift effects, which involve pure resonant frequency offsets, field inhomogeneities generally produce smooth field variations, resulting in image distortions (Figure 12.8). We can picture the full effect of image distortions similar to the way that we earlier described the effects of T_2^* variation across the image plane by considering the full image to be a sum of subimages corresponding to one value of T_2^*. Now we want to divide the full image into subimages corresponding to different field offsets. Then each of these planes is shifted along the phase-encoded axis (y) in an EPI acquisition in proportion to its field offset, and the resulting reconstructed image is then the sum of each of these separately shifted images. As described earlier, the shifts along the y-axis are proportional to the data acquisition time T_{acq} and also to the main magnetic field strength B_0. Magnetic susceptibility differences between tissues create magnetic field offsets that are proportional to B_0, so it is convenient to define a dimensionless number ν, such that the field offset $\Delta B = B_0 \nu$. Typical field offsets in the brain due to inhomogeneous tissues are on the order of 1 ppm, and so ν is expressed in parts per million. With B_0 expressed in Tesla and the acquisition time T_{acq} expressed in seconds, the local signal is shifted Δy pixels in an EPI image (assuming one pixel is equal to the true resolution) given by

$$\Delta y \text{(pixels)} = 42.6 \, B_0 \, (T) \, v \, \text{(ppm)} \, T_{acq} \, \text{(s)} \qquad [12.2]$$

The magnitude of the distortions in EPI images is proportional to the main magnetic field and to the total data acquisition time. The magnitude of v is determined by the shape and composition of the human head and is not affected by field strength. Equations [12.1 and 12.2] illustrate the central conflict involved in trying to achieve both high SNR and minimal distortions. The distortions can be minimized by decreasing T_{acq}, but this also decreases SNR. Similarly, increasing the magnetic field strength increases the intrinsic SNR but also increases the magnitude of the distortions. Thus, there is always a trade-off between SNR and image distortion, and the optimal balance depends on the part of the brain being imaged. In the parietal and occipital lobes, the field is reasonably uniform, so SNR in these regions can be improved with a longer T_{acq} at the expense of increased distortions in the frontal and temporal lobes.

One further complication results from these distortions of the image. In the preceding thought experiment of adding up a stack of shifted subimages each corresponding to a different field offset, each subimage is a complex image. With a gradient echo acquisition, the signal from each subimage also develops a phase offset proportional to the field offset and the echo time. When the subimages are added back together, these phase offsets can produce signal cancellation, and thus affect how the net signal mapped to one pixel location evolves in time. This effect on the net signal at a point is described as a T_2^* effect, but this argument emphasizes that the nature of T_2^* effects is subtle. The signals that are combined in one pixel of the image and interfere to cause T_2^* signal loss do not necessarily arise from the same location! Field inhomogeneities thus affect both image distortions and T_2^* effects in a complicated way.

Figure 12.9 illustrates how field inhomogeneities lead to distortions, signal dropouts, and T_2^* effects. It shows simulations for a simple spherical object, representing the head, containing a smaller spherical cavity near the bottom, representing a sinus cavity. The cavity creates a dipole field distortion throughout the head, and the upper left figure shows contours of the field offset ΔB. The strength of the dipole field was chosen to give $\Delta B = 1$ ppm of B_0 at the upper pole of the cavity. This is a modest field distortion, and for conventional imaging the distortions are minor. But for EPI the distortions are substantial, as shown in the simulated images. In these simulations, it was assumed that the x- and z-coordinates of the local signal are accurately mapped, and it is only the y-position that is mismapped. In each example, images are shown for an SE acquisition and a GRE acquisition, to bring out the two distinct effects of field distortions: (1) signals are mapped to the wrong locations in both SE and GRE acquisitions; and (2) in GRE imaging, there is an additional T_2^* effect due to phase cancellation of signals from different locations mapped to the same voxel. In these simulations, we have neglected any T_2^* effects due to slice thickness, such as those illustrated in Figure 12.7, to show the effects that come just from the mismapping in y. In these examples, the intrinsic signal is uniform, and any variations of intensity in the SE images are due to a bunching or spreading of the mapped locations of the individual signals (i.e., a distortion of the voxel shape). In the GRE images, the additional effects of phase cancellation are included. The com-

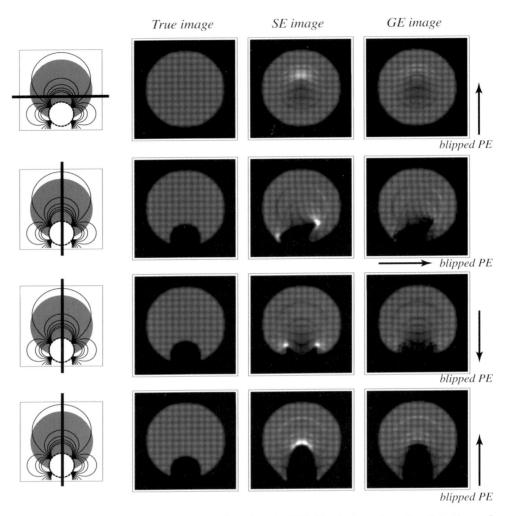

Figure 12.9. Simulation of off-resonance distortions in EPI. Simulations show the distortions of EPI images of a sphere (representing the head) with a smaller off-center spherical air space inside (representing a sinus cavity). The magnetic field distribution and imaging plane are shown in the first column, the second column is the true (undistorted) image, the third column is the spin echo image, and the fourth column is the gradient echo image. The distorted maps were calculated by appropriately shifting each local signal along the blipped phase-encoded direction, indicated by the arrows. For the GRE images, the phase of each local signal was included in the calculations, so the GRE image shows signal dropouts in addition to the distortions exhibited by the SE images. Grid lines indicate the distortions of the local voxel shapes.

mon pattern is that the field distortions will create some bright spots in the SE images where signals are bunched together, but these same areas will often show signal reductions in the GRE image because spins from a wider range of fields are interfering. There are thus two sources of signal dropouts in GRE images illustrated here: a dispersion of the signal into a wider area, which lowers the intensity of both SE and GRE images, and a T_2^* effect due to phase variations within the voxel.

The nature of the distortion is quite simple in principle but rather complicated in appearance. For a positive field offset, the signal is shifted toward the positive end of the y-gradient axis, so the distortion depends on the direction of the gradient and also its sign (i.e, the order of collection of k-space samples in k_y). The top row shows axial images collected just above the cavity. At all points, the field offset is positive, and the central points are shifted the most. The second and third lines show the distortions when the blipped gradient is horizontal and vertical, respectively, and the fourth row shows the effect of reversing the gradient. Note that reversing the sign of the gradient has a significant effect. In the GRE image in the third row, the regions near the sinus cavity are distorted but measurable because the dominant displacement is down, spreading out the signals. But with the sign of the gradient reversed (bottom row), the regions near the sinus cavity are shifted up, bunching the signals together, and the net signal is largely gone due to phase cancellation.

If the image signal is not lost due to signal dropouts, it is possible to unwarp the spatial distortions in EPI images by measuring a magnetic field map for each slice with a GRE pulse sequence and using Equation [12.2] to estimate the expected shift. With a GRE sequence, the phase evolution due to field offsets is not refocused, so the phase change between images with two different echo times directly reflects the field offset. Because the distortion is directly related to the local field offset, this provides the needed information to unwarp the EPI images (Jezzard and Balaban, 1995; Reber et al., 1998). However, it should be noted that there are limits to what can be corrected. If the signals from two regions are mapped to the same voxel, it will not be possible to separate the two contributions. Often, however, the distortion is a smooth local stretching, and unwarping works reasonably well.

The preceding arguments emphasize the trade-offs between SNR and image distortions in EPI acquisitions. Increasing the acquisition time can improve SNR, but this beneficial effect must be balanced against the costs of increased distortions and signal dropouts. The latter may entirely offset the nominal SNR gain, just as increasing the slice thickness will increase SNR in a uniform field, but the decrease of T_2^* due to broad field gradients across the voxel may nullify the SNR improvement. For fMRI at higher fields, the problems of distortions and signal dropouts are a serious concern.

Motion Artifacts

Any motion during the acquisition of an MR image will produce artifacts (Wood and Henkelman, 1985). Such motions include subject movement, such as head motion, coughing or swallowing, and physiological motions such as pulsatile blood flow, CSF motions, and respiratory motions. In a conventional MR image motion artifacts appear as a ghosting or diffuse blurring that extends along the phase-encoded direction over the full FOV of the image. Note that this is distinctly different from motion artifacts in other imaging settings, such as photography. With a camera, any motion while the shutter is open produces a blurred image on the film, but the blurring extends only over the range of motion of the object, not over the whole frame.

In MRI, any motion during the image acquisition means that the different samples in k-space are inconsistent with one another. If a subject tips his head slightly in the middle of a scan, the early k-space samples are appropriate for an image of the head in the first position, but the later samples are consistent with the new position. Each k-space sample describes a wave extending across the entire image plane, and so inconsistencies in the sampling can lead to artifacts over the full FOV. For example, with a consistent set of k-space samples, the contributions of all the different wave patterns cancel outside the head and add constructively inside the head to give a clear brain image. But if the samples are inconsistent, the cancellation outside the head is incomplete, and so the artifacts can appear far removed from the moving tissues themselves.

In conventional MRI, motion artifacts are spread out in the phase-encoded direction. The reason the frequency-encoded direction is little affected is that each data line in k_x is collected quickly (i.e., in about 8 ms), so most motions are frozen during this short interval, and all the collected samples are consistent with the same image. But the time between k_y samples (i.e., the time TR between phase-encoding steps) is much longer, and so the inconsistencies that arise in the k-space data are between different k_y-lines.

If the motion is periodic, such as pulsatile flow in blood vessels, the artifacts can appear as distinct ghosts rather than just as a blurring. Figure 12.10 shows an example of a conventional axial FLASH image with TR = 0.25 s, windowed to expose the line of ghosts arising from the sagittal sinus. The two largest ghosts are about 80 resolution elements on either side of the sagittal sinus. The spatial shift of the ghosts depends on how the heart rate compares to the repetition time TR. To see how such ghosts arise, consider again how the sampling in k-space is done in conventional imaging. Each k_x-line is measured after a separate RF excitation pulse, and the lines at different values of k_y are measured in order from $-k_{max}$ to $+k_{max}$ with a time interval TR between each measurement. Suppose that the signal from a blood vessel varies sinusoidally with the frequency of the heart rate. If the heart beats once per second, then the measured samples in k-space representing the image of the vessel will have an additional sinusoidal modulation in the k_y-direction. For example, with a TR of 0.5 s, the modulation is very rapid, alternating with each k_y-line. If the TR is 1.0 s, the scanning is effectively gated to the heart rate and so there is no modulation of the k-space samples. But if the TR is 1.1 s, there is a slow modulation of the k_y samples because the sampling is slightly off in frequency from the heart rate. If the first k_y sample is synchronous with a heartbeat, the next sample 1.1 s later will occur 1/10 of the way into the next heart cycle, and each subsequent sample will occur an additional 1/10 of the way into the heart cycle. The modulation period for the k_y samples is then 10 s, because that is how long it will take for another measured sample to fall on the same phase of the heart cycle. This is another example of *aliasing*, in which a high-frequency oscillation appears to be a much lower frequency in a set of measured samples because the sampling frequency was too low. (Aliasing also leads to the wraparound effect associated with the field-of-view, as described in Chapter 10.) The critical sampling frequency, called the Nyquist frequency, required to detect accurately a maximum frequency f_{max} is $2f_{max}$. In this example, the TR of

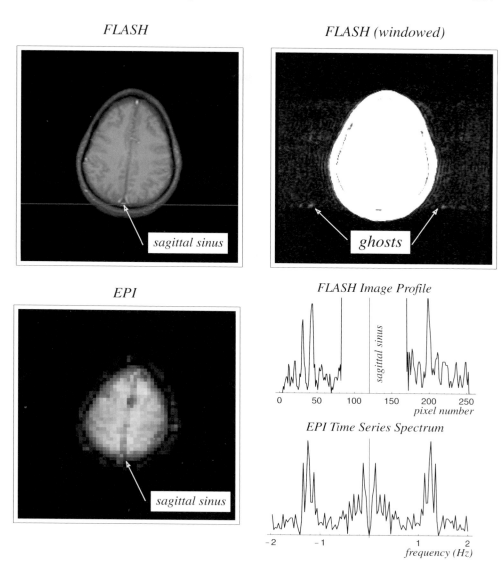

Figure 12.10. Physiological motion artifacts. Pulsatile flow in the sagittal sinus creates ghost images of the vessel in a conventional FLASH image acquired in 32 s with TR = 250 ms, 128 phase-encoding steps (along a left/right axis), and reconstructed as a 256 matrix (so one resolution element is 2 pixels) (top). The spectrum of a dynamic time series of EPI images of the same section acquired with the same TR for an equal period of time show strong cardiac components at about 1.2 Hz. The ghosting pattern in the FLASH image is directly related to the spectrum of the fluctuations (bottom right).

0.5 s (2-Hz sampling rate) critically samples the heart rate with a period of 1 s (1 Hz), but in the other cases, the heart frequency is aliased to a lower frequency. When the TR is the same as the heart period, the apparent heart rate in the data is shifted to zero frequency, and when TR is 1.1 s the apparent heart rate is shifted from a frequency of 1 Hz to a frequency of 0.1 Hz.

The effect of a periodic signal variation during a conventional MRI acquisition is, thus, to create a periodic modulation of the k-space samples. But a periodically varying signal looks exactly like a constant signal arising from a displaced position along y. We can look at this effect in the same way we looked at distortions in EPI images due to field inhomogeneities. The signals from two voxels separated by one resolution element will acquire a phase difference of 360° between the first k_y-line and the last. So any signal varying periodically will be shifted in the image by one resolution element for each 360° of phase evolution during data acquisition. Note, though, that this phase evolution is between k-space samples, so the apparent periodicity with aliasing taken into account is important (e.g., if TR is equal to the heart period, there are no artifacts). The practical result of these arguments is a simple rule for the displacement of the ghost. If the period of the pulsation is T, and there are N phase-encoding steps separated by a time TR in the image acquisition, then the shift of the ghost image in resolution elements is N TR/T. This relation holds, even if the heart rate is not critically sampled, if the shift is understood to mean the total number of pixels shifted, such that a shift past the edge of the FOV is wrapped around to the other side (aliased). Returning to the example of Figure 12.10, a shift of 40 pixels out of a FOV of 128 pixels with TR = 250 ms is consistent with a heart period of 0.8 s (a heart rate of 75 beats/min).

In this simple example, we considered the blood signal to consist of a constant average term plus one oscillatory term. In fact, these are just the first two terms of the Fourier series expansion of the blood signal in terms of temporal frequencies. The contributions of higher harmonics of the signal could also be included, and these terms would create additional ghosts. These terms correspond to higher frequency modulation of the k-space samples, and each will be shifted in proportion to the frequency (i.e., the ghost from the second harmonic is shifted twice as far as the ghost from the first harmonic of the fundamental frequency). The result is that the temporal FT of the local signal during data collection is transformed into a string of ghost images in the image domain. The correspondence between the pattern of ghosts and the Fourier spectrum of the time variations is illustrated in Figure 12.10. In addition to the conventional image showing the ghosting pattern from the sagittal sinus, a set of dynamic EPI images were also acquired in the same subject. The FT of the temporal variation of the sagittal sinus signal agrees reasonably well with a profile through the conventional FLASH image showing the ghosting pattern. (The EPI and the FLASH data were acquired in separate runs, so the spectrum of fluctuations is not identical.)

In this example, we considered the case in which the signal variation is characterized by a fundamental frequency and its harmonics, which produces distinct ghosts. But neither cardiac pulsations nor respiration are truly periodic, and so we would expect that the more general case of signal variation is described by a Fourier series with contributions from many frequencies. The ghosting pattern is then a more diffuse spread of signal along y. This same effect, in which the signal from a voxel is spread out in space in the image depending on the temporal FT of the local signal, happens for every point in the image, and the net image is then the sum of the spread-out image of each of the local signals.

In fact, this brings us back to the same way of looking at imaging and image artifacts that we have used throughout this chapter. The effect of any process on an MR image can be analyzed by looking at how the k-space representation of the true image is modified. Earlier we used this idea to understand the effects of finite k-space sampling, smoothing the images in postprocessing, and distortions due to field offsets. This is simply the generalization of that idea to any temporal variation of the signal during data acquisition that modifies the k-space samples. But it is important to remember that with motion artifacts, as with distortions due to field inhomogeneity, we are no longer dealing with a global windowing function applied to the full image data. Instead, the image of each point in the object is spread out in a way that depends on the FT of the signal from that point. The signal from another point, with a different temporal pattern of signal variation, will produce a different pattern of ghosts. The full image with motion artifacts is then the sum of the spread-out signals from each of these points. Understandably, the resulting image can be severely degraded, and even though the source of the ghosting patterns can sometimes be easily recognized (such as pulsatile flow artifacts), motion artifacts are often uninterpretable in practice.

Physiological Noise

The previous section dealt with the nature of the motion artifacts that can occur in conventional imaging. Such artifacts can completely destroy the diagnostic value of the image, and this has been a primary motivating factor in the development of fast imaging techniques. If the total acquisition time is short, it is easier for the subject to hold still. And if the imaging time is short enough, the most problematic physiological motions (cardiac and respiratory) are essentially frozen. With EPI and total data acquisition times of 30–50 ms, there are virtually no motion artifacts.

But fMRI studies are based on dynamic imaging, so a single image is not sufficient. With contrast agent studies, rapidly repeated images are required to follow the kinetics of the contrast agent. In Blood Oxygenation Level Dependent (BOLD)-fMRI studies, dynamic images are acquired over several minutes while a subject alternates between task and control states. In these applications, we must deal with a time series of images, and although each image is free of motion artifacts, fluctuations in the local signal over time now appear directly as shot-to-shot variations of the local signal (as in Figure 12.10). In other words, the temporal variation of the local signal in a time series of EPI images will have a noise component due to physiological motions in addition to the standard thermal noise discussed earlier (Glover and Lee, 1995).

In the broadest sense, this physiological noise includes outright subject movement in addition to effects of cardiac and respiratory motions. Movement of the subject's head during a BOLD-fMRI run is a critical problem. In BOLD studies, the signal changes associated with brain activation are only a few percent. But head movement of only a small fraction of a voxel can produce signal changes of this order, particularly when the voxel is at the border of two regions with different signal intensities (i.e., an edge in the image). Then a small shift of the location of the voxel across this boundary due to motion can create substantial changes in the voxel signal. If the motion is correlated with the stimulus (e.g., if the subject tips her head slightly each time a visual stimulus is presented), this can create large apparent activations that are purely artifactual (Hajnal et al., 1994).

For this reason, the subject's head is tightly restrained, and a bite-bar system is often used to further stabilize the head. In addition, after the data are collected, the images are processed with a motion correction algorithm that applies small translations and rotations to the images to produce the best mutual alignment (Cox, 1996; Friston et al., 1995; Woods, Mazziota, and Cherry, 1993). However, even with preventive measures and postprocessing corrections such as this, head movement remains one of the most common problems in BOLD studies, particularly in patient populations (Friston et al., 1996).

Assuming that head motion can be prevented and/or corrected, the more physiological sources of noise still remain. If physiological data (e.g., heart beats and respiration) are recorded during the fMRI experiment, these data can be used to estimate retrospectively and remove the physiological fluctuations from the fMRI time series (Hu et al., 1995). This approach can considerably improve the fMRI data, but it is not always feasible to perform the necessary physiological monitoring. The effect of physiological noise is that the standard deviation of the local signal over time is larger than what one would estimate from the variation of the background of a single image, which is an estimate of the thermal noise alone. In fact, the temporal noise in images of the brain is often several times larger than the thermal noise, suggesting a strong contribution from physiological noise. If one maps the standard deviation of the temporal noise in different regions of the brain, the distribution correlates strongly with brain structures; indeed, a map of the noise standard deviation often looks much like a map of CSF.

In addition to increasing the magnitude of the noise, physiological fluctuations can also introduce temporal and spatial correlations in the noise. For example, respiratory motions have periods of several seconds and are likely to affect large regions in a similar way. Indeed, respiratory motions can affect the signal from the brain even if the head is still. Noll (1995) concluded that signal variations at the respiratory frequency arise from magnetic field variations in the brain on the order of a few parts per billion, likely due to changes in the shape of the body with respiration. As a result of such effects with long temporal correlations and broad spatial patterns, the noise component of the signal from a voxel in one image may not be independent of the noise in the next image in a time series. In addition, the noise in the signal from one voxel may not be independent of the noise in nearby voxels.

The presence of temporal and spatial noise correlations substantially complicates the analysis of the statistical significance of detected activations. The problem of correlated noise is the problem outlined earlier: how much does the noise go down with averaging? The detection of an activated voxel essentially depends on detecting a signal difference between the task and control states, but the statistical significance of any measured average signal difference depends on the number of degrees of freedom, the number of independent measurements involved. The temporal correlations of the noise may significantly reduce the degrees of freedom. Spatial correlations of the noise affect spatial smoothing and the statistical significance of clusters of activated pixels (Friston et al., 1994). Often the statistical threshold for defining activations is relaxed for clusters of adjacent pixels, on the theory that clusters of random apparent activation are unlikely to occur if the noise is independent. But stimulus-correlated motion regularly produces many contiguous, artifactually activated pixels at the edge of the brain. So the statistical significance of clusters of activation critically depends on the spatial correlations. Unfortunately, however, physiological noise is still not understood in a quantitative way, and the full significance of noise correlations in BOLD studies is still being investigated. These issues will be taken up again in Chapter 18.

REFERENCES

Cox, R. W. (1996) AFNI: Software for analysis and visualization of functional magnetic resonance neuroimages. *Comput. Biomed. Res.* **29,** 162–73.

Friston, K. J. (1996) Statistical parametric mapping and other analyses of functional imaging data. In: *Brain Mapping: the Methods,* pp. 363–86. Eds. A. W. Toga and J. C. Mazziota. Academic: New York.

Friston, K. J., Ashburner, J., Frith, C. D., Poline, J.-B., Heather, J. D., and Frackowiak, R. S. J. (1995) Spatial registration and normalization of images. *Human Brain Mapping* **2,** 165–89.

Friston, K. J., Williams, S., Howard, R., Frackowiak, R. S. J., and Turner, R. (1996) Movement related effects in fMRI time-series. *Magn. Reson. Med.* **35,** 346–55.

Friston, K. J., Worsley, K. J., Frackowiak, R. S. J., Mazziota, J. C., and Evans, A. C. (1994) Assessing the significance of focal activations using their spatial extent. *Human Brain Mapping* **1,** 210–20.

Glover, G. H., and Lee, A. T. (1995) Motion artifacts in fMRI: Comparison of 2DFT with PR and spiral scan methods. *Magn. Reson. Med.* **33,** 624–35.

Grant, P. E., Vigneron, D. B., and Barkovich, A. J. (1998) High resolution imaging of the brain. *MRI Clinics of North America* **6,** 139–54.

Hajnal, J. V., Myers, R., Oatridge, A., Schwieso, J. E., Young, I. R., and Bydder, G. M. (1994) Artifacts due to stimulus correlated motion in functional imaging of the brain. *Magn. Reson. Med* **31,** 283–91.

Hoult, D. I., and Richards, R. E. (1979) The signal to noise ratio of the nuclear magnetic resonance experiment. *J. Magn. Reson.* **24,** 71–85.

Hu, X., Le, T. H., Parrish, T., and Erhard, P. (1995) Retrospective estimation and correction of physiological fluctuation in functional MRI. *Magn. Reson. Med.* **34,** 201–12.

Jezzard, P., and Balaban, R. S. (1995) Correction for geometric distortion in echo planar images from B_0 field distortions. *Magn. Reson. Med.* **34,** 65–73.

Lange, N. (1996) Statistical approaches to human brain mapping by functional magnetic resonance imaging. *Statistics in Medicine* **15,** 389–428.

Macovski, A. (1996) Noise in MRI. *Magn. Reson. Med.* **36,** 494–7.

Noll, D. C. (1995) Methodologic considerations for spiral k-space functional MRI. *Int. J. Imag. Syst. Tech.* **6,** 175–83.

Parker, D. L., and Gullberg, G. L. (1990) Signal to noise efficiency in magnetic resonance imaging. *Med. Phys.* **17,** 250–7.

Poline, J.-B., Worsley, K. J., Evans, A. C., and Friston, K. J. (1997) Combining spatial extent and peak intensity to test for activations in functional imaging. *NeuroImage* **5,** 83–96.

Reber, P. J., Wong, E. C., Buxton, R. B., and Frank, L. R. (1998) Correction of off-resonance related distortion in EPI using EPI based field maps. *Magn. Reson. Med.* **39,** 328–30.

Wood, M. L., and Henkelman, R. M. (1985) MR image artifacts from periodic motion. *Med. Phys.* **12,** 143–51.

Woods, R. P., Mazziota, J. C., and Cherry, S. R. (1993) MRI-PET registration with automated algorithm. *J. Comput. Assist. Tomogr.* **17,** 536–46.

PRINCIPLES OF FUNCTIONAL MAGNETIC RESONANCE IMAGING

IIIA

Perfusion Imaging

13

Principles of Tracer Kinetics

INTRODUCTION

The previous chapters considered magnetic resonance imaging (MRI) as a sensitive technique for depicting human anatomy. The magnetic resonance (MR) signal is intrinsically sensitive to several properties of tissues, such as relaxation times and diffusion, and the flexibility of pulse sequence design makes possible a variety of imaging techniques. Within the last decade, the field of MRI has expanded to include studies of tissue function in addition to anatomy. The remaining chapters describe how subtle MR effects are exploited to measure different aspects of the perfusion state of tissue. Although the Blood Oxygenation Level Dependent (BOLD) effect is most often used in brain activation studies, a drawback of this technique is that it only provides information on the change in activity between one state and another. For example, measurements made while a subject alternates between a control state and a task state reveal regions of the brain showing a significant signal difference between the two states. But BOLD techniques provide no information on the resting or chronic perfusion state.

In the next three chapters, we describe two classes of MRI techniques that do provide measures of the resting perfusion state. The first class is based on the use of intravascular contrast agents that alter the magnetic susceptibility of blood, and so affect the MR signal. The second class of techniques is *arterial spin labeling* (ASL), in which arterial blood is magnetically tagged before it arrives in the tissue, and the amount delivered to the tissue is then measured. These two approaches are quite different, and, as we will see, the two techniques essentially measure different aspects of the perfusion state of the tissue. The contrast agent techniques provide a robust measurement of cerebral blood volume (CBV), whereas the ASL techniques measure cerebral blood flow (CBF).

In the healthy brain, CBF and CBV are believed to be closely correlated, in the sense that an increase in CBF is accompanied by an increase in CBV (Grubb et al., 1974). However, as discussed in Chapter 3, it is best to view this relationship simply as a correlation, rather than as a tight link. Blood flow is controlled by changes in the caliber of the arterioles, but the small blood volume changes associated with arteriolar dilitation are likely much smaller than the measured total CBV changes. Furthermore, recent studies using some of the techniques described here have found that the blood volume increase associated with brain activation resolves more slowly than the CBF increase (Mandeville et al., 1998), suggesting that the large CBV increase is not controlling the CBF increase. Furthermore, there is substantial evidence that the correlation between CBF and CBV found in the healthy brain is disrupted in disease. For example, ischemic states are often marked by a reduced CBF but an elevated CBV, a situation described as a reduced perfusion reserve (Gibbs et al., 1984; Kluytmans, Groud, and Viergever, 1998).

For these reasons, measurements of both CBF and CBV have important clinical roles. Both contrast agent techniques and ASL techniques draw heavily on ideas of tracer kinetics developed over the last 50 years, and so, to lay the groundwork for understanding how these techniques work, this chapter is a review of the principles of tracer kinetic methods.

BASIC CONCEPTS OF TRACER KINETICS

Time/Activity Curves

Tracer kinetic modeling has a long history in the study of physiology (Axel, 1980; Lassen and Perl, 1979; Meier and Zierler, 1954; Zierler, 1962). In a tracer study, an agent is injected into the blood, and the kinetics of the agent as it passes through the tissue are monitored. Radioactive labels make possible a direct measurement of the tissue concentration of the agent, as in position emission tomography (PET) studies. Technically speaking, a tracer study usually means that the agent is a labeled version of a metabolic substrate (e.g., ^{11}C-glucose or $^{15}O_2$), and the agent then traces the fate of that substrate. However, the same principles apply to other agents that are not a modified form of a metabolic substrate (e.g., ^{133}Xe or nitrous oxide) but nevertheless distribute through the tissue in a way that reflects some underlying physiological parameter, such as blood flow. In fact, the question of whether a particular agent acts as a tracer of a particular metabolic substrate can be subtle. Deoxyglucose is a different molecule than glucose; yet it is used as a tracer of the early stages of glucose metabolism (Sokoloff et al., 1977). The differences between the two molecules appear in a correction factor called the lumped constant, as described in Chapter 1. In contrast, $^{11}CO_2$ *is* a labeled form of carbon dioxide; yet this agent does *not* act as a tracer of CO_2 in the body because intrinsic CO_2 is not only delivered to tissue by blood flow, like the labeled agent, but is also created in the tissue by oxidative metabolism, unlike the agent (Buxton et al., 1984).

In the following, we will take the broad view of tracer kinetics as a description of the dynamic tissue concentration of any agent that is delivered to the tissue by blood flow. The essential data in a tracer study then are the tissue concentration of the agent measured over time and the agent concentration measured in arterial blood. These curves are described as *time/activity curves,* where activity refers to concentration of the agent, often measured as an amount of radioactivity, and not to neural activity. In fact, a basic assumption of tracer studies is that the physiological system is in a steady state during the measurement so that neural activity and flow are constant. The arterial concentration $C_A(t)$ is the driving function of the system, and the tissue concentration $C_T(t)$ is the output. Connecting the input and the output is a model for the kinetics of the agent that involves several physiological parameters, and the goal of tracer kinetic analysis is to estimate these parameters from the data.

Volume of Distribution of the Agent

For MR applications of tracer kinetics, we are primarily concerned with agents that are not metabolized in the brain so that they are simply passively distributed. For these agents, the two physiological parameters that directly affect the kinetics are the local cerebral blood flow and the *partition coefficient,* or *volume of distribution,* of the agent. The local CBF is most often expressed as the volume of arterial blood delivered per minute to 1 g of tissue. But for imaging applications, the natural unit for an element of tissue is volume, rather than mass, because an image voxel refers to a volume of tissue. Expressed in these terms, the local CBF, which we will abbreviate as f, is the milliliters of arterial blood delivered per milliliter of tissue per minute. The units of f are simply inverse time, and we can often think of f as a rate constant governing the delivery of metabolic substrates. A typical value for the human brain is $f = 0.6$ min^{-1} (or 60 ml/min-100 ml of tissue or 0.01s^{-1}).

The partition coefficient λ describes how the agent would naturally distribute between blood and tissue if allowed to equilibrate. Specifically, if the concentration of the agent in blood is held constant for a very long time at a value C_0, the total tissue concentration of the agent will approach a value $C_T(\infty)$ such that $\lambda = C_T(\infty)/C_0$. The dimensions of λ (and the concentrations) must be defined in a way that is consistent with the dimensions of f. If f is expressed as milliliters of blood per minute for each gram of tissue, then λ has the dimensions milliliters per gram (ml/g) (i.e., volume of distribution per gram of tissue), arterial concentration is expressed as moles per milliliter (moles/ml), and tissue concentration is expressed as moles per gram (moles/g). But if instead f is defined as milliliters of blood per minute for each milliliter of tissue, so that its dimensions are simply inverse time, then λ is dimensionless (volume of distribution per volume of tissue). We will use the latter definition, so that f is expressed as inverse time, λ is dimensionless, and all concentrations are expressed in moles per milliliter.

In the simplest case, the agent freely diffuses into the tissue until the extravascular concentration matches the intravascular concentration, so that $\lambda = 1$. On the other hand, if the agent only distributes through a part of the tissue space, the partition coefficient is less than one. For example, if the agent freely diffuses into the interstitial space, but not the intracellular space, at equilibrium the interstitial concentration will be equal to the arterial concentration, but the intracellular concentration will be zero. The total tissue concentration will be proportional to the interstitial plus blood volume fractions, which is typically about 20%, and so λ will be about 0.2. This is the reason why the partition coefficient is often described as the volume of distribution of the agent, and for many agents this is a useful way to interpret λ.

But thinking of λ as a tissue/blood partition coefficient, rather than a volume of distribution, is a more general description that applies to any agent. An agent could have a partition coefficient greater than one or much less than one even though it has access to the full volume of the tissue. For example, O_2 diffuses throughout the tissue space but is more soluble in lipids than in water (Kassissia et al., 1995). At equilibrium, there is a higher concentration in the tissue space than in the blood plasma due to the greater concentration of cell membranes, and so λ is greater than one. But the case of O_2 is even more complicated because most of the O_2 in blood is bound to hemoglobin, and so if the partition coefficient is defined in terms of the *total* arterial blood content, rather than the plasma content, λ is much less than one. Another example is CO_2, which freely enters all the tissue spaces but also combines with water to form bicarbonate ions. If labeled CO_2 is introduced into the blood, the label will distribute between dissolved gas and bicarbonate ions, and this distribution depends on the local pH. The partition coefficient for labeled CO_2 then depends on the arterial and tissue pH values (Buxton et al., 1984) and can be greater or less than one despite the fact that the CO_2 enters all the tissue space.

These examples indicate that the interpretation of λ can involve some subtleties. But for the agents of interest in MRI, it is reasonable to think of λ as a measure of the fraction of the total tissue volume that the agent can enter. Then a diffusible tracer, such as tagged water, that enters the full tissue space, has $\lambda = 1$. In contrast, an intravascular tracer, such as Gd-DTPA, that remains confined to the vasculature in the healthy brain, has $\lambda = CBV$ (typically about 4% in the brain). Furthermore, if the agent readily fills this volume, in the sense that there is no impediment to the agent (i.e., it freely diffuses into its volume of distribution), then a useful time constant is $\tau = \lambda/f$. This time constant is the characteristic time required for the tissue to come into equilibrium with the blood. (Literally, an agent delivered at a constant rate f into a tank with volume λ will fill the available space in a time τ.) In other words, for the same flow, the volume of distribution of an intravascular agent is quickly filled because the blood volume is only a small fraction of the total volume, while the volume of distribution of a freely diffusible agent requires a much longer time to fill.

For example, with a CBF of 60 ml/min-ml of tissue (0.01 s^{-1}), the equilibrium time for an intravascular tracer with a CBV of 4% is about 4 s, but for a diffusible tracer τ is about 100 s. As we will see, this huge difference in the time constants is critical for interpreting tissue time/activity curves in terms of local physiological parameters. The kinetics of an agent, as reflected in the local tissue concentration curve, depend on both the local blood flow f and the local volume of distribution λ. The goal in analyzing such curves is to derive a measurement of one or both of these physiological quantities, and the quality of these measurements will depend on how sensitive the tissue curve is to each quantity.

INTERPRETING THE TISSUE CONCENTRATION CURVE

Dependence on Flow and Volume of Distribution

As the simplest example, suppose that the arterial concentration of the agent is maintained at a constant level C_A for a long time, after which the concentration drops abruptly to zero (see Figure 13.1). What will the tissue time/activity curve look like? Initially, the tissue curve will smoothly increase as flow delivers the agent to the tissue element, and the slope can be directly quantified in terms of the local flow f. In a short time Δt, the volume of blood delivered per milliliter of tissue is $f\Delta t$, and because each unit volume of blood carries C_A moles of the agent the change in the tissue concentration of the agent is $\Delta C_T = fC_A \Delta t$. Thus, the slope of the initial portion of the tissue curve is simply proportional to the local blood flow and the arterial concentration. In this initial linear period, before any of the agent has had a chance to leave the tissue volume, the tissue concentration depends only on the local flow and is independent of the volume of distribution of the agent. As time goes on, some of the agent that arrived early will begin to clear from the tissue by venous flow, and the linear rise of the tissue curve will begin to taper off. Eventually, if the duration of the arterial input curve is long enough, the tissue curve will reach an equilibrium plateau. From this time on, the volume of distribution of the agent is filled to the same concentration as in the artery, and the rate of delivery of new agent by arterial flow is matched to the rate of clearance by venous flow. Within the volume of distribution of the agent, the concentration is equal to the arterial concentration, C_A, but since this volume only occupies a fraction λ of the total volume of the tissue element, the net tissue concentration at the plateau is λC_A. Thus, on the plateau, the tissue concentration directly reflects the local volume of distribution and is independent of flow.

After the arterial concentration is reduced to zero, with no more delivery of new agent, the tissue concentration will decrease over time as the agent is cleared by venous flow. The exact shape of this portion of the curve will depend on details of the particular agent and its volume of distribution. But a simple model that is often used is to assume that the agent passes rapidly from the blood throughout its volume of distribution, so that the venous blood remains in equilibrium with the rest of the tissue even as the total concentration is decreasing. That is, the venous concentration C_v quickly adjusts so that it is always equal to C_T/λ as the tissue concentra-

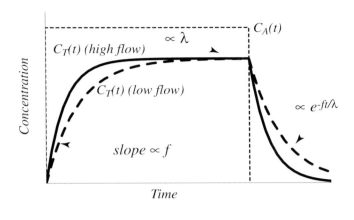

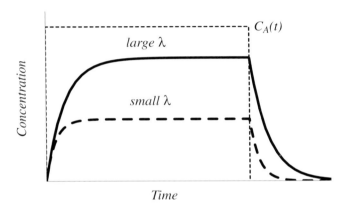

Figure 13.1. Tracer kinetics. Idealized examples of tracer kinetic curves are shown, with the arterial concentration $C_A(t)$ represented as a perfectly rectangular bolus. The top plot shows two tissue concentration curves $C_T(t)$ for different flows (f) but the same volume of distribution (λ). The second plot shows tissue curves for the same f but different λ. The agent is delivered in proportion to f, so the slope of the early part of $C_T(t)$ depends just on f. After a steady-state plateau is reached, $C_T(t)$ is proportional to λ and independent of f. Finally, after delivery stops, the clearance of the agent depends on the ratio f/λ.

tion C_T decreases. In each short time interval Δt, the amount of the agent carried out is $fC_v\,\Delta t = (f/\lambda)\,C_T\Delta t$, so the fraction of the tissue concentration removed in Δt is $f\Delta t/\lambda$. This produces an exponential decay of the tissue concentration, $e^{-t/\tau}$, with $\tau = \lambda/f$. Thus, the clearance of the agent does not depend on the exact value of either the flow or the volume of distribution but only on their ratio.

To summarize, then, the tissue curve depends on the local flow and the volume of distribution of the agent to different degrees at different times. The initial upslope of the tissue curve depends only on f, the plateau depends only on λ, and the clearance portion depends on the ratio f/λ. During the upslope portion of the curve, the tissue concentration provides a pure measurement of local flow, independent of λ. Because none (or very little) of the delivered agent has cleared, the agent is acting essentially like a microsphere, which is delivered to the tissue in proportion to flow and then remains trapped in the capillary bed. On the plateau, the tissue concentration provides no information on the local flow and, instead, provides a direct measurement of the local volume of distribution of the agent. The clearance portion of the curve again provides information on flow, but only in the form of f/λ. That is, from a clearance measurement alone, only the ratio $\lambda/f = \tau$ can be measured, and to extract a measurement of flow alone, the volume of distribution must be known or measured separately.

Measuring CBF and CBV

With these arguments in mind, the essential difference between the kinetics of a diffusible agent and an intravascular agent can be understood. The time to reach the plateau and the time required for clearance are both on the order of $\tau = \lambda/f$. For an intravascular tracer this is only about 4 s, but for a diffusible tracer it is over 1 min. For an intravascular tracer, the transition periods before and after the equilibrium plateau are very short and thus difficult to measure. And because these are the only times when the curve is sensitive to flow, it is difficult to measure flow with an intravascular agent. On the other hand, because the plateau is quickly reached and can be maintained for a long time, the volume of distribution is readily measured. And λ for an intravascular agent is simply the local blood volume, CBV. In contrast, for a diffusible agent the transition regions when the tissue curve depends strongly on flow are much longer and so are much more easily measured.

In practice, a complete tissue concentration curve such as this is rarely measured. Instead, different techniques focus on different aspects of the tissue curve. In ^{133}Xe studies, the radioactive xenon is an inert gas that freely diffuses into the tissue (Obrist et al., 1967). After breathing in the gas, the clearance of the agent from the subject's brain is monitored with external detectors that measure the gamma rays emitted by the radioactive xenon. By placing an array of detectors around the head, the clearance from local regions can be measured. However, this is not the same thing as a true measurement of tissue concentration. The sensitivity pattern of a single detector is indeed localized, so each activity measurement can be taken as being proportional to the local tissue concentration of the agent, but it is difficult to turn this into an absolute tissue concentration. However, for measuring a decay time for the tissue activity, this type of proportional measurement is sufficient. If the clearance is indeed exponential, then the measured activity will drop by a factor of $1/e$ during the time $\tau = \lambda/f$. To convert a measurement of τ into an estimate of local flow, λ must be known, or a value must be assumed. Clearance studies with ^{133}Xe can thus provide a robust measurement of f/λ, but uncertainties in the value of λ and how it might vary from one tissue to another (e.g., gray matter compared with white matter) make this a less robust measurement of blood flow.

With PET and $H_2^{15}O$, however, the local concentration of the agent is accurately measured, and so it is possible to focus on the early part of the tissue time/activity curve. In the bolus administration method, data are collected over the first 40 s following a rapid injection of the tracer (Raichle, 1983). Because the tissue concentration during this period is dominated by delivery by arterial flow, the measured PET counts in each image voxel are primarily sensitive just to local CBF and are only weakly sensitive to λ. For longer data acquisition times, the signal-to-noise ratio (SNR) would improve, but the signal would become more dependent on λ. The method is, thus, designed to provide a robust measurement of flow independent of any uncertainties about λ.

These principles were developed in the context of analyzing radioactive tracer studies. However, the physical principles and the mathematical modeling underlying MRI techniques for perfusion imaging based on arterial spin labeling are similar, as will be developed in Chapter 15.

The General Form of the Tissue Concentration Curve

The preceding examples have assumed an ideal arterial concentration curve that rises immediately to a plateau value, stays constant at that value for a time, and then drops immediately back to zero. The delivery, plateau, and clearance portions of the curve were shown to be determined by f, λ, and $\tau = \lambda/f$, respectively. However, in practice, the arterial concentration curve is never a rectangular function, and so for a real tissue concentration curve the borders between delivery, plateau, and clearance regions become blurred, and it is more difficult to see directly how sensitive the tissue curve is to these three physiological parameters. In Box 13, a more general mathematical treatment of tracer kinetics is developed for an arbitrary arterial concentration $C_A(t)$. Based on this treatment, it is possible to draw some general conclusions about how blood flow, blood volume, and the mean transit time τ affect the tissue curve. In general, the tissue concentration curve can be written as (from Equation [B13.1])

$$C_T(t) = C_A(t) * [f\, r(t)] \qquad\qquad [13.1]$$

where the * indicates convolution, $C_T(t)$ is the tissue concentration curve, $C_A(t)$ is the arterial concentration curve, f is the local CBF, and $r(t)$ is the local residue function (Figure 13.2). The residue function $r(t)$ contains most of the details of the distribution and kinetics of the agent. Specifically, $r(t_2 - t_1)$ is the fraction of the number of moles of the agent that entered the tissue at time t_1 that are still in the tissue at time t_2. Then $r(t) = 1$ for $t = 0$ because there has been no time for any of the agent to leave, and with increasing t, it must decrease monotonically. As shown in more detail in Box 13, based on the definition of $r(t)$, the integral of $r(t)$ over all t is equal to the mean transit time τ. Using Equation [13.1], one can show that for *any* shape of $r(t)$, the mean transit time, flow, and volume of distribution are always related by the central volume principle (CVP) as $\tau = \lambda/f$.

It is useful to look at Equation [13.1] in the context of linear systems, such that the arterial concentration curve is the input function and the combination $fr(t)$ is the impulse response (the term in brackets in Equation [13.1]). Then the output (the tissue concentration curve) is the convolution of the input function (the arterial concentration curve) with the impulse response, as illustrated in Figure 13.2. From the definition of $r(t)$, we can see two important characteristics of the local impulse response of the tissue. First, the initial amplitude is f, because $r(0) = 1$. Second,

BOX 13. A GENERAL MODEL FOR TRACER KINETICS

The goal in tracer kinetic modeling is to develop a mathematical relation between the arterial concentration of the agent $C_A(t)$ and the resulting tissue concentration $C_T(t)$. One can think of $C_A(t)$ as the driving function of the system, the input function, and $C_T(t)$ as the output. For the agents of interest for MRI (both diffusible and intravascular tracers), the kinetic model will depend primarily on just two local physiological parameters: the local cerebral blood flow f and the partition coefficient (or volume of distribution) of the agent λ. We can construct a general expression for the tissue curve at time t by adding up the amount of agent delivered up to t weighted by the probability that the agent is still in the tissue voxel at t. To do this, we define a residue function $r(t-t')$, the probability that a molecule of the agent that entered the tissue voxel at time t' is still there at time t. We assume that the underlying physiology is in a steady state (e.g., constant flow throughout the experiment) so that r only depends on the interval $t - t'$ and not the absolute values of t or t'. Then the number of molecules of the agent delivered during a short interval between t' and $t' + dt'$ is $fC_A(t')dt'$, and the probability that they are still in the tissue element at time t is $r(t - t')$. The net tissue concentration at time t is then

$$C_T(t) = \int_0^t f\, C_A(t')\, r\,(t - t')\, dt' = f\, C_A(t) * r(t) \tag{B13.1}$$

Where the * symbolizes convolution as defined by this equation. The essential condition required for the validity of Equation [B13.1] is that when each molecule of the agent enters the capillary bed it has the same possible fates as every other molecule of the agent. This condition could break down if the underlying physiology is not in a steady state (e.g., a changing f during the experiment). Or, this equation could break down if the agent is present in such a high concentration that there is competition for a saturable transport system, such as glucose extraction from the capillary bed in the brain, which has a limited capacity. In the latter case, a molecule that enters when the agent concentration is low would have a higher probability of being extracted than one that entered when the concentration is high. But for most MRI studies, Equation [B13.1] is appropriate as a general expression for the tissue concentration of the agent as a function of time.

Equation [B13.1] applies to a wide range of agents, but we have achieved this generality by lumping all the details of transport and uptake of the agent into the single function $r(t)$. In particular, Equation [B13.1] hides the full dependence of the tissue curve on perfusion because $r(t)$ depends on f as well. A more detailed consideration of the form of $r(t)$ for different agents is necessary to clarify how the measured kinetics of an agent can be used to measure the local perfusion. By definition, $r(t)$ is the probability that a molecule of the agent that entered the capillary bed at $t = 0$ is still there at time t, so $r(0) = 1$ since there has been no time for any of the agent to leave. Furthermore, $r(t)$ must monotonically decrease with increasing time because the probability that a particular molecule is still present cannot be higher at a later time than at an earlier time.

The residue function is closely related to the distribution of transit times through the tissue voxel, $h(t)$. If many particles enter the tissue at the same moment, the fraction that will stay in the tissue voxel for a total time between t and $t + dt$ is $h(t)dt$. But this fraction that leaves at time t is also the change in the fraction that remains at time t, which is *(dr/dt)dt.* Therefore, the relation between the residue function and the distribution of transit times is

$$\frac{dr}{dt} = -h(t) \tag{B13.2}$$

The mean transit time, τ, is then

$$\tau = \int_0^\infty t\, h(t)\, dt = \int_0^\infty r(t)\, dt \tag{B13.3}$$

From Equation [B13.1], we can derive an important general relationship called the central volume principle, which was introduced in Chapter 2. Suppose that the arterial concentration is maintained at a constant value C_A for a very long time t. As t approaches infinity, the tissue concentration must approach its equilibrium value λC_A. From Equations [B.13.1] and [B13.3], as t approaches infinity with C_A held constant, C_T approaches $f\tau C_A$, and so equating this with the equilibrium condition requires

$$\tau = \frac{\lambda}{f} \tag{B13.4}$$

This simple relationship between the flow, the volume of distribution, and the mean transit time is completely general, regardless of the exact form of $r(t)$. And it also shows how the form of $r(t)$ is constrained by our two local physiological variables f and λ, such that the integral of $r(t)$ must be equal to λ/f.

The distinction between $h(t)$ and $r(t)$ can be confusing because both appear in the literature of tracer kinetics, but they actually play different roles, depending on the nature of the experiment. In animal experiments, particularly those done before imaging techniques became available, the measured quantity is often the venous outflow concentration of the agent rather than the tissue concentration. The venous concentration can be modeled as the convolution of $h(t)$ with the arterial curve $C_A(t)$ because $h(t)$ directly describes how long it is likely to take for a molecule of the agent delivered to the vascular bed to transit the bed and show up in the venous concentration. But for imaging studies, the *tissue* concentration is measured, and this is modeled as the convolution of $C_A(t)$ with $fr(t)$ rather than $h(t)$.

To put this another way, we are treating the system as linear so that both the venous concentration and the tissue concentration result from a convolution of the arterial input function with an appropriate impulse response function. For the venous concentration, the impulse response is $h(t)$; for the tissue concentration, the impulse response is the product $fr(t)$. The tissue impulse response depends on both flow and the volume of distribution, with an initial amplitude of f and an area equal to λ. In contrast, $h(t)$ depends primarily on the mean transit time τ, which is the ratio λ/f. For this reason, the difference in the impulse responses for the venous concentration and the tissue concentration is not a simple difference in form; the tissue curve actually carries more information than the venous curve because the impulse response depends on the values of both f and λ and not just on their ratio.

A common approach to modeling tracer kinetic curves is *compartmental modeling*, and it is useful to consider how such models fit into the more general framework developed here. For example, suppose that the tissue is modeled as a single well-mixed com-

(continued)

BOX 13, continued

partment. The rate of delivery of agent to the tissue compartment is $fC_A(t)$, and the rate of clearance of the agent from tissue is $fC_v(t)$, where $C_v(t)$ is the concentration of the agent in venous blood. If the exchange of the agent between blood and tissue is very rapid, so that the two pools stay in equilibrium even as the overall concentration is changing, then we can equate $C_T = \lambda C_v$, and the rate of clearance then is $C_T f/\lambda$. The rate of change of the tissue concentration is then the difference between the rate of delivery and the rate of clearance:

$$\frac{dC_T(t)}{dt} = f\, C_A(t) - \frac{f}{\lambda}\, C_T(t) \qquad\qquad [B13.5]$$

The solution of this differential equation is given by Equation [B13.1] with $r(t) = e^{-ft/\lambda}$. In other words, a single-compartment model is described by the general model with an exponential form for $r(t)$.

Compartmental models are often useful in analyzing tracer kinetic data, but it is important to determine which results strongly depend on the restrictive assumptions of compartmental models and which follow from the more general model and are thus more robust. An important example concerns the interpretation of kinetic curves for an intravascular agent in terms of local CBV. Suppose that an agent is delivered in a bolus form so that the arterial concentration drops back down to zero after a time. The integral of the arterial curve is then finite, and the integral of the tissue curve will also be finite. What is the relation between these two integrated values? To answer this, we can turn to the general model. Mathematically, the integral of a convolution of two functions is the product of the separate integrals of the two functions. Then from Equation [B13.1] we have

$$\int_0^\infty C_T(t)\, dt = \lambda \int_0^\infty C_A(t)\, dt \qquad\qquad [B13.6]$$

In other words, for any agent that is not metabolized, the integral of the local tissue curve over all time is proportional to the local partition coefficient times the integral of the arterial curve. And if the agent remains confined to the vasculature, λ = CBV. So for an intravascular agent, the integrated tissue curve provides a robust measurement of CBV, regardless of the exact form of either the tissue curve or the arterial curve. The arterial curve is global, rather than local, so a map of the local integrated tissue activity is, in fact, directly proportional to a map of CBV.

An aspect of tracer studies that we have not yet addressed is the decay of the tracer. For example, in the $H_2{}^{15}O$ bolus administration PET technique, the radioactive decay of the ^{15}O must be taken into account. More of the originally labeled water is present in the image voxel than the current level of ^{15}O activity would indicate because some has decayed during the measurement time. But this is a simple correction because the half-life (2 min) of ^{15}O is well known. However, there is another rather different strategy for measuring CBF that makes use of the fact that the agent decays away over time (Frackowiak et al., 1980). This technique was originally developed for use with $H_2{}^{15}O$, but as we will see in Chapter 15, the same idea is applied in one type of ASL imaging. In this steady-state technique, the short half-life of ^{15}O is a key component of the flow sensitivity, rather than just a decay term requiring correction as in the bolus administration technique. Because the label is decaying away, there is another way for the agent to "clear" from the voxel in addition to venous flow. The water itself does not clear any faster, but the radioactive tracer marking the water disappears, so for practical purposes the agent can be cleared from the tissue by two mechanisms. The $H_2^{15}O$ is administered continuously until a steady state is reached in which the tissue concentration of ^{15}O depends on a balance between delivery by arterial flow and clearance by a combination of venous flow and radioactive decay. As a result, the tissue concentration curve is changed in an interesting way from the preceding descriptions. Without radioactive decay, the plateau of the tissue curve results when delivery of the agent by arterial flow is balanced by clearance by venous flow. The rate of delivery is fC_A, the rate of clearance by venous flow is $fC_V = fC_T/\lambda$, and so the plateau tissue concentration is $C_T = \lambda C_A$, as discussed earlier. But now we also include the rate of clearance by radioactive decay, C_T/t_d, where t_d is the characteristic decay time of the radioactive nucleus. The tissue concentration reaches a steady state when the delivery rate is equal to the *net* clearance rate (venous flow plus radioactive decay), and the resulting tissue concentration is

$$C_T(\text{steady state}) = \frac{f\,C_A}{f/\lambda + 1/t_d} \qquad\qquad [B13.7]$$

Note that when the decay time is very long, so that clearance is dominated by venous flow, only the first term in the denominator matters, and the plateau concentration becomes $C_T = \lambda C_A$. The tissue concentration is then a direct measure of the volume of distribution, independent of the local flow, as argued earlier. On the other hand, if the decay time is very short, only the second term in the denominator matters, and the plateau concentration is $C_T = ft_d\,C_A$. The tissue concentration directly reflects the local CBF and is independent of the volume of distribution. In this case, virtually all the clearance is by decay rather than venous flow. With a decay constant $t_d = 2$ min for ^{15}O, clearance by flow and decay are comparable. The steady-state tissue concentration then depends on both CBF and the volume of distribution.

For MRI arterial spin labeling studies, relaxation of the tagged spins plays the same role as radioactive decay in nuclear medicine studies, so we need a more general formulation of Equation [B13.1] to include decay of the agent. The essential derivation of Equation [B13.1] was simply to add up all the molecules of the agent that had arrived in the past weighted with the probability that they are still in the tissue. Originally, this probability was $r(t)$, but now we must include the possibility that the agent left by decay. Let $m(t)$ be the fraction of the agent that has not decayed away by time t. Then the probability that a molecule is still in the tissue and has not decayed away is $r(t)m(t)$, so the general expression for the tissue curve is (Buxton et al., 1998)

$$C_T(t) = \int_0^t f\,C_A(t')\,r(t-t')\,m(t-t')\,dt' = f\,C_A(t)*[r(t)\,m(t)] \qquad\qquad [B13.8]$$

For exponential decay Equation [B13.8] produces Equation [13.7] for constant C_A. We will use Equation [B13.8] in Chapter 15 to analyze ASL experiments.

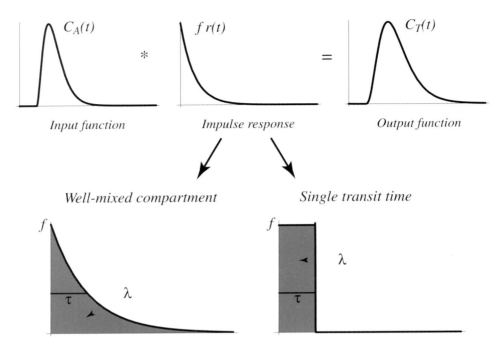

Figure 13.2. General form of the tissue concentration curve. From Equation [13.1], for any agent, the tissue concentration curve $C_T(t)$ is the convolution of the arterial concentration curve $C_A(t)$ with the local impulse response, which is the product of the local flow f and $r(t)$, the probability that a molecule of the agent entering the tissue element at $t = 0$ will still be there at time t. The peak of the impulse response is f, and the area under the impulse response is λ, the volume of distribution of the agent. Two examples of the impulse response are shown at the bottom. For a well-mixed compartment, $r(t)$ is an exponential, and for an intravascular agent with plug flow through identical capillaries, so that the transit time is identical for all molecules of the agent, $r(t)$ is a rectangle. For either case, the mean transit time is $\tau = \lambda/f$.

because the integral of $r(t)$ is τ ($= \lambda/f$), the area under the impulse response is λ. The extent to which a tissue concentration curve depends on f or λ will then depend on whether it depends on the peak value of the impulse response or just the area under it. We will use this approach to analyze the sensitivity of the tissue curve of an intravascular agent to CBF and CBV in a later section.

The Residue Function $r(t)$

The form of Equation [13.1] may seem remarkably simple for a general description of tracer kinetic curves, but we have achieved this simplicity by hiding all the complexities of the transport and distribution of the agent in the shape of $r(t)$. The shape of $r(t)$ is constrained such that $r(0) = 1$ and the integral is λ/f, but within these constraints a wide range of shapes is possible. To give a sense of what $r(t)$ looks like under different conditions, we can examine several examples (Figure 13.3). To begin with, consider the classic case of microsphere studies introduced in Chapter 3. Labeled microspheres are injected in an artery and delivered to a capillary bed, but because the spheres are designed to be too large to fit through the capillaries,

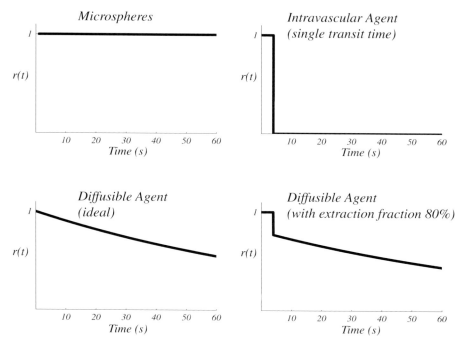

Figure 13.3. The shape of the residue function. The impulse response of the tissue curve is $fr(t)$, and several shapes for the residue function $r(t)$ are illustrated. Microspheres are trapped in the tissue, so $r(t) = 1$ (top left). For an intravascular agent traversing identical capillaries with plug flow, there is only one transit time, so $r(t)$ is a narrow rectangle. For the ideal diffusible tracer, $r(t)$ is an exponential (lower left), and for a partially extracted diffusible tracer, $r(t)$ must describe the fact that a fraction of the agent quickly traverses the capillary bed and is cleared, while the remaining extracted fraction has a much longer transit time (lower right).

they remain lodged in the tissue. For this agent, $r(t) = 1$ for all time (since the microspheres never leave the tissue), and so by Equation [13.1] the measured tissue concentration is simply the perfusion f times the integral of the arterial concentration. This is a robust method for measuring f and is usually considered the gold standard for perfusion measurements. The integrated arterial curve can be measured from any convenient artery and need not be measured locally. [The form $r(t) = 1$ does satisfy the CVP because both the integral of $r(t)$ and the partition coefficient λ are infinite. In other words, a microsphere behaves as if it is filling an infinite volume of distribution so that none of it ever leaves because the mean transit time is also infinite.]

A diffusible tracer is one that freely crosses the blood brain barrier and enters the extravascular space, such as an inert gas (e.g., ^{133}Xe) or labeled water (e.g., $H_2{}^{15}O$). A simple form for $r(t)$ that satisfies the CVP and is commonly used to model the kinetics of these agents is $r(t) = e^{-ft/\lambda}$. This exponential form naturally arises in compartmental models in which the rate of transport out of a compartment is taken to be a rate constant times the concentration in the compartment.

This simple form is equivalent to modeling the tissue as a single well-mixed compartment (see Box 13).

This example shows how the local flow affects the tissue curve in two distinct ways: the amount of agent delivered to the tissue is directly proportional to f, and the clearance of the agent depends on f through the form of $r(t)$. So either delivery or clearance of the agent can be used as the basis for a measurement of f, as discussed earlier. With the $H_2^{15}O$ method, the tracer is administered rapidly, and the initial concentration in the tissue (averaged over the first 40 s) is measured locally with PET, directly yielding a measurement proportional to f based on the delivery of the agent. The concentration maps can be calibrated by also measuring the arterial curve. In the ^{133}Xe method, the agent is administered by inhalation, and the clearance curve is measured with an external detector. The measured tissue curve can then be fit to a decaying exponential, and the time constant for clearance is λ/f. Provided that λ is known (and for diffusible tracers it is near one), f can be measured directly from the clearance curve.

Although perfusion can be measured with a diffusible tracer either from delivery or from clearance of the agent, measurements based on delivery are more robust. Delivery is always proportional to flow, as with microspheres, and is independent of $r(t)$. That is, for delivery f enters directly as a multiplicative factor in Equation [13.1], regardless of the form of $r(t)$. But to model clearance, a form of $r(t)$ must be assumed, and calculated perfusion will always be somewhat model-dependent. For example, consider measuring f in a voxel that contains two types of tissue with different values of perfusion (e.g., gray and white matter). Delivery of the tracer is then governed simply by the average value of f in the voxel, but clearance is now more complicated than the simple exponential form, and $r(t)$ should be modeled as a biexponential form.

An exponential form for $r(t)$ is often used to model diffusible tracers, but what is an appropriate form for an intravascular agent? One could use an appropriate exponential (e.g., with $\lambda = 0.04$ instead of $\lambda = 1$). But a single well-mixed compartment seems to be a poor approximation for blood flow through a vascular tree. As a counterexample, suppose that the capillary bed consists of identical capillaries, with plug flow at the same velocity in each one. Then the transit time τ through the tissue is identical for all molecules of the agent, with each molecule spending precisely a time τ in the tissue, and $r(t)$ is rectangular with a width τ (Figures 13.2 and 13.3). This also is an extreme form for $r(t)$, and the true form likely lies somewhere between the rectangle and the exponential.

Even for a diffusible tracer with $\lambda = 1$, the exponential form of $r(t)$ will only apply if the agent rapidly enters its volume of distribution. What happens if, instead, there is an impediment to rapid filling? For example, if the permeability of the capillary wall to the agent is low, some of the agent delivered to the capillary bed will not even leave the blood and will be carried away by venous flow. For example, labeled water is not fully extracted in the brain so that, even though its volume of distribution is the whole tissue volume, it can require some time to diffuse into it. This leads to systematic errors in the estimation of CBF in PET studies with $H_2^{15}O$. A useful measure of this effect is the unidirectional extraction fraction E, the fraction of the delivered agent that leaves the blood during its passage through the capillary bed. If E is close to 100%, then the exponential form for $r(t)$ is likely to be accurate. But if E is only 80%, then 20% of the agent will clear much more rapidly. To describe the effects of limited extraction, we must modify the form of $r(t)$. Figure 13.3 illustrates what $r(t)$ would look like if 20% of the delivered agent passes through without entering the tissue, with each unextracted molecule having a capillary transit time of 4 s. The remaining 80% of the delivered agent is extracted and follows the exponential behavior of a diffusible tracer.

This example illustrates the importance of having a more general model for tracer kinetics than what is provided by compartmental models alone. The assumptions of compartmental models are often not true in practice, and the more general treatment makes possible more accurate modeling and analysis of errors in the techniques. These examples also serve as a reminder that even though we often adopt a model in which the kinetics of the agent are described just by f and λ, the shape of $r(t)$ is also important.

Sensitivity of the Tissue Curve to f and λ

In tracer studies, or contrast agent studies in MRI, the goal is to derive estimates of f or λ from the measured concentration curves. With a diffusible agent, λ is about equal to one, and so the goal is to measure f. With an intravascular agent, such as Gd-DTPA in MR studies of the brain, $\lambda = CBV$, so it is desirable to extract estimates of both f and λ from the kinetic curves. The precision of any estimate of these physiological parameters depends on how sensitive the shape and magnitude of the tissue curve are to these parameters. For example, if we can change CBF by a factor of 2 and this produces a negligible change in the tissue curve of an agent, then we have no hope of measuring f from such data. Furthermore, for an intravascular agent, the curve is affected by both f and λ, and we are concerned with how well we can separate these effects to produce accurate measurements of each.

Equation [13.1] provides the basis for drawing some general conclusions about the sensitivity of the tissue concentration curve to f and λ. In Equation [13.1], the tissue concentration curve is represented as a convolution of the arterial input function $C_A(t)$ and the tissue impulse response function $fr(t)$. For any agent, the tissue impulse response has an initial amplitude equal to f and an area of λ. So we can look in a general way at how the convolution of two functions depends on the peak amplitude and the area of each of the functions to clarify the sensitivity to f and λ.

Accurately measuring the shape of the tissue curve requires high temporal resolution and a good signal-to-noise ratio. However, a relatively straightforward quantity to measure is the area under the tissue curve, and we can use a mathematical property of convolutions to derive an important conclusion about how the tissue curve depends on λ (see Box 13 for details). The integral of a convolution over all time is equal to the product of the separate integrals of the two functions. The integral of the impulse response is λ, so this means that the integral of the tissue curve over all time is simply λ times the integral of the arterial concentration curve, *independent of f or the shape of r(t)*. This means that λ can be measured in a very robust way from the integral of the tissue curve, and this is the basis for using Gd-DTPA to measure CBV. Furthermore, even without any measurements of the arterial curve, just the integral of the tissue curve alone is directly proportional to local CBV because the integrated arterial curve should be the same for all capillary beds.

How sensitive is the tissue curve to f? From the preceding argument, we can already draw an important conclusion. If the area under the tissue curve depends only on λ, then varying f for constant λ will change the *shape* of the curve but not the area. Figure 13.4 shows examples for an intravascular agent, illustrating how f affects the initial slope of the tissue curve and the time of the peak but does not change the area. We can further define the limits to sensitivity to f by returning to Equation [13.1]. Imagine convolving two functions, one broad in time and one narrow. One can think of this as smoothing the broad function with a set of local weights defined by the narrow function, as we considered in Chapter 10 in the context of image smoothing. Whenever a broad curve is smoothed with a narrow curve, the resulting smoothed curve is similar to the original broad curve but scaled by the area of the narrow curve. For example, in standard curve smoothing, the area of the smoothing kernel (the narrow function) is kept equal to one to preserve the local mean of the curve being smoothed. Returning to our tissue curve, if the arterial concentration curve is much broader than the impulse response function, the tissue curve will be a slightly smoothed version of the arterial curve multiplied by the area of the impulse response (λ). In this case, the resulting curve does not depend much on the amplitude of the impulse response, so the tissue curve is only weakly sensitive to flow. On the other hand, if the arterial bolus is much narrower than the impulse response, the resulting tissue curve will be a slightly smoothed version of the impulse response multiplied by the area of the arterial curve. The shape of the impulse response then carries over into the tissue curve, and the peak of the tissue curve reflects f. These effects can be seen in the curves in Figure 13.4.

Another way to think about this is to note that the mean transit time τ is also the characteristic time required for the tissue to come into equilibrium with the blood. As discussed at the beginning of the chapter, the tissue curve is only sensitive to flow during the approach to equilibrium, and at equilibrium the curve just depends on λ. So for a broad bolus, such that the arterial curve changes very slowly, the tissue concentration of the agent quickly equilibrates with the current value of the arterial concentration. The result is that the tissue curve is essentially a replica of the arterial curve scaled by λ and carries no information on flow. On the other hand, with a very narrow bolus, the arterial concentration is changing so fast that the tissue concentration cannot catch up. The tissue curve then reflects how fast the local tissue concentration can change, which depends on τ and thus depends on flow.

Because τ for a diffusible agent is very long, nuclear medicine techniques all employ diffusible tracers to measure flow; it is easy to produce an arterial bolus that is much shorter than τ so that the local tissue curve will be sensitive to flow. To use an intravascular agent for a flow measurement requires a much sharper arterial bolus because τ is so short (about 4 s). Indeed, it was suggested in the nuclear medicine literature that measurement of CBF with an intravascular tracer is not possible (Lassen, 1984). The slight delay in the peak of the tissue curve relative to the arterial curve is difficult to measure, and unless the arterial bolus is only a few seconds wide,

Sensitivity to λ

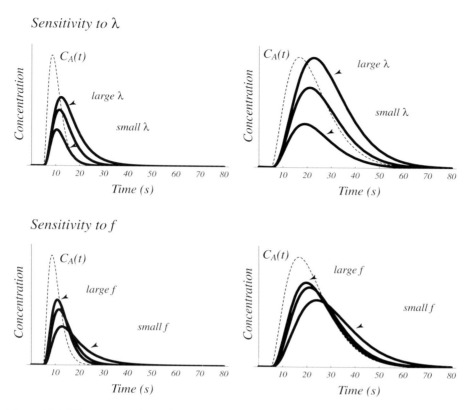

Figure 13.4. Tissue curves for an intravascular agent. The curves illustrate the sensitivity of the tissue concentration curves to the volume of distribution λ (top row) and the local blood flow f (bottom row) for a narrow arterial bolus (left column) and a broader arterial concentration curve $C_A(t)$ (right column). In each plot, the central curve was calculated for λ = 0.04 and f = 0.01 s^{-1} with an assumed exponential form for $r(t)$. The other two curves show the effects of increasing and decreasing one parameter by 50% (λ is varied in the top plots, and f is varied in the bottom plots). The area under the tissue concentration curve is λ times the area under the arterial concentration curve. For an intravascular agent λ = CBV, so the area under the curve provides a robust measurement of local blood volume. The tissue curve is only weakly sensitive to flow increases, particularly with a broader arterial curve, but is somewhat more sensitive to a decreased flow (ischemia). Note that the peak of the tissue curve is shifted in proportion to the mean transit time $\tau = \lambda/f$.

the amplitude of the tissue curve will depend primarily only on CBV and not CBF. However, with current MR imagers, it is possible to collect full images at rates faster than one image per second. Furthermore, with a rapid venous injection, it is possible to create an arterial bolus with a width of 4–8 s, which is comparable to τ for an intravascular agent in the resting human brain. Even though this is not sufficiently narrow to enter the regime where the peak of the curve depends only on CBF, it does produce a sensitivity of the tissue curve to the local CBF.

From the foregoing arguments, we should expect that the tissue curve of an intravascular agent would be more sensitive to ischemia (reduced flow) than to activation (increased flow), as can be seen in Figure 13.4. With a large flow increase, τ is shortened, and we move closer to the regime where the peak of the curve depends primarily on CBV and less on CBF. In contrast, with a reduction in flow, τ becomes longer, increasing the sensitivity to CBF.

The central problem in measuring CBF from a dynamic curve of an intravascular tracer is that the influence of CBF on the shape of the curve cannot be cleanly separated from the effects of CBV. This is in sharp contrast to the task of measuring CBV: the area under the tissue curve is directly proportional to CBV regardless of the local value of CBF. In other words, varying CBF with a constant CBV changes the shape of the tissue curve but does not change the area under it. Furthermore, the shift in the peak of the tissue curve depends on local delays in the arrival of the arterial bolus in addition to τ, so the time of the peak alone also is not a reliable indicator of CBF. Nevertheless, the fact that the shape of the tissue curve for a very sharp bolus does depend on the local CBF means that there is hope of extracting a measurement of CBF. This requires an analysis using both the arterial curve and the tissue curve and is discussed in Chapter 14.

In summary, measurements of the kinetics of an intravascular agent provide a robust measurement proportional to CBV based on the area under the tissue curve. That is, the area under the local tissue curve is a direct reflection of CBV, lacking only a global scaling factor, the area under the arterial curve. However, extracting an estimate of CBF from such data is more difficult, requiring rapid imaging, a narrow arterial bolus of the agent, and a measurement of the arterial concentration curve. The CBF estimate is likely to be more accurate in states of reduced flow than in states of increased flow; consequently, it is more useful in ischemia studies than in activation studies.

REFERENCES

Axel, L. (1980) Cerebral blood flow determination by rapid-sequence computed tomography: A theoretical analysis. *Radiology* **137**, 679–86.

Buxton, R. B., Frank, L. R., Wong, E. C., Siewert, B., Warach, S., and Edelman, R. R. (1998) A general kinetic model for quantitative perfusion imaging with arterial spin labeling. *Magn. Reson. Med.* **40**, 383–96.

Buxton, R. B., Wechsler, L. R., Alpert, N. M., Ackerman, R. H., Elmaleh, D. R., and Correia, J. A. (1984) The measurement of brain pH using 11-CO_2 and positron emission tomography. *J. Cereb. Blood Flow Metabol.* **4**, 8–16.

Frackowiak, R. S. J., Lenzi, G. L., Jones, T., and Heather, J. D. (1980) Quantitative measurement of cerebral blood flow and oxygen metabolism in man using ^{15}O and PET: Theory, procedure and normal values. *J. Comput. Assist. Tomogr.* **4**, 727–36.

Gibbs, J. M., Wise, R. J., Leenders, K. L., and Jones, T. (1984) Evaluation of cerebral perfusion reserve in patients with carotid artery occlusion. *Lancet* **1**, 310–14.

Grubb, R. L., Raichle, M. E., Eichling, J. O., and Ter-Pogossian, M. M. (1974) The effects of changes in PCO_2 on cerebral blood volume, blood flow, and vascular mean transit time. *Stroke* **5**, 630–9.

Kassissia, I. G., Goresky, C. A., Rose, C. P., Schwab, A. J., Simard, A., Huet, P. M., and Bach, G. G. (1995) Tracer oxygen distribution is barrier-limited in the cerebral microcirculation. *Circ. Res.* **77**, 1201–11.

Kluytmans, M., Grond, J. v. d., and Viergever, M. A. (1998) Gray matter and white matter perfusion imaging in patients with severe carotid artery lesions. *Radiology* **209**, 675–82.

Lassen, N. A. (1984) Cerebral transit of an intravascular tracer may allow measurement of regional blood volume but not regional flow. *J. Cereb. Blood Flow Metabol.* **4**, 633–4.

Lassen, N. A., and Perl, W. (1979) *Tracer Kinetic Methods in Medical Physiology.* Raven Press: New York.

Mandeville, J. B., Marota, J. J. A., Kosofsky, B. E., Keltner, J. R., Weissleder, R., Rosen, B. R., and Weisskoff, R. M. (1998) Dynamic functional imaging of relative cerebral blood volume during rat forepaw stimulation. *Magn. Reson. Med.* **39**, 615–24.

Meier, P., and Zierler, K. L. (1954) On the theory of the indicator-dilution method for measurement of blood flow and volume. *J. Appl. Physiol.* **6**, 731–44.

Obrist, W. D., Thompson, H. K., King, C. H., and Wang, H. S. (1967) Determination of regional cerebral blood flow by inhalation of 133-xenon. *Circ. Res.* **20**, 124–35.

Raichle, M. E. (1983) Brain blood flow measured with intravenous H2-O-15: Implementation and validation. *J. Nucl. Med.* **24**, 790–8.

Sokoloff, L., Reivich, M., Kennedy, C., Rosiers, M. H. D., Patlak, C. S., Pettigrew, K. D., Sakurada, O., and Shinohara, M. (1977) The [14-C]deoxyglucose method for the measurement of local cerebral glucose utilization: Theory, procedure, and normal values in the conscious and anesthetized albino rat. *J. Neurochem.* **28**, 897–916.

Zierler, K. L. (1962) Theoretical basis of indicator-dilution methods for measuring flow and volume. *Circ. Res.* **10**, 393–407.

14

Contrast Agent Techniques

BOLUS TRACKING STUDIES

The Beginning of fMRI

In clinical magnetic resonance imaging (MRI) studies contrast agents are used to alter local relaxation times (Lauffer, 1996). Gadolinium-DTPA is the most commonly used contrast agent. Gadolinium (Gd) is a lanthanide metal ion with the unique property of having seven unpaired electrons. In most atoms, electrons in an orbital pair up with opposite spin so that the net magnetic moment due to the electrons is zero. Unpaired electrons create a strong, fluctuating magnetic field in their vicinity that promotes relaxation of nuclear magnetic moments. When gadolinium reaches a tissue water pool, the T_1 of the local water protons is reduced, increasing the signal in a T_1-weighted image. In the healthy brain, Gd-DTPA does not cross the blood brain barrier, and because the agent remains confined to the vasculature, there is little relaxivity effect. The T_1 of the intravascular component is reduced, so the blood signal increases, but the extravascular spins are unaffected. The typical blood volume in brain tissue is only about 4%, so the net signal increase due to the presence of gadolinium is small. But in a tumor with leaky capillaries, the gadolinium readily diffuses into the extravascular space, and the tumor enhances on the magnetic resonance (MR) image.

In the late 1980s, Villringer and co-workers discovered an additional effect of gadolinium that forms the basis for using contrast agents in functional magnetic resonance imaging (fMRI) (Villringer et al., 1988). By observing the healthy brain with rapid dynamic MRI, they were able to track the bolus of Gd-DTPA as it passed through the brain in a rat model. The surprising result was that the MR signal *dropped* transiently as the bolus passed through. Given the common use of Gd-DTPA as a relaxivity agent to *enhance* the signal from specific tissues, it was clear that this effect was due to something other than the relaxation effect. The source of the effect is that gadolinium also possesses a large magnetic moment, which alters the local magnetic susceptibility (Fisel et al., 1991; Rosen et al., 1990). Because the gadolinium is confined to the blood vessels, the susceptibility difference between the intravascular and extravascular spaces creates microscopic field gradients in the tissue. As spins precess at different rates in the inhomogeneous field, their signals get out of phase with one another, and the net signal in a gradient recalled echo (GRE) image is reduced. This is described as a shortening of T_2^*. Furthermore, the signal is also reduced in a spin echo (SE) image because diffusion through the microscopic field gradients causes the spin echo to be less effective in refocusing the phase offsets due to field inhomogeneities (see Chapter 9). The magnetic susceptibility effect of gadolinium requires a sharp bolus to produce a high-enough concentration of gadolinium in the vessels to produce a significant susceptibility change, and it also requires an intact blood brain barrier to produce a susceptibility difference between the intravascular and extravascular spaces.

The discovery of this magnetic susceptibility effect and the development of techniques to follow the passage of an agent through the brain marked the beginning of fMRI, opening the door to physiological studies in addition to anatomy (Rosen, Belliveau, and Chien, 1989). The first demonstration of brain activation with MRI used serial injections of Gd-DTPA to measure the increased blood volume in the visual cortex when subjects viewed a flashing light (Belliveau et al., 1991). In the activated state, the signal drop as the gadolinium passed through the brain was deeper and shifted slightly earlier. For brain activation studies, BOLD techniques have superceded these contrast agent techniques, but as newer long-lasting agents are developed and approved for human use, we are likely to see a resurgence in interest in using contrast agents for fMRI studies. Dynamic contrast agent studies are now a standard clinical tool for investigating a number of disease states involving altered perfusion (Edelman et al., 1990; Rosen et al., 1991).

Measuring CBV with a Bolus Tracking Experiment

The signal drop as gadolinium passes through the microvasculature is transient, but can be measured with fast imaging techniques such as echo planar imaging (EPI). In qualitative terms, we expect that the larger the concentration of the agent within the voxel, the greater the field gradients produced, and the larger the signal dip will be. The underlying events in a dynamic contrast agent study are shown schematically in Figure 14.1. After a rapid venous injection, the agent passes through the heart and produces an arterial bolus, shown as a plot of the time-dependent arterial concentration $C_A(t)$. This bolus is delivered to each tissue ele-

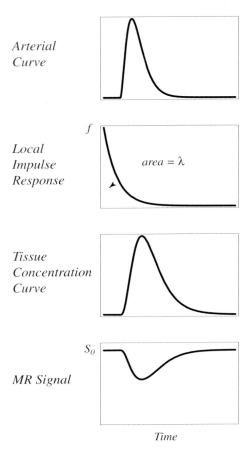

Arterial
Curve

Local
Impulse
Response

f

area $= \lambda$

Tissue
Concentration
Curve

MR Signal

S_0

Time

Figure 14.1. Dynamics of MR contrast agents. The effects of an agent such as Gd-DTPA are illustrated. A rapid venous injection produces an arterial bolus of the agent. The local tissue curve is the convolution of the arterial curve with a local impulse response function that depends on the local cerebral blood flow f and the cerebral blood volume λ. As the agent passes through the tissue, T_2^* is shortened, creating a dip in the local signal measured with dynamic MRI.

ment, creating a local tissue concentration curve $C_T(t)$. The tissue concentration curve is the convolution of the arterial curve with a local impulse response function that depends on the local cerebral blood flow (CBF) and cerebral blood volume (CBV) (see Chapter 13). The tissue concentration curve, in turn, shortens the local T_2^*, creating a dip in the MR signal curve measured over time. The MR signal curve is usually measured with a rapid EPI technique, with a typical temporal resolution of one image per second on each slice.

To extract a quantitative measurement of blood volume or blood flow from such data the signal must be modeled in more detail based on the principles of tracer kinetics introduced in Chapter 13. Tracer kinetics is based on modeling the dynamic curve of agent concentration in tissue as a function of time, but with MR studies, the measured quantity is the MR signal over time. So the modeling requires two steps: (1) relating agent concentration $C_T(t)$ to MR signal $S(t)$ and (2) relating physiological parameters such as blood flow and blood volume to $C_T(t)$. The first stage is modeling the biophysics of MR signal loss due to magnetized blood vessels, and the second stage is modeling the kinetics of how inflow and outflow control the tissue concentration of an injected agent.

In the first stage of modeling, the change in the MR signal $S(t)$ is related to the change in the gadolinium concentration. The general question of modeling the MR signal effects due to altered susceptibility of blood has received a great deal of attention (Boxerman et al., 1995; Kennan, Zhoug, and Gore, 1994; Weisskoff et al., 1994; Yablonsky and Haacke, 1994). The question is important not only for the interpretation of contrast agent curves but also for the interpretation of BOLD contrast due to altered blood oxygenation. The MR signal depends on the pulse sequence used, but for this application, the effect we are analyzing is an altered transverse relaxation, so the essential difference between pulse sequences is whether it is a gradient echo or spin echo acquisition. For a GRE acquisition, the additional signal loss due to gadolinium is primarily due just to the fact that the microscopic field distortions create an inhomogeneous field, and the additional dephasing of precessing spins reduces T_2^*. But with an SE pulse sequence, the effects of an inhomogeneous field are refocused, so naively we would expect an SE measurement to be insensitive to these field distortions. If the spatial scale of these distortions were macroscopic, like the broad field distortions created by the sinus cavities, the SE sequence would indeed correct for these effects. But because the spatial scale of the field distortion, the size of a capillary, is comparable to the distance moved by a diffusing water molecule during TE, the spin echo only partly refocuses these effects. The result is that an SE experiment, although less sensitive than a GRE experiment, nevertheless also shows a signal drop due to gadolinium. Furthermore, the spin echo is more effective at refocusing the effects of field gradients around larger vessels because the diffusion distance is then much shorter than the vessel radius. As a result, the SE signal is more sensitive to changes in the capillary magnetic susceptibility (see Chapter 9).

For SE and GRE experiments, we can model the dynamic MR signal as

$$S_{SE}(t) = S_0\, e^{-\text{TE}\, R_2(t)}$$
$$S_{GRE}(t) = S_0\, e^{-\text{TE}\, R_2^*(t)}$$

[14.1]

where TE is the echo time. The transverse relaxation rates can be expressed as

$$R_2(t) = R_2(0) + \Delta R_2(C_T(t))$$
$$R_2^*(t) = R_2^*(0) + \Delta R_2^*\,(C_T(t))$$

[14.2]

The local gadolinium concentration in tissue is $C_T(t)$, and the initial relaxation rates, $R_2(0)$ and $R_2^*(0)$, are simply the inverses of T_2 and T_2^* when there is no gadolinium present. The essential connection between the MR signal and the gadolinium concentration then depends on how ΔR_2 and ΔR_2^* depend on $C_T(t)$. This question is complicated because the answer depends on the size of the blood vessels involved. For the smallest vessels, with diameters comparable to the distance a water molecule moves randomly during an experiment, diffusion effects are important. As a result, this relationship is likely to be nonlinear for ΔR_2 (Boxerman et al., 1995). But for GRE studies, a simple approximation appears to be reasonably accurate: ΔR_2^* is proportional to the gadolinium concentration in the imaging voxel. We can then write

$$\Delta R_2^*(t) = k\, C_T(t) \qquad\qquad [14.3]$$

where k is a constant of proportionality.

The first step in analyzing dynamic contrast agent data is to use Equations [14.1]–[14.3] to convert the local MR signal measured over time $S(t)$ into a curve proportional to the tissue concentration $C_T(t)$ (Figure 14.2). This is done by normalizing the MR signal intensities to the initial intensity S_0 prior to injection and taking the natural logarithm

$$\Delta R_2^*(t) = -\frac{1}{TE}\ln\left(\frac{S(t)}{S_0}\right) = k\, C_T(t) \qquad\qquad [14.4]$$

With this connection between the dynamic MR curve and the local concentration of the agent, we can now apply the principles of tracer kinetics. In particular,

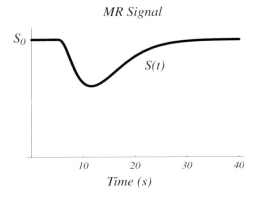

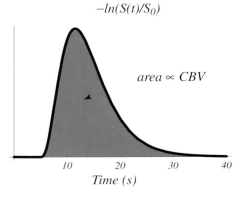

Figure 14.2. Analysis of dynamic contrast agent data. The MR signal over time $S(t)$ is first converted to a measure proportional to ΔR_2^* by normalizing each measured value $S(t)$ to the mean value S_0 before injection, and taking the natural logarithm. The area under this curve is then directly proportional to local CBV.

from Equation [B13.6] in Box 13, the integral of the tissue concentration curve is equal to λ times the integral of the arterial concentration, where λ is the volume of distribution of the agent. In the healthy brain, Gd-DTPA is an intravascular agent, so $\lambda = CBV$. Combining this with Equation [14.4],

$$\int_0^\infty \Delta R_2^*(t)\, dt \propto CBV \tag{14.5}$$

The missing constant of proportionality is k times the integral of the arterial concentration curve. The constant k is generally unknown, and the arterial curve is usually not measured. Nevertheless, a pixel-by-pixel map of the integral of ΔR_2^* is a map of CBV, lacking only a global scaling factor to convert the image intensities into units of absolute blood volume (i.e., milliliters of blood per milliliter of tissue).

The preceding arguments specifically applied to GRE studies, for which we can assume that ΔR_2^* varies approximately linearly with the local gadolinium concentration. But for SE studies, this relationship is likely to be nonlinear, and so we cannot assume that ΔR_2 is a linear function of the gadolinium concentration. Nevertheless, Boxerman and co-workers have argued that the integrated R_2 curve should still yield an accurate measurement proportional to local CBV as long as the form of this nonlinearity is reasonably uniform across the brain (Boxerman et al., 1995). In practice, dynamic SE data are analyzed in the same way as dynamic GRE data.

In a typical implemention of a CBV measurement from Gd-DTPA kinetics, dynamic images are collected for 40–60 s after rapid injection of the agent. To optimize the signal-to-noise ratio (SNR) of the CBV measurement, it is important that a sufficiently long period of baseline images be collected before the bolus of the agent arrives in the imaging voxel, so it is best to start the imaging series well before the agent is injected (Boxerman, Rosen, and Weisskoff, 1997). If the imaging is continued for 30–60 s after the arrival of the initial bolus, a broad but weaker second signal dip sometimes occurs due to recirculation of the agent. In principle, recirculation of the agent and reappearance in tissue is not a concern for the preceding analysis. This just makes the arterial curve have a more complicated shape, but the integrated tissue curve should still be simply proportional to the integral of this arterial curve including the second pass. However, if there is any leakage of the agent into the extravascular space, as might occur in tumors, or any tendency for the agent to bind to the endothelium and remain in the voxel, then recirculation poses a problem for accurate measurements of CBV. Furthermore, the integral of the arterial curve (or the tissue curve) is only a well-defined number if the curve returns to zero before the end of the experiment because otherwise it will depend on local transit delays as well. In practice, the tissue signal is often reduced at the end of the dynamic imaging, indicating that the agent is still circulating through the tissue. For these reasons, a useful approach is to fit the early part of the tissue concentration curve, covering the initial first-pass bolus, to an assumed shape and use the parameters of that fit to determine the area. The shape that is usually used is a gamma-variate function (Belliveau et al., 1991; Boxerman et al., 1997):

$$\Delta R_2^*(t) = K(t - t_0)^\alpha\, e^{-(t - t_0)/\beta} \tag{14.6}$$

where the amplitude K, the time of first arrival of the agent t_0, and the dimensionless parameters α and β are the free parameters adjusted to give the best fit to the data. The area under the first-pass part of the curve is then

$$\text{Area} = K\, \Gamma(1 + \alpha)\, \beta^{(1 + \alpha)} \qquad\qquad\qquad [14.7]$$

where $\Gamma(x)$ is the gamma function. The gamma-variate fitting approach generally works well when the SNR is reasonably high, but for very noisy data, it may actually make the SNR worse (Boxerman et al., 1997).

MEASURING CBF

The Sensitivity of the Tissue Curve to CBF

An intravascular agent such as Gd-DTPA provides a robust measurement of blood volume from the integrated tissue concentration curve. But is the shape of the curve sensitive enough to the local flow to provide a measurement of CBF as well? This has been a significant challenge, and progress has been made in recent years. To understand the problem, we must look more closely at the tissue curve that results from a bolus injection of an intravascular agent. The initial intravenous injection may require only a few seconds, but this initial bolus is broadened as it passes through the heart and lungs to enter the arterial blood, so the width of the arterial bolus as it arrives at the tissue capillary bed is typically about 4–10 s. We can explore the dependence of the resulting tissue curve on CBF with numerical simulations based on the general mathematical treatment of tracer kinetics developed in Box 13.

In Chapter 13 the tissue concentration curve of an agent was described in terms of the local CBF, which we will abbreviate as f for simplicity, and the local volume of distribution of the agent λ. By the central volume principle, these two quantities are always related to the mean transit time τ as $\tau = \lambda/f$. For the case of an intravascular agent, $\lambda = \text{CBV}$. In addition to these parameters, the tissue curve also depends on a function $r(t)$, the residue function that gives the probability that a molecule of the agent that arrived in the image voxel at $t = 0$ is still there at time t. The integral of $r(t)$ over all time is equal to τ, the mean transit time of the agent through the tissue. The tissue concentration curve $C_T(t)$ was modeled as a convolution of the arterial concentration curve with the local impulse response function, and the impulse response is the product $fr(t)$. Thus, the initial amplitude of the impulse response is equal to f, and the integrated area under the impulse response is λ [because the integral of $r(t)$ is τ, and $f\,\tau = \lambda$]. The impulse response must have these two properties to satisfy mass conservation, but the shape of the impulse response is unknown within these constraints.

We can appreciate the range of possible tissue curves by considering two extreme models for the impulse response that likely bracket the true shape for an intravascular agent. The first model is an exponential form, with $r(t) = e^{-ft/\lambda}$. This form arises in compartmental models and is often used to model freely diffusible tracers that fill the full tissue volume. In applying this form to an intravascular agent,

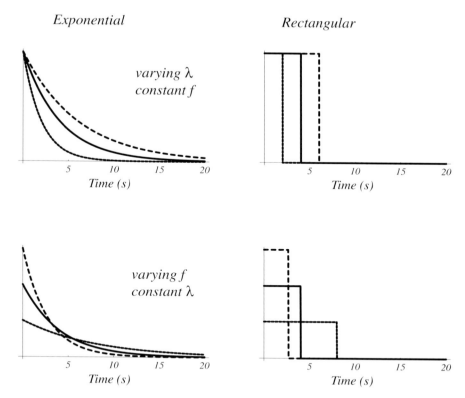

Figure 14.3. The shape of the impulse response function. The true shape of the impulse response function for an intravascular agent is not known, but it probably lies somewhere in between the two extremes shown here, an exponential and a rectangle. The only constraint on the impulse response function is that the initial value is f and the area is λ. The different curves show how the shape of the impulse response varies when one or the other of these parameters is varied.

we are treating the blood as a well-mixed single compartment. A well-mixed pool may seem like a poor model for a vascular bed, so the second model is appropriate for flow down identical pipes. Suppose that the capillaries are all identical, with equal length and blood velocity, and that the flow pattern is plug flow rather than laminar flow. Then every molecule of the agent will have the same transit time τ, and $r(t)$ is a rectangle with amplitude equal to one and a width τ (i.e., the probability for a molecule to still be in the tissue is one until $t = \tau$, and then it drops to zero). The two models are illustrated in Figure 14.3, showing how the shape of the impulse response changes when λ is varied with constant f and vice versa. Note that, as required, changing λ with constant f alters the area without changing the initial amplitude, while changing f with constant λ alters the initial amplitude but keeps the area constant.

Figure 14.4 illustrates the sensitivity of the tissue curve to the local parameters f and λ in a manner similar to Figure 13.4. In Figure 13.4 the focus was on the importance of producing a narrow arterial bolus for retaining sensitivity to flow. The goal with Figure 14.4 is to illustrate how the sensitivity to flow also involves a sensitivity

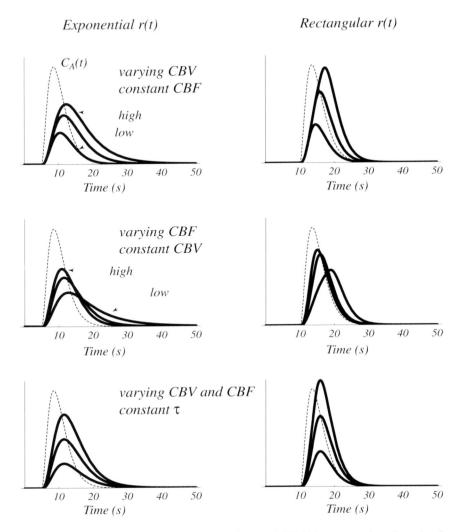

Figure 14.4. Sensitivity of the tissue curve to CBF and CBV. The curves show how the tissue concentration changes for different values of CBF and CBV for the two impulse response shapes shown in Figure 14.3. The top row shows the changes due to 50% changes (plus and minus) in CBV, producing corresponding changes in the area under the curve. The sensitivity to 50% changes in CBF (middle row) is more subtle, changing the shape of the curves without changing the area under them. The tissue curve is more sensitive to a decrease in CBF than an increase, and the shift of the peaks of the curves depends on the shape of the impulse response. When CBV and CBF change by the same amount (bottom row) so that the mean transit time τ remains constant, the curves are scaled replicas of one another.

to the unknown shape of $r(t)$. For all simulations, the arterial curve was the same narrow bolus, shown as a dotted line. In each plot, tissue curves are shown for three values of one of the parameters, with the other held fixed. The central curve in each plot was calculated for $f = 0.01$ s^{-1} (equivalent to 60 ml/100 g-min) and $\lambda = 0.04$, typical values for the healthy human brain. The tissue curves were calculated using

Equation [B13.1], with the two forms of the residue function $r(t)$ as described earlier: an exponential and a rectangle. The first row shows the effect of a 50% change in λ (plus and minus) with the flow held constant. The result is a dramatic change in the tissue curve, with the area under the curve directly proportional to λ. Note also that increasing λ also increases τ, and this broadens the curve and shifts the peak to a slightly later time by a few seconds. For the same delivery rate (f = constant), a larger volume of distribution takes longer to fill, although, because the intravascular volume is still a small fraction of the total volume, the additional time required is only a few seconds. Note also that the curves with a rectangular form of $r(t)$ have a substantially larger peak amplitude for the same values of f and λ.

The second row of plots shows the effect of 50% changes in f with λ held constant. For flow changes, the tissue curves are more similar in amplitude, differing only in the shape and timings. Indeed, the area under each curve is proportional to λ, regardless of the flow, so the differences in these curves are just shape changes with constant area. With increased flow, the tissue curve is narrower and peaks earlier. However, note that the tissue curve for a 50% increase in flow is very similar to the resting curve, particularly for the case of a rectangular $r(t)$. In short, the tissue curve is not very sensitive to flow increases above the normal level, so activation studies to measure the change in CBF using an intravascular tracer are likely to suffer from poor SNR. However, for a flow decrease, there is more of a change in the tissue curve, so the measurement of flow changes in ischemia is more feasible. The reason for the different sensitivity to a flow increase than a flow decrease is due to the change in τ. As discussed in Chapter 13, the tissue curve of any agent becomes insensitive to f when the width of the arterial bolus is much wider than τ. With a flow increase, τ becomes shorter, and the tissue curve moves closer to the regime where it is independent of f. But a decreased flow lengthens τ and so makes the tissue curve more sensitive to f.

The third row of plots shows curves in which f and λ are both changed by 50% so that the mean transit time $\tau = \lambda/f$ remains constant. The interesting result is that the three tissue curves are identical scaled replicas of each other. This illustrates the fact that the shape of the tissue curve is determined by τ, with the area scaled in proportion to λ.

From the curves in Figure 14.4, we can draw two conclusions: with an intravascular tracer, a measurement of CBV is quite robust, but a measurement of CBF is much more difficult. The area under the tissue curve is directly proportional to CBV, regardless of the value of CBF or the shape of $r(t)$. However, the tissue curve is intrinsically much less sensitive to CBF, and the nature of this sensitivity is more complex than the sensitivity to CBV. The value of the local CBF affects τ and through τ affects the width of the tissue curve and the timing of the peak. But these timing parameters are also strongly affected by the shape of the arterial curve. That is, τ affects how much the tissue curve is broadened and delayed compared with the arterial curve, so $C_A(t)$ must be measured to interpret these timing parameters of the tissue curve. The amplitude of the peak of the tissue curve is also affected by CBF, but this sensitivity also depends strongly on the shape of $r(t)$ (compare the two columns in Figure 14.4). To interpret the amplitude of the tissue curve in terms of

CBF, the form of $r(t)$ must be known or estimated from the data. In short, estimation of CBF from dynamic curves of an intravascular agent requires an additional measurement of the arterial curve and careful modeling of the data. We consider these questions in more detail in the following sections.

The Mean Transit Time

The mean transit time τ through a tissue element is equal to λ/f, as described by the central volume principle. But in the analysis of Gd-DTPA kinetic curves, a different parameter has been introduced and called the "mean transit time," abbreviated as MTT. This quantity is the time from injection of the bolus to the mean of the tissue concentration curve and so is distinctly different from τ. The MTT parameter is readily measured from the MR data and is routinely calculated. Furthermore, MTT is lengthened in ischemia, so the measurement has important value in assessing low flow states. However, it is unfortunate that this quantity is called the mean transit time because it creates confusion with the true mean transit time τ (Weisskoff et al., 1993). In the following, we will continue to use the standard terminology of MTT for this quantity and consider how it is related to τ.

The MTT has several physiological contributions. The first, of course, is the mean time of the arterial curve itself. The mean time of the tissue curve cannot be earlier than the mean time of the arterial curve. In addition, the relevant arterial curve is the curve at the imaging voxel, and this is delayed from the time of the injection due to the transit time Δt required for the agent to reach the tissue. Because the transit delays to different parts of the brain are different, Δt should be considered a local variable rather than a global variable such as the shape of the arterial curve. Finally, there is an additional broadening of the tissue curve due to the local kinetics. This term is of primary interest because it depends on the local blood flow.

Mathematically, calculating the MTT amounts to treating the tissue curve as a probability distribution and calculating the mean. In fact, also thinking of the arterial curve and the impulse response as probability functions is a fruitful way to see how these factors contribute to the final MTT of the tissue curve. The convolution of the arterial curve with the impulse response is analogous to the convolution of two probability functions. For example, if x and y are two independent random numbers, the probability distribution for $x+y$ is the convolution of the separate probability distributions for x and y, and the mean of $x+y$ is the sum of the mean x and the mean y. In other words, because of the convolution structure of the tissue curve, the final MTT is simply the sum of the individual MTTs of the arterial curve and the impulse response (Figure 14.5). Putting these contributions together with the initial transit delay, we can write

$$\text{MTT} = \Delta t + \text{MTT}_{art} + \text{MTT}_{tissue} \tag{14.7}$$

where MTT_{art} is the MTT of the arterial curve and MTT_{tissue} is the MTT of the impulse response function.

If the time of the first arrival of the agent, Δt, is estimated and subtracted from the full MTT, then the remainder is directly related to the MTT values of the arterial curve and of the tissue impulse response. It is tempting to assume at this point that

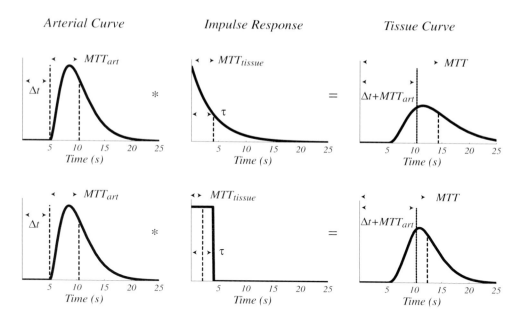

Arterial Curve   *Impulse Response*   *Tissue Curve*

Figure 14.5. The "mean transit time" (MTT). The quantity called MTT is not the true mean transit time τ but rather the mean time of the tissue concentration curve. For this reason, MTT includes transit delays Δt, the MTT of the arterial bolus (MTT_{art}), and the MTT of the tissue (MTT_{tissue}). Note, however, that even MTT_{tissue} is not necessarily equal to the true mean transit time τ. For an exponential impulse response function, $MTT_{tissue} = \tau$ (top row), but for a rectangular impulse response function, $MTT_{tissue} = \tau/2$ (bottom row).

the term MTT_{tissue} should be the true mean transit time τ, but this is still not correct, as illustrated in Figure 14.5. The figure shows the mean times for the arterial curve, the tissue curve, and the two forms of the impulse response we introduced earlier. For the exponential impulse response, MTT_{tissue} is indeed equal to τ, but for the rectangular impulse response, MTT_{tissue} is equal to $\tau/2$. The effect of this difference in MTT_{tissue} for the two models can also be seen in the tissue curves in this example. For the rectangular impulse response, the MTT is less than the MTT for the exponential model, despite the fact that the arterial curve and the local values of CBF and CBV are identical. These two forms of the impulse response function likely bracket the possible shapes in a real capillary bed, so we can conclude that MTT_{tissue} is always on the order of τ (within a factor of 2), but we cannot define the precise relationship between MTT_{tissue} and τ unless we know the form of $r(t)$.

The measured MTT is thus difficult to interpret in a rigorous quantitative way. But it is, nevertheless, a useful measurement. In ischemic states, several factors may combine to create a lengthened MTT. A partial stenosis of a major artery feeding the local capillary bed may result in a longer transit delay Δt in addition to a reduced perfusion. Collateral circulation feeding the affected area may also lead to a longer Δt because the blood follows a longer route in getting to the tissue capillary bed. A decrease in local CBF will increase τ, and so this will lengthen MTT_{tissue}. In addition, based on PET studies, it has been suggested that tissue at risk of infarction also has an elevated CBV (Gibbs et al., 1984), and this would further increase τ and MTT_{tissue}. Although the terminology is potentially confusing, the MTT, nevertheless, is likely to be a sensitive indicator of ischemia.

Measuring CBF

The preceding arguments and the simulations in Figure 14.4 suggest that the effects of CBF on the tissue concentration of an intravascular agent are subtle. Not only does the MTT depend on CBF, but it also depends on the width of the arterial bolus, the transit delays to the tissue vascular bed, and the shape of $r(t)$ in addition to τ. For this reason, the MTT does not provide a reliable way of measuring CBF, although it does provide a qualitative indication of CBF.

A possible approach to resolving these ambiguities, and obtaining a measurement of CBF from measurements of the tissue curve alone, is to measure the initial slope as the agent first arrives in the tissue. During the initial delivery phase, before any of the agent has had time to clear from the tissue, the quantity present in the tissue *is* directly proportional to how much has been delivered and so is proportional to local CBF. However, the measurement of this initial slope is difficult. The first arrival of the agent in a voxel must be estimated, and the slope must be estimated over a narrow time window smaller than τ (after a delay of τ, much of the initially delivered agent will have cleared from the voxel). In the healthy brain, with $\tau = 4$ s, only a small part of the measured tissue curve can be used. In ischemia, this measurement becomes more feasible because τ is substantially lengthened. With this approach, the measured quantity is proportional to local CBF, and the unknown proportionality constant depends on the early shape of the arterial input curve. In other words, a map of the initial slope would be a quantitative map of CBF, lacking only a global calibration factor to convert the map values into units of absolute CBF, in the same sense that a map of the integral of $\Delta R_2^*(t)$ is a quantitative map of CBV.

Given that CBF does have some effect on the shape of the entire tissue curve, a more general approach is to measure the arterial curve in addition to the tissue curve and then to model the tissue curve as a convolution of the arterial curve with an unknown impulse response function. The goal is to deconvolve the measured tissue curve to produce an estimate of the impulse response (Østergaard et al., 1996a, 1996b; Rempp et al., 1994). From the foregoing modeling considerations, the impulse response is $fr(t)$, so the initial amplitude is the local CBF.

Measuring the arterial input function presents some technical challenges. One approach is to draw arterial blood samples, as is done in quantitative PET studies, to measure the arterial concentration of the agent directly. Understandably, this is an undesirable approach for most human studies because of its invasiveness. An approach to estimating the arterial curve from dynamic imaging data is to look for pixels showing both the earliest arrival times of the agent and strong signal changes, which are presumably voxels dominated by arteries (Rempp et al., 1994). The average of the tissue curves for these voxels is then an estimate of the arterial curve. In an early application of this approach, Rempp and co-workers found reasonable average CBF values for human gray matter and white matter of 69.7 ± 29.7 and 33.6 ± 11.5 ml/100 g/min, respectively (Rempp et al., 1994). Part of the variance in the CBF measurements could be attributed to an effect of the age range of the subjects

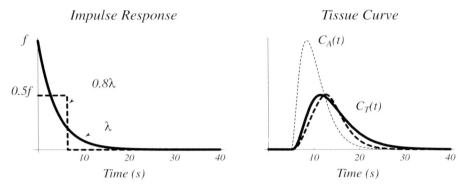

Figure 14.6. Ambiguities in estimating CBF from the tissue curve. The essential difficulty in estimating CBF from the tissue concentration curve of an intravascular agent is that different values of flow with different shapes of the impulse response function can nevertheless produce similar tissue concentration curves. The two impulse response shapes describe local flow values that differ by a factor of two (left), yet the tissue curves are nearly identical (right).

($n = 12$, with an age range of 20–64 yr), so the precision of the measurement is likely better than these variances would suggest.

Østergaard and co-workers have analyzed in depth the problem of deconvolving the arterial curve from the tissue curve to estimate the local impulse response function (Østergaard et al., 1996a, 1996b). The difficulty in any deconvolution problem is that two different impulse response functions may produce similar output curves when convolved with the same input curve (an example is shown in Figure 14.6). This makes the deconvolution process very sensitive to noise in that a small change in the data leads to a radically different estimate of CBF. One approach to deconvolution is to assume a form for the impulse response described by a few parameters, such as an exponential, and then to fit the data to determine these parameters. However, the correct form to use is not known, and in disease the local shape of $r(t)$ may change dramatically. An alternative, model-independent approach is to try to estimate the full shape of $r(t)$ from the data. This essentially amounts to modeling $r(t)$ at a finite set of times t, and finding the linear least squares best estimate of each of these amplitudes. Østergaard and co-workers found that a singular value decomposition (SVD) computational approach yielded the most reliable estimates of CBF (Østergaard et al., 1996b).

The work of Østergaard and co-workers shows that this approach can work, but deriving reliable routine measurements of CBF from the dynamics of an intravascular agent remains a challenging task. In particular, resolving ambiguities such as the one illustrated in Figure 14.6 requires high SNR measurements and accurate estimates of the arterial input function. As our understanding of the shape of the impulse response function in health and disease improves our ability to estimate CBF from contrast agent data will improve.

Other Contrast Agents

The foregoing description of contrast agent studies is shaped around a bolus injection of Gd-DTPA, and this is the standard approach. But a number of variations have also been developed. Gadolinium has a T_1 effect in addition to the T_2^* or

T_2 effect, and potentially this can complicate the quantitative analysis of the dynamic data, particularly in tumor studies in which there may be some leakage of the agent out of the vasculature. Dysprosium agents have been used as an alternative to gadolinium agents because dsyprosium creates a stronger T_2^* effect for the same dose but has no T_1 effect (Lev et al., 1997; Zaharchuk et al., 1998).

A limitation of Gd-DTPA studies is the short lifetime of the agent in the blood. Measurements of CBF with an intravascular agent are only possible when the agent is delivered as a sharp bolus, but simpler measurements of CBV could be done with an agent that remains in the blood for a longer time. If the agent exerts a susceptibility effect, then the signal difference before and after the administration of the agent would provide a direct measure of the local CBV. In contrast, with a dynamic injection, the tissue curve must be integrated over time, requiring fast dynamic imaging. And the cost of fast imaging is reduced image resolution and SNR. For this reason, a blood pool agent that creates a T_2^* effect could be used for higher resolution imaging of CBV.

Furthermore, with a long-lasting blood pool, agent another strategy is possible. The approach to the measurement of CBV with Gd-DTPA described earlier is based on the susceptibility effect of gadolinium, which alters local tissue T_2 and T_2^*. However, gadolinium also decreases the T_1 of blood, and so in a T_1-weighted image this will increase the blood signal. This is the basis for using a bolus of Gd-DTPA to enhance the signal of blood and improve MR angiography images. But this can also serve as the basis for measuring CBV with T_1-weighted images (Lin et al., 1997). Note that with this approach the echo time (TE) is kept short to minimize the T_2^* effect on the images, which has the opposite effect: a shorter T_1 increases the signal, but a shorter T_2 or T_2^* decreases the signal. However, T_1-based studies are potentially more sensitive to the effects of water exchange between blood and tissue because T_1 relaxation is much slower than T_2 relaxation (Donahue, Weisskoff, and Burstein, 1997).

If the blood concentration of the agent remains constant, dynamic changes in the CBV can be measured during activation studies with dynamic imaging. With a single injection of Gd-DTPA, we cannot measure dynamic changes in CBV because we interpret the dynamic signal curve as the result of a changing delivery of the agent to a constant local CBV. Multiple injections are required to measure CBV in different physiological states (Belliveau et al., 1991). However, multiple injections can have overlapping effects, even if the injections are tens of minutes apart (Levin et al., 1995). But if the agent remains at the same concentration in the blood, then after a brief adjustment time (a few seconds) the local concentration of the agent in the voxel will change to match a change in CBV, so dynamic signal changes will reflect changes in CBV. Contrast agent development is still an active field, and in recent years several approaches have been developed for producing a longer lasting blood pool agent, including gadolinium label of albumin (Schmiedl et al., 1987), red blood cells (Johnson et al., 1998), and dextran (Wang et al., 1990).

Another promising approach is the use of agents based on superparamagnetic iron oxide crystals (Majumdar, Zoghbi, and Gore, 1988; Weissleder et al., 1989, 1990). These particles are small (4–25 nm) and structurally similar to magnetite.

The term superparamagnetic describes the fact that the magnetic properties of these crystals lie between paramagnetism and ferromagnetism. As described in Chapter 7, in paramagnetism individual magnetic moments tend to align with an externally applied magnetic field. However, this alignment is due just to the independent interaction of each magnetic moment with the field; there is little interaction between the magnetic moments. In ferromagnetism, however, there is a strong interaction among the individual magnetic moments so that neighboring particles align together. This ordering extends over a certain range of distance and defines a domain of magnetization. A large crystal contains a number of domains, each with a different local orientation of the magnetization. At the domain boundaries, there is a sharp change in the magnetization orientation. When placed in a magnetic field, the domains aligned with the field grow at the expense of the other domains, producing a net magnetization that remains after the magnetic field is removed. Superparamagnetic crystals are sufficiently small that they only contain one domain and so do not display all the ferromagnetic properties of a larger crystal. Because of the iron spins, they become strongly magnetized in a magnetic field but do not retain the magnetization when the field is removed. Superparamagnetic iron agents produce strong T_2^* effects when confined to the vasculature, similar to gadolinium and dysprosium.

Most of the alternative blood pool agents already described are currently used only in animal studies (Forsting et al., 1994; Kent et al., 1990; Mandeville et al., 1996; 1998; Simonsen et al., 1999). But when similar agents are approved for human studies, they will provide a potentially powerful alternative to Blood Oxygenation Level Dependent (BOLD) techniques for activation studies.

CLINICAL APPLICATIONS

Contrast agent techniques have been applied to the study of a variety of disease states, including stroke, vascular stenosis, arteriovenous malformation, and cerebral neoplasm (Edelman et al., 1990). For example, several studies have shown that dynamic CBV measurements are diagnostically useful in determining the grade of gliomas, the most common primary neoplasms in the brain (Aronen et al., 1994; Maeda et al., 1993b; Sugahara et al., 1998). Both the treatment and the prognosis for gliomas depend on assessing the tumor grade, so this is a primary goal of diagnostic imaging. High-grade tumors are generally associated with disruption of the blood brain barrier and so enhance on T_1-weighted images with Gd-DTPA. But high-grade tumors are also associated with increased vascularity, which produces a larger signal dip with a dynamic Gd-DTPA study due to the larger CBV. At first glance, these two effects of gadolinium, T_1 enhancement and a susceptibility-related signal drop, appear to be mutually contradictory. The susceptibility effect depends on the gadolinium being confined to the vascular space, whereas the T_1 enhancement depends on the gadolinium leaving the blood. But both effects are possible if the gadolinium slowly leaks out of the blood. Then the first pass of the agent is dominated by susceptibility effects, particularly if the flip angle of a GRE pulse sequence is reduced to suppress T_1 sensitivity. After a few minutes, a T_1-weighted image shows enhancement.

MR contrast agent techniques have been used in many studies of ischemic disease and have helped to establish the current view of the evolution of stroke (Baird and Warach, 1998; Hossman and Hoehn-Berlage, 1995; Kucharczyk et al., 1991). In embolic stroke, the blockage of an artery reduces flow to a region of brain. If flow is not restored, an infarction will develop. However, stroke hardly ever results in complete ischemia, and collateral vessels can often provide some flow to parts of the ischemic territory. The current view of stroke is that there is often an ischemic core in which the flow is reduced to such a low level that cellular ionic levels cannot be maintained, leading over time to irreversible neuronal damage. However, surrounding this ischemic core is a region called the *ischemic penumbra,* characterized by reduced flow that is unable to supply sufficient metabolic energy to maintain electrical activity but is above the threshold for breakdown of cellular ionic gradients (Obrenovitch, 1995). This tissue is at risk of infarction but potentially can be saved; consequently, it is the target for therapeutic intervention. Tissue with reduced flow often has an elevated CBV, which is most likely a compensatory response to maintain flow by lowering cerebrovascular resistance in the face of a reduced driving pressure (Gibbs et al., 1984). As flow decreases further, the oxygen extraction fraction increases, a condition that has been called "misery perfusion" (Derdeyn et al., 1999).

The therapeutic window for acute stroke is the first few hours, before irreversible damage is done (Brott et al., 1992). However, with standard MRI, the first evidence of a stroke is not until several hours later, when blood brain barrier breakdown leads to accumulation of extravascular water, and this edema produces an enhancement in T_2-weighted images (Yuh et al., 1991). Two MR techniques have proven useful in assessing the early stages of stroke: diffusion imaging and contrast agent techniques. As described in Chapter 9, the earliest change in stroke detectable with MR is a reduction in the apparent diffusion constant (ADC) (Minterovich et al., 1991). Perfusion studies in animal models with MR contrast agents also reveal early changes (Kucharczyk et al., 1991; Maeda et al., 1993a). Human studies with contrast agent techniques have found reduced CBV in the infarct core (Rother et al., 1996; Sorensen et al., 1996) but elevated CBV in the peri-infarct zone has also been reported (Tsuchida et al., 1997).

Contrast agent techniques have also been used in studies of patients at risk for stroke to assess changes in tissue perfusion. Occlusive artery disease puts patients at greater risk of major stroke. With partial or complete occlusion of a major artery, the reduction of blood flow to an affected territory by normal circulation routes may be partially compensated by collateral pathways. Collateral flow in large vessels can be measured with angiographic techniques, but the pattern of collateral flow does not correlate well with increased oxygen extraction fraction measured with PET, an indication of local misery perfusion (Derdeyn et al., 1999). However, contrast agent studies provide a direct measure of compromised local hemodynamics, including increased CBV and lengthened MTT (Kluytmans et al., 1999; Kluytmans, Groud, and Viergever, 1998).

REFERENCES

Aronen, H. J., Gazit, I. E., Louis, D. N., Buchbinder, B. R., Pardo, F. S., Weisskoff, R. M., Harsh, G. R., Cosgrove, G. R., Halpern, E. F., Hochberg, F. H., and Rosen, B. R. (1994) Cerebral blood volume maps of gliomas: Comparison with tumor grade and histologic finding. *Radiology* **191,** 41–51.

Baird, A. E., and Warach, S. (1998) Magnetic resonance imaging of acute stroke. *J. Cereb. Blood Flow Metabol.* **18,** 583–609.

Belliveau, J. W., Kennedy, D. N., McKinstry, R. C., Buchbinder, B. R., Weisskoff, R. M., Cohen, M. S., Vevea, J. M., Brady, T. J., and Rosen, B. R. (1991) Functional mapping of the human visual cortex by magnetic resonance imaging. *Science* **254,** 716–19.

Boxerman, J. L., Hamberg, L. M., Rosen, B. R., and Weisskoff, R. M. (1995) MR contrast due to intravascular magnetic susceptibility perturbations. *Magn. Reson. Med.* **34,** 555–66.

Boxerman, J. L., Rosen, B. R., and Weisskoff, R. M. (1997) Signal-to-noise analysis of cerebral blood volume maps from dynamic NMR imaging studies. *J. Magn. Reson. Imag.* **7,** 528–37.

Brott, T. G., Haley, E. C., Levy, D. E., Barsan, W., Broderick, J., Sheppard, G. L., Spilker, J., Kongable, G. L., Massey, S., and Reed, R. (1992) Urgent therapy for stroke I: Pilot study of tissue plasminogen activator administered within 90 minutes. *Stroke* **23,** 632–40.

Derdeyn, C. P., Shaibani, A., Moran, C. J., Cross, D. T., Grubb, R. L., and Powers, W. J. (1999) Lack of correlation between pattern of collateralization and misery perfusion in patients with carotid occlusion. *Stroke* **30,** 1025–32.

Donahue, K. M., Weisskoff, R. M., and Burstein, D. (1997) Water diffusion and exchange as they influence contrast enhancement. *J. Magn. Reson. Imag.* **7,** 102–10.

Edelman, R. R., Mattle, H. P., Atkinson, D. J., Hill, T., Finn, J. P., Mayman, C., Ronthal, M., Hoogewoud, H. M., and Kleefield, J. (1990) Cerebral blood flow: Assessment with dynamic contrast-enhanced T^*_2-weighted MR imaging at 1.5 T. *Radiology* **176,** 211–20.

Fisel, C. R., Ackerman, J. L., Buxton, R. B., Garrido, L., Belliveau, J. W., Rosen, B. R., and Brady, T. J. (1991) MR contrast due to microscopically heterogeneous magnetic susceptibility: Numerical simulations and applications to cerebral physiology. *Magn. Reson. Med.* **17,** 336–47.

Forsting, M., Reith, W., Dorfler, A., von Kummer, R., Hacke, W., and Sartor, K. (1994) MRI in acute cerebral ischemia: Perfusion imaging with superparamagnetic iron oxide in a rat model. *Neuroradiology* **36,** 23–6.

Gibbs, J. M., Wise, R. J., Leenders, K. L., and Jones, T. (1984) Evaluation of cerebral perfusion reserve in patients with carotid artery occlusion. *Lancet* **1,** 310–14.

Hossman, K.-A., and Hoehn-Berlage, M. (1995) Diffusion and perfusion MR imaging of cerebral ischemia. *Cerebrovascular and Brain Metabolism Reviews* **7,** 187–217.

Johnson, K. M., Tao, J. Z., Kennan, R. P., and Gore, J. C. (1998) Gadolinium bearing red cells as blood pool MRI contrast agents. *Magn. Reson. Med.* **40,** 133–42.

Kennan, R. P., Zhong, J., and Gore, J. C. (1994) Intravascular susceptibility contrast mechanisms in tissues. *Magn. Reson. Med.* **31,** 9–21.

Kent, T., Quast, M., Kaplan, B., Lifsey, R. S., and Eisenberg, H. M. (1990) Assessment of a superparamagnetic iron oxide (AMI-25) as a brain contrast agent. *Magn. Reson. Med.* **13,** 434–43.

Kluytmans, M., Grond, J. v. d., Everdingen, K. J. v., Klijn, C. J. M., Kappelle, L. J., and Viergever, M. A. (1999) Cerebral hemodynamics in relation to patterns of collateral flow. *Stroke* **30,** 1432–9.

Kluytmans, M., Grond, J. v. d., and Viergever, M. A. (1998) Gray matter and white matter perfusion imaging in patients with severe carotid artery lesions. *Radiology* **209**, 675–82.

Kucharczyk, J., Mintorovitch, J., Asgari, H. S., and Moseley, M. (1991) Diffusion/perfusion MR imaging of acute cerebral ischemia. *Magn. Reson. Med.* **19**, 311–15.

Lauffer, R. B. (1996) MR contrast agents: Basic principles. In: *Clinical Magnetic Resonance Imaging, Vol. 1,* pp. 177–91. Eds. R. R. Edelman, J. R. Hesselink, and M. B. Zlatkin. Saunders: Philadelphia.

Lev, M. H., Kulke, S. F., Sorensen, A. G., Boxerman, J. L., Brady, T. J., Rosen, B. R., Buchbinder, B. R., and Weisskoff, R. M. (1997) Contrast-to-noise ratio in functional MRI of relative cerebral blood volume with sprodiamide injection. *J. Magn. Reson. Imag.* **7**, 523–7.

Levin, J. M., Kaufman, M. J., Ross, M. H., Mendelson, J. H., Maas, L. C., Cohen, B. M., and Renshaw, P. F. (1995) Sequential dynamic susceptibility contrast MR experiments in human brain: Residual contrast agent effect, steady state, and hemodynamic perturbation. *Magn. Reson. Med.* **34**, 655–63.

Lin, W., Paczynski, R. P., Kuppusamy, K., Hsu, C. Y., and Haacke, E. M. (1997) Quantitative measurements of regional cerebral blood volume using MRI in rats: Effects of arterial carbon dioxide tension and mannitol. *Magn. Reson. Med.* **38**, 420–8.

Maeda, M., Itoh, S., Ide, H., Matsuda, T., Kobayashi, H., Kubota, T., and Ishii, Y. (1993a) Acute stroke in cats: Comparison of dynamic susceptibility-contrast MR imaging with T_2- and diffusion-weighted MR imaging. *Radiology* **189**, 227–32.

Maeda, M., Itoh, S., Kimura, H., Iwasaki, T., Hayashi, N., Yamamoto, K., Ishii, Y., and Kubota, T. (1993b) Tumor vascularity in the brain: Evaluation with dynamic susceptibility-contrast MR imaging. *Radiology* **189**, 233–8.

Majumdar, S., Zoghbi, S. S., and Gore, J. C. (1988) Regional differences in rat brain displayed by fast MRI with superparamagnetic contrast agents. *Magn. Reson. Imag.* **6**, 611–15.

Mandeville, J. B., Marota, J., Keltner, J. R., Kosovsky, B., Burke, J., Hyman, S., LaPointe, L., Reese, T., Kwong, K., Rosen, B., Weissleder, R., and Weisskoff, R. (1996) CBV functional imaging in rat brain using iron oxide agent at steady state concentration. In: *ISMRM, Fourth Scientific Meeting,* pp. 292: New York.

Mandeville, J. B., Marota, J. J. A., Kosofsky, B. E., Keltner, J. R., Weissleder, R., Rosen, B. R., and Weisskoff, R. M. (1998) Dynamic functional imaging of relative cerebral blood volume during rat forepaw stimulation. *Magn. Reson. Med.* **39**, 615–24.

Minterovich, J., Moseley, M. E., Chileuitt, L., Shimizu, H., Cohen, Y., and Weinstein, P. R. (1991) Comparison of diffusion- and T_2-weighted MRI for the early detection of cerebral ischemia and reperfusion in rats. *Magn. Reson. Med.* **18**, 39–50.

Obrenovitch, T. P. (1995) The ischaemic penumbra: Twenty years on. *Cerebrovascular and Brain Metabolism Reviews* **7**, 297–323.

Østergaard, L., Sorensen, A. G., Kwong, K. K., Weisskoff, R. M., Gyldensted, C., and Rosen, B. R. (1996a) High resolution measurement of cerebral blood flow using intravascular tracer bolus passages. Part II: Experimental comparison and preliminary results. *Magn. Reson. Med.* **36**, 726–36.

Østergaard, L., Weisskoff, R. M., Chesler, D. A., Gyldensted, C., and Rosen, B. R. (1996b) High resolution measurement of cerebral blood flow using intravascular tracer bolus passages. Part I: Mathematical approach and statistical analysis. *Magn. Reson. Med.* **36**, 715–25.

Rempp, K. A., Brix, G., Wenz, F., Becker, C. R., Guckel, F., and Lorenz, W. J. (1994) Quantification of regional cerebral blood flow and volume with dynamic susceptibility contrast-enhanced MR imaging. *Radiology* **193**, 637–41.

Rosen, B. R., Belliveau, J. W., Aronen, H. J., Kennedy, D., Buchbinder, B. R., Fischman, A., Gruber, M., Glas, J., Weisskoff, R. M., Cohen, M. S., Hochberg, F. H., and Brady, T. J. (1991) Susceptibility contrast imaging of cerebral blood volume: human experience. *Magn. Reson. Med.* **22,** 293–9.

Rosen, B. R., Belliveau, J. W., and Chien, D. (1989) Perfusion imaging by nuclear magnetic resonance. *Magn. Reson. Quart.* **5,** 263–81.

Rosen, B. R., Belliveau, J. W., Vevea, J. M., and Brady, T. J. (1990) Perfusion imaging with NMR contrast agents. *Magn. Reson. Med.* **14,** 249–65.

Rother, J., Guckel, F., Neff, W., Schwartz, A., and Hennerici, M. (1996) Assessment of regional cerebral blood volume in acute human stroke by use of single-slice dynamic susceptibility contrast-enhanced magnetic resonance imaging. *Stroke* **27,** 1088–93.

Schmiedl, U., Ogan, M., Paajanen, H., Marotti, M., Crooks, L. E., Brito, A. C., and Brasch, R. C. (1987) Albumin labeled with Gd-DTPA as an intravascular blood pool enhancing agent for MR imaging: Biodistribution and imaging studies. *Radiology* **162,** 205–10.

Simonsen, C. Z., Østergaard, L., Vestergaard-Poulsen, P., Rohl, L., Bjornerud, A., and Gyldensted, C. (1999) CBF and CBV measurements by USPIO bolus tracking: reproducibility and comparison with Gd-based values. *J. Magn. Reson. Imag.* **9,** 342–7.

Sorensen, A. G., Buonanno, F. S., Gonzalez, R. G., Schwamm, L. H., Lev, M. H., Huang-Helliger, F. R., Reese, T. G., Weisskoff, R. M., Davis, T. L., Suwanwela, N., Can, U., Morreira, J. A., Copen, W. A., Look, R. B., Finklestein, S. P., Rosen, B. R., and Koroshetz, W. J. (1996) Hyperacute stroke: Evaluation with combined multisection diffusion-weighted and hemodynamically weighted echo-planar MR imaging. *Radiology* **199,** 391–401.

Sugahara, T., Korogi, Y., Kochi, M., Ikushima, I., Hirai, T., Okuda, T., Shigematsu, Y., Liang, L., Ge, Y., Ushio, Y., and Takahashi, M. (1998) Correlation of MR imaging-determined cerebral blood volume maps with histologic and angiographic determination of vascularity of gliomas. *Am. J. Radiol.* **171,** 1479–86.

Tsuchida, C., Yamada, H., Maeda, M., Sadato, N., Matsuda, T., Kawamura, Y., Hayashi, N., Yamamoto, K., Yonekura, Y., and Ishii, Y. (1997) Evaluation of peri-infarcted hypoperfusion with T^*_2-weighted dynamic MRI. *J. Magn. Reson. Imag.* **7,** 518–22.

Villringer, A., Rosen, B. R., Belliveau, J. W., Ackerman, J. L., Lauffer, R. B., Buxton, R. B., Chao, Y.-S., Wedeen, V. J., and Brady, T. J. (1988) Dynamic imaging with lanthanide chelates in normal brain: Contrast due to magnetic susceptibility effects. *Magn. Reson. Med.* **6,** 164–74.

Wang, S. C., Wikstrom, M. G., White, D. L., Klaveness, J., Holtz, E., Rongved, P., Moseley, M., and Brasch, R. C. (1990) Evaluation of Gd-DTPA labelled dextran as an intravascular MR contrast agent: Imaging characteristics in normal rat tissue. *Radiology* **175,** 483–8.

Weisskoff, R. M., Chesler, D., Boxerman, J. L., and Rosen, B. R. (1993) Pitfalls in MR measurements of tissue blood flow with intravascular tracers: Which mean transit time? *Magn. Reson. Med.* **29,** 553–9.

Weisskoff, R. M., Zuo, C. S., Boxerman, J. L., and Rosen, B. R. (1994) Microscopic susceptibility variation and transverse relaxation: Theory and experiment. *Magn. Reson. Med.* **31,** 601–10.

Weissleder, R., Elizondo, G., Wittenberg, J., Rabito, C. A., Bengele, H. H., and Josephson, L. (1990) Ultrasmall paramagnetic iron oxide: Characterization of a new class of contrast agents for MR imaging. *Radiology* **175,** 489–93.

Weissleder, R., Stark, D. D., Engelstad, B. L., Bacon, B. R., Compton, C. C., White, D. L., Jacobs, P., and Lewis, J. (1989) Superparamagnetic iron oxide: Pharmokinetics and toxicity. *AJR* **152,** 167–73.

Yablonsky, D. A., and Haacke, E. M. (1994) Theory of NMR signal behavior in magnetically inhomogenous tissues: The static dephasing regime. *Magn. Reson. Med* **32,** 749–63.

Yuh, W. T. C., Crain, M. R., Loes, D. J., Greene, G. M., Ryals, T. J., and Sato, Y. (1991) MR imaging of cerebral ischemia: Findings in the first 24 hours. *Am. J. Neuroradiol.* **12,** 621–9.

Zaharchuk, G., Bogdanov, A. A., Marota, J. J. A., Shimizu-Sasamata, M., Weisskoff, R. M., Kwong, K. K., Jenkins, B. G., Weissleder, R., and Rosen, B. R. (1998) Continuous assessment of perfusion by tagging including volume and water extraction (CAPTIVE): A steady-state contrast agent technique for measuring blood flow, relative blood volume fraction, and the water extraction fraction. *Magn. Reson. Med.* **40,** 666–78.

15

Arterial Spin Labeling Techniques

INTRODUCTION

Bolus tracking studies with intravascular contrast agents provide a robust measurement of blood volume, but as discussed in Chapter 14 a measurement of cerebral blood flow (CBF) is more difficult. The kinetic curve of an intravascular contrast agent is more sensitive to decreases in CBF than increases, making these techniques a useful tool for clinical studies of ischemia but less useful for measurements of CBF changes with activation in the healthy brain. In recent years, a different class of techniques for measuring local tissue perfusion with MRI has been developed based on arterial spin labeling (ASL) (Alsop and Detre, 1996; Detre et al., 1992; Edelman et al., 1994; Helpern et al., 1997; Kim, 1995; Williams et al., 1992; Wong, Buxton, and Frank, 1998a).

ASL techniques provide noninvasive images of local CBF with better spatial and temporal resolution than any other technique, including nuclear medicine methods. The development of ASL techniques is an active area of research, and although they are not yet widely available on standard MR imagers, ASL applications are steadily growing. The standard technique for mapping patterns of activation in the healthy brain is still Blood Oxygenation Level Dependent (BOLD) imaging, but questions remain about the accuracy of localization of BOLD changes and the quantitative interpretation of the magnitude of BOLD signal changes (see Part IIIB). ASL techniques have already become a standard tool for investigations of the mechanisms underlying the BOLD effect (Buxton, Wong, and Frank, 1998b; Hoge et al., 1999a, 1999b, 1999c; Kim and Ugurbil, 1997), and the applications of ASL to more routine activation studies are likely to continue to expand. One limitation of the BOLD technique is that it is sensitive only to changes in perfusion associated with a particular task and insensitive to chronic alterations of perfusion. Because ASL provides a direct measurement of CBF, these methods are likely to find wider clinical applications in studies of disease progression, in the evaluation of pharmacological treatments, and perhaps in routine diagnosis of diseases marked by altered CBF (Alsop, Detre, and Grossman, 2000).

The principle behind ASL techniques is relatively simple (Figure 15.1). The goal is to measure CBF, the rate of delivery of arterial blood to a local brain voxel in an imaged slice of interest. Before acquiring the image, a 180° radiofrequency (RF) inversion pulse is applied to flip the magnetization of the water in arterial blood before the blood reaches the image slice. The water molecules carrying the labeled magnetization flow into each tissue element in proportion to the local CBF. After a sufficient delay TI to allow the tagged blood to reach the slice of interest, the tag image is made. The experiment is then repeated without labeling the arterial blood to create a control image, and the two images are subtracted to produce the ASL difference image. In the difference image, the signal from static spins subtracts out, leaving just the signal of arterial blood delivered to each voxel during the time interval TI.

More quantitatively, the delivered arterial blood carries an intrinsic magnetization M_{0A} in the control image, the fully relaxed arterial blood equilibrium magnetization. In the ideal case (e.g., neglecting relaxation and other factors), the arterial blood carries a magnetization $-M_{0A}$ in the tag image because of the inversion. Furthermore, the amount of blood delivered during the interval TI is fTI, where f is the local CBF. Then for the ideal case, the signal in the ASL difference image is due to a change in net magnetization $\Delta M = 2M_{0A} f$TI. For a CBF of 60 ml/min-100 ml of tissue ($= 0.01$ s^{-1}) and a typical experiment time of TI $= 1$ s, ΔM is on the order of 1% of M_{0A}, so the ASL difference signal is small compared to the raw image signal. Nevertheless, the signal intensity in the ASL difference image is directly proportional to local CBF, and with sufficient averaging CBF can be mapped reliably.

This is the basic idea behind all ASL techniques. In the context of tracer kinetics, the "agent" used here is labeled water, a diffusible tracer, and these ASL techniques closely parallel PET techniques using $H_2^{15}O$ (Frackowiak et al., 1980; Raichle, 1983). However, an important difference is that in ASL the water is labeled magnetically, rather than by injection of a tracer, and the ASL experiment can be repeated many times to improve the signal-to-noise ratio (SNR) or to follow the dynamics of CBF change with activation. Although the basic idea behind ASL is simple, the implementation of this idea requires careful attention to the details of the experimental design and a number of confounding factors that must be taken into account

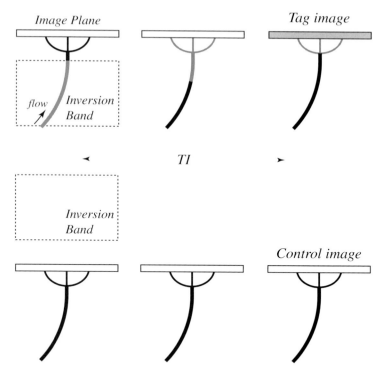

Figure 15.1. Arterial spin labeling. The basic principle of ASL is to acquire two images of a slice through the brain, a *tag* image following inversion of the magnetization of arterial blood and a *control* image in which the magnetization of arterial blood is not inverted. The illustration shows one implementation of this idea in which a 180° inversion pulse is applied to a band below the image plane (top row), and after a delay TI to allow the tagged arterial blood (shown as a gray vessel) to be delivered to the slice, the tag image is acquired. For the control image, the inversion band is applied above the slice so that blood is not tagged (but off-resonance effects on the static spins in the image plane are balanced), and the control image is also collected after a delay TI. If the control experiment is carefully designed, the static tissue subtracts out from the ASL difference signal (control – tag) leaving a direct image of the amount of arterial blood delivered to each voxel of the slice in the time interval TI.

for the measurement to be a quantitative reflection of CBF. The various ASL techniques differ in how the tagging is done, how the control image is acquired, and how potential systematic errors are handled.

Historically, two basic approaches to ASL perfusion imaging have been developed, which can be classified as pulsed ASL (PASL) and continuous ASL (CASL). Initially, these two approaches seemed quite distinct. But over time it has become clear that for human studies both of the original approaches suffer from systematic errors due to physiological factors other than CBF that affect the measurement, in particular the transit delay from the tagging region to the slice. For quantitative perfusion measurements, these techniques have been modified to deal with this problem, and with these changes the two approaches in fact are converging, as is discussed more fully later. But for now, it is helpful to understand the original approaches. A related approach, called the T_1-method, is discussed in Box 15.

BOX 15. THE T_1 METHOD

The description of ASL methods in the main text focused on the signal difference between an image with tagged arterial blood and a control image without tagging, isolating the signal from delivered blood from the static tissue signal. But there is a related technique that instead focuses on how flow affects the local longitudinal relaxation, called the T_1 method (Chesler and Kwong, 1995; Kwong et al., 1992; Schwarzbauer, Morrissey, and Haase, 1996). The method uses many of the same key ideas as the ASL techniques, but the viewpoint is different, and it can be difficult to see precisely how the two approaches are connected.

The T_1 method involves the same measured data as in the FAIR experiment: inversion recovery (IR) signals measured at different inversion times TI with selective and nonselective inversion pulses. If we were to analyze this data as a FAIR experiment, we would treat the data collected with a nonselective inversion as the tagged images and the data collected with the selective inversion as the control images, and for each TI we would calculate the ASL difference signal (control – tag). This difference signal as a function of TI would be treated as the concentration of a delivered "agent" and analyzed as though it were from a tracer kinetic study. But to understand the T_1 method, we need to switch viewpoints and think of the data as two sets of data measuring longitudinal relaxation after an inversion pulse, one with a slice-selective inversion and the other with a non-selective inversion. Each of these two sets of data is analyzed separately to measure the apparent relaxation time T_1.

To make this concrete, suppose that we have an ideal physiological and experimental scenario: (1) each tissue voxel has a uniform tissue composition (e.g., not a mixture of gray matter and white matter); (2) water freely diffuses through the entire tissue space; (3) water is 100% extracted in its passage through the capillary bed; and (4) the slice-selective inversion pulse has a perfectly rectangular slice profile so that there are no transit delays. Now consider how tissue relaxation is affected in the slice-selective inversion recovery experiment. After the inversion pulse, the tissue magnetization begins to relax back toward equilibrium with a time constant T_1. At the same time, blood flow carries away inverted spins and delivers fully relaxed spins because we assume that arterial spins just outside the edge of the voxel are not affected by the selective inversion pulse. The total water content remains the same, so effectively inverted spins are exchanged one for one for fully relaxed spins, which looks just as if they have relaxed back to equilibrium. Thus, flow appears as an enhanced longitudinal relaxation.

To see quantitatively how flow affects the apparent relaxation rate, it is helpful to think about the magnetization difference from equilibrium, $M_0 - M(t)$, where M_0 is the tissue equilibrium magnetization, and $M(t)$ is the tissue magnetization at time t. Longitudinal relaxation is simply an exponential attenuation of this difference. In a short interval between t and $t + dt$, the change in the longitudinal magnetization due to relaxation is

$$dM_{relax} = [M_0 - M(t)] \frac{dt}{T_1} \qquad \text{[B15.1]}$$

In the same time interval dt, flow delivers a magnetization $fM_{0A}dt$ and clears a magnetization $fM_v(t)dt$, where $M_v(t)$ is the venous magnetization. We now make two assumptions about the relationship between the blood and tissue magnetizations. The first assumption is that the tissue can be treated as a single, well-mixed compartment, so that $M_v = M/\lambda$, where λ is the classical partition coefficient for water. The second assumption is that the blood equilibrium magnetization M_{0A} is equal to M_0/λ. Then the net change in the magnetization due to flow is

$$dM_{flow} = fM_{0A} - fM_v = [M_0 - M(t)]\frac{fdt}{\lambda} \qquad [B15.2]$$

This has precisely the same form as true T_1 decay (i.e., the change is proportional to the current value, which produces exponential decay), and so the net relaxation curve including flow is again a simple exponential, but with an effective time constant T_{1app} given by

$$\frac{1}{T_{1app}} = \frac{1}{T_1} + \frac{f}{\lambda} \qquad [B15.3]$$

This is the essential relationship underlying the T_1 method: with a selective inversion pulse, the apparent T_1 depends on local flow. By measuring a relaxation curve with multiple TIs, the data can be fit to determine T_{1app}. If T_1 can be measured separately, then f/λ can be calculated directly. However, T_1 is a local tissue property, and the difference between T_1 and T_{1app} is very small: $1/T_1$ is about 1 s^{-1}, whereas f/λ is about 0.01 s^{-1}. Because of this small difference, it is necessary to measure the true T_1 locally with high precision to make an accurate estimate of f/λ. And this is where the difficulty comes in for the T_1 method: how do we measure the true T_1 of tissue without any flow contribution?

The approach employed is to measure a similar relaxation curve with a nonselective inversion pulse. Then the arterial blood is also inverted, so we no longer have an exchange of inverted spins for fully relaxed spins. If we further assume that the T_1 of blood is the same as the T_1 of tissue, then the inverted arterial spins and the inverted tissue spins relax at the same rate, and in this case flow has no effect on the relaxation curve. The measured T_1 is then the true T_1 of tissue. In a sense, this provides the control experiment, showing what relaxation would be like without flow. But here we see some of the confusion between the T_1 method and the ASL methods. The FAIR experiment uses essentially the same data, yet we described the nonselective inversion experiment as the tag experiment, and the selective inversion experiment as the control experiment based on whether the arterial blood was inverted. Furthermore, we argued earlier that the ASL techniques are sensitive to f, independent of λ, but Equation [B15.3] clearly shows that the T_1 method is only sensitive to the ratio f/λ. How can this be if both FAIR and the T_1 method work with the same data?

In fact, the presence of the form f/λ in Equation [B15.3] is somewhat subtle, and ultimately misleading. In Chapter 13, λ was introduced as the partition coefficient (or volume of distribution) of an agent. In tracer kinetics studies, the form f/λ arises in the description of the clearance of the agent from tissue. For example, in a ^{133}Xe study, the exponential clearance of the agent is monitored with external detectors, and the time constant for clearance is $\tau = \lambda/f$, the mean transit time through the tissue. In Equation [15.1], λ was introduced in just this way in the venous clearance term. So it is natural to assume that the source of the factor f/λ in Equation [B15.3] is simply the factor f/λ that

(continued)

BOX 15, continued

appears in Equation [15.1]. This would imply that the T_1 method is somehow sensitive to the clearance of the tagged spins, as in a ^{133}Xe study. However, this is not correct, despite previous arguments to the contrary by the present author (Buxton et al., 1998a).

In fact, because the duration of a PASL experiment is very short, we would expect that clearance of the tagged spins by venous flow should be negligible during the course of the experiment so that the measured data are independent of the classical partition coefficient λ. For example, suppose that we examined two hypothetical capillary beds, one in which water freely diffuses into the tissue space and one in which the capillary wall is completely impermeable to water. In the first case λ is about 1.0, and in the second case λ is about 0.04, the blood volume fraction. This is a huge difference in the local value of λ, and yet the signals measured for multiple TIs in the range of 0–1.5 s with both selective and nonselective inversions would be nearly identical. For these short experiments, there is no time for any appreciable fraction of the tagged spins to clear by venous flow. So despite the form of Equation [B15.3], the change in the apparent relaxation rate cannot really depend on the classical partition coefficient λ.

The source of the expression f/λ in Equation [B15.3] is not the clearance term from Equation [15.1] but rather the second assumption we made about λ preceding Equation [B15.2]. There we assumed that $M_0/M_{0A} = \lambda$. To emphasize that this is an assumption, we will define this ratio as λ', and the assumption that led to Equation [B15.3] is then $\lambda' = \lambda$. It is really λ' that enters into Equation [B15.3]. To see this, consider an example in which λ' is not equal to λ. Suppose that we compare two voxels, one filled with gray matter (GM) and one half-filled with GM and half with cerebrospinal fluid (CSF). Let the CBF and the partition coefficient of the full GM voxel be f and λ, respectively. What would different techniques measure in the voxel half-filled with gray matter? For the sake of the argument, assume that there is an impenetrable barrier between the CSF and the GM so that water delivered to the gray matter by flow does not have access to the adjoining CSF space. Then the net flow to the half-filled voxel is $f/2$, but the classical partition coefficient is $\lambda/2$ because the delivered water would only fill half of the voxel. Because of this, nuclear medicine techniques would give different results depending on whether they were sensitive to delivery or clearance of the agent. For example, a microsphere study, which depends only on delivery, would measure the flow to be $f/2$ in the voxel half full of gray matter. However, a ^{133}Xe study, which is sensitive only to clearance of the agent, would measure f/λ to be identical in the two voxels because both f and λ are reduced by a factor of two in the half-filled voxel. In other words, the clearance time is unchanged.

What would MR measurements show for the same half-filled voxel? With the ASL approach, the tagged spins are treated essentially as microspheres because there is little time for clearance. So analyzing the data as a FAIR experiment, the measured flow would be $f/2$. But what would the T_1 method find? From Equation [B15.3], it would appear that the calculated value of f/λ should be identical to that for the voxel filled with GM. But in fact the relaxation curve is now more complicated because the measured curve is really the sum of two separate relaxation curves for GM and CSF. To clarify the argument, suppose that the equilibrium magnetizations of CSF and GM are identical, and that the T_1s of GM, CSF, and blood are all the same (this is a poor assumption, but it makes the argument simpler). Then CSF relaxes with a rate constant $1/T_1$ for both the nonselective and selective inversions, whereas GM relaxes with a rate constant $1/T_1$ for the nonselective inversion and $1/T_1 + f/\lambda$ for the selective inversion. The data are the average of these two curves, so the measured relaxation rate for the nonselective inversion would be $1/T_1$, but the relaxation rate for the selective inversion would be about $1/T_1 + 0.5f/\lambda$. In other words, the T_1 method would measure a value of f/λ only half as large for the voxel half-filled with GM, just as the ASL calculation from the same data would also find f reduced by a factor of 2.

The reason these two measurements come out the same is that λ' is not equal to λ in this example, and λ' really should be in Equation [B15.3]. Because the voxel is still full of water, the ratio M_0/M_{0A} is unchanged, even though λ is cut in half. To avoid confusion, then, the basic relationship for the T_1 method (Equation [B15.3]) should be more clearly written as

$$\frac{1}{T_{1app}} = \frac{1}{T_1} + f\frac{M_{0A}}{M_0}$$ [B15.4]

For the case of a voxel uniformly filled with GM, Equation [B15.3] and [B15.4] are identical; however, for more general examples such as our half-filled voxel, Equation [B15.3] is not correct.

In short, the T_1 method and the ASL approach deal with the same data and yield the same results, despite the apparent differences in the form of the equations. However, the conceptual framework is very different for the two approaches. With the ASL approach, flow is viewed as affecting the MR signal by delivering tagged spins to the voxel, whereas flow is viewed as altering the longitudinal relaxation time with the T_1 method. For the ideal case, these two conceptual frameworks lead to the same results. However, the problem with the T_1 method is that this conceptual framework breaks down when we try to deal with practical applications in which there is exchange of spins between blood and tissue with different T_1s, and transit delays from the tagging region to the slice. As soon as we depart from the ideal case, the basic assumption of the T_1 method (Equation [B15.4]) is no longer true, and we can no longer think of the effect of flow as simply a change in the relaxation rate.

For example, the apparent relaxation rate measured with the nonselective inversion does not give the true T_1 of tissue if the T_1 of blood is different from the T_1 of tissue (Chesler and Kwong, 1995; Schwarzbauer et al., 1996). That is, the T_1 measured with a nonselective inversion is still somewhat flow-dependent: there is a net change in magnetization as one tissue spin is replaced by one arterial spin in the voxel because the two sets of spins are relaxing at different rates. The effect of this is that the T_1 method will systematically overestimate the correct value of f. Because blood has a longer T_1 than tissue, the entering arterial spins will always be more inverted (less relaxed) than the tissue spins that are removed. The tissue then appears to be relaxing more slowly, so $1/T_1$ is underestimated. When this too small value is subtracted from the measured $1/T_{1app}$, flow is overestimated. This systematic overestimation of flow will be worse for white matter because the T_1 difference with blood is greater.

(continued)

BOX 15, continued

For quantitative perfusion imaging with CASL and PASL, it is critical to control for transit delay effects. The T_1 method also suffers from problems related to transit delays, although these have not been explored to the same extent as for ASL methods. The nature of the problem for the T_1 method is the assumption that flow affects the apparent relaxation rate throughout the TI period. However, because the selective inversion slice profile is imperfect, it is usually made wider than the imaged slice. This means that the first arterial spins to enter the voxel after the inversion are partly inverted, rather than fully relaxed. Effectively, this means that flow does not begin to have its full effect on the apparent relaxation rate until after the fully relaxed spins begin to enter the voxel. One approach to controlling for these effects would be to use only TI values that are long enough to allow the relaxed arterial spins to reach the voxel. The measurement of T_1 would then be a bit more complicated because the local magnetization would be starting at an unknown initial magnetization M_1. Normally, the magnetization is assumed to start at $-M_0$ and relax toward $+M_0$ with time constant T_1. There are then two parameters to fit, M_0 and T_1, so at least two TI values are required. But with transit delay problems, the relaxation rate shortly after the inversion is unknown and possibly variable. So we must measure the relaxation starting at an unknown value M_1 measured at the first TI, and relaxing to M_0. Now there are three parameters to fit, so measurements with at least three TIs are required. The time efficiency is thus drastically reduced compared to the ASL approach, which can produce quantitative measurements with as few as two measurements (e.g., one tag and one control image with QUIPSS II).

In short, dealing with the normal confounding factors that affect CBF measurements in the context of the T_1 method requires a substantial departure from the basic concept of flow altering the relaxation rate. That is, the fundamental equation of the T_1 method (Equation [B15.3], or more correctly [B15.4]) is only true for an ideal case that does not occur in practice. In contrast, dealing with these confounding effects is more straightforward with the ASL approach used in the rest of the chapter. Transit delays and different relaxation rates in blood and tissue can be incorporated into the analysis through Equation [15.3] without departing from the basic kinetic picture of the delivery of a bolus of tagged blood.

ARTERIAL SPIN LABELING TECHNIQUES

Continuous ASL

The original demonstrations of ASL were based on CASL (Detre et al., 1992; Williams et al., 1992). In this approach, the magnetization of arterial blood is continuously inverted in the neck using a continuous RF pulse (Figure 15.2). This technique of adiabatic inversion of flowing blood was originally introduced as a blood labeling technique for MR angiography applications (Dixon et al., 1986). The essential idea of adiabatic inversion is that the effective RF field in the rotating frame is slowly swept from off-resonance to on-resonance and back to off-resonance again (see Chapter 7). When the effective field reaches resonance, the magnetization

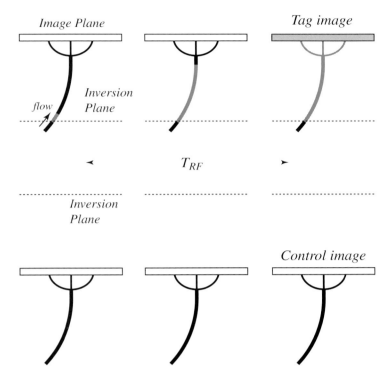

Image Plane   *Tag image*

flow   *Inversion*
              Plane

T_{RF}

Inversion
Plane

                                                          Control image

Figure 15.2. Continuous arterial spin labeling. In the original ASL technique, the magnetization of arterial blood is inverted continuously while an RF pulse is applied in the presence of a magnetic field gradient along the flow direction. As the blood passes through the location where the RF pulse is on-resonance (the inversion plane), the magnetization is inverted. A continuous stream of tagged arterial blood is created as long as the RF field is applied (T_{RF}), typically 3–4 s. For the control image the same RF is applied with the inversion plane symmetrically placed above the slice, so that no arterial blood is tagged.

begins to follow it and so can be cleanly inverted. In imaging applications, long adiabatic inversion pulses (e.g., 20–30 ms in length) are used to produce sharp slice profiles by varying the RF during the pulse. But in adiabatic inversion of flowing blood, the motion of the blood itself produces a sweep of the effective field while the RF is constant. This is done by applying a constant field gradient in the flow direction while the RF pulse is on. Then as the blood flows along the gradient axis, the local resonant frequency changes, causing the effective field to sweep through resonance and invert the magnetization of the blood.

The inversion of the magnetization of the arterial blood occurs over a small spatial region located at the position along the gradient axis where the RF pulse is on-resonance. That is, we can think of the combination of the RF and the gradient field as defining an inversion plane. As flowing blood crosses this plane, its magnetization is inverted. For example, for brain imaging, the tagging plane is a transverse plane cutting through the major arteries at the base of the brain. This process of adiabatic inversion of flowing blood creates a continuous stream of tagged blood originating at the inversion plane for as long as the RF pulse is turned on (Figure 15.2). For a CASL experiment, the duration T_{RF} of the RF pulse is typically several seconds (Alsop and Detre, 1996). This creates an arterial bolus of tagged blood with a duration $T_A = T_{RF}$. After the end of the RF pulse, the tag image is acquired.

In all ASL experiments, the way the control image is acquired is a critical factor that affects the quantitative accuracy of the CBF measurement. Because the ASL signal difference (control–tag) that carries the CBF information is only about 1% of the control image intensity, a systematic error of 1% in the control image would produce a 100% error in the CBF measurement. The control experiment must satisfy two conditions: (1) the arterial blood is not tagged, so that it enters the tissue fully relaxed; and (2) the static spins within the image slice should generate precisely the same signal as they did in the tag image, so that a subtraction (control–tag) leaves nothing but the difference signal of the spins delivered by arterial flow. The long RF pulse in the tag part of the CASL experiment is off-resonance for the slice of interest and so ideally should have no effect on the image slice. But as discussed in Chapter 7, off-resonance pulses can produce a slight tipping of the magnetization directly, and through magnetization transfer effects the magnetization in the image slice can be affected even more strongly (McLaughlin et al., 1997; Pekar et al., 1996; Zhang et al., 1992). These off-resonance effects of the RF pulse alter the longitudinal magnetization of the static spins in the image independently of any flow effect, so the control experiment must reproduce these effects as closely as possible. A typical control image in CASL is acquired by applying a similar long RF pulse but with the frequency of the RF or the sign of the gradient switched so that blood entering from *above* the slice would be tagged rather than arterial blood entering from below. In this way, the off-resonance effects on the slice are approximately balanced, and because the inversion plane for the control image is often outside the head, nothing is tagged.

One problem with this scheme for the control pulse is that only one image plane is properly controlled. That is, to control for magnetization transfer effects, the control RF pulse must be off-resonance by the same amount as the tagging RF pulse, so the inversion planes of the two RF pulses must be symmetrically placed around the image slice. For multislice acquisitions, there will be systematic errors for all but the center slice. A promising alternative approach is to use a separate small coil to do the inversion, and if the coil is far enough from the image slice, there will be minimal contamination by magnetization transfer effects (Zhang et al., 1995). The control image then can be acquired exactly like the tag image, but with no RF pulse applied, and this control would be appropriate for multiple slices. However, this approach requires a hardware configuration that is not generally available on MR scanners.

In practice, several other factors need to be taken into account to make a quantitative measurement of CBF, and these will be considered in more detail later in the chapter. For example, the tagged magnetization decays during the experiment, and a correction must be made for spatial variations in T_1. Other confounding factors include incomplete inversion of the arterial blood (Zhang, Williams, and Koretsky, 1993), relaxation during the transit from the inversion region to the slice (Alsop and Detre, 1996; Zhang, et al., 1992), and signal contributions from large vessels (Ye et al., 1997). When these effects are taken into account, CASL provides a quantitative measurement of local perfusion. Initial animal studies involving CBF alterations by altering PCO_2 showed excellent agreement between CBF measured with arterial spin labeling and with microspheres (Walsh et al., 1994). The CASL technique was successfully applied in human subjects by Roberts and co-workers (1994) and more recently in several studies (Alsop and Detre, 1996; Alsop et al., 2000; Talagala and Noll, 1998; Ye et al., 1996, 1997, 1998).

Pulsed ASL

The basic description of ASL at the beginning of the chapter was essentially an ideal version of PASL (see Figure 15.1). Instead of a continuous RF pulse to invert blood as it flows through the inversion plane, a single 180° RF pulse is applied as a spatially selective pulse that tips over all spins in a thick band below the slice of interest. After a delay to allow the tagged blood to flow into the slice, the tag image is acquired. As with CASL, collecting a high-quality control image is critical for the accuracy of ASL. As noted previously, the goal is to acquire a control image in which arterial blood is not inverted but the signal from static spins in the slice is precisely the same as it was in the tagged image. The second part of this goal is hard to accomplish. For example, a slice-selective inversion slab, even when constructed to have as rectangular a profile as possible, will nevertheless have small wings that can extend into the imaging slice.

In EPISTAR (echo planar imaging and signal targeting with alternating radiofrequency), the tagging band is typically 10-cm thick with a gap of 1 cm between the edge of the band and the edge of the imaged slice (Edelman et al., 1994) (Figure 15.3). The control image is acquired with the same strategy used in CASL. An identical inversion pulse is applied on the other side of the imaging slice, inverting a band of spins above the image slice. Ideally the control pulse does not tag any arterial blood that will flow into the image slice but produces effects on the static spins due to the wings of the slice profile that are similar to the off-resonance effects of the tagging pulse. In a CASL experiment, the tag and control RF inversion planes typically are several centimeters from the image plane, so the control plane may even be outside the head. However, with EPISTAR, the near edges of the tagging band and the control band are only about 1 cm from the edge of the image slice. An artifact that can result from this scheme is that venous blood entering from above will actually be tagged by the control pulse and so will appear as focal dark spots in the subtraction image (Figure 15.4).

In FAIR (flow-sensitive alternating inversion recovery), the tag image is acquired with a nonselective inversion pulse, and the control image is acquired with a slice-selective inversion pulse centered on the image slice (Kim, 1995). If the two types of inversion pulse are carefully designed to have the same effect on the static spins in the image slice, then the entering arterial blood is inverted with the nonselective RF pulse but fully relaxed with the selective RF pulse. The static spins in the image slice are identically inverted (ideally) in both experiments, so their signal subtracts out.

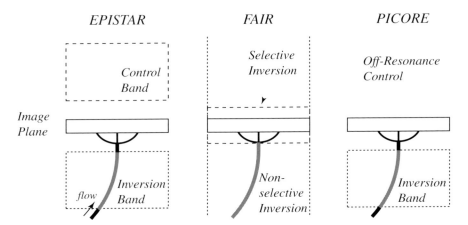

Figure 15.3. Pulsed arterial spin labeling. In PASL the arterial magnetization is inverted all at once, and three variations of PASL are shown. In EPISTAR (left), the tag is created with a spatially selective inversion slab below the image plane, and the control is the same inversion slab applied above the slice. In FAIR (middle), the tag is created with a nonselective inversion that inverts everything within the RF coil, and the control is a selective inversion on the image plane. In PICORE (right), the tag is done as in EPISTAR, but the control is the same RF pulse applied off-resonance to the slice and with no gradient on, so nothing is inverted. All these schemes ideally invert the arterial magnetization for the tag image and leave it fully relaxed for the control image.

As with all ASL experiments, the quality of the control experiment is critical. The difficulty in performing a FAIR experiment is to ensure that the slice-selective inversion produces a clean 180° pulse over the entire thickness of the imaged slice that matches the nonselective inversion. Because the slice profile is not perfectly rectangular, the spatial width of the selective inversion pulse is typically twice the width of the imaged slice so that the width of the image plane falls under the uniform center of the selective inversion (Kim, 1995). Improvements in the design of slice-selective pulses may help to alleviate this problem (Yongbi, Branch, and Helpern, 1998), moving the technique closer to the ideal experiment of perfectly matched selective and nonselective inversions over the imaged slice. However, it is likely that the selective inversion will always have to be larger than the imaged slice thickness.

In comparison with the EPISTAR technique, instead of a tagging band with a set width, FAIR attempts to invert all spins outside the image plane with the nonselective inversion pulse. In practice, of course, there is a limit to the spatial extent of an RF pulse set by the size of the coil even if no field gradients are applied. One can think of the FAIR experiment as making the tagging band as large as the RF coil will allow to tip over the maximum number of arterial spins. Also, with this scheme, blood entering from either side of the slice is tagged, and so this technique is likely to be more robust when the imaging slice is fed by arterial flow from both directions. On the other hand, artifacts due to tagged veins will appear bright, rather than dark as in EPISTAR (Figure 15.4).

EPISTAR   FAIR   PICORE

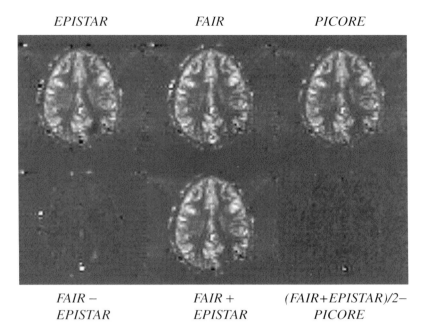

FAIR −   FAIR +   (FAIR+EPISTAR)/2−
EPISTAR   EPISTAR   PICORE

Figure 15.4. Venous artifacts with PASL techniques. One artifact in PASL is that venous blood entering from above the slice appears negative because it is inverted by the control pulse in EPISTAR (top left) and appears positive because it is inverted by the nonselective tagging pulse in FAIR (top middle). In PICORE (top right), nothing above the slice is tagged. This is illustrated in the bottom row by subtracting the EPISTAR image from the FAIR image so that all spins entering from above the slice appear bright (bottom left). The PICORE image is essentially identical to the average of the EPISTAR and FAIR images (bottom right). (Data courtesy of E. Wong.)

A third technique, PICORE (proximal inversion with a control for off-resonance effects), uses a tag similar to that of EPISTAR (Wong, Buxton, and Frank, 1997). For the control image, the same RF inversion pulse is applied as in the tag image with two exceptions: no field gradients are turned on, and the frequency of the RF pulse is shifted so that the image plane experiences the same off-resonance RF pulse in both tag and control images. Because there are no gradients applied, the RF pulse is off-resonance for all spins, so nothing is inverted. This technique has the advantage that venous blood entering from the superior side of the image plane is not tagged, in contrast to EPISTAR and FAIR (Figure 15.4).

It is important to note that, in these PASL experiments, the flow information is carried in the *difference* signal (control − tag) and not in the intrinsic tissue signal. For this reason, the raw images may have quite different intrinsic contrast, as in the EPISTAR and FAIR images shown in Figure 15.5, but the ASL difference images are very similar. Because the goal with ASL imaging is that the intrinsic tissue signals should subtract out, leaving only the signal difference of delivered blood, there is a useful trick to improve the accuracy of the subtraction. The essential problem is that the intrinsic tissue signal is much larger than the arterial blood signal, so we are subtracting two large numbers to estimate a small difference. If the intrinsic tissue

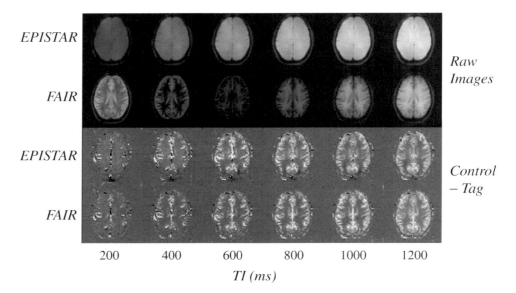

Figure 15.5. The ASL difference signal is independent of the raw image contrast. Image series for a range of TI values are shown for EPISTAR and FAIR to demonstrate that the CBF information is carried in the ASL difference image (control – tag). Despite the very different intrinsic contrast in EPISTAR and FAIR, the difference images are quite similar. (Data courtesy of E. Wong.)

signal can be reduced, the subtraction should be more robust. This is done by applying a 90° saturation pulse on the imaged slice just after the 180° tagging pulse (Edelman et al., 1994; Wong et al., 1997). In this way, the static tissue signal recovers from zero and so is weaker at the time of measurement, but the ASL difference signal due to delivered arterial blood is unaffected.

These PASL techniques also suffer from potential systematic errors that make quantification of CBF more difficult. As with CASL, off-resonance effects are a potential problem, although the source of these effects is likely dominated by imperfect slice profiles rather than magnetization transfer effects (Frank, Wong, and Buxton, 1997). For all these PASL approaches, we would ideally like to have the tagging band flush against the edge of the imaged slice. But because neither the slice profile of the inversion pulse nor the imaging excitation pulse are perfectly sharp, there must be a gap between the edge of the inversion band and the edge of the image slice. If there is a gap, then there will necessarily be a transit delay before the tagged blood arrives in the voxel. The transit delay in PASL is shorter than with CASL because the tagging band is usually closer, but this is still an important problem affecting quantitative measurements of CBF and will be discussed further later.

In addition, these approaches to PASL also suffer from a subtler problem related to the duration of the tagged bolus in the arterial blood. To understand this problem, and in preparation for the more quantitative discussion in the next section, it is helpful to think about ASL as an example of an experiment in tracer kinetics, as discussed in Chapters 13 and 14. In any such study, the tissue concentration of an agent is driven by the arterial input function. For ASL experiments, the "agent" is the inverted magnetization carried by the arterial blood, and the "tissue concentration" corresponds to the measured ASL signal difference at different delays after the RF pulse. Indeed, ASL is somewhat like a microsphere experiment in which the agent is delivered to the tissue but never leaves. The net amount in each tissue element after the arterial bolus has entered is simply f times the integral of the arterial concentration curve. We will develop this idea further in the next section, but for now the important question is: what is the arterial input function in ASL? For the CASL experiment, the answer is clear: the arterial "concentration of magnetization" is proportional to the equilibrium magnetization of blood M_{0A}, and the duration of the arterial bolus T_A is simply the duration T_{RF} of the RF tagging pulse (Figure 15.6). Then for the ideal CASL experiment, the arterial bolus reaching the tissue voxel is

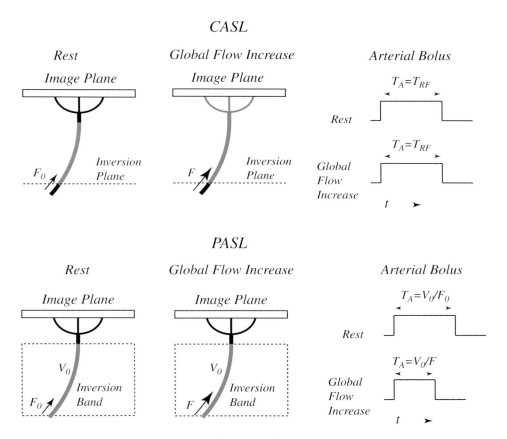

Figure 15.6. Arterial bolus curves for PASL and CASL. A fruitful approach to modeling the ASL signal is to treat the magnetically tagged arterial blood as an "agent" delivered to the tissue. The driving function of such a kinetic model is the arterial concentration of the agent, the arterial bolus of tagged spins. Ideally, the arterial bolus has a well-defined time width T_A. The figure illustrates what happens when there is a global flow increase that increases the flow rate F through the large tagged vessels. For CASL, inverted blood is continuously produced for as long as the RF is turned on, so $T_A = T_{RF}$ independent of F. But for PASL, a volume V_0 of spins is tagged (the arterial blood within the tagging band), and so the time width of the arterial bolus is set by V_0/F, the time required for the tagged blood to leave the inversion band, which depends on the physiological state. For this reason, T_A is not a well-defined quantity in a standard PASL experiment.

rectangular with a time width $T_A = T_{RF}$ (we will neglect any broadening of the bolus as it travels to the capillary bed for the purposes of this argument).

But what is the corresponding arterial bolus width T_A in the PASL experiment? In the PASL experiment, the arterial tagging is done in *space* rather than in *time*. The duration of the arterial bolus in a PASL experiment is the average transit time of arterial blood out of the tagging band. For example, suppose that the arterial volume within the tagging band is V_0, and the net arterial flow through the tagging band is F_0, and to keep the argument simple, suppose that the arterial flow is plug flow. Then the duration of the arterial bolus is $T_A = V_0/F_0$. But this means that the duration of the arterial input function is determined by the physiological state and has been taken out of the experimenter's hands.

For example, suppose that flow to the brain increases globally (e.g., as in a CO_2 inhalation experiment). Then F_0 would increase in proportion to the change in CBF, and so the duration T_A of the arterial bolus would be decreased in proportion to the flow change. This could lead to the surprising effect of a resting CBF measurement producing a reasonable map of perfusion, but a similar map made with globally increased flow showing no change in perfusion at all. If the delay after the tagging pulse is sufficiently long for all the tagged spins to be delivered to the tissue slice at rest, then the distribution of the tagged spins will accurately reflect local CBF. But then, with a global activation so that the local flow at every point in the brain is increased, the number of tagged spins is still the same because the same volume V_0 of blood is inverted. These tagged spins are delivered in proportion to flow as before, and so the same number of tagged spins will be delivered to each voxel, yielding an identical perfusion map. Note that this effect would not happen in a CASL experiment. In both PASL and CASL, the number of tagged spins leaving the tagging region is proportional to $F_0 T_A$. But in PASL, $T_A = V_0/F_0$ so the number of tagged spins is fixed, but with CASL, T_A is determined by the experimenter and so is constant, independent of the physiological conditions. With CASL, a global increase in flow and F_0 then increases the number of tagged spins produced, and the measured signal difference is larger, reflecting the global flow increase.

Another effect of a physiologically dependent T_A in a PASL experiment is that the local value of T_A may vary from one region of the brain to another. The reason for this is that the tagging band will contain several arteries, and each will have a different T_A depending on the volume of the artery within the tagging band and the flow through that artery. The local width of the arterial input function may then vary between tissue regions fed by different arteries. In short, with PASL the duration T_A of the arterial bolus is poorly defined and varies with location in the brain and with the physiological state, but with CASL the duration T_A is a well-defined experimental parameter (T_{RF}). We will return to this problem later.

Modeling the ASL Experiment

To extract a quantitative measurement of perfusion from ASL data, a detailed model of the process combining kinetics and relaxation is needed. Detre and co-workers (1992) introduced a modeling approach based on combining single compartment kinetics with the Bloch equations, and this approach was extended to the FAIR experiment by Kim (1995) and Kwong and co-workers (1992, 1995). In this approach, the Bloch equation for the longitudinal magnetization is modified to include delivery and clearance terms proportional to the local flow f:

$$\frac{dM(t)}{dt} = \frac{M_0 - M(t)}{T_1} + f M_A(t) - \frac{f}{\lambda} M(t) \qquad [15.1]$$

where M_0 is the equilibrium longitudinal magnetization of tissue, λ is the partition coefficient (or volume of distribution) for water, and M and M_A are the time-dependent longitudinal magnetizations of tissue and arterial blood, respectively. The flow-dependent parts of this equation are similar to compartmental models used in tracer kinetics studies, and the implicit assumption is that water distribution in the brain can be treated as a single well-mixed compartment.

Equation [15.1] has served as the basis for most of the quantitative analyses of ASL. However, this equation is based on a restrictive premise, that labeled water delivered to the brain immediately mixes with the large pool of tissue water. This is the standard assumption used in positron emission tomography (PET) studies with $H_2^{15}O$, so it seems plausible to apply the same model to ASL studies. However, PET studies follow the kinetics of labeled water over a time period on the order of 1 min, while for ASL the kinetics over 1 s are important for the analysis. For example, a critical problem with quantitative ASL experiments is the transit delay of several hundred milliseconds from the tagging region to the image plane. Such small time intervals are negligible in a PET experiment but are the primary source of systematic errors in ASL. Other potential systematic errors in ASL include effects of capillary/tissue exchange of water on the relaxation of the tag and the effects of incomplete water extraction from the capillary bed.

A more general treatment is possible based on the kinetic model described in Box 13 (Buxton et al., 1998a), and we will use this approach here for describing both the pulsed and the continuous labeling techniques. With appropriate assumptions, this general model reproduces the earlier modeling work but is flexible enough to include the systematic effects described previously. The first question in applying the general kinetic model developed in Box 13 to ASL is: what precisely corresponds to agent concentration in the ASL experiment?

Assuming that the control experiment is well designed, the magnetization difference $\Delta M(t)$ (control – tag) measured with ASL can be considered to be a quantity of magnetization that is carried into the voxel by arterial blood. That is, we treat ΔM as a concentration of a tracer that is delivered by flow and then apply tracer kinetics principles as in Box 13. The amount of this magnetization in the tissue at a time t will depend on the history of delivery of magnetization by arterial flow and clearance by venous flow and longitudinal relaxation. These physical processes can be described by defining three functions of time: (1) the delivery function $c(t)$ is the normalized arterial concentration of magnetization arriving at the voxel at time t; (2) the residue function $r(t)$ is the fraction of tagged water molecules that remain at a time t after their arrival; and (3) the magnetization relaxation function $m(t)$ is the fraction of the original longitudinal magnetization tag carried by the water molecules that remains at a time t after their arrival in the voxel. The arterial input function $c(t)$ is defined to be equal to one if the blood arrives fully inverted in the tag experiment and fully relaxed in the control experiment. As an example, if there is no transit delay between the tagging region and the image plane, $c(t) = \exp[-t/T_{1A}]$ for pulsed ASL, where T_{1A} is the longitudinal relaxation time of arterial blood. That is, $c(t)$ is reduced from one because as time goes on the magnetization of the arriving blood in the tag experiment is partly relaxed. If the clearance of water from the tissue follows single compartment kinetics, $r(t)$ is a single exponential. And if the labeled water immediately exchanges into the tissue space so that further decay occurs with the time constant T_1 of the tissue space, $m(t)$ is a decaying exponential with time constant T_1.

With these definitions, $\Delta M(t)$ can be constructed as a sum over the past history of delivery of magnetization to the tissue weighted with the fraction of that magnetization which remains in the voxel. Following the inversion pulse, the arterial magnetization difference is $2M_{0A}$, where M_{0A} is the equilibrium magnetization of arterial blood. The amount delivered to a particular voxel between t' and $t' + dt'$ is $2M_{0A}fc(t')dt'$, where f is the cerebral blood flow (expressed in units of milliliters of blood per milliliter of voxel volume per second). The fraction of the magnetization that remains at time t is $r(t - t')m(t - t')$. Then, as in Box 13, we simply add up the contributions to $\Delta M(t)$ over the full course of the experiment:

$$\Delta M(t) = 2M_{0A}f \int_0^t c(t')\, r(t-t')\, m(t-t')\, dt'$$

$$= 2M_{0A}f\, c(t) * [r(t)\, m(t)] \tag{15.2}$$

$$= f\, A_{eff}$$

where $*$ denotes convolution as defined in Equation [15.2]. In the final line of Equation [15.2], all the complexities of the kinetics have been combined into the term A_{eff}. Physically, this term is the effective area of the arterial bolus. For example, if the delivered magnetization behaved like microspheres so that whatever is delivered to the voxel never leaves and never decays away, then A_{eff} is simply the integral of the arterial curve. For this ideal case $r(t) = m(t) = 1$, and the convolution in Equation [15.2] reduces to the integral of $c(t)$.

The formulation in Equation [15.2] emphasizes the central role of the flow f in determining the ASL signal. The measured magnetization difference is equal to the product of f and A_{eff}, and so we can think of A_{eff} as a calibration factor that converts the local flow into a measured magnetization difference. This has two important consequences. The first is that A_{eff} controls the SNR of the experiment; for a larger A_{eff}, the same local flow will produce a larger ASL signal difference. The second critical aspect is that the extent to which the ASL signal reflects *only* local flow is described by the sensitivity of A_{eff} to other factors such as transit delays and relaxation times. Ideally, A_{eff} would only depend on global factors so that it would be the same for all voxels. Then even if A_{eff} is not known precisely, a map of the ASL difference signal would still be a quantitative reflection of the local CBF, lacking only the global scaling factor to convert image difference measurements into appropriate units for CBF.

To understand the potential systematic errors in ASL experiments with Equation [15.2], we must first choose appropriate forms for the three functions $c(t)$, $r(t)$, and $m(t)$. Two effects that we want to include are a transit delay Δt from the tagging region to the image slice and a delay T_{ex} after the labeled water arrives in the voxel before it exchanges into the extravascular space. The transit delay describes the fact that the tagged spins require some time to travel from the tagging region to the image plane. When the tagged spins enter the voxel, they must continue down the vascular tree until they reach the capillary bed before they can exchange into the tissue. While they are still in blood, they relax with the longitudinal relaxation time of blood, T_{1A}, and after exchange they relax with T_1, the tissue relaxation time. This is modeled in a very simple way by assuming that the spins leave the capillary and enter the tissue space at a time T_{ex} after they enter the voxel. The mathematical forms of the functions that describe these processes are

$$c(t) = \begin{cases} 0 & 0 < t < \Delta t \\ \alpha e^{-t/T_{1A}} \ (PASL) & \Delta t < t < \Delta t + T_A \\ \alpha e^{-\Delta t/T_{1A}} \ (CASL) & \Delta t < t < \Delta t + T_A \\ 0 & \Delta t + T_A < t \end{cases} \qquad [15.3]$$

$$r(t) = e^{-ft/\lambda}$$

$$m(t) = \begin{cases} e^{-t/T_{1A}} & t < T_{ex} \\ e^{-T_{ex}/T_{1A}} \ e^{-(t-T_{ex})/T_1} & t > T_{ex} \end{cases}$$

For completeness, the expression for $c(t)$ includes a factor α that describes the inversion efficiency of the experiment (Alsop and Detre, 1996; Zhang et al., 1993). Specifically, α is the achieved fraction of the maximum possible change in longitudinal relaxation between the tag and control experiments. This describes the fact that the $180°$ inversion may not be complete (i.e., less than $180°$) or that the longitudinal magnetization in the control image may not be fully relaxed. For PASL experiments, α is usually very close to one, but for CASL experiments this can be an important correction. Figure 15.7 shows example kinetic curves of $\Delta M(t)$ based on Equation [15.3].

With these model functions, we can now examine how A_{eff} depends on different confounding factors. We will use the notation TI for the time of the measurement in analogy with an inversion recovery experiment, even though the way we interpret the data is in terms of delivery and decay of the tag. The kinetic curves shown in Figure 15.7 are essentially plots of how A_{eff} varies with the inversion time TI. We can further illustrate how various factors influence A_{eff} by defining a function $a(t)$ as the contribution of magnetization that entered the voxel at time t to the final net magnetization difference measured at TI. From Equation [15.2], this function is

$$a(t) = 2M_{0A} \ c(t) \ r(TI - t) \ m(TI - t) \qquad [15.4]$$

and the integral of $a(t)$ is A_{eff}. By plotting $a(t)$ for each time t between the beginning of the experiment ($t = 0$) and the measurement time ($t = TI$), we can visualize A_{eff} directly as the area under the curve. The area A_{eff} is our primary interest because

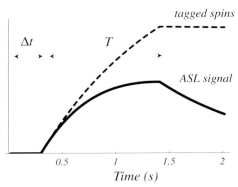

PASL Signal

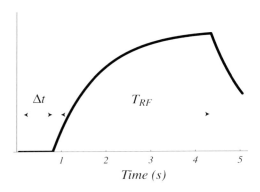

CASL Signal

Figure 15.7. ASL kinetic curves. Illustration of the ideal ASL difference signal as a function of time (TI) for a PASL experiment (top) and a CASL experiment (bottom) calculated with Equation [15.3]. Labeled spins begin to arrive in the voxel after a transit delay Δt and continue to arrive for the duration of the bolus (T for PASL and T_{RF} for CASL). For the PASL experiment, the concentration of delivered spins (i.e., ignoring relaxation) is shown as a dashed line.

this is what affects quantitative measurements of CBF, but it is often helpful to see in detail how a particular systematic error affects the contribution of spins entering at different times to the final measured signal.

   This approach is illustrated in Figure 15.8 for several examples of a PASL experiment with TI = 1 s and a CASL experiment with a tagging time T_{RF} = 3 s. For the ideal case of a perfect inversion with no relaxation ($m(t)$ = 1) and no venous clearance ($r(t)$ = 1), all time points contribute equally to the final magnetization in the voxel, so $a(t)$ is a rectangle and A_{eff} is large. Because of the longer tagging time with CASL, A_{eff} is larger and so the SNR is larger than for PASL. In practice, of course, this ideal form could not occur because relaxation does occur, but it serves to illustrate the meaning and interpretation of $a(t)$ and A_{eff}.

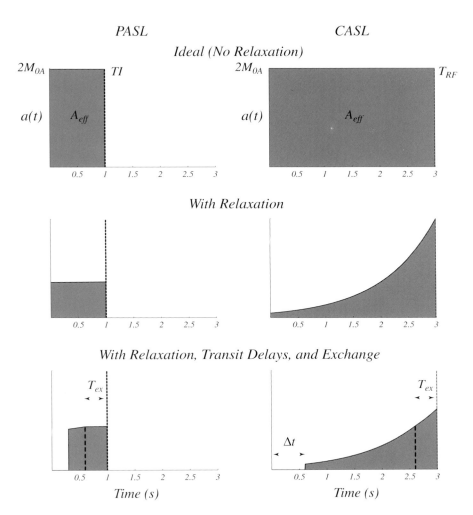

Figure 15.8. The calibration factor A_{eff}. The ASL difference signal is modeled as $\Delta M = f A_{eff}$, where A_{eff} is the effective area under the arterial curve. This is illustrated by plotting $a(t)$, the contribution of the spins arriving in the voxel at time t to the measured signal at time TI. The calibration factor A_{eff} is the shaded area under $a(t)$. If there were no relaxation, all delivered spins would contribute equally to the measured signal (top). With relaxation, the signal from all the delivered spins is attenuated in PASL (middle left), whereas the signal from recently arrived spins has decayed less for CASL (middle right). The more general case including a transit delay Δt and a delay to exchange of the tagged water with tissue water T_{ex} is shown on the bottom.

The second example in Figure 15.8 was calculated with a simplified form of Equation [15.3]. The assumptions were that tagged water molecules begin to enter the voxel immediately after the inversion ($\Delta t = 0$), that water molecules exchange into tissue and begin to relax with the T_1 of tissue immediately after they enter the voxel ($T_{ex} = 0$), and that clearance by venous flow is described by a single exponential. As we will see in later sections, these three assumptions are in order of decreasing importance for quantifying CBF: transit delays create the largest errors, relaxation rate differences have a lesser effect, and venous clearance is usually negligible. In Figure 15.8 (second row), the effect of these assumptions is that spins that arrived earlier contribute less to the final magnetization, as we would expect when relaxation effects are included. Note also that relaxation significantly decreases A_{eff} compared to the ideal form, and so relaxation strongly affects the SNR.

The third example in Figure 15.8 shows a more realistic model that illustrates the effects of the two parameters Δt and T_{ex}. The transit delay shifts $a(t)$, and when the delay is long, the area A_{eff} is significantly reduced. The time of exchange has a more subtle effect, altering the slope of $a(t)$ at a time T_{ex} before the image acquisition. This affects the area A_{eff}, but by a smaller amount than the transit delay effect. In the following sections, we use Equations [15.2]–[15.4] and plots like those in Figure 15.8 to illustrate the effects of potential systematic errors on the scaling factor A_{eff}.

CONTROLLING SYSTEMATIC ERRORS

Transit Delay Effects

A key local variable that affects the ASL signal is the transit delay Δt from the tagging region to the imaged voxel, introduced in the previous section (Alsop and Detre, 1996; Buxton et al., 1998a; Wong et al., 1997; Wong, Buxton, and Frank, 1998b; Zhang et al., 1993). If the transit delays to different parts of the imaged slice were all similar, Δt would affect the magnitude of A_{eff} but would not cause it to vary across the brain. The ASL signal would then accurately reflect CBF differences between brain regions, although the effect of Δt would have to be taken into account in determining the value of A_{eff} to calibrate the flow measurement. Unfortunately, however, this is not the case (Figure 15.9). The transit delay can vary by several tenths of a second across a single image plane (Wong et al., 1997). Furthermore, Δt decreases with activation (Buxton et al., 1998a). For these reasons, transit delays are a significant confounding factor for the interpretation of the ASL signal in terms of CBF.

The effect of a transit delay on A_{eff} for CASL is illustrated in Figure 15.10. Curves of $a(t)$, the contribution to the measured ΔM from spins arriving in the voxel at time t, are shown for two transit delays (0.5 and 0.9 s). For the tissue with the longer transit delay, A_{eff} is significantly reduced because many of the tagged spins have not reached the voxel by the time of the image. The solution to this problem proposed by Alsop and Detre (1996) is also illustrated in Figure 15.10. Instead of applying the long tagging pulse for a duration T_{RF} and then immediately acquiring an image, a delay δt is inserted after the end of tagging before the image acquisition. The effect of this is to create nearly equal values of A_{eff}, despite the large difference in transit delay. If the inserted delay is greater than the longest transit delay ($\delta t > \Delta t$), all the tagged arterial bolus will be delivered to all the image voxels. The only remaining effect of the different transit times is due to different relaxation rates in blood and tissue. The tagged spins in the voxel with the longest transit delay spend more time in the blood and so relax somewhat less than spins that quickly exchange into tissue. However, this residual dependence of the local transit delay is small, and the trick of inserting a delay is effective in controlling for variability of Δt.

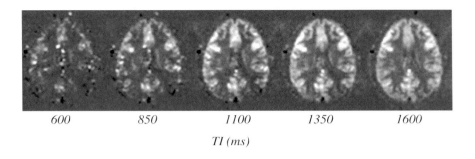

600   850   1100   1350   1600

TI (ms)

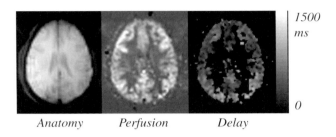

1500 ms

0

Anatomy   *Perfusion*   *Delay*

Figure 15.9. Variable transit delays. PASL images made at different times TI after the inversion pulse show early delivery in large vessels for short TI and a slower spread of the signal to the brain parenchyma. Note, however, that the occipital region takes substantially longer to fill in due to a longer transit delay. The calculated map of transit delays is shown on the lower right. (Data courtesy of E. Wong.)

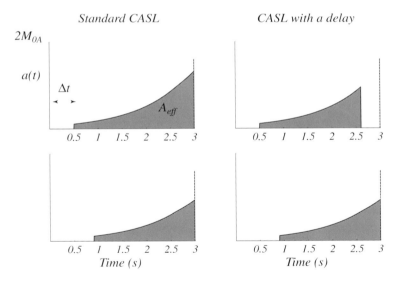

Figure 15.10. Controlling for transit delay effects in CASL. The problem posed by variable transit delays from the tagging plane to the image plane is illustrated on the left. The calibration factor A_{eff} depends strongly on the delay because fewer of the tagged spins have reached the voxel with the longer transit delay Δt (0.9 s compared to 0.5 s in the upper plot) and so creates a large systematic error in the measurement of CBF. The solution to the problem is to insert a delay δt after the end of the RF pulse (T_{RF}) before imaging to allow complete delivery of the arterial bolus to all the image voxels. The plots on the right show $a(t)$ for $T_{RF} = 2.1$ s and $\delta t = 0.9$ s.

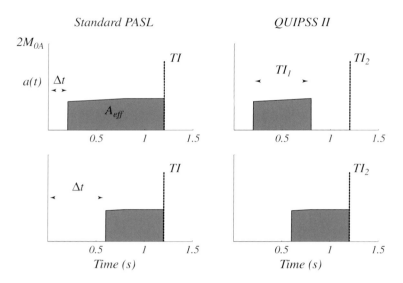

Figure 15.11. Controlling for transit delay effects in PASL. As with CASL, variable transit delays severely affect the calibration factor A_{eff}, producing systematic errors in the measurement of CBF (left). In this example, the image is measured at TI = 1.2 s, and the two illustrated delays Δt are 0.2 and 0.6 s, creating a large difference in A_{eff}. The solution to this problem in QUIPSS II is to create a well-defined arterial bolus width by applying a saturation pulse to the tagging band after a delay TI_1 and then to acquire the image at a time TI_2 after the arterial bolus has been delivered to all the voxels (right). Slight differences remain in A_{eff} for the two cases due to different relaxation times in blood and tissue, but these differences have a small effect on the CBF measurement.

Figure 15.11 shows the effect of transit delays in a PASL experiment. In these examples, smaller transit delays were used (0.2 and 0.6 s) because the tagging region is generally closer to the imaged slice with PASL than with CASL. Nevertheless, the area A_{eff} is still strongly affected by Δt. The solution to the problem is similar to the CASL solution. By waiting sufficiently long so that all the tagged arterial bolus reaches all the voxels in the image, the only remaining sensitivity to the transit delay will be a small relaxation effect similar to that in CASL. However, there is a problem in applying this idea to PASL: the duration of the arterial bolus T_A is not a well-defined quantity. As described earlier, an essential difference between CASL and PASL is that CASL tags spins in time so that the arterial bolus has a well-defined width $T_A = T_{RF}$ set by the duration of the tagging pulse. But PASL tags in space, inverting all spins in a fixed volume, so the duration of the arterial curve depends on the flow in the large tagged arteries. For this reason, the duration of the arterial bolus can vary across the brain.

To apply the idea of adding a delay to the pulse sequence to allow all the tagged spins to arrive, the duration of the arterial bolus must be controlled. The technique QUIPSS II (Quantitative Imaging of Perfusion with a Single Subtraction, version II) is designed to provide this needed control over the arterial bolus width (Wong et al., 1998a). The QUIPSS II modification to PASL is to add between the inversion pulse and the imaging pulse a 90° saturation pulse that hits the same tagging band as the inversion pulse. For example, with EPISTAR/QUIPSS II, the selective inversion pulse is applied in a tagging band below the slice at $t = 0$, a saturation pulse is applied in the same band at $t = TI_1$, and the image is made at $t = TI_2$. The control image is done with the inversion band above the slice so that arterial blood is not tagged, but again the saturation pulse is applied to the original tagging band at $t = TI_1$ (i.e., the saturation pulse is applied to the same spatial region in both the tag and control experiments).

The effect of the saturation pulse is to snip off the end of the arterial bolus and produce a well-defined bolus with duration $T_A = TI_1$. To see this, it is helpful to follow the fate of the arterial magnetization within the tagging band in the two parts of the experiment. For the tag image, all the arterial magnetization in the tagging band is initially inverted, and it then begins to flow out of the tagging band. But before all the labeled blood has had a chance to leave, the saturation pulse is applied. The magnetization of the originally tagged spins remaining in the tagging band is then flipped into the transverse plane, leaving a longitudinal magnetization of zero. Now consider the same spins in the control experiment. The initial inversion pulse has no effect on the arterial spins in the tagging band, so they remain fully relaxed and begin to flow out of the band carrying full magnetization. But the saturation pulse reduces the longitudinal magnetization of the remaining arterial spins to zero at time TI_1, just as in the tag experiment. The difference between the tag and control signals then drops to zero after a time TI_1.

For QUIPSS II to yield a quantitative flow image, two conditions must be satisfied: (1) the saturation pulse must be applied before all of the tagged spins have left the tagging band, and (2) the delay after the saturation pulse must be long enough for all the arterial tagged spins to reach the tissue voxel. If the natural duration of the tag is T_0, set by the volume and flow rate of the arterial blood in the tagging band, then these conditions for QUIPSS II to be accurate are $TI_1 < T_0$ and $TI_2 - TI_1 > \Delta t$. In practice, with the tagging band only 1 cm away from the image slice, typical values are $TI_1 = 700$ ms – and $TI_2 = 1400$ ms. With the QUIPSS II modification, the quantitation problems of the original PASL techniques can be corrected. For example, with global flow changes the number of tagged spins is increased because more will flow out of the tagging band before the saturation pulse is applied, so the number of tagged spins delivered to a voxel will be proportional to the local flow. In other words, the QUIPSS II modification changes PASL from tagging in space to tagging in time, like CASL.

If these conditions are satisfied, the calibration factor for ΔM in the QUIPSS II experiment is approximately

$$A_{eff} \cong 2M_{0A}\, TI_1\, e^{-TI_2/T_{1A}} \qquad\qquad [15.5]$$

The reason that this expression is only approximate is that the relaxation term really depends on the time of exchange T_{ex}. Equation [15.5] is accurate if $T_{ex} > TI_2 - \Delta t$ so that all the spins relax with the T_1 of blood during the experiment. If this is not true, then the amount of decay will depend on precisely when the spins were extracted into the tissue, and this will depend on Δt as well as T_{ex}. We will consider these relaxation effects further in the next section.

In practice, a potential source of error with QUIPSS II is the quality of the saturation pulse applied to the tagging band. Ideally, the edges of the 90° saturation pulse should precisely match the edges of the 180° inversion pulse. The quality of the saturation can be improved by replacing the single saturation pulse with a periodic train of thin-slice saturation pulses at the distal end of the tagging band to create a well-defined arterial bolus (Luh et al., 1999).

In their original forms, CASL and PASL approaches seemed quite different, with one a steady-state technique and the other a dynamic technique. With these modifications to control for transit delays and improve the quantitative accuracy, the two approaches are converging. With the insertion of a delay, CASL has taken on more of the character of a pulsed technique with long pulses. The difference between QUIPSS II and CASL with a delay is really just technical differences in how the arterial bolus of tagged spins is produced. In fact, to optimize CASL for SNR, it is advantageous to shorten the RF pulse further so that CASL becomes more pulselike and less of a steady-state measurement (Wong et al., 1998b). Still, because CASL creates freshly inverted arterial magnetization throughout the duration of the pulse, whereas PASL is a single inversion at the beginning, the SNR can be greater with CASL.

Relaxation Effects

For both CASL and PASL, the cost of controlling for transit delays is reduced sensitivity. As can be seen in Figures 15.10 and 15.11, with the added delays, there is more relaxation and a reduction in the calibration factor A_{eff}. Furthermore, because the T_1s of white matter and gray matter are significantly different, we must consider the role of variations in the local relaxation rate on A_{eff}. In the earlier sections, the relaxation of the tagged spins was likened to the radioactive decay of a tracer such as ^{15}O. For dynamic measurements radioactive decay is a simple correction for loss of the agent, and for steady-state measurements it figures directly in the measured concentration of the agent (see Box 13). For these radioactive agents the decay time is simply a well-known physical constant, but in ASL experiments the situation is more complicated. Initially, the tagged magnetization decays with the T_1 of blood, but as the tagged water molecules enter the extravascular space, they decay with the T_1 of tissue. In a CASL experiment, accounting for T_1 decay is even more complicated because of magnetization transfer (MT) effects. In the presence of an off-resonance RF field, MT effects alter the apparent T_1 of the tissue, so the relevant apparent T_1 for CASL experiments must include these MT effects (Zhang et al., 1992).

The time of exchange T_{ex} of labeled water molecules into the tissue space is not well known. This question has been addressed experimentally with MRI by partly destroying the signal from blood with diffusion-weighting gradients. The motion of blood leads to rapid dephasing of the transverse magnetization, even for relatively weak diffusion-sensitizing gradients. In effect, the apparent diffusion coefficient of water molecules in blood appears to be much higher than the apparent diffusion coefficient in the extravascular space. Studies in a rat model using CASL with a 3.5 s tagging time found that about 90% of the tagged spins exhibited an apparent diffusion coefficient similar to tissue, indicating that these spins had left the blood and

joined the tissue water pool (Silva, Williams, and Koretsky, 1997). In a human experiment using CASL with diffusion-weighting gradient pulses to destroy the blood signal, the mean time to exchange with tissue was found to be 0.94 s for a tagging plane
3 cm below the center of the imaged slice (Ye et al., 1997). This delay is really T_{ex} +
Δt as we have defined the terms, suggesting that T_{ex} may be on the order of a few
tenths of a second.

Figure 15.12 illustrates the sensitivity of the calibration factor A_{eff} to differences
in the tissue relaxation times for PASL. The curves show examples for assumed
relaxation times (T_1) of 1.0 s for gray matter, 0.7 s for white matter, and 1.2 s for
blood. Clearly, if T_{ex} is long enough, the local relaxation time will have no effect on
A_{eff} because the tagged spins always remain in blood during the experiment. Two
values of the exchange time were used in the examples in Figure 15.11, $T_{ex} = 0.2$ s
and $T_{ex} = 0.7$ s, with a measurement time TI = 1.1 s and a transit delay $\Delta t = 0.2$ s. In
these examples for a standard PASL experiment, the fractional difference of A_{eff} for
white matter compared with gray matter is 6.5% when $T_{ex} = 0.2$ s and 0.6% when
$T_{ex} = 0.7$ s. For the extreme case of $T_{ex} = 0$ (curves not shown), A_{eff} differs between
white matter and gray matter by only 10%. With PASL, even for the worst case of
rapid exchange into tissue, variations in the local T_1 have a relatively weak effect on
the calibration factor A_{eff}.

For the CASL experiment, the examples in Figure 15.13 were calculated with
$T_{RF} = 2.6$ s and $\Delta t = 0.4$ s, and the sensitivity of A_{eff} to differences in the relaxation

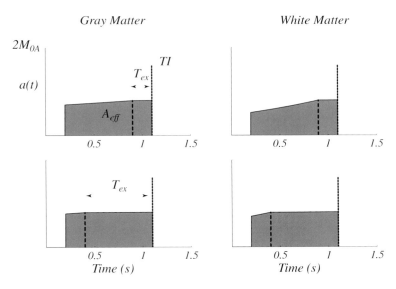

Figure 15.12. Effects of relaxation on A_{eff} with PASL. The tag is assumed to relax with the T_1 of
blood (about 1.2 s) while the labeled spins are still in the vasculature and to relax with the T_1 of tissue (about 1.0 s for gray matter and 0.7 s for white matter) after the spins have exchanged into the
tissue. The calibration factor A_{eff} then depends somewhat on the local value of T_1 (e.g., gray matter
or white matter), but the magnitude of the effect also depends on T_{ex}, the time after arrival in the
voxel when spins exchange from blood to tissue. For the top row $T_{ex} = 0.2$ s, and for the bottom row
$T_{ex} = 0.6$ s. For all these examples, relaxation effects have a relatively minor impact on A_{eff}.

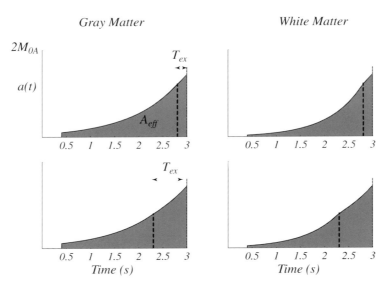

Figure 15.13. Effects of relaxation on A_{eff} with CASL. Plots for CASL similar to those in Figure 15.12 show a stronger effect of relaxation rate in the CASL experiment. Because the duration of the tagging (several seconds) is much longer with CASL, there is more time for tagged spins to exchange into tissue. The calibration factor A_{eff} then depends more strongly on the local T_1, and a correction for spatial variations in T_1 is usually required.

times is quite a bit greater because of the long duration of the experiment. The fractional difference of A_{eff} for white matter compared with gray matter is 32% when $T_{ex} = 0.2$ s and 21% when $T_{ex} = 0.7$ s. For the extreme case of $T_{ex} = 0$, the fractional difference is 37%. For this reason, it is more critical to measure a T_1 map along with the ASL data in a CASL experiment to correct for the variability in A_{eff} caused by variations in local T_1.

Other Issues in Quantifying CBF

In addition to the transit delay effects and relaxation effects described previously, there are a few other systematic factors that affect the accuracy of CBF measurements with ASL (Buxton et al., 1998a; Wong et al., 1997). The first is the issue of tagged spins in large vessels that are simply flowing through the image voxel. The meaningful definition of perfusion is the amount of arterial blood delivered to a capillary bed within a voxel. Tagged spins in an artery within a voxel that are destined for a capillary bed in another region should not be counted as perfusing that voxel. For example, PASL experiments with short TI often show focal bright spots in arteries because there has not been sufficient time for the tagged spins to reach the brain parenchyma.

With both QUIPSS II and CASL with a delay, this flow-through effect is likely to be small because both approaches use long delays to allow the tagged blood to distribute to the tissues. The effect can be further reduced by applying diffusion-weighting to spoil the signal from large vessels (Ye et al., 1997). One might imagine that the best approach for ensuring that we do not suffer from this problem would be to apply large gradient pulses to destroy all vascular signal so that only spins that have exchanged into tissue will contribute to the ASL signal. But, in fact, this would be overkill. The signal from tagged blood in small arteries that are feeding capillary beds within the voxel does not need to be destroyed because such spins are properly counted as contributing to the perfusion of that voxel. In effect, excessive diffusion-weighting would increase the transit delay, in the sense that the tagged spins do not contribute to the voxel signal until a later time after they have reached the capillary bed and exchanged with tissue. In other words, for practical purposes, the transit delay is the time from the beginning of the experiment to the first appearance of the signal from tagged spins in the voxel. So excessive diffusion weighting will decrease the sensitivity of the measurement because fewer spins are measured and will exacerbate the problem of transit delays without improving the accuracy.

Off-resonance excitation effects are always a potential problem with quantitative ASL. For PASL, the problem is primarily that the RF pulses do not have perfectly sharp slice profiles (Frank et al., 1997). The essential effect of this is that the arterial input function is then not a simple rectangle. For example, in EPISTAR the rounded edge of the tag slice profile on the distal side means that the first tagged spins to arrive in the voxel were not fully inverted, producing a rounded leading edge to the arterial curve. The same effect happens in FAIR, but here it occurs because the slice-selective control slice profile has a rounded edge. In both cases, the difference (control – tag) is important, so in both cases the effect is a rounded arterial input function. Effectively, this means that less tagged magnetization is delivered during the earlier part of the bolus than if the arterial curve had an ideal rectangular shape, and this could lead to an underestimate of CBF.

APPLICATIONS

Multislice ASL

Multislice perfusion imaging with ASL presents two problems: (1) acquiring a suitable control image for each of the slices, and (2) handling increased transit delays for the slices farther from the tagging region. To achieve a good subtraction of the static signal in the slice, the unwanted effects of the tagging pulse on the slice must be carefully matched in the control experiment. In CASL, the primary source of the tagging pulse effects on the image slice is magnetization transfer, whereas for PASL it is primarily slice profile effects (Frank et al., 1997). Balancing the off-resonance effects of the tagging pulse on the image slice is more critical for the CASL experiment because of the longer duration of the tagging RF pulse. For example, consider the standard CASL experiment in which the control image is acquired with the inversion plane placed symmetrically above the image plane. This balances magnetization transfer effects of the tagging RF pulse on the spins in the slice, so their signal subtracts out. But this type of control only works for one slice. A second slice must necessarily be closer to either the tagging band or the control band.

As noted earlier, one direct approach to solving this problem for CASL is to use a second, small coil to apply the tag in the neck (Silva et al., 1995). If the coil is sufficiently far away, the effects of the continuous RF are localized and do not affect the image slice, so a simple control image without the RF inversion works for all slices. Alsop and co-workers proposed a novel control pulse to allow multislice perfusion imaging without the additional hardware required for an extra RF coil (Alsop and Detre, 1998). The control pulse is the same as the tagging pulse, except that it is modulated at 250 Hz. This amplitude modulation creates two closely spaced inversion planes so that flowing blood is first inverted and then almost immediately flipped back. The RF power used in the tagging pulses is the same, and the resonant frequency offset for any image plane is then the same for the two pulses, so the MT effects should be similar. However, one cost of this approach is that the tagging efficiency is reduced, which cuts into the potential SNR advantage of CASL techniques over PASL techniques (Wong et al., 1998b).

Recently Edelman and Chen (1998) proposed a similar solution for the EPISTAR control experiment, which uses properties of the adiabatic inversion pulse used for tagging. With this pulse, the RF power used is not directly related to the final flip angle (180°) because of the nature of the adiabatic inversion, but the RF power combined with the frequency offset and duration determine the MT effects. The new control experiment is done with two sequential inversion pulses separated by a small time interval (for a combined flip angle of 360°) and applied to the tagging band, rather than symmetrically above the slice. The power of the single tagging pulse is increased to match the combined power of the two control pulses (yet still produce a 180° inversion) so that the magnetization of arterial blood is flipped through 180° in the tag experiment and 360° in the control experiment. Furthermore, the RF power and duration of the two pulses are the same, and for any image slice the offset frequency is also identical for the two pulses. Consequently, MT effects are balanced, although there may be some residual slice profile differences between the tag and control pulses. As with the CASL approach, this provides an appropriate control for multiple slices.

In FAIR, the limitation on multislice imaging is the integrity of the selective inversion across all the slices. This is again a slice profile problem; however, instead of the wings, it is now the flatness of the center that causes the problem. The magnitude of these slice profile effects is sensitive to exactly how the inversion pulse is created, and optimization to improve the flatness of the center and minimize the wings reduces the control problem substantially (Frank et al., 1997). Applying an initial saturation pulse to the image plane in both the tag and control experiments further reduces the problem by minimizing the intrinsic tissue magnetization so that errors in the subtraction of these signals are smaller (Wong et al., 1997). Multislice images can then be acquired with rapid single-shot imaging (Yang et al., 1998) or with volume-imaging techniques (Kao, Wan, and MacFall, 1998).

However, in addition to the problem of producing a good control image for all the slices, a second concern for quantitative imaging is that the transit delay becomes progressively longer the farther each slice is from the tagging region. Based on studies with different gaps between the tagging band and the slice, a rough estimate is that the transit delay increases by about 150 ms for each additional 1-cm gap (Wong et al., 1997). For this reason, it is essential for quantitative multislice

PASL to use a technique that controls for transit delay effects on the measured signal, such as QUIPSS II.

In a typical multislice implementation of QUIPSS II, five to seven slices are imaged in rapid succession with a single-shot EPI acquisition after a single tagging pulse is applied below the block of images (Wong et al., 1997). After a delay TI_1 the saturation pulse is applied to cut off the end of the arterial bolus, and after another delay TI_2 the image of a slice is acquired. The imaging rate is about one image every 80 ms, so if the image time (TI_2) for the first slice is 1200 ms, it is 1520 ms for the last slice. To control for transit delays, $TI_2 - TI_1$ should be longer than the delay from the tagging band to the slice, so the most distal slice with the longest delay should be collected last to allow time for the tagged spins to arrive. This proximal to distal order of slice collection could potentially create a problem if some of the tagged bolus destined for a more distal slice is still in a larger artery in a more proximal slice when the latter is imaged. It is thus important that TI_2 is sufficiently long that all tagged spins in large vessels that are simply flowing through the slice have had sufficient time to clear. Each imaging excitation pulse also alters the magnetization of the arterial blood within the slice, and so effectively retags the blood, which also could create a problem if this newly tagged blood reaches more distal slices. However, with sufficiently rapid image acquisition, there is not enough time for the blood saturated in one image acquisition to reach the next slice before the next image is acquired.

Activation Studies with ASL

Cerebral blood flow changes during simple motor and sensory tasks were first demonstrated with ASL techniques by Kwong and co-workers and reported in the same seminal paper that described human brain activations measured with the BOLD effect (Kwong et al., 1992). Subjects viewed a flashing array of lights while slice-selective inversion recovery images were collected. These flow-sensitive images showed small signal increases of a few percent, which correlated with the stimulus. Since then, human brain activation has been demonstrated with EPISTAR (Edelman et al., 1994; Siewert et al., 1996), FAIR (Kim, 1995; Kim and Tsekos, 1997; Yang et al., 1998), QUIPSS II (Buxton et al., 1998b; Wong et al., 1997), and CASL (Talagala and Noll, 1998; Ye et al., 1998).

In a typical activation mapping experiment, the subject alternates between blocks of task and control (e.g., 30 s on/30 s off) while a dynamic series of images is collected. Each pixel time course is then examined to see if there is a significant correlation between the local MR signal and the stimulus pattern. The same design can be adapted to a flow activation study with ASL by collecting a dynamic series of alternating control and tag images. From this data set, a time series of the flow signal (control – tag) is generated and analyzed in the same way as the BOLD signal is analyzed in a standard fMRI experiment. Because the ASL activation is a change in arterial flow to a region, whereas the BOLD signal is primarily a change in venous oxygenation in a region, the ASL activation map should be a more accurate representation of the site of activity. That is, ASL measurements should not suffer from the draining vein problem, which can produce an apparent BOLD activation in a brain region downstream from the actual site of neural activity.

A powerful feature of ASL is that it is possible to map flow and BOLD activation patterns simultaneously and independently with an appropriately modified ASL sequence. This has made ASL a primary tool for investigating the underlying mechanisms of the BOLD effect (Buxton et al., 1998b). The basic idea is that in an ASL data set, alternating between tag and control images, the time course of signal *differences* (control − tag) is flow-weighted, whereas the time course of signal *averages* (control + tag) is BOLD-weighted. For example, by collecting the tag and control images of the ASL sequence with a GRE-EPI pulse sequence with TE = 30 ms, each individual image is BOLD weighted. From the raw image time series of a voxel, a BOLD-weighted time series is calculated by averaging the signal at each time point with the mean of the signals just before and just after. For each time point, this is equivalent to adding a control and a tag signal. From the raw time series, a flow-weighted time series is calculated by subtracting the mean of the two nearest neighbors from the signal at each time point. This is equivalent to subtracting a control and a tag signal at each time point. To produce a consistent time course, the sign must be flipped for alternate time points to correct for the fact that they alternate between control − tag and tag − control.

Another promising approach for simultaneous measurement of CBF and BOLD changes is the use of a dual-echo spiral acquisition. With a spiral trajectory through k-space, the sampling starts with $k = 0$, so the effective TE can be very short (a few milliseconds), improving the SNR of the ASL measurement. The second echo is collected with a TE more typical of a BOLD experiment (30–40 ms) to provide the BOLD time series. Figure 15.14 shows an example of simultaneous measurements of flow and BOLD changes during a simple sequential finger-tapping exercise measured with spiral QUIPSS II. The separate flow and BOLD time courses were calculated from the raw data as previously described. Note that the shapes of the two time courses are somewhat different, with the BOLD time course showing a pronounced poststimulus undershoot. Figure 15.14 also shows a simple subtraction of the images made during the tapping exercise from the images made during the rest period. The subtraction image for the flow-weighted series is much cleaner. The BOLD image shows two prominent areas of activation near the central sulcus but also shows a weaker diffuse and patchy pattern of signal change, possibly due to residual motion artifacts or slow signal drifts. In contrast, the map of CBF changes shows only two bright focal areas of activation. The alternating subtractions in the construction of the flow series tend to cancel out slow motion effects that plague BOLD time series. Finally, these two maps also show that the locations of the prominent flow and BOLD changes do not necessarily coincide, consistent with the interpretation that BOLD is primarily sensitive to draining veins, while ASL is more closely associated with the capillary bed and the brain parenchyma. This is discussed further in Chapter 16.

For the preceding analysis to accurately separate the raw time series into a BOLD-weighted and a flow-weighted time series, the two sensitivities should be truly separable so that the BOLD-weighted time series is independent of flow changes and the flow-weighted time series is independent of BOLD effects. With ASL the effect of BOLD changes on the measured flow change is small, particularly

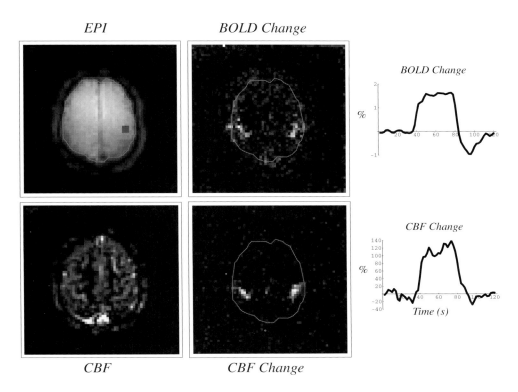

Figure 15.14. Simultaneous measurements of flow and BOLD changes with activation. Data from a combined flow and BOLD finger-tapping study at 1.5 T acquired with a spiral dual-echo acquisition are shown. The ASL pulse sequence was PICORE-QUIPSS II, with the flow time series calculated from the first echo (TE = 3 ms) and the BOLD time series calculated from the second echo (TE = 30 ms). The EPI image (upper left) shows a 3×3 region of interest (ROI), and the average time courses for the ROI are on the right (average of 16 cycles, 40 s of tapping alternated with 80 s of rest). The average flow image is on the lower left. Maps of fractional signal change with activation measured for BOLD and CBF are shown in the middle. The activation maps are similar but not identical, and the flow and BOLD time courses are distinctly different, with the BOLD signal showing a distinct poststimulus undershoot. (Data courtesy of T. Liu.)

for the dual echo spiral acquisition with short TE. But even with a longer TE, the BOLD weighting of the flow signal is minor. For example, with a GRE acquisition, both the tag and control images are BOLD-weighted, so the intensity of each may change by a few percent with activation. This means that the ASL difference signal will also change by a few percent due to BOLD effects, but this is much less than the typical flow change with activation of 50% or more. For this reason, we can assume that the flow time series is only weakly affected by BOLD changes. However, the converse is not true. In general, BOLD effects cannot be cleanly separated from flow effects in most ASL techniques. However, it is possible to modify PASL techniques to minimize the flow sensitivity of the average signal if an initial saturation pulse is applied to the slice. To see why this works, we begin by examining how flow changes affect the BOLD-weighted average time series.

For the average ASL signal (control + tag) to be independent of flow, the average magnetization of the spins delivered by flow must match the current magnetization in the tissue. Then as flow carries away a tissue spin and replaces it with an arterial spin, each on average carrying the same magnetization, there will be no change in the tissue signal due to flow. In other words, during the experiment the average relaxation curve of the delivered spins should match the relaxation curve of the tissue spins. Consider first the ideal CASL experiment. During the control experiment the arterial spins are fully relaxed, but during the tagging time arterial spins enter fully inverted (neglecting transit delay effects) and then relax back toward equilibrium. The average signal of one set of spins that remains fully relaxed and a second set that follows an inversion recovery curve is equivalent to a *saturation* recovery curve because the average magnetization starts at zero and recovers from there. The static spins in the tissue are fully relaxed throughout the experiment (neglecting off-resonance effects), and so the average arterial signal is always much less than the average signal of the tissue spins. This produces a significant negative flow weighting on the BOLD signal (i.e., the flow increase with activation would decrease the apparent BOLD increase).

In the EPISTAR experiment, the situation is similar. The tissue spins are relaxed during the experiment, while the average arterial signal follows a saturation recovery curve, so there is significant negative flow weighting on the average BOLD signal. For the FAIR experiment, with a slice-selective inversion for the control and a nonselective inversion for the tag, the arterial spins again follow a saturation recovery curve. But the spins in the tissue follow an inversion recovery curve; consequently, the average arterial spin curve is always higher than the tissue curve. This produces a positive flow weighting on the BOLD signal.

Because the average arterial signal always follows a saturation recovery curve, we can eliminate the flow weighting of the average signal if the tissue signal can be made to follow a similar saturation recovery curve (Wong et al., 1997, 1998a). This is done with the PASL techniques by applying a 90° saturation pulse to the image plane before the tagging pulse is applied. For EPISTAR, the subsequent inversion pulse has minimal effect on the tissue spins, so the tissue relaxation is a saturation recovery curve. For FAIR the inversion pulses hit the image plane, but because the longitudinal magnetization was reduced to zero by the saturation pulse, they have minimal effect. Again, the tissue spins recover with a saturation recovery curve, and flow weighting of the BOLD time series is minimized.

The example in Figure 15.14 illustrates the differences in the flow and BOLD time series calculated from the same raw data. Not only are the locations of the strongest BOLD and CBF changes somewhat different, but the time courses are different as well. The BOLD time course shows a pronounced poststimulus undershoot that is much weaker in the flow time course. Such combined measurements of flow and BOLD signal changes are a useful tool for studies of the basic mechanisms underlying the BOLD effect, and as ASL techniques improve we are likely to see more extensive use of these techniques for brain-mapping experiments.

REFERENCES

Alsop, D. C., and Detre, J. A. (1996) Reduced transit-time sensitivity in noninvasive magnetic resonance imaging of human cerebral blood flow. *J. Cereb. Blood Flow Metabol.* **16,** 1236–49.

Alsop, D. C., and Detre, J. A. (1998) Multisection cerebral blood flow MR imaging with continuous arterial spin labeling. *Radiology* **208,** 410–16.

Alsop, D. C., Detre, J. A., and Grossman, M. (2000) Assessment of cerebral blood flow in Alzheimer's disease by spin-labeled magnetic resonance imaging. *Ann. Neurol.* **47,** 93–100.

Buxton, R. B., Frank, L. R., Wong, E. C., Siewert, B., Warach, S., and Edelman, R. R. (1998a) A general kinetic model for quantitative perfusion imaging with arterial spin labeling. *Magn. Reson. Med.* **40,** 383–96.

Buxton, R. B., Wong, E. C., and Frank, L. R. (1998b) Dynamics of blood flow and oxygenation changes during brain activation: The balloon model. *Magn. Reson. Med.* **39,** 855–64.

Chesler, D. A., and Kwong, K. K. (1995) An intuitive guide to the T1 based perfusion model. *Intl. J. Imag. Syst. Technol.* **6,** 171–4.

Detre, J. A., Leigh, J. S., Williams, D. S., and Koretsky, A. P. (1992) Perfusion imaging. *Magn. Reson. Med.* **23,** 37–45.

Dixon, W. T., Du, L. N., Faul, D. D., Gado, M., and Rossnick, S. (1986) Projection angiograms of blood labeled by adiabatic fast passage. *Magn. Reson. Med.* **3,** 454–62.

Edelman, R. R., and Chen, Q. (1998) EPISTAR MRI: multislice mapping of cerebral blood flow. *Magn. Reson. Med.* **40,** 800–5.

Edelman, R. R., Siewert, B., Darby, D. G., Thangaraj, V., Nobre, A. C., Mesulam, M. M., and Warach, S. (1994) Qualitative mapping of cerebral blood flow and functional localization with echo-planar MR imaging and signal targeting with alternating radio frequency (STAR) sequences: applications to MR angiography. *Radiology* **192,** 513–20.

Frackowiak, R. S. J., Lenzi, G. L., Jones, T., and Heather, J. D. (1980) Quantitative measurement of cerebral blood flow and oxygen metabolism in man using 15O and PET: Theory, procedure and normal values. *J. Comput. Assist. Tomogr.* **4,** 727–36.

Frank, L. R., Wong, E. C. and Buxton, R. B. (1997) Slice profile effects in adiabatic inversion: Application to multislice perfusion imaging. *Magn. Reson. Med.* **38,** 558–64.

Helpern, J. A., Branch, C. A., Yongbi, M. N., and Huang, N. C. (1997) Perfusion imaging by un-inverted flow-sensitive alternating inversion recovery (UNFAIR). *Magn. Reson. Imag.* **15,** 135–9.

Hoge, R. D., Atkinson, J., Gill, B., Crelier, G. R., Marrett, S., and Pike, G. B. (1999a) Investigation of BOLD signal dependence on cerebral blood flow and oxygen consumption: The deoxyhemoglobin dilution model. *Magn. Reson. Med.* **42,** 849–63.

Hoge, R. D., Atkinson, J., Gill, B., Crelier, G. R., Marrett, S., and Pike, G. B. (1999b) Linear coupling between cerebral blood flow and oxygen consumption in activated human cortex. *Proc. Natl. Acad. Sci. USA* **96,** 9403–8.

Hoge, R. D., Atkinson, J., Gill, B., Crelier, G. R., Marrett, S., and Pike, G. B. (1999c) Stimulus-dependent BOLD and perfusion dynamics in human VI. *NeuroImage* **9,** 573–85.

Kao, Y. H., Wan, X., and MacFall, J. R. (1998) Simultaneous multislice acquisition with arterial-flow tagging (SMART) using echo planar imaging (EPI). *Magn. Reson. Med.* **39,** 662–5.

Kim, S.-G. (1995) Quantification of regional cerebral blood flow change by flow-sensitive alternating inversion recovery (FAIR) technique: Application to functional mapping. *Magn. Reson. Med.* **34,** 293–301.

Kim, S.-G., and Tsekos, N. V. (1997) Perfusion imaging by a flow-sensitive alternating inversion recovery (FAIR) technique: Application to functional brain imaging. *Magn. Reson. Med.* **37,** 425–35.

Kim, S.-G., and Ugurbil, K. (1997) Comparison of blood oxygenation and cerebral blood flow effects in fMRI: Estimation of relative oxygen consumption change. *Magn. Reson. Med.* **38,** 59–65.

Kwong, K. K., Belliveau, J. W., Chesler, D. A., Goldberg, I. E., Weisskoff, R. M., Poncelet, B. P., Kennedy, D. N., Hoppel, B. E., Cohen, M. S., Turner, R., Cheng, H.-M., Brady, T. J., and Rosen, B. R. (1992) Dynamic magnetic resonance imaging of human brain activity during primary sensory stimulation. *Proc. Natl. Acad. Sci. USA.* **89,** 5675–9.

Kwong, K. K., Chesler, D. A., Weisskoff, R. M., Donahue, K. M., Davis, T. L., Ostergaard, L., Campbell, T. A., and Rosen, B. R. (1995) MR perfusion studies with T1-weighted echo planar imaging. *Magn Reson Med* **34,** 878–87.

Luh, W.-M., Wong, E. C., Bandettini, P. A., and Hyde, J. S. (1999) QUIPSS II with thin slice TI1 periodic saturation: A method for improved accuracy of quantitative perfusion imaging using pulsed arterial spin labeling. *Magn. Reson. Med.* **41,** 1246–54.

McLaughlin, A. C., Ye, F. Q., Pekar, J. J., Santha, A. K. S., and Frank, J. A. (1997) Effect of magnetization transfer on the measurement of cerebral blood flow using steady-state arterial spin tagging approaches: A theoretical investigation. *Magn. Reson. Med.* **37,** 501–10.

Pekar, J., Jezzard, P., Roberts, D. A., Leigh, J. S., Frank, J. A., and McLaughlin, A. C. (1996) Perfusion imaging with compensation for asymmetric magnetization transfer effects. *Magn. Reson. Med.* **35,** 70–9.

Raichle, M. E. (1983) Brain blood flow measured with intravenous $H_2^{15}O$: Implementation and validation. *J. Nucl. Med.* **24,** 790–8.

Roberts, D. A., Detre, J. A., Bollinger, L., Insko, E. K., and Leigh, J. S. (1994) Quantitative magnetic resonance imaging of human brain perfusion at 1.5T using steady-state inversion of arterial water. *Proc. Nat. Acad. USA* **91,** 33–7.

Schwarzbauer, C., Morrissey, S. P., and Haase, A. (1996) Quantitative magnetic resonance imaging of perfusion using magnetic labeling of water proton spins within the detection slice. *Magn. Reson. Med.* **35,** 540–6.

Siewert, B., Bly, B. M., Schlaug, G., Darby, D. G., Thangaraj, V., Warach, S., and Edelman, R. R. (1996) Comparison of the BOLD- and EPISTAR-technique for fuctional brain imaging by using signal detection theory. *Magn. Res. Med.* **36,** 249–55.

Silva, A. C., Williams, D. S., and Koretsky, A. P. (1997) Evidence for the exchange of arterial spin-labeled water with tissue water in rat brain from diffusion-sensitized measurements of perfusion. *Magn. Reson. Med.* **7,** 232–7.

Silva, A. C., Zhang, W., Williams, D. S., and Koretsky, A. P. (1995) Multi-slice MRI of rat brain perfusion during amphetamine stimulation using arterial spin labeling. *Magn. Reson. Med.* **33,** 209–14.

Talagala, S. L., and Noll, D. C. (1998) Functional MRI using steady-state arterial water labeling. *Magn. Reson. Med.* **39,** 179–83.

Walsh, E. G., Minematsu, K., Leppo, J., and Moore, S. C. (1994) Radioactive microsphere validation of a volume localized continuous saturation perfusion measurement. *Magn. Reson. Med.* **31,** 147–53.

Williams, D. S., Detre, J. A., Leigh, J. S., and Koretsky, A. P. (1992) Magnetic resonance imaging of perfusion using spin-inversion of arterial water. *Proc. Natl. Acad. Sci. USA* **89,** 212–16.

Wong, E. C., Buxton, R. B., and Frank, L. R. (1997) Implementation of quantitative perfusion imaging techniques for functional brain mapping using pulsed arterial spin labeling. *NMR Biomed.* **10,** 237–49.

Wong, E. C., Buxton, R. B., and Frank, L. R. (1998a) Quantitative imaging of perfusion using a single subtraction (QUIPSS and QUIPSS II). *Magn. Reson. Med.* **39,** 702–8.

Wong. E. C., Buxton, R. B., and Frank, L. R. (1998b) A theoretical and experimental comparison of continuous and pulsed arterial spin labeling techniques for quantitative perfusion imaging. *Magn. Reson. Med.* **40,** 348–55.

Yang, Y., Frank, J. A., Hou, L., Ye, F. Q., McLaughlin, A. C., and Duyn, J. H. (1998) Multislice imaging of quantitative cerebral perfusion with pulsed arterial spin labeling. *Magn. Reson. Med.* **39,** 825–32.

Ye, F., Smith, A., Yang, Y., Duyn, J., Mattay, V., Ruttiman, U., Frank, J., Weinberger, D., and McLaughlin, A. (1998) Quantitation of regional cerebral blood flow during motor activation: A steady-state arterial spin tagging study. *Neuroimage* **6,** 104–12.

Ye, F. Q., Matay, V. S., Jezzard, P., Frank, J. A., Weinberger, D. R., and McLaughlin, A. C. (1997) Correction for vascular artifacts in cerebral blood flow values measured by using arterial spin tagging techniques. *Magn. Reson. Med.* **37,** 226–35.

Ye, F. Q., Pekar, J. J., Jezzard, P., Duyn, J., Frank, J. A., and McLaughlin, A. C. (1996) Perfusion imaging of the human brain at 1.5 T using a single-shot EPI spin tagging approach. *Magn. Reson. Med.* **36,** 219–24.

Yongbi, M. N., Branch, C. A., and Helpern, J. A. (1998) Perfusion imaging using FOCI RF pulses. *Magn. Reson. Med.* **40,** 938–43.

Zhang, W., Silva, A. C., Williams, D. S., and Koretsky, A. P. (1995) NMR measurement of perfusion using arterial spin labeling without saturation of macromolecular spins. *Magn. Reson. Med.* **33,** 370–6.

Zhang, W., Williams, D. S., and Koretsky, A. P. (1993) Measurement of rat brain perfusion by NMR using spin labeling of arterial water: in vivo determination of the degree of spin labeling. *Magn. Reson. Med.* **29,** 416–21.

Zhang, W., Williams, D. S., Detre, J. A., and Koretsky, A. P. (1992) Measurement of brain perfusion by volume-localized NMR spectroscopy using inversion of arterial water spins: Accounting for transit time and cross-relaxation. *Magn. Reson. Med.* **25,** 362–71.

IIIB

Blood Oxygenation Level Dependent Imaging

16

The Nature of the Blood Oxygenation
Level Dependent Effect

The BOLD Effect
The Biophysical Basis of the BOLD Effect
    Magnetic Field Distortions Shorten T_2^*
    The Moderating Effect of Diffusion on T_2^* Changes
    The Intravascular Contribution to the BOLD Signal
    Spin Echo BOLD Signal Changes

    BOX 16: MODELING THE BOLD SIGNAL

The Physiological Basis of the BOLD Effect
    The BOLD Effect Depends on Combined Changes in CBF,
        $CMRO_2$, and CBV
    Are CBF and $CMRO_2$ Changes Coupled During Activation?

THE BOLD EFFECT

The previous chapters described magnetic resonance imaging (MRI) techniques for measuring cerebral blood flow and blood volume. By introducing contrast agents or manipulating the magnetization of arterial blood before it arrives in a tissue voxel, the MR signal becomes sensitive to aspects of local tissue perfusion. Such techniques are clinically valuable for investigating disorders characterized by perfusion abnormalities, such as stroke and tumors, and these techniques have also seen limited use in investigations of normal brain function. But the functional magnetic resonance imaging (fMRI) technique that has created a revolution in research on the basic functions of the healthy human brain is based on an intrinsic sensitivity of the magnetic resonance (MR) signal to local changes in perfusion and metabolism. When neural activity increases in a region of the brain, the local MR signal produced in that part of the brain increases by a small amount due to changes in blood oxygenation. This Blood Oxygenation Level Dependent (BOLD) effect is the basis for most of the fMRI studies done today to map patterns of activation in the working human brain.

The BOLD effect is most pronounced on gradient echo (GRE) images, indicating that the effect is primarily an increase of the local value of T_2^*. The fact that the oxygenation of the blood has a measurable effect on the MR signal from the surrounding tissue was discovered by Ogawa and co-workers imaging a rat model at 7 T (Ogawa et al., 1990). They found that the MR signal around veins decreased when the oxygen content of the inspired air was reduced, and the effect was reversed when the oxygen was returned to normal values. The oxygen sensitivity of the MR signal from blood was known from previous studies that showed that T_2 depends strongly on the oxygenation of the hemoglobin (Thulborn et al., 1982). But Ogawa and co-workers demonstrated an additional feature in their rat studies. They observed that the signal reductions were not just in the blood itself but also in the tissue space around the vessels, suggesting that T_2^* was reduced in both the intravascular *and* extravascular spaces. They proposed that this effect was due to changes in the magnetic susceptibility of blood, similar to (but weaker than) the susceptibility changes caused by contrast agents. The important difference, however, is that this alteration of the susceptibility of blood is an intrinsic physiological effect. Shortly after this, a reduced MR signal was observed in an ischemia model and attributed to the same cause: a reduction of T_2^* with decreasing oxygenation of the blood (Turner et al., 1991).

These early physiological manipulations demonstrated that reductions in blood oxygenation led to a signal decrease. Kwong and co-workers (1992) demonstrated that brain activation in human subjects produced a local signal *increase* that could be used for functional brain mapping, and several other groups reported the same finding that year (Bandettini et al., 1992; Frahm et al., 1992; Ogawa et al., 1992). The discovery that activation produces a signal increase was somewhat surprising because it indicated that the T_2^* had increased, rather than decreased, suggesting that blood is more oxygenated with activation.

Earlier chapters laid the foundation for understanding how fMRI based on the BOLD effect works. The BOLD effect comes about because of two reasons, one biophysical and one physiological: (1) deoxyhemoglobin produces magnetic field gradients around and through the blood vessels that decrease the MR signal, and (2) brain activation is characterized by a drop in the local oxygen extraction fraction (OEF) and a corresponding drop in the local concentration of deoxyhemoglobin. The reduction in deoxyhemoglobin during activation then produces a small increase in the MR signal. The BOLD effect is widely used for mapping patterns of activation in the working human brain and has been applied in a number of animal models as well. However, the interpretation of the results of these studies requires a careful consideration of the nature of the BOLD response. In this chapter and the next, we will consider the origins, spatial accuracy, and time course of the BOLD response and also discuss some practicalities of doing BOLD-based fMRI experiments. The statistical analysis of BOLD data is considered in Chapters 18 and 19.

THE BIOPHYSICAL BASIS OF THE BOLD EFFECT

Magnetic Field Distortions Shorten T_2^*

The physical basis of the BOLD sensitivity of the MR signal is that deoxyhemoglobin alters the magnetic susceptibility of blood. The concept of magnetic susceptibility was discussed in Chapter 7. Whenever a material is placed in a magnetic field, it becomes slightly magnetized due to the partial alignment with the field of magnetic dipoles within the material, and magnetic susceptibility is a measure of the resulting magnetization. Specifically, the local magnetization is proportional to the magnetic field, and the constant of proportionality is the magnetic susceptibility. The effect of this magnetization is that the field within the material is slightly shifted from the main magnetic field, and the shift is proportional to the magnetic susceptibility. The full magnetic susceptibility of a material has several contributions: unpaired electron spins, orbital motions of electrons, and unpaired nuclear spins. The last is, of course, the magnetization we exploit in NMR to generate a signal, but the nuclear magnetization makes a negligible contribution to the total magnetic susceptibility. In paramagnetic materials, the unpaired electrons are the primary determinant of the magnetic susceptibility.

The magnetic properties of hemoglobin, and their dependence on the oxygenation state of the heme groups, has been known for some time (Pauling and Coryell, 1936). Deoxyhemoglobin is paramagnetic, and when oxygen binds to the heme group, the paramagnetic effect is reduced. The result is that the magnetic susceptibility of blood varies linearly with the blood oxygenation (Weisskoff and Kiihne, 1992). However, the susceptibility shift due to deoxyhemoglobin is an order of magnitude smaller than the susceptibility shift produced by a standard injection of a contrast agent such as gadolinium-DTPA, and so the magnitude of the effect on the MR signal is much smaller than the effects described in Chapter 14.

When two dissimilar materials are placed next to each other, field gradients are produced due to the difference in magnetic susceptibility. This is commonly seen on a large spatial scale in MRI, where field gradients occur in the vicinity of bone, air, and tissue interfaces. In a nonuniform field, spins precess at different rates, and the local signals gradually become out of phase with each other. For broad gradients, with spatial scales much larger than an image voxel, such susceptibility effects show up as local phase variations in a gradient recalled echo (GRE) image (Figure 16.1). In these phase maps the sharp jumps from white to black are simply due to the fact that the phase angle is cyclic (i.e., the jump corresponds to the smooth phase increase from 359° to 0°). The field distortions vary smoothly, and the black-to-white transitions are effectively contour lines of the field distribution. In the case of broad field gradients, the spins within a voxel precess reasonably coherently, but at a different rate from spins in another part of the brain. However, if the spatial scale of the field gradients is microscopic (smaller than an image voxel), then the net signal from the voxel is reduced due to the dephasing of the spins that contribute to the voxel signal. This signal drop is described as a T_2^* effect, a reduction in the apparent transverse relaxation time measured with a GRE pulse sequence.

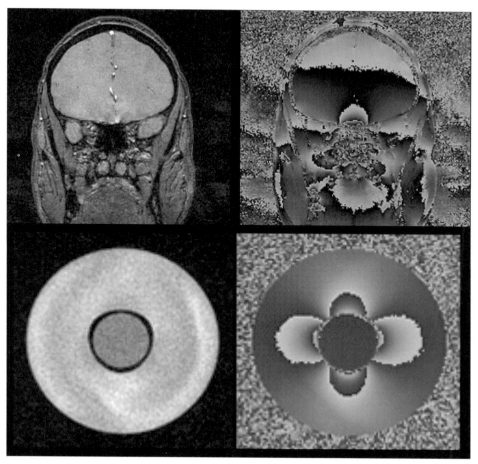

Figure 16.1. Magnetic field distortions due to magnetic susceptibility differences. Gradient echo magnitude (left) and phase (right) images of a coronal section through the brain (top) and two concentric cylinders with different susceptibilities (bottom). With a GRE acquisition, the image phase is proportional to the local magnetic field offset (the sharp transition from black to white is due to the cyclic nature of the phase angle and not a jump in field offset). In the brain image, the field is distorted by the different susceptibility of the air space in the sinus cavity. The magnetized cylinder is a model for a blood vessel containing deoxyhemoglobin, showing a dipole field distortion in the surrounding space.

An imaging voxel in the brain contains blood in arteries, capillaries, and veins. Moving down the vascular tree, the deoxyhemoglobin content steadily increases, from near zero in the arteries to about 40% of the total hemoglobin concentration in the veins. Venous blood suffers the largest change in magnetic susceptibility, but capillary blood is affected as well. The presence of deoxyhemoglobin creates magnetic field gradients around the red cells and in the tissue space surrounding the vessels. These field gradients shorten T_2^* and reduce the MR signal at rest from what it would be if there were no deoxyhemoglobin present. Based on calibration studies of the BOLD effect, described in more detail in Box 16, the signal is reduced by about 8% at 1.5 T from the

BOX 16. MODELING THE BOLD SIGNAL

The BOLD effect arises when the magnetic susceptibility of blood is altered by a change in the concentration of deoxyhemoglobin, producing field gradients around the vessels and an attenuation of the MR signal. A quantitative model of this process is important for understanding the basic mechanisms of the BOLD effect, for optimizing the image acquisition technique to maximize sensitivity, and for calibrating the BOLD signal to measure local $CMRO_2$. In this section, we will consider the gradient echo signal only, because that is the most common technique used in fMRI and the modeling is simplified because diffusion effects are not as pronounced. The simplest model of the MR signal S involves two tissue parameters, an intrinsic local signal S_0 and a transverse decay rate R_2^*:

$$S = S_0 \, e^{-TE \, R_2^*} \hspace{5cm} \text{[B16.1]}$$

where TE is the echo time. A change in the deoxyhemoglobin content alters R_2^*, and the goal of modeling the BOLD signal is to describe the dependence of R_2^* on blood volume and blood oxygenation. This physical process has been extensively studied with Monte Carlo simulations (Boxerman et al., 1995a, 1995b; Ogawa et al., 1993b; Weisskoff et al., 1994), analytical calculations (Yablonsky and Haacke, 1994), and experiments in model systems (Weisskoff and Kiihne, 1992; Weisskoff et al., 1994). A useful empirical model that has grown out of these studies has a very simple dependence on blood volume V and the deoxyhemoglobin concentration in blood [dHb] (Davis et al., 1998):

$$R_2^* \propto V[dHb]^\beta \hspace{5cm} \text{[B16.2]}$$

The transverse relaxation rate has many sources, and here we are really focusing just on the part contributed by deoxyhemoglobin. That is, Equation [B16.2] is not a full description of R_2^*, and one should imagine R_2^* as consisting of a sum of terms, with Equation [B16.2] representing just the contribution of deoxyhemoglobin.

The exponent β indicates that the dependence on blood oxygenation is not necessarily a simple proportionality. For the simplest case of looking just at the extravascular signal changes around larger veins, $\beta = 1$ would be a good approximation. In this case, R_2^* depends just on the total deoxyhemoglobin in the voxel (the product of the blood volume and the deoxyhemoglobin concentration in blood). However, this simple picture does not adequately describe two other effects. The first is diffusion of the water molecules through the field gradients around the vessels. This effect is important for the capillaries, which have a radius smaller than typical diffusion distances during an experiment. With diffusion, the exponent β is greater than one, and this is usually given as the reason for choosing $\beta > 1$.

However, a larger β also provides an approximate description for another important effect, the signal change of the blood itself. At 1.5 T, a large fraction of the BOLD signal change is due to the large change in the blood signal, due both to the increased oxygenation and the increased blood volume. To see why it is important for β to be greater than one, imagine the special case in which the increase of blood volume and the decrease of blood deoxyhemoglobin concentration are perfectly balanced to leave the total amount of deoxyhemoglobin in the voxel unchanged. Then if $\beta = 1$, the model prediction would be that there is no BOLD effect because the product V[dHb] is unchanged and so R_2^* is unchanged. This constancy of the signal would be approximately correct for the extravascular signal around larger vessels, but it would not account for the increase of the intrinsic blood signal due to the decrease in the intravascular concentration of deoxyhemoglobin. For this reason, $\beta > 1$ provides a better empirical description of the signal change.

Furthermore, if the total water content of the voxel remains fixed, then an increase of blood volume must be at the expense of a decrease of tissue water (e.g., the increased blood volume may squeeze some CSF out of the brain space). This idea is supported by experiments which found no change in M_0 with activation (Speck and Hennig, 1998). The exchange of extravascular space for intravascular space will alter the net signal, but the direction of the signal change depends on whether the intrinsic blood signal is greater than or less than the intrinsic extravascular signal. At 1.5 T, the intrinsic blood signal is stronger than that of the surrounding tissue because the resting T_2^* is longer, so the exchange of tissue space for blood would increase the MR signal, creating a positive BOLD signal change without altering the total deoxyhemoglobin. An exponent $\beta > 1$ is consistent with this effect: a decrease of [dHb] decreases the relaxation rate even though V[dHb] stays constant. Based on Monte Carlo simulations that included an intravascular contribution, $\beta = 1.5$ was found to be a good approximation for 1.5 T (Boxerman et al., 1995b). For high magnetic fields (e.g., 7 T) the T_2 of blood is short, so the increased blood signal with activation is negligible. In this regime, $\beta = 1$ is likely a better approximation (Mandeville et al., 1999; Ogawa, Lee, and Barrere, 1993a).

However, this model fails to describe the volume exchange effect for very high magnetic fields because the T_2 of blood, and thus the intrinsic signal, is less than that of the surrounding tissue. At high field, our special case of increasing V and decreasing [dHb] with no change in the product V[dHb] would produce a slight negative BOLD signal change due to the replacement of part of the extravascular volume with blood, which produces a weaker signal. This effect is not modeled with Equation [B16.2] because a decrease of the net BOLD signal with decreasing [dHb] would require the exponent β to be negative. Nevertheless, this is likely to be a small effect, and Equation [B16.2] is a reasonable approximation to an average R_2^* for fMRI studies. However, such an effect may be important for understanding the transient initial dip of the MR signal observed at higher magnetic fields.

Armed with Equation [16.2] as a model for the deoxyhemoglobin contribution to R_2^*, the difference ΔR_2^* between the activated (a) and rest (r) states is

$$\Delta R_2^* \propto (V_a[\text{dHb}]_a^\beta - V_r[\text{dHb}]_r^\beta) = \frac{1}{V_r[\text{dHb}]_r^\beta}(vc^\beta - 1) \qquad \text{[B16.3]}$$

where $v = V/V_0$ is the activated blood volume normalized to its resting value and $c = [\text{dHb}]_a/[\text{dHb}]_r$ is the normalized concentration of deoxyhemoglobin. For small signal changes, the measured fractional signal change is then

$$\frac{\Delta S}{S} = \frac{S_a - S_r}{S_r} \cong -\text{TE}\,\Delta R_2^* = S_{max}\,(1 - vc^\beta) \qquad \text{[B16.4]}$$

All the parameters in Equation [16.4] are dimensionless. If there is no change in blood volume or deoxyhemoglobin concentration, then $v = c = 1$, and there is no signal change. The constant S_{max} in front lumps together several factors and describes the

(continued)

BOX 16, continued

maximum signal change that could be observed. If blood flow increased by such an enormous amount that there is no deoxyhemoglobin left in the voxel, then $c = 0$ and the fractional signal change is S_{max}. As an example calculation, if blood volume increases by 20% ($v = 1.2$) and the deoxyhemoglobin concentration decreases by 40% ($c = 0.6$), the signal change is 0.44 S_{max}.

Equation [B16.4] represents the biophysical side of the modeling, relating the BOLD signal to the change in blood volume and blood oxygenation. The physiological side of the modeling involves relating the change in blood oxygenation to the changes in $CMRO_2$ and CBF. The oxygen metabolic rate can always be written in terms of the local CBF and the net oxygen extraction fraction E, the fraction of oxygen delivered to the capillary bed by arterial flow that is consumed by metabolism in the tissue:

$$CMRO_2 = E \, CBF \, [O_2]_{art} \qquad\qquad [B16.5]$$

where $[O_2]_{art}$ is the arterial concentration of oxygen. Nearly all this oxygen is carried in the blood bound to hemoglobin, so $[O_2]_{art}$ is proportional to the blood concentration of hemoglobin, [Hb]. When the vascular system is in a steady state, the venous concentration of deoxyhemoglobin is $[dHb]_{ven} = E \, [Hb]$. Then if we normalize $CMRO_2$ and CBF to their values at rest (as we already did with blood volume v), with $m = CMRO_2$ (act.)/$CMRO_2$ (rest) and $f = CBF$(act.)/CBF(rest), the normalized concentration of deoxyhemoglobin in venous blood is

$$c = \frac{m}{f} \qquad\qquad [B16.6]$$

Combining this with Equation [B16.4], the BOLD signal expressed in terms of the local changes in blood volume v, blood flow f, and oxygen metabolism m, is

$$\frac{\Delta S}{S} = S_{max}\left(1 - v\left[\frac{m}{f}\right]^{\beta}\right) \qquad\qquad [16.7]$$

The two model parameters, in addition to the physiological changes, are β and S_{max}. As noted earlier, for 1.5 T, $\beta = 1.5$ is a good approximation, whereas for higher fields (> 4T) β is closer to 1.0. The parameter S_{max} is likely to vary between regions of the brain due to variations in resting blood volume, and it will increase with higher field, producing a larger BOLD effect.

Equation [B16.7] offers a way to estimate local $CMRO_2$ from the BOLD signal change, if f, v, and S_{max} can be determined independently (Davis et al., 1998). The blood flow change can be measured with arterial spin labeling methods (see Chapter 15). The blood volume change is more difficult to determine directly, although it can be measured with contrast agents in animal studies (Mandeville et al., 1998). In the future, such agents will be available for human studies as well. MRI techniques to measure dynamic blood volume changes without contrast agents are in development (Wong, Buxton, and Frank, 1997), but in the absence of these techniques recent studies have assumed that the blood volume change is tightly coupled to the flow change, with $v = f^{\alpha}$. The value usually assumed is $\alpha = 0.4$ based on early, whole-brain measurements in monkeys (Grubb et al., 1974). It is not known how variable α is in the human brain.

But assuming the power law relationship, the only remaining parameter to measure is the local value of S_{max}.

To measure S_{max}, and thus calibrate the BOLD effect, a CO_2 inhalation experiment is performed, measuring both the local BOLD change and the local CBF change with ASL. Breathing CO_2 elevates CBF throughout the brain, but without any change in $CMRO_2$. For this experiment, then, $m = 1$, and from the measured BOLD change, the measured flow change, and an assumed blood volume change, S_{max} can be estimated locally using Equation [B16.7]. Following the calibration experiment, an activation study is performed, again measuring both the BOLD change and the flow change f. From these measurements and the map of S_{max} from the CO_2 experiment, the $CMRO_2$ change during activation can be calculated. If $CMRO_2$ increases with activation ($m > 1$), then for the same change in CBF, the BOLD change should be larger for the CO_2 experiment than for the activation experiment because the increased $CMRO_2$ and the corresponding increased rate of production of deoxyhemoglobin partially offsets the dilution of deoxyhemoglobin due to the large flow increase. Figure 16.2 shows curves of GRE-BOLD signal change versus the fractional CBF change calculated from Equation [B16.7] for three different assumptions about the ratio of the fractional CBF change to the fractional $CMRO_2$ change.

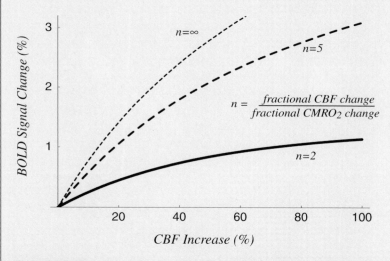

Figure 16.2. Theoretical curves of the GRE-BOLD signal as a function of the change in CBF. Curves were calculated from the model in Box 16. All curves assume that the blood volume varies as f^α, where f is the CBF and the exponent $\alpha = 0.4$. All curves also assume that the $CMRO_2$ change is coupled to the CBF change. For simplicity, this is expressed in terms of n, the ratio of the fractional change in CBF to the fractional change in $CMRO_2$ (e.g., if $n = 2$, then a 40% change in CBF is accompanied by a 20% change in $CMRO_2$). The curve for $n = 2$ corresponds to the calibrated BOLD data of (Hoge et al., 1999b), the curve for $n = 5$ corresponds approximately to the original PET data of Fox and Raichle (1986), and the curve for $n = \infty$ corresponds to the case when there is no change in $CMRO_2$, which occurs when breathing CO_2.

(continued)

BOX 16, continued

Using the calibrated BOLD technique, the fractional change in CBF was found to be two to three times larger in human subjects (Davis et al., 1998; Hoge et al., 1999b; Kim et al., 1999), and about three times larger in a rat model (Mandeville et al., 1999). These ratios are not as large as the original measurements of Fox and Raichle, but they are consistent with some other positron emission tomography (PET) results (Marrett and Gjedde, 1997). However, we should be cautious about the interpretation of these results. As discussed in Chapter 15, arterial spin labeling techniques such as flow-sensitive alternating inversion recovery (FAIR) may be inaccurate in measuring global flow changes. If the measurements of CBF change during CO_2 inhalation underestimate the true CBF change, then the $CMRO_2$ change calculated for activation will be systematically overestimated. Further work will be needed to establish the accuracy of these MR determinations of $CMRO_2$. Nevertheless, the results of Hoge and co-workers (Hoge et al., 1999b) reproduced in Figure 16.3 clearly show a simple relation between the CBF and $CMRO_2$ changes, supporting the idea that these two physiological quantities are coupled during activation.

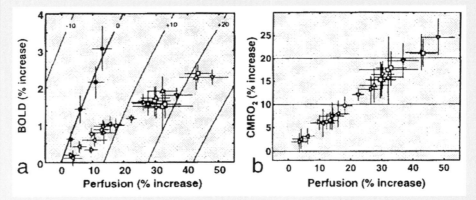

Figure 16.3. Evidence for the coupling of CBF and $CMRO_2$ during neural activation. $CMRO_2$ and CBF changes in the visual cortex were measured during a variety of visual stimuli using a calibrated BOLD technique (see Box 16). On the left, the BOLD signal is plotted versus the measured perfusion changes for all the studies. Contours of equal percent change in $CMRO_2$ (also plotted) are derived from experiments altering CO_2, which increases CBF without changing $CMRO_2$, and so define the contour of 0% change in $CMRO_2$. The remaining points show that with activation the BOLD signal change is less for the same change in flow due to increased $CMRO_2$. The CBF change was about twice as large as the $CMRO_2$ change for all conditions. (Reproduced with permission from Hoge et al. *Proc. Natl. Acad. Sci., USA* **96**:9403–9408, 1999; copyright 1999 by National Academy of Sciences, USA.).

signal with fully oxygenated blood (Davis et al., 1998). Brain activation leads to a much larger increase in blood flow than oxygen metabolism, so the net O_2 extraction fraction drops with activation. The capillary and venous blood are more oxygenated, and so there is less deoxyhemoglobin present in the voxel. With less deoxyhemoglobin, the susceptibility of the blood moves closer to the susceptibility of the surrounding tissue, and the field gradients are reduced. The T_2^* becomes longer, and the signal measured with a T_2^*-weighted pulse sequence increases by a few percent.

To see more precisely how this T_2^* effect on the extravascular spins comes about, consider the simplified picture of a long cylinder surrounded by a medium with a different magnetic susceptibility, a model for a capillary or vein containing deoxyhemoglobin. If the capillary is oriented perpendicular to the magnetic field, the z-component of the magnetic field is distorted as shown in the cross-sectional view image in Figure 16.1. The field pattern has a dipole shape, with opposite field offsets along the main field direction and perpendicular to the main field. An important feature of this pattern is that the magnitude of the field offset at the surface of the cylinder depends only on the susceptibility difference and not on the radius of the cylinder, whereas the spatial extent of the field distortion is proportional to the radius. Figure 16.4 shows the histogram of field offsets within a range of four times the vessel radius (calculated by simply sampling many random points around the vessel). We can think of the net signal from this volume as the signal measured in a single voxel. Because the rate of precession of each of the spin groups within the box is directly proportional to the field offset, this histogram is also the NMR spectrum that would be measured, and the net signal as a function of time $A(t)$ is simply the Fourier transform of this histogram. For simplicity, we neglect the true T_2 decay, so $A(t)$ represents the additional attenuation of the signal due to the difference in magnetic susceptibility between the vessel and the surrounding space.

The decay curve shown in Figure 16.4 is not a simple exponential because the distribution of field offsets has a rather irregular shape. However, this simple model is for one vessel oriented perpendicular to the magnetic field. A better model for a voxel containing many vessels is a collection of randomly oriented cylinders. When the same cylinder is tipped at an angle to the field, the same basic pattern of field offsets results but with a decreased range. Indeed, for a cylinder parallel to the field, there is no field offset outside (the range is compressed to zero). For a collection of randomly oriented cylinders, the field distribution and attenuation curve is shown in Figure 16.5. In this more realistic case, the attenuation is closer to exponential, and we can write this attenuation as

$$A(t) = e^{-t \, \Delta R_2^*} \tag{16.1}$$

where ΔR_2^* is the change in the transverse relaxation rate R_2^* $(= 1/T_2^*)$ due to the magnetic susceptibility difference between the blood and the surrounding tissue.

To a first approximation, ΔR_2^* depends just on the total venous volume of the vessels within the voxel, and not on the size of the vessels. (This conclusion will be modified when we consider the effects of diffusion next.) The reason for this is shown graphically in Figure 16.6. The first panel shows a single large vessel within the box, and the second shows four cylinders with half the radius but the same total

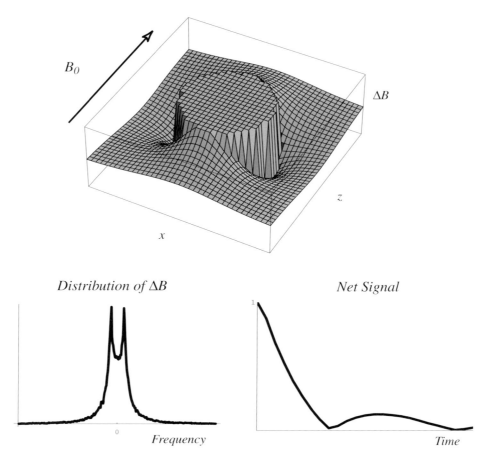

Figure 16.4. Field distortions around a magnetized blood vessel. A single magnetized cylinder oriented perpendicularly to the magnetic field B_0 creates field offsets (ΔB) in the surrounding space, with the field increased along the main field axis and decreased along a perpendicular axis (top). The distribution of fields creates a resonant frequency spectrum with two peaks (bottom left). The Fourier transform of the frequency spectrum shows how the net signal evolves in time (bottom right).

blood volume. The extent of the field distortions is scaled down in proportion to the radius for each of the smaller vessels, but the total volume affected remains the same. So the spectrum of field offsets depends just on the total blood volume and not on the vessel size. If there is no motion of the spins during the experiment, then the net signal is simply the Fourier transform of this spectrum.

The Moderating Effect of Diffusion on T_2^* Changes

The argument presented in the previous section, that the extravascular signal attenuation depends only on total blood volume and is independent of the size of the vessels holding that blood, is not strictly true due to the effects of diffusion (see Chapter 9). As a water molecule randomly moves through spatially varying fields, the precession rate of the nuclei is always proportional to the current value of the

Phase Distribution at TE

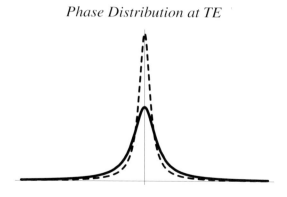

Signal Attenuation

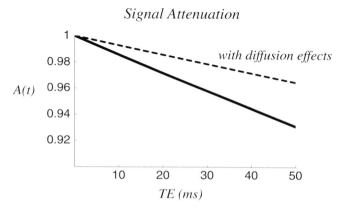

Figure 16.5. The net effect of many randomly oriented magnetized blood vessels on the GRE signal. With many cylinders the distribution of fields has only a single peak (top), producing an approximately exponential decay of the signal (bottom). When diffusion effects are included, the signal is no longer the Fourier transform of the field distribution, but for any time TE the signal attenuation A is the Fourier transform of the local *phase* distribution. Without diffusion, the phase distribution is identical to the field distribution. But with diffusion effects (dashed line), the phase distribution at any time point is narrower because the motion of the spins effectively averages over the field distribution.

field, so the precession rate for each spin will vary randomly (Figure 16.7). Because the precession rate is not constant, the attenuation is not simply the Fourier transform of the distribution of field offsets. Instead, one must follow each spin as it randomly diffuses, adjusting its precession rate as it moves to a region with a different field offset, and then adding up the net signal from each spin with its acquired phase offset. Numerical analyses of just this sort (Monte Carlo simulations) have been done to explore these effects of diffusion, and the results are in good agreement with analytical calculations and experiments in model systems with small field perturbers (Boxerman et al., 1995b; Fisel et al., 1991; Ogawa et al., 1993b; Weisskoff et al., 1994; Yablonsky and Haacke, 1994).

The effect of these diffusional motions is an averaging of the field offset felt by any one spin, resulting in a reduced phase dispersion (Figure 16.5). It is really this

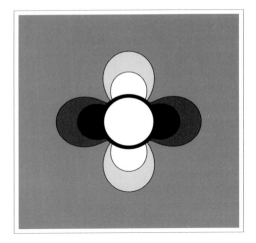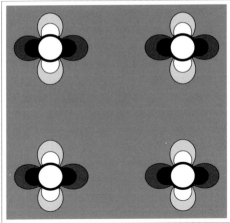

Figure 16.6. The spectrum of field offsets depends primarily on the total volume of the blood vessels containing deoxyhemoglobin. The magnetic field of a magnetized cylinder falls off inversely with the square of distance. A single large vessel creates a larger pattern of field offsets (left) than a smaller vessel (right), but the magnitude of the field offset at the surface of the cylinder is the same. For this reason, the pattern of vessels on the right, with the same total blood volume, affects the same volume of spins as the single vessel on the left. So when diffusion effects are negligible, the BOLD effect is proportional to the local venous blood volume.

dispersion of phases after the spins have evolved for a time TE that determines the attenuation at TE. One can think of this as plotting the histogram of phase offsets at time TE, and then adding up vectors with these phase offsets to produce a net signal. In the absence of diffusion, each spin sits in the same location, with its phase evolving at a rate proportional to the local field offset. For this case, the distribution of phases is simply proportional to the distribution of field offsets. But if the spins move during the experiment and sample different field offsets, the net phase at TE reflects the past history of motions of each spin. In the extreme case of very rapid diffusion, each spin feels all of the field offsets, and so each has a similar history. But if all of the spins are experiencing the same range of field offsets, then there will be very little phase dispersion and so very little attenuation, and it appears as if the range of field offsets has narrowed (Figure 16.5). In short, any diffusion of the water molecules will reduce the GRE-BOLD effect.

The magnitude of the diffusion effect on the signal depends on how far a water molecule diffuses during the experiment, and how this distance compares with the spatial scale of the field variations (Figure 16.7). As described in Chapter 9, the "average" displacement of a water molecule with diffusion coefficient D during a time interval T is given by $\Delta x^2 = 2DT$. This is the size of the expected displacement along any spatial axis, so the full displacement in space is $\Delta x^2 + \Delta y^2 + \Delta z^2 = 6DT$. For considering the diffusion effects around long magnetized blood vessels, displacement along the length of the vessel does not alter the field offset, and so these displacements do not affect the relaxation rate. For this reason, we can take as a typical diffusion distance the expected displacement in a cross-sectional plane, $\sqrt{4DT}$. A typical echo time TE in a GRE-BOLD experiment is 40 ms. In the brain, with a

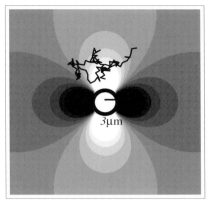
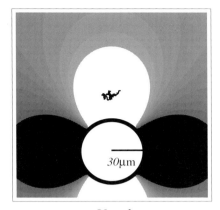

Capillary   *Venule*

Figure 16.7. Diffusion produces an averaging over field offsets that is more effective for the smallest vessels. The random walk of a diffusing water molecule is shown as a wiggly black line overlayed on the field distortion pattern around a capillary (radius 3 μm) and a venule (radius 30 μm). A molecule diffusing around a capillary will experience a larger range of field offsets, and the net phase will reflect the average of these fields. This averaging reduces the phase dispersion of all the diffusing spins. In contrast, a molecule diffusing near a larger venule or vein experiences a more constant field, and the phase dispersion among spins then reflects the full distribution of magnetic field offsets. The signal attenuation is greater around the venous vessels.

water diffusion coefficient of about $D = 1$ μm^2/ms, the typical distance moved then is about 13 μm. This distance is larger than the radius of a capillary, comparable to the radius of smaller venules, and smaller than the radius of a small vein. The variation of ΔR_2^* with vessel size is shown in Figure 16.8 (top). If the vessel is a larger venule or vein, so that the typical distance moved by a molecule due to diffusion is much smaller than the radius of the vessel, there will be little variation in the field offset felt by the spin. In this case, the GRE-BOLD effect is large, and the attenuation factor is simply the Fourier transform of the distribution of field offsets. On the other hand, for capillaries, the distance moved is larger than the radius of the vessel, and ΔR_2^* is reduced by the diffusional averaging. For a gradient echo signal, the attenuation varies smoothly between these two extremes.

The upper plot in Figure 16.9 shows calculated curves for the attenuation of the GRE-BOLD extravascular signal around capillaries and veins as a function of the oxygen saturation of the hemoglobin. The two curves are based on the numerical simulations of Ogawa et al. (1993b) for the same total blood volume (2%) and for a magnetic field strength of 1.5 T. For the same level of oxygen saturation of the hemoglobin, the attenuation around veins is typically about five times larger than the attenuation around capillaries because of the effect of diffusion. Furthermore, hemoglobin is significantly less saturated in the veins than in the capillaries. At rest, the venous oxygenation in the brain is about 60%, corresponding to a typical oxygen extraction fraction of 40%. With activation, the venous hemoglobin saturation can increase to more than 70%. For the capillaries, the changes are less dramatic. Assuming that the average capillary hemoglobin saturation is midway between the

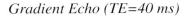

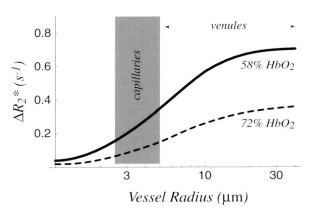

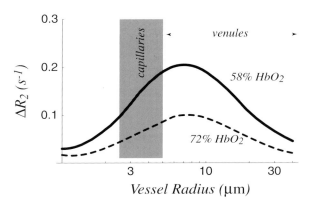

Figure 16.8. Calculated curves of the change in the extravascular transverse relaxation rate at 1.5 T as a function of vessel size. Curves are shown for two levels of hemoglobin oxygen saturation (HbO_2) for the gradient echo signal (top) and the spin echo signal (bottom). The two curves correspond approximately to the oxygenation of venous blood at rest (solid line) and during strong activation (dashed line). For the GRE signal, diffusion effects around the smallest vessels reduce the BOLD effect. For the SE signal, the BOLD effect is largest for the capillaries and smaller venules. Note that the vertical scale is three times larger for the GRE effect, reflecting the weakness of the extravascular SE-BOLD effect. (Adapted from Weisskoff, 1999.)

arterial and venous saturation levels, the same range of variation of the saturation from the resting state to the activated state is only 80–85%. It is clear that the extravascular BOLD effect is dominated by the venous side of the vasculature, due both to the reduced range of variation of the hemoglobin saturation in capillaries and to the moderating action of diffusion on the BOLD effect around capillaries. In short, GRE-BOLD experiments are primarily sensitive to the veins, and because the veins are large compared to a typical diffusion distance, diffusion effects are small.

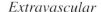

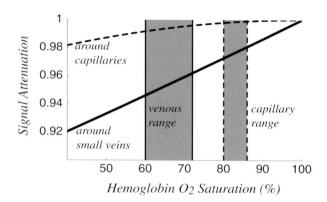

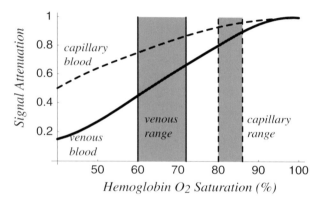

Figure 16.9. Extravascular and intravascular components of the GRE-BOLD signal change. The signal change of the extravascular (top) and intravascular (bottom) signals are plotted as a function of the oxygen saturation of hemoglobin. In each plot, the gray bars indicate the range of variation of the venous and capillary oxygenation between rest and activated states (taking the average capillary saturation to be the average of the arterial and venous saturations). Signal is plotted as the attenuation from the signal with fully oxygenated blood. The signal changes in blood itself are more than an order of magnitude larger than the extravascular signal changes so that, despite the low volume fraction occupied by blood, the intravascular and extravascular contributions to the BOLD signal at 1.5 T are comparable. At higher fields, the blood contribution diminishes. [Extravascular curves calculated from the results of Ogawa et al., (1993b); intravascular curves are adapted from Boxerman et al., (1995a.)]

The Intravascular Contribution to the BOLD Signal

The intravascular compartment is a small fraction of the total tissue volume (only about 4%), and so it is tempting to suppose that the intravascular spins would contribute a comparably small amount to the net BOLD signal change. But, in fact, the vascular contribution is comparable to the extravascular contribution at 1.5 T (Boxerman et al., 1995a). The reason for this is that the intrinsic signal change in the blood is more than an order of magnitude larger than the extravascular signal change (Figure 16.9). Within the blood, large field gradients are produced around the red blood cells carrying the deoxyhemoglobin (Thulborn et al., 1982), so that at rest the venous blood signal may be reduced by as much as 50% compared with what it would be if the blood were fully oxygenated (Boxerman et al., 1995a). This provides a much wider dynamic range for the intravascular signal change, and even though the blood occupies a small fraction of the volume, the absolute intravascular signal change is comparable to the extravascular signal change at 1.5 T.

The intravascular contribution to the BOLD signal can be measured by performing a BOLD experiment with and without bipolar gradient pulses added to the sequence. A bipolar gradient pulse is simply two matched gradient pulses with the same amplitude and duration, but opposite sign. Such pulses are commonly used to add diffusion weighting to the signal because a bipolar gradient adds sensitivity to motion (see Chapter 9). With a bipolar gradient pulse, each spin acquires a phase offset proportional to the distance it moves between the two pulses. The random motions due to diffusion create a spread of phases and an attenuation of the signal. For smaller vessels within a voxel, the uniform motion of the blood, but in randomly oriented vessels, produces a dephasing effect similar to diffusion. However, the distances moved by flowing blood are much greater than the displacements due to diffusion, so the blood signal can be destroyed with only modest diffusion weighting (although fully suppressing the signal of the slow-moving capillary blood does require significant gradient strength). So by adding a bipolar gradient pulse, most of the signal of flowing blood can be selectively suppressed with only a small effect on the extravascular signal.

Experiments comparing the BOLD signal with and without diffusion weighting have confirmed that at lower fields (1.5–3 T) a significant fraction of the BOLD signal is reduced with diffusion weighting. Boxerman and co-workers found that about 70% of the signal could be eliminated with a large degree of diffusion weighting (Boxerman et al., 1995b). At 3T, even a much more modest level of diffusion weighting reduced the BOLD signal by about 35% (Buxton et al., 1998). These data confirm that at field strengths of 1.5–3 T a substantial fraction of the GRE signal change is intravascular.

In these sections we have tried to dissect the BOLD effect into small vessel and large vessel effects, and into separate contributions from extravascular and intravascular signal changes. For practical applications, however, it is useful to combine these different sources of the BOLD effect into one empirical relationship that describes the total BOLD signal change as a function of blood volume and blood oxygenation. This relation is derived in Box 16 for the GRE-BOLD signal following (Davis et al., 1998). Using such a relationship we can model how the physiological changes in cerebral blood flow (CBF), cerebral metabolic rate of oxygen ($CMRO_2$), and cerebral blood volume (CBV) combine to produce a BOLD signal change.

Spin Echo BOLD Signal Changes

With a spin echo (SE) pulse sequence, the 180° radio frequency (RF) pulse refocuses the phase offsets due to precession in an inhomogeneous field, so at first glance it might appear that there should be no BOLD effect with SE imaging. However, a spin echo works only if the spins remain in the same field throughout the experiment. Phase offsets acquired during the first half of the echo time are reversed by the 180° pulse, and the same phase offset acquired in the second half of the echo time then precisely cancels the phase from the first half. But due to diffusion, each water molecule wanders randomly during the course of the experiment. If the spatial scale of the field inhomogeneities is smaller than the typical distance moved by a water molecule, then the spins are in different fields (and precessing at different rates) during the first and second half of the experiment. The spin echo does not refocus the phase offsets completely, and the remaining phase dispersion will produce a reduction in the net signal. As with the GRE signal, we can write this additional attenuation of the SE signal due to deoxyhemoglobin in the vessels as

$$A(t) = e^{-t\,\Delta R_2} \tag{16.2}$$

where ΔR_2 is the change in the transverse relaxation rate R_2 ($= 1/T_2$). Because of the partial refocusing effect of the spin echo, ΔR_2 is always less than ΔR_2^*, and so the SE-BOLD effect is always weaker than the GRE-BOLD effect.

In a typical SE-BOLD experiment the echo time is longer than for a GRE-BOLD experiment (e.g., TE = 100 ms compared with TE = 40 ms) to maximize the signal change due to a small change in R_2. The change in transverse relaxation rate ΔR_2 in an SE experiment is plotted in the lower panel of Figure 16.8. Not only are the changes in R_2 much smaller than the changes in R_2^*, but the dependence on vessel size is also quite different. For the larger vessels, diffusion effects are negligible, so the spin echo efficiently refocuses the field offsets that produce a large GRE-BOLD effect. The change in R_2 is minimal, so the SE-BOLD effect is negligible. As we move to smaller vessels, diffusion makes the spin echo less effective at refocusing the phase dispersion from field offsets, and ΔR_2 becomes larger. However, the SE-BOLD effect peaks for a vessel radius around 7 μm in these calculations and diminishes for smaller vessels. In this regime, the spin echo does a poor job of refocusing, but the extensive field averaging due to diffusion narrows the range of phase offsets and reduces ΔR_2 just as it reduces ΔR_2^*.

Because of this sensitivity to vessel size, SE-BOLD is more selective for the smallest vessels, the capillaries, and small venules. This has been a primary motivation for using SE-BOLD for brain mapping despite the lower sensitivity, based on the assumption that the SE signal changes would map more tightly to the capillary bed rather than draining veins. In other words, the SE pulse sequence trades sensitivity for increased specificity. In practice, an asymmetric spin echo (ASE) sequence often is used (see Chapter 8). An ASE sequence is intermediate between a GRE and an SE pulse sequence in its sensitivity to local field offsets.

However, the argument for the greater selectivity of the SE technique is based on considerations of the extravascular signal change. As with the GRE technique, the total BOLD effect has a strong contribution from the intravascular compartment. Recently, van Zijl and co-workers argued that with a SE method the BOLD effect is strongly dominated by intravascular signal changes at 1.5 T (Oja et al., 1999; Zijl et al., 1998). And because the venous blood exhibits the largest signal change with decreasing deoxyhemoglobin, the largest SE-BOLD changes are in the veins as well. This implies that SE-BOLD may be more sensitive to draining veins than GRE-BOLD, where the extravascular and intravascular contributions are closer to being equal. In other words, although the extravascular SE-BOLD signal change is likely to be more sensitive to the capillary changes, at lower fields this weak signal change is swamped by the much larger signal change in the veins. To regain the capillary selectivity, one could apply spoiler gradients to destroy the intrinsic signal of the veins. However, this would reduce an already weak signal even further, and so in practice the method would be very insensitive. However, at higher fields (7 T and higher), the blood signal is naturally reduced because the T_2 of blood shortens with increasing field. The reduced blood signal, combined with the increased signal-to-noise ratio at high field, makes SE imaging a desirable technique at high field.

In short, although early studies of SE-BOLD indicated a greater selectivity for the capillary bed compared with draining veins, it seems likely that this selectivity will not be fully attainable in practice until BOLD studies are done at much higher magnetic field strengths where the signal from blood is suppressed. A recent study in rats at 9.4 T found that the T_2 of venous blood was reduced to 9 ms and that there was no significant contribution of blood signal to the SE-BOLD effect (Lee et al., 1999). These authors estimated that if the TE used is equal to the tissue T_2, the fractional contribution of the venous blood signal change itself to the net SE-BOLD signal change is 60% at 1.5 T, 8% at 4.7 T, and 1% at 9.4 T.

THE PHYSIOLOGICAL BASIS OF THE BOLD EFFECT

The BOLD Effect Depends on Combined Changes in CBF, CMRO$_2$, and CBV

Like the PET methods that preceded fMRI, the BOLD effect is not a direct measure of neural activity. Healthy neurons exist in a state far from thermodynamic equilibrium, so that action potentials and neurotransmitter release at the synapse occur without the need to supply any additional energy. In other words, neuronal signaling depends on downhill thermodynamic processes. But after synaptic activity, the ionic gradients must be restored, and neurotransmitters must be cleared from the synapse and repackaged to prepare for the next event. This stage of recovery from neural activity requires energy metabolism. Blood flow, glucose metabolism, and oxygen metabolism all increase to supply the necessary substrates for energy metabolism to the brain. The precise mechanisms that orchestrate these metabolic changes are not well understood, although a number of chemical agents have been identified that have a strong vasodilatory effect (Villringer and Dirnagle, 1995). For example, the extracellular concentrations of potassium and nitric oxide (NO) both are increased by neural activity and cause the arterioles to dilate, increasing cerebral blood flow.

With PET studies of brain activation, the measured quantity is a well-defined physiological parameter, such as CBF, the cerebral metabolic rate of glucose (CMR-Glc), $CMRO_2$, or CBV. All these quantities increase with activation, as described in Chapters 1–3. However, the BOLD effect is not a simple reflection of any one of these physiological changes. The change in the oxygenation of the blood with activation depends on the balance of the changes in CBF and $CMRO_2$. If they change by the same fraction, the oxygen extraction fraction (E) does not change, and there is no change in the oxygenation of the venous blood. On the other hand, if CBF increases much more than $CMRO_2$, which is what is observed, then E drops, and the venous blood is more oxygenated. But the BOLD signal change is not even a pure reflection of the change in E. As described earlier, the BOLD effect depends on the total quantity of deoxyhemoglobin within a voxel and so depends on the CBV as well as the concentration within the venous blood. An increase of CBV alone, without any change in E, would increase the total deoxyhemoglobin and cause a drop in the MR signal (a negative BOLD effect).

The complexity of the BOLD response, then, is not just that it depends on the changes in several physiological parameters, but also that the expected changes with activation may have conflicting effects on the BOLD signal change. With activation, PET studies have found that CBF increases dramatically, CBV increases moderately, and $CMRO_2$ increases by a much smaller amount (see Chapters 1–3). The resulting drop in E tends to increase the MR signal, whereas the increase in CBV tends to decrease the MR signal. In the adult brain, the oxygenation change overwhelms the volume change, and the result is a positive BOLD effect (an increase of the MR signal). However, recently a few groups have reported that in infants the BOLD effect is reversed (i.e., the MR signal drops with activation) (Meek et al., 1998). If confirmed, such results could be due to larger $CMRO_2$ or larger CBV changes with activation. Furthermore, recent experiments in animal models have found that the time courses for the changes in CBF, $CMRO_2$, and CBV following activation are not the same, and that this can produce transient features in the BOLD response, such as a poststimulus undershoot of the MR signal (Mandeville et al., 1998). The important role of these different time courses in shaping the hemodynamic response are described in Chapter 17.

Are CBF and $CMRO_2$ Changes Coupled During Activation?

There is substantial experimental evidence that CBF is tightly coupled to neural activity, and some of the animal studies supporting this were described in Chapters 1–3. For human studies, there is no direct way to measure neural activity itself for direct comparison with CBF. Instead, experiments are done in which a stimulus is varied in magnitude in a way that is likely to produce a graded response of neural activity. A CBF response that varies in a systematic way with some aspect of the stimulus provides support for the idea that CBF is coupled to neural activity. Several studies of this type were done using PET to measure CBF and demonstrated a graded CBF response. For example, in primary visual cortex, the CBF response increases with increasing frequency of a flashing light for frequencies in the range 1–8 Hz (Fox and Raichle, 1984, 1985). A study in the sensorimotor cortex found that CBF increases approximately linearly with the rate of finger tapping in the range 0.5–4 Hz (Blinkenberg et al., 1996); however, another study found a plateau of CBF change for the fastest rates (Sadato et al., 1996). In several auditory areas, CBF increases approximately linearly with the presentation rate of words in the range of 10–90 words per minute (Price et al., 1992). When similar experiments have been performed with fMRI, the amplitude of the BOLD signal change also showed a graded response in the primary visual cortex (Kwong et al., 1992), the primary motor cortex (Rao et al., 1996; Sadato et al., 1997; Schlaug et al., 1996), and the primary auditory cortex (Rees et al., 1997).

The idea that CBF changes are tightly coupled to neural activity is widely accepted. However, the quantitative interpretation of the BOLD signal remains in doubt because the question of whether $CMRO_2$ changes with activity, and if so by how much, has been controversial. This question remains a central concern for the interpretation of BOLD experiments. The experimental fMRI results cited earlier lend support to the idea that the BOLD signal reflects neural activity, but a full quantitative understanding of the magnitude of the BOLD effect depends on the $CMRO_2$ change with activation.

The observed mismatch in the changes of CBF and $CMRO_2$ with activation was originally termed an uncoupling, in the sense that it appeared that the CBF increased much more than was necessary to support the small change in $CMRO_2$ (Fox and Raichle, 1986). But if they are truly uncoupled, so that they vary independently, then the quantitative interpretation of BOLD signal changes as a reflection of the degree of neural activity is problematic. Indeed, if CBF and $CMRO_2$ vary independently, then it is possible that the BOLD effect would be a poor indicator of the level of activity. For example, suppose that the blood flow increase is like a switch, so that once some threshold level of neural activity is reached CBF increases by some large but fixed amount. Further suppose that this CBF change is sufficient to support a large $CMRO_2$ change, but the actual local change in $CMRO_2$ is matched to the neural activity. Now consider two regions, one that is strongly activated and one that is only weakly activated. In both regions, the CBF change is the same, but the $CMRO_2$ change is larger in the more strongly activated region. However, because higher $CMRO_2$ generates more deoxyhemoglobin, the BOLD effect is stronger in the less activated region! Indeed, by this scenario the most strongly activated regions might not show a BOLD change at all if the $CMRO_2$ change were comparable to the CBF change. The possibility that CBF changes are truly uncoupled from $CMRO_2$ changes clearly presents a major problem for the interpretation of BOLD experiments.

The change in $CMRO_2$ would not be a problem for the interpretation of the BOLD effect if the change is always negligible. In the seminal work of Fox and Raichle, the change in $CMRO_2$ was only 5%, compared with a CBF change of 30%. Another early study found no change in $CMRO_2$ (Kuwabara et al., 1992). However, more recent PET studies in humans have consistently found significant changes in $CMRO_2$, although when the change in CBF was also measured it was always at least twice as large as the change in $CMRO_2$ (Marrett and Gjedde, 1997; Seitz and Roland, 1992; Vafaee et al., 1998, 1999). These studies show that the change in $CMRO_2$ is not negligible, so a potential uncoupling of CBF and $CMRO_2$ poses an important problem for the interpretation of BOLD signal changes.

Two ideas have been proposed for how such a mismatch of CBF and $CMRO_2$ changes could occur even though the two are coupled. The first possibility is that blood flow is controlled on a coarse spatial scale, but the changes in $CMRO_2$ occur on a finer spatial scale. Then the change in $CMRO_2$ averaged over the broader region in which flow is increased produces a smaller average change in $CMRO_2$ compared to CBF. This idea has been described as "watering the garden for the sake of one thirsty flower" (Malonek and Grinvald, 1996). If this effect is the primary cause of the observed mismatch, then the scenario outlined earlier could be important. Imagine that $CMRO_2$ increases in patches smaller than an imaging voxel, but that CBF is controlled only over a spatial scale of a few millimeters. Then the more patches which have a $CMRO_2$ change, the weaker the BOLD signal will be, and again any quantitative interpretation of BOLD signal changes is difficult.

An alternative idea is that the large CBF change is necessary to support a small change in $CMRO_2$ (Buxton and Frank, 1997) (see Chapter 3). The basis of this idea is the hypothesis that oxygen delivery is limited at rest, so that there is no reserve of oxygen in the tissue to draw on to increase $CMRO_2$ (Gjedde et al., 1991; Kassissia et al., 1995). To increase $CMRO_2$, the flux of O_2 from the capillary to the tissue must be increased, and this flux is proportional to the average pO_2 in the capillary. Because the O_2 as dissolved gas and the O_2 bound to hemoglobin are in rapid equilibrium, an increase of capillary pO_2 requires an increase of hemoglobin saturation as well. An increased oxygen saturation level in the capillary is only possible if the venous saturation is increased, and this requires a reduction in the net oxygen extraction fraction. In other words, by this model the oxygen extraction fraction E must drop to raise the capillary pO_2 and increase the availability of oxygen to the tissue for metabolism. To decrease E, the flow must increase much more than the $CMRO_2$. A more mathematical model for this effect predicts that the CBF change must be several times larger than the $CMRO_2$ change (Buxton and Frank, 1997). With this model, the CBF and $CMRO_2$ changes are coupled without being equal, and the result is that regions with a larger change in CBF and $CMRO_2$ should show a larger BOLD effect.

Recent experiments support the idea of a close coupling of CBF and $CMRO_2$. Ideally, this can be tested by comparing the changes in CBF, $CMRO_2$, and the BOLD signal associated with different levels of activity. However, for practical reasons there is very little data comparing all three measurements. A number of PET studies have shown a graded response of CBF with a graded magnitude of the stimulus, as described earlier. However, measuring $CMRO_2$ with PET is a much more complicated procedure, requiring multiple agents and measurements to account properly for blood flow and blood volume effects, so there are fewer studies of $CMRO_2$ and CBF. Recently, MRI techniques for measuring CBF and $CMRO_2$ have been developed, and these methods have the promise of providing these essential comparisons for establishing the physiological basis of the BOLD method.

Recently Hoge and colleagues used this MRI technique to collect the most compelling evidence to date for a close relationship between CBF and $CMRO_2$ changes with activation in the visual cortex (Hoge et al., 1999a, 1999b) (Figure 16.3). They combined BOLD measurements and arterial spin labeling measurements of CBF to calibrate the BOLD signal with a CO_2 inhalation experiment and make possible a measurement of $CMRO_2$ (see Box 16). They produced graded levels of activation with various visual stimuli, including diffuse isoluminant chromatic displays and high spatial frequency achromatic luminance gratings as well as checkerboards modulated at different rates. The result was an impressively tight and linear relationship between the CBF change and the $CMRO_2$ change, with the fractional change in CBF about twice as large as the fractional change in $CMRO_2$. These data strongly support the idea that CBF and $CMRO_2$ are tightly coupled during activation, despite the fact that the CBF change is larger than the $CMRO_2$ change. Other investigators using variations of this MR technique have found a similar, but somewhat larger, ratio of fractional CBF change to fractional $CMRO_2$ change in humans (Davis et al., 1998; Kim et al., 1999) and in rats (Mandeville et al., 1999). These ratios measured with MRI are smaller than the original PET result of Fox and Raichle (about $6:1$). Some of the variability in these ratios could be due to systematic errors in the CBF measurements with ASL, but all these results support the idea of a tight coupling between CBF and $CMRO_2$ during activation, with the CBF increase at least twice as large as the $CMRO_2$ increase.

Despite the broad agreement of the results of these calibrated BOLD experiments, the question of how much $CMRO_2$ changes during activation is still controversial. Hyder and co-workers have used a different MR technique based on ^{13}C spectroscopy to estimate $CMRO_2$ changes based on the cycling of labeled carbon through the TCA cycle (Hyder et al., 1996, 1997). Using this technique, they found very large changes in $CMRO_2$ in a rat model, much larger than those estimated with the calibrated BOLD method in a similar study (Mandeville et al., 1999). When combined with ASL measurements of flow, they found $CMRO_2$ changes to be similar to the CBF changes in different levels of anesthesia. They have proposed a modification to the oxygen limitation model to account for such large $CMRO_2$ changes by including a parameter to describe changes in the diffusivity of oxygen with activation (Hyder, Shulman, and Rothman, 1998). If this parameter is large enough, the increased delivery of oxygen during activation can be accomplished with a smaller increase of flow. At this time, the source of the conflicting results of calibrated BOLD measurements and nuclear magnetic resonance (NMR) spectroscopy measurements is unknown, and a thorough reexamination of the basic assumptions and experimental corrections used in the two techniques will be critical for resolving this controversy.

In summary, current evidence supports the idea that $CMRO_2$ and CBF changes are coupled during neural activity, but with the CBF change always larger than the $CMRO_2$ change. If this is true, then we can expect that a drop in the oxygen extraction fraction and the resulting positive BOLD signal change should be a reliable indicator of neural activity. However, further work is needed to understand the coupling between CBF and $CMRO_2$, and how this coupling is disrupted in disease and potentially in anesthetized states.

REFERENCES

Bandettini, P. A., Wong, E. C., Hinks, R. S., Tikofsky, R. S., and Hyde, J. S. (1992) Time course EPI of human brain function during task activation. *Magn. Reson. Med.* **25**, 390–7.

Blinkenberg, M., Bonde, C., Holm, S., Svarer, C., Andersen, J., Paulson, O. B., and Law, I. (1996) Rate dependence of regional cerebral activation during performance of a repetitive motor task: A PET study. *J. Cereb. Blood Flow Metabol.* **16**, 794–803.

Boxerman, J. L., Bandettini, P. A., Kwong, K. K., Baker, J. R., Davis, T. L., Rosen, B. R., and Weisskoff, R. M. (1995a) The intravascular contribution to fMRI signal change: Monte Carlo modeling and diffusion-weighted studies in vivo. *Magn. Reson. Med.* **34**, 4–10.

Boxerman, J. L., Hamberg, L. M., Rosen, B. R., and Weisskoff, R. M. (1995b) MR contrast due to intravascular magnetic susceptibility perturbations. *Magn. Reson. Med.* **34**, 555–66.

Buxton, R. B., and Frank, L. R. (1997) A model for the coupling between cerebral blood flow and oxygen metabolism during neural stimulation. *J. Cereb. Blood Flow Metabol.* **17**, 64–72.

Buxton, R. B., Luh, W.-M., Wong, E. C., Frank, L. R., and Bandettini, P. A. (1998) Diffusion weighting attenuates the BOLD peak signal change but not the post-stimulus undershoot. In: *Sixth Meeting, International Society for Magnetic Resonance in Medicine*, p. 7: Sydney, Australia.

Davis, T. L., Kwong, K. K., Weisskoff, R. M., and Rosen, B. R. (1998) Calibrated functional MRI: Mapping the dynamics of oxidative metabolism. *Proc. Natl. Acad. Sci. USA* **95**, 1834–9.

Fisel, C. R., Ackerman, J. L., Buxton, R. B., Garrido, L., Belliveau, J. W., Rosen, B. R., and Brady, T. J. (1991) MR contrast due to microscopically heterogeneous magnetic susceptibility: Numerical simulations and applications to cerebral physiology. *Magn. Reson. Med.* **17**, 336–47.

Fox, P. T., and Raichle, M. E. (1984) Stimulus rate dependence of regional cerebral blood flow in human striate cortex, demonstrated by positron emission tomography. *J. Neurophysiol.* **51**, 1109–20.

Fox, P. T., and Raichle, M. E. (1985) Stimulus rate determines regional brain blood flow in striate cortex. *Ann. Neurol.* **17**, 303–305.

Fox, P. T., and Raichle, M. E. (1986) Focal physiological uncoupling of cerebral blood flow and oxidative metabolism during somatosensory stimulation in human subjects. *Proc. Natl. Acad. Sci. USA* **83**, 1140–4.

Frahm, J., Bruhn, H., Merboldt, K.-D., Hanicke, W., and Math, D. (1992) Dynamic MR imaging of human brain oxygenation during rest and photic stimulation. *J. Magn. Reson. Imag.* **2**, 501–5.

Gjedde, A., Ohta, S., Kuwabara, H., and Meyer, E. (1991) Is oxygen diffusion limiting for blood-brain transfer of oxygen? In: *Brain Work and Mental Activity*, pp. 177–84. Eds. N. A. Lassen, D. H. Ingvar, M. E. Raichle, and L. Friberg. Alfred Benzon Symposium: Copenhagen.

Grubb, R. L., Raichle, M. E., Eichling, J. O., and Ter-Pogossian, M. M. (1974) The effects of changes in PCO_2 on cerebral blood volume, blood flow, and vascular mean transit time. *Stroke* **5**, 630–9.

Hoge, R. D., Atkinson, J., Gill, B., Crelier, G. R., Marrett, S., and Pike, G. B. (1999a) Investigation of BOLD signal dependence on cerebral blood flow and oxygen consumption: The deoxyhemoglobin dilution model. *Magn. Reson. Med.* **42**, 849–63.

Hoge, R. D., Atkinson, J., Gill, B., Crelier, G. R., Marrett, S., and Pike, G. B. (1999b) Linear coupling between cerebral blood flow and oxygen consumption in activated human cortex. *Proc. Natl. Acad. Sci. USA* **96,** 9403–8.

Hyder, F., Chase, J., Behar, K., Mason, G., Siddeek, M., Rothman, D., and Schulman, R. (1996) Increased tricarboxylic acid cycle flux in rat brain during forepaw stimulation detected with $^1H[^{13}C]NMR$. *Proc. Natl. Acad. Sci. USA* **93,** 7612–17.

Hyder, F., Rothman, D. L., Mason, G. F., Rangarajan, A., Behar, K. L., and Shulman, R. G. (1997) Oxidative glucose metabolism in rat brain during single forepaw stimulation: A spatially localized $^1H[^{13}C]$ nuclear magnetic resonance study. *J. Cereb. Blood Flow Metabol.* **17,** 1040–7.

Hyder, F., Shulman, R. G., and Rothman, D. L. (1998) A model for the regulation of cerebral oxygen delivery. *J. Appl. Physiol.* **85,** 554–64.

Kassissia, I. G., Goresky, C. A., Rose, C. P., Schwab, A. J., Simard, A., Huet, P. M., and Bach, G. G. (1995) Tracer oxygen distribution is barrier-limited in the cerebral microcirculation. *Circulation Res.* **77,** 1201–11.

Kim, S. G., Rostrup, E., Larsson, H. B. W., Ogawa, S., and Paulson, O. B. (1999) Determination of relative $CMRO_2$ from CBF and BOLD changes: Significant increase of oxygen consumption rate during visual stimulation. *Magn. Reson. Med.* **41,** 1152–61.

Kuwabara, H., Ohta, S., Brust, P., Meyer, E., and Gjedde, A. (1992) Density of perfused capillaries in living human brain during functional activation. *Prog. Brain Res.* **91,** 209–15.

Kwong, K. K., Belliveau, J. W., Chesler, D. A., Goldberg, I. E., Weisskoff, R. M., Poncelet, B. P., Kennedy, D. N., Hoppel, B. E., Cohen, M. S., Turner, R., Cheng, H.-M., Brady, T. J., and Rosen, B. R. (1992) Dynamic magnetic resonance imaging of human brain activity during primary sensory stimulation. *Proc. Natl. Acad. Sci. USA.* **89,** 5675–9.

Lee, S. P., Silva, A. C., Ugurbil, K., and Kim, S. G. (1999) Diffusion-weighted spin-echo fMRI at 9.4 T: Microvascular/tissue contribution to BOLD signal changes. *Magn. Reson. Med.* **42,** 919–28.

Malonek, D., and Grinvald, A. (1996) Interactions between electrical activity and cortical microcirculation revealed by imaging spectroscopy: Implications for functional brain mapping. *Science* **272,** 551–4.

Mandeville, J. B., Marota, J. J. A., Ayata, C., Moskowitz, M. A., Weisskoff, R. M., and Rosen, B. R. (1999) MRI measurement of the temporal evolution of relative $CMRO_2$ during rat forepaw stimulation. *Magn. Reson. Med.* **42,** 944–51.

Mandeville, J. B., Marota, J. J. A., Kosofsky, B. E., Keltner, J. R., Weissleder, R., Rosen, B. R., and Weisskoff, R. M. (1998) Dynamic functional imaging of relative cerebral blood volume during rat forepaw stimulation. *Magn. Reson. Med.* **39,** 615–24.

Marrett, S., and Gjedde, A. (1997) Changes of blood flow and oxygen consumption in visual cortex of living humans. *Adv. Exp. Med. Biol.* **413,** 205–8.

Meek, J. H., Firbank, M., Elwell, C. E., Atkinson, J., Braddock, O., and Wyatt, J. S. (1998) Regional hemodynamic response to visual stimulation in awake infants. *Pediatric Res.* **43,** 840–3.

Ogawa, S., Lee, T.-M., Nayak, A. S., and Glynn, P. (1990) Oxygenation-sensitive contrast in magnetic resonance image of rodent brain at high magnetic fields. *Magn. Reson. Med.* **14,** 68–78.

Ogawa, S., Lee, T. M., and Barrere, B. (1993a) The sensitivity of magnetic resonance image signals of a rat brain to changes in the cerebral venous blood oxygenation. *Magn. Reson. Med.* **29,** 205–10.

Ogawa, S., Menon, R. S., Tank, D. W., Kim, S.-G., Merkle, H., Ellerman, J. M., and Ugurbil, K. (1993b) Functional brain mapping by blood oxygenation level-dependent contrast magnetic resonance imaging: a comparison of signal characteristics with a biophysical model. *Biophy. J.* **64,** 803–12.

Ogawa, S., Tank, D. W., Menon, R., Ellermann, J. M., Kim, S.-G., Merkle, H., and Ugurbil, K. (1992) Intrinsic signal changes accompanying sensory stimulation: Functional brain mapping with magnetic resonance imaging. *Proc. Natl. Acad. Sci. USA* **89,** 5951–5.

Oja, J. M. E., Gillen, J., Kaupinnen, R. A., Kraut, M., and Zijl, P. C. M. v. (1999) Venous blood effects in spin-echo fMRI of human brain. *Magn. Reson. Med.* **42,** 617–26.

Pauling, L., and Coryell, C. D. (1936) The magnetic properties and structure of hemoglobin, oxyhemoglobin, and carbonmonoxyhemoglobin. *Proc. Natl. Acad. Sci. USA* **22,** 210–16.

Price, C., Wise, R., Ramsay, S., Friston, K., Howard, D., Patterson, K., and Frackowiak, R. (1992) Regional response differences within the human auditory cortex when listening to words. *Neurosci. Lett.* **146,** 179–82.

Rao, S. M., Bandettini, P. A., Binder, J. R., Bobholz, J., Hammeke, T. A., Stein, E. A., and Hyde, J. S. (1996) Relationship between finger movement rate and functional magnetic resonance signal change in human primary motor cortex. *J. Cereb. Blood Flow Metabol.* **16,** 1250–4.

Rees, G., Howseman, A., Josephs, O., Frith, C. D., Friston, K. J., Frackowiak, R. S. J., and Turner, R. (1997) Characterizing the relationship between BOLD contrast and regional cerebral blood flow measurements by varying the stimulus presentation rate. *NeuroImage* **6,** 270–8.

Sadato, N., Ibanez, V., Campbell, G., Deiber, M. P., Bihan, D. L., and Hallett, M. (1997) Frequency-dependent changes of regional cerebral blood flow during finger movements: Functional MRI compared to PET. *J. Cereb. Blood Flow Metabol.* **17,** 670–9.

Sadato, N., Ibanez, V., Deiber, M. P., Campbell, G., Leonardo, M., and Hallett, M. (1996) Frequency-dependent changes of regional cerebral blood flow during finger movements. *J. Cereb. Blood Flow Metabol.* **16,** 23–33.

Schlaug, G., Sanes, J. N., Tahngaraj, V., Darby, D. G., Jancke, L., Edelman, R. R., and Warach, S. (1996) Cerebral activation covaries with movement rate. *NeuroReport* **7,** 879–83.

Seitz, R. J., and Roland, P. E. (1992) Vibratory stimulation increases and decreases the regional cerebral blood flow and oxidative metabolism: A positron emission tomography (PET) study. *Acta Neurol. Scand.* **86,** 60–7.

Speck, O., and Hennig, J. (1998) Functional imaging by I_0- and T^*_2-parameter mapping using multi-image EPI. *Magn. Reson. Med.* **40,** 243–8.

Thulborn, K. R., Waterton, J. C., Matthews, P. M., and Radda, G. K. (1982) Oxygenation dependence of the transverse relaxation time of water protons in whole blood at high field. *Biochim. Biophys. Acta* **714,** 265–70.

Turner, R., LeBihan, D., Moonen, C. T. W., Despres, D., and Frank, J. (1991) Echoplanar time course MRI of cat brain oxygenation changes. *Magn. Reson. Med.* **27,** 159–66.

Vafaee, M., Marrett, S., Meyer, E., Evans, A., and Gjedde, A. (1998) Increased oxygen consumption in human visual cortex: response to visual stimulation. *Acta Neurol. Scand.* **98,** 85–9.

Vafaee, M. S., Meyer, E., Marrett, S., Paus, T., Evans, A. C., and Gjedde, A. (1999) Frequency-dependent changes in cerebral metabolic rate of oxygen during activation of human visual cortex. *J. Cereb. Blood Flow Metabol.* **19,** 272–7.

Villringer, A., and Dirnagle, U. (1995) Coupling of brain activity and cerebral blood flow: Basis of functional neuroimaging. *Cerebrovascular and Brain Metabolism Reviews* **7,** 240–76.

Weisskoff, R. M., and Kiihne, S. (1992) MRI susceptometry: Image-based measurement of absolute susceptibility of MR contrast agents and human blood. *Magn. Reson. Med.* **24,** 375–83.

Weisskoff, R. M., Zuo, C. S., Boxerman, J. L., and Rosen, B. R. (1994) Microscopic susceptibility variation and transverse relaxation: Theory and experiment. *Magn. Reson. Med.* **31,** 601–10.

Wong, E. C., Buxton, R. B., and Frank, L. R. (1997) A method for dynamic imaging of blood volume. In: *Fifth Meeting, International Society for Magnetic Resonance in Medicine,* pp. 372: Vancouver.

Yablonsky, D. A., and Haacke, E. M. (1994) Theory of NMR signal behavior in magnetically inhomogenous tissues: The static dephasing regime. *Magn. Reson. Med* **32,** 749–63.

Zijl, P. C. M. v., Eleff, S. E., Ulatowski, J. A., Oja, J. M. E., Ulug, A. J., Traystman, R. J., and Kauppinen, R. A. (1998) Quantitative assessment of blood flow, blood volume and blood oxygenation effects in functional magnetic resonance imaging. *Nature Med.* **4,** 159–67.

17

Mapping Brain Activation with BOLD-fMRI

Introduction
The BOLD Hemodynamic Response
> Location of BOLD Signal Changes
> The Relationship Between the BOLD Effect and
> > Neural Activity
> Linearity of the BOLD Response
> Dynamics of the BOLD Response
> Biomechanical Sources of the Poststimulus Undershoot
> The Fast Response (the Initial Dip)

Optimizing BOLD Image Acquisition
> Magnetic Field Dependence
> Image Acquisition Parameters
> Motion Artifacts
> Image Distortions

INTRODUCTION

Functional magnetic resonance imaging (MRI) based on the Blood Oxygenation Level Dependent (BOLD) effect is now a widely used tool for probing the working brain. The goal of fMRI studies is to map patterns of local changes in the magnetic resonance (MR) signal in the brain as an indicator of neural activity associated with particular stimuli. The prototypical fMRI experiment alternates blocks of stimulus and control periods while a series of dynamic images is collected with an echo-planar imaging (EPI) pulse sequence. The signal time course for each voxel of the image is analyzed to test whether there is a significant correlation of the signal with the stimulus (i.e., whether the signal increased during the stimulus). The statistical analysis of BOLD fMRI data is a critical component of the experiment, and the ideas behind the different approaches are described in Chapter 18. For now we want to consider the BOLD hemodynamic response itself in more detail.

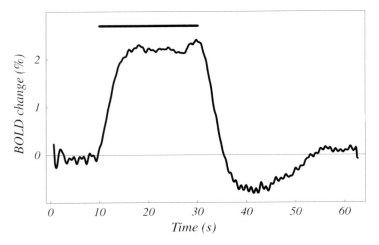

Figure 17.1. The BOLD signal. Sample BOLD response in the visual cortex measured at 3 T. Subjects wore goggles that flashed a grid of red lights at 8 Hz. The stimulus (indicated by a horizontal bar) lasted for 20 s, followed by 40 s of darkness. The data show the average response of 32 cycles of stimulus/rest for three subjects. Characteristic features of the BOLD response are a delay of a few seconds after the start of the stimulus, a ramp of about 6 s up to a plateau, and a poststimulus undershoot before the signal returns to baseline.

Figure 17.1 shows an example of the BOLD signal response in the visual cortex during a simple visual stimulus. The imaging used EPI on a 3-T scanner with a repetition time of 2 s between images on the same slice and a resolution (voxel dimensions) of $3.75 \times 3.75 \times 5$ mm (Buxton et al., 1998a). Subjects wore goggles that flashed a rectangular grid of red LED lights at a rate of 8 Hz, with the flashing lights on for 20 s followed by 40 s of darkness. This cycle was repeated eight times to make an 8-min run; the run was repeated four times, and the data were averaged for each of three subjects. The dynamic MR images provided a time course for the signal from each voxel, and those voxels showing a significant correlation with the stimulus pattern were selected and averaged to form the time course in Figure 17.1.

The average response in Figure 17.1 is fairly typical of BOLD responses to a number of stimuli. There is an initial delay of 1–3 s after the initiation of the stimulus, followed by a ramp of 5–8 s before a plateau signal change is reached (Bandettini et al., 1993). After the end of the stimulus, the BOLD signal ramps down over several seconds and often undershoots the original baseline. The poststimulus undershoot in these data has about half the magnitude of the peak itself, and the undershoot takes about 20 s to resolve. Although the poststimulus undershoot is not always evident, numerous examples can be found in the fMRI literature (Hu, Le, and Ugurbil, 1997; Menon et al., 1995; Merboldt et al., 1995; Ogawa et al., 1992; Turner et al., 1993). In fact, the first demonstration of the use of the BOLD effect for mapping activations shows evidence for a poststimulus undershoot as a lowering of the baseline after the first stimulus block (Kwong et al., 1992). Frahm and co-workers reported examples of pronounced undershoots that take more than a minute to resolve (Frahm et al., 1996; Fransson et al., 1998, 1999; Kruger, Kleinschmidt, and Frahm,

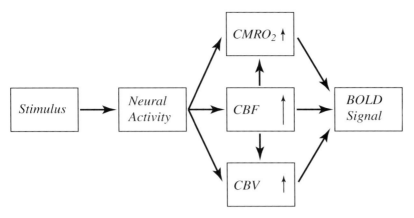

Figure 17.2. The chain of events leading to the BOLD signal. A stimulus triggers local neural activity, which in turn triggers metabolic activity in the form of a large increase of cerebral blood flow, a small increase of cerebral metabolic rate of oxygen, and a moderate increase of cerebral blood volume. The combined changes in CBF, $CMRO_2$ and CBV create the BOLD signal change.

1996). In addition, several groups have observed an initial dip in the BOLD signal lasting 1–2 s before the up ramp of the primary positive signal change (Ernst and Hennig, 1994; Hu et al., 1997; Menon et al., 1995). The initial dip has excited considerable interest because it may map more precisely to the spatial location of the neural activity.

As described in Chapter 16, the BOLD effect is a somewhat complicated process, depending on changes in cerebral blood flow (CBF), cerebral blood volume (CBV), and cerebral metabolic rate of oxygen ($CMRO_2$). In fact, the chain of events between an applied stimulus and the measured BOLD signal involves several distinct steps, as illustrated in Figure 17.2. The stimulus first induces local changes in neural activity. The neural activity then triggers increased energy metabolism with accompanying changes in CBF, CBV, and $CMRO_2$, and these physiological changes then combine to alter the MR signal. In this section, we will examine the BOLD hemodynamic response in more detail to address three key questions:

1. Does the BOLD signal change accurately reflect the location of neural activity change?
2. Does the BOLD signal change accurately reflect the magnitude of the neural activity change?
3. Do transients in the dynamic BOLD response reflect transients of neural activity or a temporal mismatch of the changes in CBF, CBV, or $CMRO_2$?

THE BOLD HEMODYNAMIC RESPONSE

Location of BOLD Signal Changes

An important issue in the interpretation of BOLD studies is the accuracy of the localization. Because the venous vessels undergo the largest changes in deoxyhemoglobin content, the largest BOLD signal changes are likely to occur around draining veins (Lai et al., 1993). Such veins may be removed from the area of neuronal activation, so the location of the BOLD change could differ by as much as a centimeter or more from the area of increased neural activity. The dominant role of veins is confirmed by several experiments. In BOLD experiments the voxel size is typically greater than 30 mm^3, and at 1.5 T the BOLD activations are a few percent or less. However, when the voxel size of the images is reduced, the amplitude of the largest BOLD signal changes increases dramatically (to 20% and larger) (Frahm, Merboldt, and Hanicke, 1993), suggesting that the changes are localized to a region smaller than 1–2 mm. This is consistent with the much larger change in the signal of venous blood described in Chapter 16, suggesting that high spatial resolution creates voxels that are largely filled with blood. Furthermore, comparison of the locations of BOLD signal changes with MR angiograms designed to reveal the venous vasculature shows a good correspondence between the two. A recent study with submillimeter resolution concluded that the activated areas were predominantly found to be in the sulci in the location of venous vessels with diameters on the order of the pixel size (Hoogenraad et al., 1999).

Arterial spin labeling (ASL) experiments show that the locations of the largest CBF change and the locations of the largest BOLD signal change do not always coincide. Figure 17.3 shows an example of a finger-tapping experiment performed with QUIPSS II (Quantitative Imaging of Perfusion with a Single Subtraction, version II), an arterial spin labeling technique that makes possible a simultaneous measurement of both the flow and BOLD signal changes (Wong, Buxton, and Frank, 1997) (see Chapter 15). The technique alternates tag images, in which the magnetization of the arterial blood is inverted before reaching the image plane, and control images, in which the blood is not inverted. Subtraction of tag from control then gives an image that directly reflects the amount of blood delivered to each voxel, and so is proportional to cerebral blood flow. All images were acquired with a gradient echo (GRE) EPI pulse sequence with TE = 30 ms so that each image also carries some BOLD weighting. From the raw time series for each pixel, a flow-sensitive and a BOLD-sensitive time series were constructed by calculating the difference signal (control – tag) over time and the average signal (control + tag) over time, respectively (see Chapter 15). These two time series, calculated from the same raw data, can be used to map independently the locations of the flow and BOLD changes.

Figure 17.3 shows that the peaks of the flow and BOLD changes do not precisely coincide in this example made at 1.5 T. On the right side, the BOLD change appears to lie directly in the sulcus, consistent with the signal being dominated by a draining vein. But the flow change appears to be displaced to either side of the sulcus, consistent with a CBF change that is more localized to the parenchyma. On the left side, the focus of BOLD activity and the focus of flow activity are shifted by about 1 cm.

The localization of the BOLD signal changes can be improved, but at the expense of sensitivity. At higher magnetic field strengths, the voxels with the largest signal changes can simply be ignored, and only the weaker signal changes used for

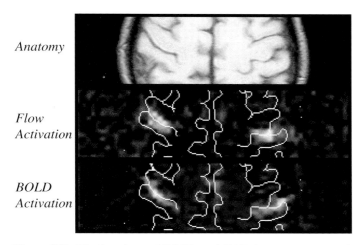

Anatomy

Flow Activation

BOLD Activation

Figure 17.3. The locations of BOLD and CBF changes. An example of an arterial spin labeling study of the sensorimotor area during a finger-tapping experiment at 1.5 T, showing an anatomical image (top), a map of flow change (middle), and a map of BOLD change (bottom). An outline of the sulci is added to the activation maps. The foci of activation for BOLD and CBF are similar but not identical, consistent with the idea that BOLD changes are dominated by veins, and a larger draining vein may be displaced from the site of neural activity.

mapping (Menon et al., 1993). For 1.5-T experiments, however, the signal changes are initially small enough that discarding the strongest signals would severely decrease the sensitivity. Given this constraint on lower field fMRI, the experimental strategy should be governed by the goals of the experiment. If the goal is simply to test whether a brain region is activated, then the displacements due to draining veins are not likely to be critical. On the other hand, for detailed mapping studies in which the precise anatomical location is critical, an ASL experiment may be more appropriate than a BOLD experiment.

As discussed in Chapter 16, the spin echo (SE) experiment has been proposed as a better localized measurement because the extravascular signal change with SE is more sensitive to the smallest vessels due to diffusion effects. For this reason, an SE or an asymmetric SE (which is intermediate between a standard SE and GRE signal in terms of sensitivity to small vessels) should reveal changes at the capillary level. However, the large changes in the intravascular signal in an SE experiment suggest that at 1.5 T the SE signal, like the GRE signal, is dominated by signal changes in the veins (Oja et al., 1999; Zijl et al., 1998). For this reason, the greater selectivity of the SE pulse sequence may not be effective until the main field strength is quite high so that the blood signal is suppressed by the shortened T_2 (Lee et al., 1999). Alternatively, diffusion-weighting gradients could be applied with an SE experiment at any field to destroy selectively the blood signal, leaving just the extravascular signal change. This would restore the spatial selectivity of the SE experiment, but at the expense of a great deal of sensitivity. These concerns with the trade-off of spatial selectivity and sensitivity are an important reason for doing BOLD experiments at higher magnetic fields.

The Relationship Between the BOLD Effect and Neural Activity

In most BOLD experiments for mapping activation in the brain, the investigator is interested in the pattern of neural activation rather than the pattern of blood flow and energy metabolism changes that follow. So a critical question is: how reliably does the BOLD effect reflect the underlying neural activity? We have already discussed the issue of the location of the BOLD activation and the problem of draining veins, and now we want to address the amplitude of the response. Does the magnitude of the BOLD response accurately reflect the magnitude of the neural activity change? In every fMRI mapping experiment we assume that it does and that, if one area has a larger BOLD signal change than another, then the change in neural activity is correspondingly larger. The agreement of the results of numerous fMRI experiments with other techniques and with the well-established body of literature on the functional organization of the brain clearly suggests that BOLD signal changes do reflect some aspect of neural activity. However, a full quantitative answer to this question is lacking for several reasons.

To begin with, the "magnitude of neural activity" must be clarified. For example, two natural ways to quantify neural activity are: (1) the average rate of generation of action potentials within a region of the brain, and (2) the average rate of neurotransmitter recycling within the region. These two definitions reflect different aspects of neural activity. Focusing on action potentials emphasizes the neural output, the rate at which incoming impulses are able to generate new impulses in the region. In contrast, focusing on neurotransmitter release and recycling at the synapse emphasizes the neural input, the synaptic activity. Because of this different focus, the two definitions in fact define two distinct rates of activity. For excitatory activity, the two rates may be similar because a greater rate of release of neurotransmitter would produce a greater rate of generation of action potentials. But with inhibitory activity, these two rates of neural activity will change in opposite directions, with greater synaptic activity decreasing the rate of spiking of the local neurons.

So, does the BOLD signal reflect synaptic activity or the generation of action potentials? The answer is critical for interpreting deactivations in BOLD data. Occasionally areas of the brain show a decreased signal (a negative BOLD effect) during particular tasks. A deactivation clearly suggests that excitatory activity has decreased, but does it mean that inhibitory activity has increased to suppress the generation of action potentials or that inhibitory inputs have decreased along with the excitatory inputs? The answer is still uncertain, but a plausible argument can be made that the changes in energy metabolism are primarily sensitive to synaptic activity (Sokoloff, 1991). Ultimately, the answer depends on the energy cost of different processes involved in neural activity. At the synapse, the neurotransmitter must be cleared and repackaged in vesicles in the presynaptic neuron. Fluctuating pre- and postsynaptic potentials are driven by ion fluxes, so the resting ion concentrations must be restored by active transport. Detailed studies of the precise location of changes in glucose metabolism measured with the deoxyglucose technique in animals found the activity to be concentrated in the regions with a high density of synaptic connections rather than associated with the cell body itself (Kadekaro, Crane, and Sokoloff, 1985). A full answer to these questions requires the combination of fMRI and direct electrode recording in the same animal, and such experiments have only recently become feasible with the demonstration of fMRI in awake, behaving nonhuman primates (Dubowitz et al., 1998; Stefanacci et al., 1998; Logothetis et al., 1999). These important, but difficult, experiments should provide a much firmer foundation for the interpretation of BOLD signal changes in terms of the underlying neural activity.

Linearity of the BOLD Response

In the absence of any direct measure of neural activity to compare with the BOLD response, a number of investigators have examined the quantitative relationship between simple stimuli and the resulting BOLD response. In Chapter 16, several reports of a graded BOLD response to a graded stimulus were mentioned. We can think of these studies as varying the stimulus magnitude. Another approach is to vary the stimulus duration with a constant stimulus magnitude, and the central question asked is whether the BOLD response behaves linearly with stimulus duration. For example, if the BOLD response to a 2-s stimulus is shifted and added to construct a simulated response to a 6-s stimulus, does this agree with the true response measured with a 6-s stimulus? In mathematical terms, this question is equivalent to asking whether the BOLD response is a linear convolution of the stimulus with a fixed hemodynamic response function. This idea is at the heart of most of the data processing schemes designed to pull weak signals out of a noisy background, so it is an important question.

Several studies have been done experimentally comparing the response to brief stimuli to the response to longer stimuli. Many of these have used visual stimuli with different durations (Boynton et al., 1996; Dale and Buckner, 1997; Vasquez and Noll, 1998), but auditory stimuli (Glover, 1999; Robson, Dorosz, and Gore, 1998) and motor tasks (Glover, 1999) also have been used. The consistent result of these studies is that, even though the response is roughly linear, there is a definite nonlinear component. The nature of the nonlinearity is that the response to a brief stimulus (e.g., <4 s) appears stronger than would be expected given the response to a longer stimulus.

There are several possible explanations for this nonlinearity, and it is helpful to think about the process that leads from the stimulus to the BOLD response as consisting of three steps, as illustrated in Figure 17.2. The first step is the translation of the stimulus pattern into a temporal sequence of local neural activity. The second step is the translation of the neural activity time course into changes in blood flow, blood volume, and oxygen metabolism. And the third step is the translation of the CBF, $CMRO_2$, and CBV time courses into the BOLD response. Each of these steps could be either linear or nonlinear.

The first step, from a stimulus time course to a neural activity time course is likely to be nonlinear. In recordings of the electrical activity of neurons, a common pattern of response to a sustained stimulus is an initial peak of activity (firing rate) followed by a reduction to a plateau level over a few seconds. This pattern of adaptation has been observed in many systems and is a general feature of the spiking activity of neurons (Adrian, 1926; Bonds, 1991; Maddess et al., 1988). In their original study of the nonlinearity of the BOLD signal, Boynton et al. (1996) suggested that this could be a natural explanation for the larger BOLD signal for brief stimuli.

If all the nonlinearity comes in during this first step, then the BOLD response could be a simple linear convolution with the neural activity.

However, nonlinearities could also enter in the remaining two steps. In particular, the step from metabolic changes to BOLD changes is likely to involve two types of nonlinearity. The first source of nonlinearity comes directly from the nature of the BOLD effect. There is a maximum signal that could be measured in a BOLD experiment, corresponding to full oxygenation of hemoglobin. Thus any BOLD signal increase is an approach toward this ceiling. The result is that if we plot the BOLD change as a function of the flow change, the curve will bend over for large flow changes (see Figure 16.8). Then any extrapolation of the BOLD change measured with a small flow change will overestimate the BOLD change for a large flow change. If the flow change in response to a brief stimulus is less than the fully developed flow change to a longer stimulus, this would produce a nonlinearity in the BOLD response with the same general trend as the observed nonlinearity.

A second potential source of nonlinearity is that the metabolic changes follow different time courses, with the CBV change lagging behind the CBF change (Buxton, Wong, and Frank, 1998c; Mandeville et al., 1998). For this reason, the volume change may be disproportionately smaller for a brief stimulus than for a more extended stimulus. Because a volume increase tends to reduce the BOLD signal, this effect could also contribute to making the response to a brief stimulus larger than that to a more extended stimulus.

In summary, the BOLD response is nonlinear with respect to stimulus duration. There are several plausible sources for this nonlinearity, but the full role of each has not been established. A likely source of nonlinearity is the neural response itself, which often begins with an initial peak of activity before settling down to a sustained plateau. A second likely source of nonlinearity is the transformation from CBF change to BOLD signal response, due to the flattening of the BOLD response at high flows. Given these likely sources of nonlinearity at the two ends of the chain from stimulus to BOLD response, it is possible that the middle step from neural activity to CBF response *is* a simple linear convolution, but there is no direct data to support this.

Despite these nonlinearities, it is common in the analysis of BOLD data to assume linearity. This undoubtedly introduces some error into the analysis, but in many applications the error is likely to be small. However, the full impact of these nonlinearities, particularly in newer event-related experimental paradigms that involve the separation of overlapping responses, has not been explored. Further studies designed to pinpoint the sources of the nonlinearities will be important for assessing the significance of nonlinearity in typical BOLD experiments.

Dynamics of the BOLD Response

In fMRI experiments, stimuli are often presented in a block design, so the temporal stimulus pattern is simply a square wave. To a first approximation, the BOLD response in many areas of the brain looks like a delayed and smoothed version of the stimulus pattern. However, one of the interesting features of the BOLD response is that a number of transient patterns have been reported to occur at the transitions between rest and active states. These dynamic aspects include signal overshoots and undershoots at both the beginning and end of the stimuli.

Transients in the BOLD response could be an accurate reflection of transients in the neural activity itself. However, because the BOLD signal depends on the combined changes in CBF, CBV, and $CMRO_2$, such transients also can arise if the respective time courses for these physiological changes differ. For example, if the $CMRO_2$ increases before the CBF begins to change, the BOLD response could show an initial dip due to the increase of deoxyhemoglobin. The same effect could arise if the venous blood volume increases rapidly at the onset of the stimulus, which would also increase the local deoxyhemoglobin content. A poststimulus undershoot could occur if flow transiently drops below the baseline level, or if the flow returns quickly to baseline but the blood volume returns more slowly. Because of this dependence of the BOLD signal on multiple physiological changes, it is not possible to identify the sources of these transients from BOLD measurements alone.

A useful approach for testing whether the transients of the BOLD response are neural in origin or result from mismatches in the timing of the metabolic changes is to measure the CBF change directly with arterial spin labeling techniques. If a BOLD transient is not present in the flow dynamics, then the source is likely to be in the relative time courses of the metabolic changes. If the CBF dynamics also shows the transient feature, then it is more likely to be a reflection of a transient in the underlying neural activity. Such experiments combining BOLD and ASL data have been performed to investigate several of these transient features, and both types of result have been reported.

Hoge and co-workers used a range of different visual stimuli to compare the flow and BOLD responses in the visual cortex (Hoge et al., 1999). They found that some stimuli showed initial overshoots and poststimulus undershoots of the BOLD signal whereas other stimuli did not. For those stimuli that evoked transients, the flow signal showed a corresponding pattern of transients, although less pronounced than those in the BOLD signal. They concluded that these features represented the temporal pattern of neural activity, which differed for different stimuli, rather than time lags of the physiological changes.

Other studies have found that the poststimulus undershoot is not present in the flow signal (Buxton et al., 1998c; Davis et al., 1994). Figure 17.4 shows an example from a 1.5-T study in a single subject (Buxton et al., 1999). In this study, the subject simultaneously tapped his fingers and observed a flashing black-and-white checkerboard for 20 s, followed by 100 s of rest to allow full recovery of the poststimulus undershoot. Flow and BOLD signals in both the motor cortex and the visual cortex were measured simultaneously with an ASL technique (QUIPSS II). Both the motor and visual areas showed pronounced poststimulus undershoots, but there was no evidence of an undershoot in the flow signal.

In short, we should expect that a sustained stimulus often will not elicit a uniform level of neural activity, and variations of the BOLD signal during the stimulus may reflect such variations in neural activity. A simultaneous measurement of the flow response can provide support for such an interpretation. But the fact that transients such as a poststimulus undershoot have been found to occur in the BOLD sig-

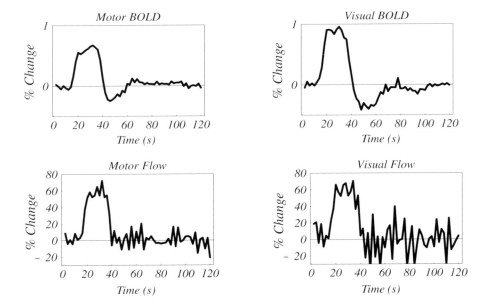

Figure 17.4. The poststimulus undershoot. A common feature of the BOLD signal is an under-shoot of the baseline after the end of the stimulus. The data shown are from a study at 1.5 T of a sin-gle subject who tapped his fingers while observing a checkerboard pattern reversing at 4 Hz. The stimulus lasted 20 s, followed by a 100-s rest period to allow visualization of the undershoot. An ASL pulse sequence (QUIPSS II) was used to measure flow and BOLD changes simultaneously in an oblique plane cutting through both the visual and motor areas of the brain. Both areas showed a pronounced poststimulus undershoot in the BOLD signal (top row), but there was no evidence of an undershoot of flow (bottom row).

nal but not in the flow signal suggests that one should be cautious about interpreting transient features of the BOLD signal without also measuring the flow response. With this in mind, we turn to the question of how the poststimulus undershoot can occur even though the flow returns to baseline.

Biomechanical Sources of the Poststimulus Undershoot

The cause and significance of the poststimulus undershoot has been a source of speculation since the beginning of fMRI. From the basic theory of the BOLD effect, a signal change is observed when the local deoxyhemoglobin content is altered, so there are two ways in which the BOLD signal could show an undershoot even though the flow signal does not. Either the $CMRO_2$ remains elevated after flow has returned to baseline, requiring an increased oxygen extraction fraction (Frahm et al., 1996; Kruger et al., 1996), or the CBV remains elevated (Buxton et al., 1998c; Mandeville et al., 1998). Both effects would cause the deoxyhemoglobin content to remain elevated after flow has returned to the resting level. These two hypotheses differ in their implications for the coupling of blood flow, blood volume, and oxygen metabolism during activation. The lag of the $CMRO_2$ change behind the return of flow to baseline would imply an uncoupling of the two, in the sense that the elevated

$CMRO_2$ does not require an elevated CBF. The lag of the CBV change behind the flow change would reflect a biomechanical phenomenon rather than a metabolic effect.

Experiments by Mandeville and co-workers have provided considerable support for the hypothesis that CBV recovery lags behind CBF recovery. In studies in a rat model, they used a long-lasting intravascular contrast agent to monitor the blood volume dynamics during activation and laser doppler flowmetry to measure CBF with a similar experimental protocol. Combining these data, the dynamic curves show a reasonably prompt return of CBF to baseline, but an elevated CBV with a time lag that matches well with the duration of the poststimulus undershoot (Mandeville et al., 1998) (Figure 17.5). In a subsequent set of experiments, these investigators directly addressed the question of the dynamics of the $CMRO_2$ change using a variation of the calibrated BOLD technique (see Box 16). Combining dynamic measurements during activation with calibration data acquired after inhalation of CO_2, the estimated dynamic curve of $CMRO_2$ closely followed the CBF curve, but with a smaller fractional change (Mandeville et al., 1999a). These data strongly support the idea that $CMRO_2$ is tightly coupled to CBF and that CBV recovery after activation lags behind CBF recovery.

Two similar biophysical models have been proposed to explain how such lags in the recovery of blood volume could occur, the balloon model (Buxton et al., 1998c) and the delayed compliance model (Mandeville et al., 1999b). Both models attribute the effect to the biomechanical properties of the vessels. To illustrate how this

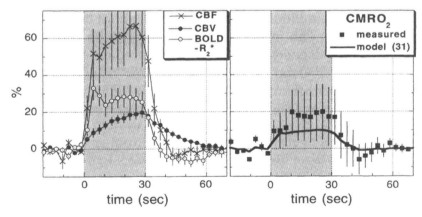

Figure 17.5. Dynamics of CBV and BOLD signal changes in a rat model. During forepaw stimulation, the changes in CBF were measured with laser doppler flowmetry, the changes in CBV were measured with MRI using a long-lasting intravascular contrast agent, and the BOLD signal change was measured with MRI. The CBV change resolves more slowly than the CBF change after the stimulus, with a good correspondence between the duration of elevated CBV and the poststimulus undershoot of the BOLD signal (left). By calibrating the BOLD change with a CO_2 experiment (see Box 16) the dynamic change in $CMRO_2$ also can be calculated (right). (The solid curve is the prediction of the oxygen limitation for the measured flow change.) (Reproduced with permission from Mandeville et al., *Magn. Reson. Med.* **42:**944–951, 1999; copyright 1999 by Wiley-Liss, a subsidiary of John Wiley & Sons, Inc.)

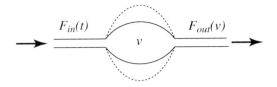

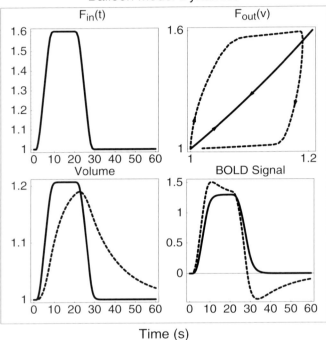

Figure 17.6. The balloon model. Two similar biomechanical models have been proposed to explain how the BOLD signal can show a pronounced poststimulus undershoot that is not present in the flow signal if CBV is slow to return to baseline (Buxton et al., 1998c; Mandeville et al., 1999b). The idea is illustrated here in terms of the balloon model, in which the venous vessels are treated as a balloon that expands with increasing CBF. The inflow $F_{in}(t)$ is the CBF response, and the outflow $F_{out}(v)$ is modeled as a function of the volume of the balloon v. The function $F_{out}(v)$ is analogous to a stress/strain curve, and for different forms of $F_{out}(v)$ the dynamics of the BOLD response can vary substantially for identical patterns of flow change. The bottom plots show dynamic curves for a simple power law form of $F_{out}(v)$, which produces a simple BOLD response, and a form showing hysteresis, which produces a pronounced poststimulus undershoot.

works, we consider the balloon model. In the balloon model, the venous compartment is modeled as an expandable balloon, with an inflow rate F_{in} and an outflow rate F_{out} (Figure 17.6). At steady state, $F_{in} = F_{out}$. During dynamic changes, the two flows are different, and the balloon inflates when $F_{in} > F_{out}$ and deflates when $F_{in} < F_{out}$. The inflow rate $F_{in}(t)$ is taken as the driving function of the system, and the outflow rate is taken to be a function of the volume of the balloon, $F_{out}(v)$. As the balloon expands the pressure inside increases, increasing the rate of outflow. The curve of $F_{out}(v)$ is then analogous to a stress/strain curve and depends on the biomechanical properties of the balloon. The dynamic quantities of interest are the total deoxyhemoglobin content and the blood volume. The equations for the time evolution of these quantities are derived simply from mass balance (Buxton et al., 1998c).

The dynamics of the balloon model are primarily governed by the shape of $F_{out}(v)$. Figure 17.6 shows the BOLD signal that results for two forms of $F_{out}(v)$ but identical CBF responses [$F_{in}(t)$]. The first is a simple power law relationship (solid line) of the form $f = v^{1/\alpha}$, with $\alpha = 0.4$ as found by Grubb and co-workers in their study of the steady-state relationship between CBF and CBV (Grubb et al., 1974). The second form of $F_{out}(v)$ (dashed line) assumes the same steady-state relationship (the Grubb law) but includes a viscoelastic resistance to rapid volume changes (Buxton et al., 1998b). The first form of $F_{out}(v)$ produces a simple BOLD response without any transient features, but the second form produces a pronounced post-stimulus undershoot. Furthermore, the viscoelastic behavior with the second form produces hysteresis, with $F_{out}(v)$ following a different curve on inflation and deflation of the balloon. This produces a slow increase of blood volume and a slow return to the resting state, creating an initial BOLD overshoot in addition to a poststimulus undershoot. Note that if instead F_{out} followed the same shallow curve on inflation that it does on deflation, the BOLD signal could show an initial dip. That is, if the curve initially has a shallow slope, so that with a sharp increase of F_{in} the first effect is a rapid filling of the balloon because F_{out} is slow to increase, then the deoxyhemoglobin content initially *increases* due to the increased venous volume, creating an initial dip in the BOLD signal (Buxton et al., 1998c). After a few seconds, the reduction in deoxyhemoglobin concentration in the blood would overwhelm the increased blood volume to create a net decrease in deoxyhemoglobin, the standard BOLD response. For all the simulations in Figure 17.6, the inflow itself [$F_{in}(t)$] is assumed to have a simple trapezoidal shape with no transients, emphasizing that these BOLD transients have a purely biomechanical origin.

The Fast Response (the Initial Dip)

The initial dip is potentially one of the most important aspects of the BOLD response, but it is also one of the most controversial. The interest in the initial dip stems from studies using intrinsic optical signals that are sensitive to oxyhemoglobin and deoxyhemoglobin (Malonek and Grinvald, 1996). In these studies, the brain of a cat was exposed, and the reflectance spectrum from the exposed surface was measured. The reflectance spectra are composed of several sources, including characteristic spectra for oxyhemoglobin and deoxyhemoglobin and a less specific scattering component. The measured spectra can be modeled to extract separate signals reflecting the deoxyhemoglobin and oxyhemoglobin concentrations, and these signals are used to map local changes in the oxygenation state of hemoglobin with a spatial resolution of 50 μm. This study was performed with visual stimuli, oriented full-field moving gratings, designed to excite differentially the orientation columns in the cat visual cortex. Functional maps were calculated by taking the difference between the responses to moving gratings with orthogonal orientations. The result-

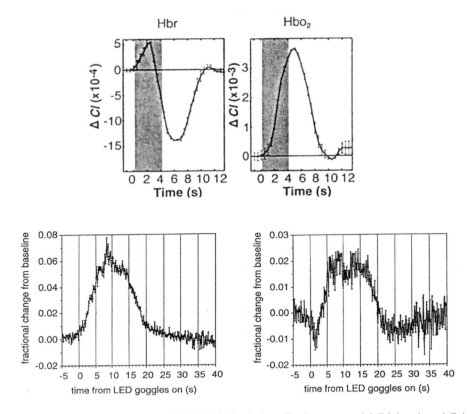

Figure 17.7. The fast response (initial dip). Optical studies in a cat model (Malonek and Grinvald, 1996) (top) and human fMRI studies (Menon et al., 1995) (bottom) have reported an early small initial increase in local deoxyhemoglobin prior to the larger and later decrease that is the primary signal mapped with fMRI. These studies suggest that the initial dip may map more tightly to the areas of neural activity than the deoxyhemoglobin decrease. The initial dip is usually interpreted as an initial increase in $CMRO_2$ prior to the CBF increase, but a similar observation could also arise from an initial increase in CBV. (Top figure reproduced with permission from Malonek and Grinvald, *Science* **272**:551–554, 1996; copyright 1996 by the American Association for the Advancement of Science. Bottom figure reproduced with permission from Menon et al., *Magn. Reson. Med.* **33**:453–459, 1995; copyright 1995 by Wiley-Liss, a subsidiary of John Wiley & Sons, Inc.)

ing dynamic curves showed a biphasic response for deoxyhemoglobin, with an initial increase in deoxyhemoglobin peaking about 2 s after the stimulus onset, followed by a later decrease of deoxyhemoglobin that was about three times larger (Figure 17.7). The delayed decrease of deoxyhemoglobin corresponds to the usual BOLD effect, but the initial increase of deoxyhemoglobin should cause an initial dip of the BOLD signal.

In addition to the demonstration of an initial deoxyhemoglobin increase, a key result of this optical study was that this fast response provided a better delineation of the orientation column structure than did the later deoxyhemoglobin decrease. The authors hypothesized that the explanation of this result is that blood flow is controlled only on a coarse spatial scale, so that activity in one set of orientation columns nevertheless increases flow to all columns. They further suggested that the fast response is the result of a rapid increase in $CMRO_2$ before the flow has begun to increase. Because this early $CMRO_2$ change is better localized to the activated column, the fast response yields a better map of the columnar structure. If this interpretation is correct, then the fast response of the BOLD signal could provide a much more accurate map of neural activity in fMRI experiments.

The initial dip of the BOLD response was first detected using a rapid spectroscopic acquisition in which the MR signal from a single large voxel was measured (Ernst and Hennig, 1994; Hennig et al., 1995). The original measurements were done at 2 T with a $2 \times 2 \times 2$ cm voxel located in the visual cortex, and the data showed a weak but significant dip in the BOLD signal at 0.5 s after the onset of a brief visual stimulus. The subsequent positive BOLD signal several seconds after the start of the stimulus was about 2.5 times larger in magnitude than the initial dip.

The initial dip was first observed in an imaging experiment by Menon and co-workers (1995). They used an EPI acquisition at 4 T, measuring the response in the visual cortex while subjects wore goggles that flashed red lights at a flicker rate of 8 Hz. They found that the later positive BOLD change was rather widespread in the visual cortex, including areas that could be identified as veins on higher resolution images. However, voxels that exhibited an initial dip mapped more accurately to gray matter. The average signal time courses for voxels that showed the initial dip and those that showed only the later positive BOLD signal showed some interesting differences. For the voxels with the initial dip, the late BOLD response was about twice as large as the initial dip (a 2% signal increase compared with a 1% signal dip), and there was a weak poststimulus undershoot. In contrast, the voxels without the initial dip showed a larger average late BOLD change of about 6% and no poststimulus undershoot. These data suggested that the initial dip maps more accurately to the site of neural activity than does the later positive BOLD signal, which includes contributions from draining veins.

A subsequent study by Hu and co-workers at 4 T investigated the dependence of the initial dip on stimulus duration, using a similar visual stimulus (Hu et al., 1997) (Figure 17.7). They found that both the initial dip and the poststimulus undershoot were reduced for the shortest stimulus tested (1.5 s) but that the magnitude of the initial dip remained approximately constant for longer stimuli (3.6 and 4.8 s) despite the observation that the late BOLD response and the poststimulus undershoot continued to increase. The initial dip reached its maximum excursion of 1–2% at 2–3 s after the stimulus onset. Additionally, the late positive BOLD response was about three times larger than the initial dip. These results were similar to the results of optical studies in the cat brain (Malonek and Grinvald, 1996).

A much weaker initial dip has also been detected at 1.5 T, with an amplitude only about 10% of the amplitude of the late positive response (Yacoub and Hu, 1999). This suggests that the initial dip scales much more strongly with the magnetic field than does the late positive response. Such a superlinear dependence on field strength would be expected if the BOLD effect is primarily occurring around the capillaries, where diffusion effects are important (see Chapter 16).

However, the initial dip is not always seen, and this has led to controversy over its existence. As noted earlier, it is very weak at 1.5 T and so is rarely seen in human studies at this field strength. Furthermore, the initial dip has not been found in studies in the rat even at high field, suggesting that the effect may differ among species (Marota et al., 1999). It has been suggested that the initial dip could be an artifact arising from using too short an interstimulus interval to allow full recovery of the hemodynamic response (Fransson et al., 1998). In both fMRI and optical studies, the final dynamic curves are the average response to many stimuli presented in succession. With a short off period between stimuli, the poststimulus undershoot will wrap around to the beginning of the stimulus when the data from a long series of stimuli is broken into single stimulus periods and averaged. However, a recent study addressing this concern with a series of experiments at 4 T found no change in the magnitude of the initial dip when the interstimulus interval was increased, suggesting that the observations of an initial dip are unlikely to be artifactual (Yacoub et al., 1999).

The nature of the initial dip is also controversial because of concerns about the optical methods themselves. The separation of the signals from deoxyhemoglobin and oxyhemoglobin requires the estimation of a scattering component that also contributes to the net reflectance spectrum, and the original studies have been criticized for using an inaccurate method (Mayhew et al., 1999). Another study by Malonek and co-workers using the same optical techniques concluded that there was an initial increase in deoxyhemoglobin, but without a corresponding decrease in oxyhemoglobin, suggesting an early blood volume increase (Malonek et al., 1997). However, a later MR study in rats found no initial rapid volume increase, and no initial dip in the BOLD signal (Marota et al., 1999). For these reasons, there is no clear consensus on whether there is an initial increase in deoxyhemoglobin with activation, and if so whether this fast response is species specific.

Finally, even taking the initial dip of the BOLD signal as an experimental fact, the interpretation of this effect is still not clear. The usual interpretation is that this represents an early increase of $CMRO_2$ before flow increases, with a corresponding increase in oxygen extraction. But an early increase of blood volume could also produce an initial dip (as suggested at the end of the previous section), similar to the way that a slowly resolving blood volume can cause a poststimulus undershoot (Buxton et al., 1998c; Hathout, Varjavand, and Gopi, 1999). In the context of the balloon model, if the initial increase in blood flow leads to an initial swelling of the venous balloon, rather than an increased outflow, the deoxyhemoglobin content would initially increase. Later, as the flow increases more, the change in oxygenation of the venous blood would begin to dominate the increased blood volume, and the total deoxyhemoglobin would decrease, producing the usual later BOLD response. Furthermore, this effect would depend strongly on field strength because the initial dip would reflect the balance between two potentially conflicting effects. These two effects are a decreased intrinsic extravascular signal due to the increased deoxyhemoglobin and the exchange of extravascular space for blood due to the increased blood volume. The first effect will always decrease the intrinsic extravascular signal, but the second effect could either decrease or increase the net signal, depending on whether the intrinsic intravascular signal is greater or less than the intrinsic extravascular signal. At 1.5 T the blood signal typically is stronger than the tissue signal, so the increased intravascular signal would offset the decreased extravascular signal, weakening the initial dip. At higher fields, the intrinsic blood signal is much weaker, and the increased blood volume at the expense of the extravascular volume then tends to reinforce the extravascular signal decrease and create a deeper initial dip. This would produce a superlinear dependence of the magnitude of the initial dip on field strength, consistent with the experimental observations.

Finally, it should be noted that at higher fields, where the blood signal is weak, an initial dip could occur due to an early volume increase even if the net deoxyhemoglobin content remains unchanged. In Box 16 the special case of a simultaneous increase of blood volume and decrease of blood oxygenation that keeps the net deoxyhemoglobin concentration balanced at a constant level was introduced as a thought experiment for understanding the BOLD signal. With constant deoxyhemoglobin, the intrinsic extravascular signal would remain the same, but the expanded blood volume would replace some of the extravascular signal with blood generating a much weaker signal, so the BOLD signal would show an initial dip despite the constancy of the deoxyhemoglobin concentration.

The origin and significance of the initial dip is an active area of current research. Further experiments with both BOLD and optical techniques are required to understand the dynamic changes in $CMRO_2$ and CBV with activation and to establish the physiological limits on spatial resolution with fMRI.

OPTIMIZING BOLD IMAGE ACQUISITION

Magnetic Field Dependence

A critical aspect of the BOLD effect is that the fractional signal changes are larger with larger main magnetic fields. A larger magnetic field creates a larger magnetization within a body, and so the field gradients due to magnetic susceptibility differences increase in proportion to the field. On top of this, the intrinsic signal-to-noise ratio (SNR) also increases with increasing field, for a similar reason. A larger field produces a more pronounced alignment of the nuclear spins and creates a larger equilibrium magnetization M_0. With any MRI pulse sequence, the signal is proportional to M_0, so the SNR increases with increasing field. The field dependence of the BOLD effect has spurred much of the recent interest in moving MRI to higher fields. At the time of writing, a number of 3-T imagers are installed or planned, several 4-T imagers are in operation, and a 7-T and an 8-T human imager have recently been installed.

The primary effect of increasing the magnetic field B_0 is an increase of the magnitude of the BOLD effect, which naturally increases the SNR of a BOLD experiment. However, other factors that conflict with this SNR increase also change and partially offset the increase in practice. Two intrinsic tissue time constants that affect the timing parameters in an MRI experiment are T_2^* and T_1. The time available for measuring a signal after it is created by an RF pulse is governed by the local T_2^*, which is determined by the magnitude of local field inhomogeneities. Just as with the BOLD effect, the field offsets due to large-scale magnetic susceptibility effects (e.g., near air/tissue boundaries) are proportional to B_0, so T_2^* is decreased with increasing field. Furthermore, in addition to T_2^* effects, these field offsets produce distortions in the images (see Chapter 12). To compensate for these larger effects at higher field, the data acquisition time T_{acq} can be reduced, but this also reduces SNR. However, even if some of the potential increase in SNR is sacrificed to compensate for increased distortion and T_2^* effects due to field inhomogeneities, there is still a net gain in SNR with increasing B_0.

The longitudinal relaxation time T_1 also increases with increasing B_0. To produce the same degree of recovery of the magnetization between radiofrequency (RF) pulses, the repetition time TR must be increased in proportion to T_1, lengthening the duration of a study. Other factors being equal, if fewer images are collected during a given time frame, the SNR per unit time is reduced. This issue is considered in more detail later.

At 4 T and higher, another effect that affects the quality of the images comes into play in human imaging. When imaging at 1.5 T, the wavelength of the RF pulse is larger than the human head. However, at 4 T this wavelength is comparable to the size of the head, and at 7 T it is smaller. This difference creates a more complicated coupling between the RF coil and the head. Consequently, it is difficult to design an RF coil that produces a uniform RF field over the whole brain. This leads to variable flip angles across the brain when the coil is used as a transmitter, and a nonuniform sensitivity pattern for detection when it is used as a receiver. In short, this effect makes uniform imaging of the entire brain more problematic at high fields.

Despite these potential limitations of high field imaging, it is clear that the step from 1.5 to 3–4 T produces a substantial increase in the SNR, and thus in the sensitivity, of BOLD experiments.

Image Acquisition Parameters

The signal-to-noise ratio of the image acquisition is a critical factor in determining the sensitivity of BOLD imaging, and the SNR depends on several parameters in addition to the main magnetic field strength. As we will see, the choice of experimental parameters usually involves a trade-off between SNR and a systematic artifact. Most BOLD studies use a GRE EPI single-shot acquisition, so we will focus on this technique in considering how to optimize the acquisition, but the basic ideas apply to other techniques as well. The primary pulse sequence parameter that makes the MR signal sensitive to the BOLD effect is the echo time TE. If TE is very short, the signal is insensitive to T_2^*, and so the signal change with activation is minimal. If TE is very long, most of the signal decays away before it is measured, so again the sensitivity is low because the signal is lost in the noise. To maximize the SNR, we must maximize the signal change due to the change in T_2^*. If the noise is purely additive so that the magnitude of the noise fluctuations in a voxel is independent of the intrinsic resting signal in the voxel, then the optimal TE is about equal to the local T_2^*. In the brain at field strengths of 1.5–3 T, typical T_2^* values are in the range of 40–60 ms, and most BOLD studies use echo times in this range.

The voxel dimensions strongly affect the SNR. In general, the SNR is proportional to the number of spins that contribute to the signal from a voxel, and so for a uniform tissue the SNR is proportional to the voxel volume (see Chapter 12). If the voxel volume is larger than the activated area in a BOLD experiment, then the measured signal change will be diluted by partial volume averaging. From this argument alone, the optimal voxel size for maximizing SNR should be relatively large, just small enough to resolve the activated area but no smaller. However, in practice another factor comes into play: magnetic field inhomogeneities. Field variations within a voxel lead to different precession rates and phase dispersion, so the net signal can be drastically reduced from what it would be if all the spin signals added coherently. In this case, increasing the voxel size can decrease the net signal by bringing in a wider range of field variations. The microscopic field distortions due to the BOLD effect should be independent of voxel size, but for broader field gradients due to macroscopic susceptibility differences (e.g., near sinus cavities) the range of field variations is directly proportional to voxel size. The effect on an image is a signal dropout (as discussed in Chapter 12).

For these reasons, the choice of voxel size is a trade-off between SNR and the need for sufficient spatial resolution to reduce signal dropout problems to an acceptable level. The SNR decreases with small voxels because there are fewer spins contributing to the signal; it also decreases with very large voxels because of magnetic field variations within the voxel. At 1.5 T, typical voxel volumes for fMRI range from about 20 to 100 mm^3. The optimum voxel size depends on the magnitude of the field variations in the area of the brain under investigation. In regions of the brain prone to field distortions, such as the frontal and temporal lobes, smaller voxels may produce better SNR.

The sensitivity of a BOLD signal measurement depends on the ratio of the absolute signal change to the added noise amplitude. A change in blood oxygenation produces a corresponding *fractional* change in the MR signal; consequently, we should maximize the resting MR signal to maximize the absolute signal change. The resting signal primarily depends on two pulse sequence parameters, the repetition time TR and the flip angle α. The repetition time has two practical effects that govern the SNR. The first effect is that TR controls how much longitudinal (T_1) relaxation occurs between RF pulses, which then affects the measured signal when the magnetization is flipped back into the transverse plane. In other words, with repeated images with TR shorter than T_1 there is a saturation effect. This saturation effect also is controlled partly by the flip angle: a smaller α leaves some of the magnetization along the longitudinal axis and produces less saturation.

In addition to the saturation effect, the TR also controls how many separate measurements can be made in a fixed time. The statistical analysis of BOLD voxel time series can be quite involved (see Chapter 18), but the detection of a BOLD signal change essentially amounts to comparing the average signal during the stimulus intervals with the average signal during the control intervals. If the noise in each measured image is independent, then the SNR will be proportional to $\sqrt{N}$, where N is the number of measurements that go into the average. And N, in turn, is proportional to 1/TR: a shorter TR allows more averages to be done in the same total experiment time. We can combine this factor with the equation for the intrinsic GRE signal from Chapter 8 to write

$$SNR \propto \frac{1}{\sqrt{T_1}} \left[\sqrt{\frac{T_1}{TR}} \sin\alpha \frac{1 - e^{-TR/T_1}}{1 - \cos\alpha \, e^{-TR/T_1}} \right]$$ [17.1]

Written in this way, the term in brackets depends only on the ratio TR/T_1 and the flip angle α.

For any given local T_1, there is an optimum choice of TR/T_1 and α that maximizes the term in brackets. However, the T_1 term in front indicates that the SNR with this optimal combination will be reduced for longer T_1. Figure 17.8 shows a contour plot of how SNR varies with the choice of TR/T_1 and α, calculated from the term in brackets. For any TR, there is an optimum flip angle that maximizes the available SNR. When TR is long compared to T_1, the optimum flip angle is 90°, which flips all the longitudinal magnetization into the transverse plane, but the maximum SNR is less than what can be achieved with a shorter TR. As TR is reduced, the optimum flip angle also reduces. With very short TR, the available SNR plateaus at a maximum level with small flip angles. So shortening TR until it is about equal to

Signal to Noise Ratio

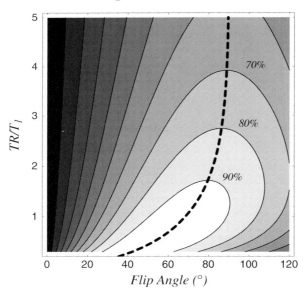

Figure 17.8. Optimizing TR and flip angle to maximize SNR. For a GRE pulse sequence, the SNR that can be achieved in a given total imaging time is shown as a contour plot. The contours indicate the percentage of the maximum possible SNR for each combination of the ratio of the repetition time to the longitudinal relaxation time (TR/T_1) and the flip angle. The dashed line shows the optimal flip angle for each value of TR/T_1. Using a long TR is costly in terms of SNR, but when the TR is reduced to approximately the value of T_1 there is little gain in SNR in shortening it further provided that the flip angle is appropriately adjusted.

T_1 is desirable, but making it even shorter does not produce much further improvement. It is helpful to consider some examples. For gray matter with $T_1 \approx 1$ s, a TR of 1 s with a flip angle of 68° achieves 96% of the theoretical maximum SNR, whereas a TR of 4 s and a 90° flip angle produces only 69% of the maximum SNR. This is a large difference. To improve the SNR of the longer TR experiment to the same level as the shorter TR experiment by averaging longer runs would nearly double the total imaging time.

It is important to note that these examples are based on the assumption that the relevant T_1 is that of gray matter. However, because GRE images are primarily sensitive to veins, and the largest field gradients occur in the perivascular space, the relevant T_1 for SNR optimization at lower fields may be that of cerebrospinal fluid (CSF), which is about 3–5 sec. The plot in Figure 17.8 still applies because the shape of the curves depends only on the ratio TR/T_1. That is, if the relevant T_1 is 4 s, then TR = 4 s and $\alpha = 68°$ would yield 96% of the available SNR, just as in the preceding example. However, the maximum available SNR also depends on T_1, decreasing as $1/\sqrt{T_1}$. If the TR is increased in proportion to the T_1, the signal generated with each repetition will be the same, but fewer signals are generated for averaging during the same fixed total imaging time. So the maximum available SNR for CSF is about half ($1/\sqrt{4}$) of the maximum SNR for gray matter. In practice, the GRE-BOLD signal is likely a combination of gray matter and perivascular CSF signal changes.

In practice, reducing the TR to about 1 s creates a conflict with coverage of the brain. Most modern scanners have a maximum image acquisition rate of about 10/s. These images could be repeated images on the same slice or cycling through a number of different slice locations to cover the whole brain. For example, 30 sagittal slices 5 mm thick will cover nearly all human brains, but if the maximum imaging rate is 10/s, the minimum TR that is possible is 3 s, longer than the optimum for gray matter SNR. For more focal studies, covering only a limited part of the brain, more optimal TRs are possible.

Motion Artifacts

The simplest interpretation of a dynamic series of MR images is that each image is measuring the net signal from an array of spatially defined voxels. In other words, the time course of a particular voxel is the average signal in a small volume of space centered at position (x, y, z). Ideally, this position also corresponds to a fixed location in the brain. For this reason, a persistent problem in BOLD experiments is subject motion. Any slight movement of the subject's head will move parts of the subject's brain to different voxel locations. If there are sharp edges in the intensity pattern of the image, such as near the edge of the brain, then movements much smaller than a voxel dimension can produce a signal change larger than the expected signal change due to the BOLD effect. This effect is particularly troublesome if the motion is correlated with the stimulus (Friston et al., 1996; Hajnal et al., 1994). For example, if the subject tips his head slightly when a visual stimulus is presented or if his head slides out of the coil slightly during a motor task, the result can be signal changes that nicely correlate with the stimulus but that are entirely artifactual. A useful check is to be sure that activations are not right at a sharp boundary in the image. Often stimulus-correlated motion will present as a positive correlation on one side of the brain and a negative correlation on the other side. But this is not the only possible pattern. For example, superior axial slices at a level where the cross section of the brain is significantly different from one slice to the next could show symmetric artifactual activation around the edge of the brain due to motion in the slice selection direction.

There are several approaches to dealing with motion artifacts. The best is perhaps to try to prevent motion as much as possible by carefully coaching the subject about the importance of remaining still and by using head restraints. These could include foam pads between the coil and the head and restraining straps. A number of groups have found that a bite bar molded to the subject's teeth with dental plastic is very effective in stabilizing the head.

After data collection, motion effects can be somewhat corrected with postprocessing software (Ashburner and Friston, 1999; Cox, 1996; Friston et al., 1995; Woods, Mazziota, and Cherry, 1993). The primary goal of such techniques is realignment of the individual images. If the motion is in the plane of the images, then a two-dimensional (2D) registration is adequate. For example, if the subject's motion is a tipping forward of the head, with no rotational component, and the images are sagittal in orientation, then the motion is entirely within the plane of the image. The correction is then a translation and rotation to align optimally the image with a reference image (e.g., the first image in the dynamic series or the average image of the series). The corrections required are subpixel shifts, so the new image matrix is an appropriate interpolation of the original image onto the new registered grid. If the motion does not lie in the image plane, then a three-dimensional (3D) registration is required. In addition to being a more time-consuming calculation, a problem for 3D registration is that the 2D images are acquired sequentially in time. This means that at any one time point we do not have a complete 3D image of the brain to compare with the 3D image at another time point. Nevertheless, 3D registration schemes have been developed to deal with these problems.

However, there are a few other problems due to motion that need to be corrected in addition to image registration (Ashburner and Friston, 1999). The first is the spin history effect. With a reasonably short TR, the MR signal is not fully relaxed, but if everything is repeated exactly the same, a steady state develops such that with each repetition the signal generated is the same. If motion causes a group of spins to move out of the selected slice, then these spins will not feel the next RF pulse. If they are later moved back into the slice, their spin history, the combined effects of RF pulses and relaxation, will be different from that of spins that remained within the selected slice. This disrupts the steady-state signal in a way that depends on the past motion. This effect can be estimated by using the history of the motion estimated from the image registration algorithm (i.e., the translations and rotations necessary to put each image into alignment).

A more subtle motion-related problem is that the basic picture – that MRI measures the signal from a set of fixed voxels in space – is not correct. Magnetic field variations within the head distort the images, as discussed in Chapter 12. This creates problems in aligning EPI images with higher resolution anatomical images that are less sensitive to these distortions. Because the source of the distortions is the head itself, any motion will also shift the pattern of distortions. In other words, the location in space corresponding to a particular voxel is not fixed. This fact adds another layer of complexity to motion correction that investigators are just beginning to address (Jezzard and Clare, 1999). The nature of these distortions and approaches for correction are described in the next section.

Image Distortions

Localization with EPI is based on the frequency of the local signal in the presence of field gradients. The key assumption is that if no gradients are applied, all spins resonate at precisely the same frequency. This is not true in general because the inhomogeneities of the head create magnetic field variations, and the resulting image is distorted. Consider a small sample of tissue in the brain in which the magnetic field is offset due to these field variations. The primary distortion of the image is that this signal will be displaced along the phase-encoded axis by a distance proportional to the field offset (see Chapter 12). Note that this effect is in addition to the signal dropout effect described earlier, which also results from local field gradients. The apparent location of the signal from a small element of tissue is shifted in the reconstructed image in proportion to the mean field offset. If there is a large spread in the field offsets within the tissue element, the signal will be reduced as well.

The basic approach to correcting image distortions due to field inhomogeneity is to first map the field distribution within the brain. This is done with a series of gradient echo images with a progression of closely spaced echo times, reconstructing the phase images in addition the magnitude images. At each voxel, the phase change between one echo time and the next is proportional to the local field offset. The echo spacing must be short enough to prevent phase ambiguities due to precession greater than 360°. At 1.5 T, a 1-ppm field offset (64 Hz) will produce a phase change of 23° if TE is changed by 1 ms, so the echo time spacing should be no more than a few milliseconds. Field maps can be made using standard 2D or 3D imaging techniques, which are not strongly distorted, or with EPI images themselves. With the first approach, the true distribution of fields is calculated, and from this map the location of where each tissue element will appear in the distorted EPI image can be calculated (Jezzard and Balaban, 1995). With EPI field maps, the locations are distorted, but from the measured field offset one can calculate where that signal must have originated (Reber et al., 1998).

With subject motion, the pattern of field offsets changes, creating a different pattern of distortions in the EPI image. In this case, a single field map collected before the fMRI experiment will not be adequate for correcting the distortions of all the images. To deal with this motion problem, which produces a dynamically changing pattern of distortions, Jezzard and Clare suggested using the phase changes of the individual EPI images in the time series to make the additional dynamic distortion corrections necessary in addition to realignment (Jezzard and Clare, 1999).

Correction for distortions with field mapping is often very helpful, particularly when overlaying functional EPI images on higher resolution structural images. However, it is important to note that such distortions cannot always be corrected. The nature of these distortions is that signals from two different regions can be added within the same distorted voxel. This can happen if the imaging gradients and the intrinsic field inhomogeneity combine to produce the same field in two separate regions. In this case, all we can measure is the combined signal, and we have no way of knowing how much came from one region and how much from the other. Because only the phase-encoded axis is strongly distorted in an EPI image, the pattern of distortions can be altered radically by changing the orientation of the phase-encoding axis. So for different parts of the brain, some imaging orientations may work much better than others for minimizing the distortions and for making the distortions more correctable.

The magnitude of image distortions depends on the total acquisition time for each image. For an EPI acquisition, the total data collection time typically is in the range of $T_{acq} = 40$–100 ms. There is a simple rule for how far the signal from an area with an offset field will be displaced in the reconstructed image: for each additional phase evolution of $360°$ during the data acquisition time due to the field offset, the signal is shifted one pixel along the y-axis. The shift is thus directly proportional to the data acquisition time, and minimizing T_{acq} will thus minimize the distortions. The acquisition time can be reduced and still allow sampling of the same points in k-space by increasing the readout gradient strength (see Chapter 12). This spreads the signal from the head over a larger range of frequencies, and so is described as increasing the bandwidth of the acquisition.

However, the problem with this approach is that the SNR of the acquisition is proportional to $\sqrt{T_{acq}}$ (one can think of the data acquisition time as equivalent to averaging a continuous signal over that interval, and SNR increases with the square root of the number of averages). So minimizing distortions also minimizes SNR, and again we are faced with a trade-off between maximizing SNR and minimizing artifacts. Note that the argument that SNR increases with increasing T_{acq} does not hold when T_{acq} becomes much larger than T_2^*. With such a long acquisition time, most of the signal has decayed away, so additional measurements are simply adding noise. The optimal choice for SNR is to have T_{acq} approximately equal to T_2^* so that the full available signal is used.

As with many aspects of MRI, optimizing the imaging protocol is a matter of balancing the trade-offs between SNR and systematic artifacts, and this depends on the goals of the study. For imaging a small region of the brain, more severe distortions in other parts of the brain may be tolerable. But distortions in the EPI images always complicate detailed comparisons with other images. It is common practice to display areas of activation calculated from the EPI images as a color overlay on a higher resolution anatomical image. High resolution MR images are not as distorted as the EPI images, so correction for distortions is critical for accurate localization. Furthermore, correction for distortions and motion artifacts is important if the images of individual subjects are to be warped into a common brain atlas (Woods et al., 1999).

REFERENCES

Adrian, E. D. (1926) The impulses produced by sensory nerve endings. *J. Physiol. (London)* **61,** 49–72.

Ashburner, J., and Friston, K. J. (1999) Image registration. In: *Functional MRI,* pp. 285–99. Eds. C. T. W. Moonen and P. A. Bandettini. Springer: Berlin.

Bandettini, P. A., Jesmanowicz, A., Wong, E. C., and Hyde, J. S. (1993) Processing strategies for time-course data sets in functional MRI of the human brain. *Magn. Reson. Med.* **30,** 161–73.

Bonds, A. B. (1991) Temporal dynamics of contrast gain in single cells of the cat striate cortex. *Vis. Neurosci.* **6,** 239–55.

Boynton, G. M., Engel, S. A., Glover, G. H., and Heeger, D. J. (1996) Linear systems analysis of functional magnetic resonance imaging in human V1. *J. Neurosci.* **16,** 4207–21.

Buxton, R. B., Luh, W.-M., Wong, E. C., Frank, L. R., and Bandettini, P. A. (1998a) Diffusion weighting attenuates the BOLD peak signal change but not the poststimulus undershoot. In: *Sixth Meeting, International Society for Magnetic Resonance in Medicine,* p. 7: Sydney, Australia.

Buxton, R. B., Miller, K., Frank, L. R., and Wong, E. C. (1998b) BOLD signal dynamics: The balloon model with viscoelastic effects. In: *Sixth Meeting, International Society for Magnetic Resonance in Medicine,* p. 1401: Sydney, Australia.

Buxton, R. B., Miller, K. L., Wong, E. C., and Frank, L. R. (1999) Application of the balloon model to the BOLD response to stimuli of different duration. In: *7th Scientific Meeting of the International Society for Magnetic Resonance in Medicine,* p. 1735: Philadelphia.

Buxton, R. B., Wong, E. C., and Frank, L. R. (1998c) Dynamics of blood flow and oxygenation changes during brain activation: The balloon model. *Magn. Reson. Med.* **39,** 855–64.

Cox, R. W. (1996) AFNI: Software for analysis and visualization of functional magnetic resonance neuroimages. *Comput. Biomed. Res.* **29,** 162–73.

Dale, A. M., and Buckner, R. L. (1997) Selective averaging of rapidly presented individual trials using fMRI. *Human Brain Mapping* **5,** 329–40.

Davis, T. L., Weisskoff, R. M., Kwong, K. K., Savoy, R., and Rosen, B. R. (1994) Susceptibility contrast undershoot is not matched by inflow contrast undershoot. In: *SMR, 2nd Annual Meeting,* p. 435: San Francisco.

Dubowitz, D. J., Chen, D.-Y., Atkinson, D. J., Grieve, K. L., Gillikan, B., Bradley, W. G., and Andersen, R. A. (1998) Functional magnetic resonance imaging in macaque cortex. *NeuroReport* **9,** 2213–18.

Ernst, T., and Hennig, J. (1994) Observation of a fast response in functional MR. *Magn. Reson. Med.* **32,** 146–9.

Frahm, J., Krüger, G., Merboldt, K.-D., and Kleinschmidt, A. (1996) Dynamic uncoupling and recoupling of perfusion and oxidative metabolism during focal activation in man. *Magn. Reson. Med.* **35,** 143–8.

Frahm, J., Merboldt, K.-D., and Hanicke, W. (1993) Functional MRI of human brain activation at high spatial resolution. *Magn. Reson. Med.* **29,** 139–44.

Fransson, P., Kruger, G., Merboldt, K. D., and Frahm, J. (1998) Temporal characteristics of oxygenation-sensitive MRI responses to visual activation in humans. *Magn. Reson. Med.* **39,** 912–19.

Fransson, P., Kruger, G., Merboldt, K. D., and Frahm, J. (1999) Temporal and spatial MRI responses to subsecond visual activation. *Magn. Reson. Imag.* **17,** 1–7.

Friston, K. J., Ashburner, J., Frith, C. D., Poline, J.-B., Heather, J. D., and Frackowiak, R. S. J. (1995) Spatial registration and normalization of images. *Human Brain Mapping* **2**, 165–89.

Friston, K. J., Williams, S., Howard, R., Frackowiak, R. S. J., and Turner, R. (1996) Movement related effects in fMRI time-series. *Magn. Reson. Med.* **35**, 346–55.

Glover, G. H. (1999) Deconvolution of impulse response in event-related fMRI. *NeuroImage* **9**, 416–29.

Grubb, R. L., Raichle, M. E., Eichling, J. O., and Ter-Pogossian, M. M. (1974) The effects of changes in PCO_2 on cerebral blood volume, blood flow, and vascular mean transit time. *Stroke* **5**, 630–9.

Hajnal, J. V., Myers, R., Oatridge, A., Schwieso, J. E., Young, I. R., and Bydder, G. M. (1994) Artifacts due to stimulus correlated motion in functional imaging of the brain. *Magn. Reson. Med.* **31**, 283–91.

Hathout, G. M., Varjavand, B., and Gopi, R. K. (1999) The early response in fMRI: A modeling approach. *Magn. Reson. Med.* **41**, 550–4.

Hennig, J., Janz, C., Speck, O., and Ernst, T. (1995) Functional spectroscopy of brain activation following a single light pulse: examinations of the mechanism of the fast initial response. *Int. J. Imag. Syst. Tech.* **6**, 203–8.

Hoge, R. D., Atkinson, J., Gill, B., Crelier, G. R., Marrett, S., and Pike, G. B. (1999) Stimulus-dependent BOLD and perfusion dynamics in human V1. *NeuroImage* **9**, 573–85.

Hoogenraad, F. G. C., Hofman, M. B. M., Pouwels, P. J. W., Reichenbach, J. R., Rombouts, S. A. R. B., and Haacke, E. M. (1999) Sub-millimeter fMRI at 1.5T: Correlation of high resolution with low resolution measurements. *J. Magn. Reson. Imag.* **9**, 475–82.

Hu, X., Le, T. H., and Ugurbil, K. (1997) Evaluation of the early response in fMRI in individual subjects using short stimulus duration. *Magn. Reson. Med.* **37**, 877–84.

Jezzard, P., and Balaban, R. S. (1995) Correction for geometric distortion in echo planar images from B_0 field distortions. *Magn. Reson. Med.* **34**, 65–73.

Jezzard, P., and Clare, S. (1999) Sources of distortion in functional MRI data. *Human Brain Mapping* **8**, 80–5.

Kadekaro, M., Crane, A. M., and Sokoloff, L. (1985) Differential effects of electrical stimulation of sciatic nerve on metabolic activity in spinal cord and dorsal root ganglion in the rat. *Proc. Natl. Acad. Sci. USA* **82**, 6010–13.

Kruger, G., Kleinschmidt, A., and Frahm, J. (1996) Dynamic MRI sensitized to cerebral blood oxygenation and flow during sustained activation of human visual cortex. *Magn. Reson. Med.* **35**, 797–800.

Kwong, K. K., Belliveau, J. W., Chesler, D. A., Goldberg, I. E., Weisskoff, R. M., Poncelet, B. P., Kennedy, D. N., Hoppel, B. E., Cohen, M. S., Turner, R., Cheng, H.-M., Brady, T. J., and Rosen, B. R. (1992) Dynamic magnetic resonance imaging of human brain activity during primary sensory stimulation. *Proc. Natl. Acad. Sci. USA* **89**, 5675–9.

Lai, S., Hopkins, A. L., Haacke, E. M., Li, D., Wasserman, B. A., Buckley, P., Friedman, L., Meltzer, H., Hedera, P., and Friedland, R. (1993) Identification of vascular structures as a major source of signal contrast in high resolution 2D and 3D functional activation imaging of the motor cortex at 1.5T: Preliminary results. *Magn. Reson. Med* **30**, 387–92.

Lee, S. P., Silva, A. C., Ugurbil, K., and Kim, S. G. (1999) Diffusion-weighted spin-echo fMRI at 9.4 T: Microvascular/tissue contribution to BOLD signal changes. *Magn. Reson. Med.* **42**, 919–28.

Logothetis, N., Guggenberger, H., Peled, S., and Pauls, J. (1999) Functional imaging of the macaque brain. *Nature Neurosci.* **2**, 555–62.

Maddess, T., McCourt, M. E., Blakeslee, B., and Cunningham, R. B. (1988) Factors governing the adaptation of cells in area 17 of the cat visual cortex. *Biol. Cybern.* **59,** 229–36.

Malonek, D., Dirnagl, U., Lindauer, U., Yamada, K., Kanno, I., and Grinvald, A. (1997) Vascular imprints of neuronal activity: Relationships between the dynamics of cortical blood flow, oxygenation and volume changes following sensory stimulation. *Proc. Natl. Acad. Sci. USA* **94,** 14826–31.

Malonek, D., and Grinvald, A. (1996) Interactions between electrical activity and cortical microcirculation revealed by imaging spectroscopy: Implications for functional brain mapping. *Science* **272,** 551–4.

Mandeville, J. B., Marota, J. J. A., Ayata, C., Moskowitz, M. A., Weisskoff, R. M., and Rosen, B. R. (1999a) MRI measurement of the temporal evolution of relative $CMRO_2$ during rat forepaw stimulation. *Magn. Reson. Med.* **42,** 944–51.

Mandeville, J. B., Marota, J. J. A., Ayata, C., Zaharchuk, G., Moskowitz, M. A., Rosen, B. R., and Weisskoff, R. M. (1999b) Evidence of a cerebrovascular post-arteriole Windkessel with delayed compliance. *J. Cereb. Blood Flow Metabol.* **19,** 679–89.

Mandeville, J. B., Marota, J. J. A., Kosofsky, B. E., Keltner, J. R., Weissleder, R., Rosen, B. R., and Weisskoff, R. M. (1998) Dynamic functional imaging of relative cerebral blood volume during rat forepaw stimulation. *Magn. Reson. Med.* **39,** 615–24.

Marota, J. J. A., Ayata, C., Moskowitz, M. A., Weisskoff, R. M., and Rosen, B. R. (1999) Investigation of the early response to rat forepaw stimulation. *Magn. Reson. Med.* **41,** 247–52.

Mayhew, J., Zheng, Y., Hou, Y., Vuksanovic, B., Berwick, J., Askew, S., and Coffey, P. (1999) Spectroscopic analysis of changes in remitted illumination: the response to increased neural activity in brain. *NeuroImage* **10,** 304–26.

Menon, R. S., Ogawa, S., Strupp, J. P., Anderson, P., and Ugurbil, K. (1995) BOLD based functional MRI at 4 tesla includes a capillary bed contribution: echo-planar imaging correlates with previous optical imaging using intrinsic signals. *Magn. Reson. Med.* **33,** 453–9.

Menon, R. S., Ogawa, S., Tank, D. W., and Ugurbil, K. (1993) 4 tesla gradient recalled echo characteristics of photic stimulation-induced signal changes in the human primary visual cortex. *Magn. Reson. Med.* **30,** 380–7.

Merboldt, K. D., Kruger, G., Hanicke, W., Kleinschmidt, A., and Frahm, J. (1995) Functional MRI of human brain activation combining high spatial and temporal resolution by a CINE FLASH technique. *Magn. Reson. Med.* **34,** 639–44.

Ogawa, S., Tank, D. W., Menon, R., Ellermann, J. M., Kim, S.-G., Merkle, H., and Ugurbil, K. (1992) Intrinsic signal changes accompanying sensory stimulation: Functional brain mapping with magnetic resonance imaging. *Proc. Natl. Acad. Sci. USA* **89,** 5951–5.

Oja, J. M. E., Gillen, J., Kaupinnen, R. A., Kraut, M., and Zijl, P. C. M. v. (1999) Venous blood effects in spin-echo fMRI of human brain. *Magn. Reson. Med.* **42,** 617–26.

Reber, P. J., Wong, E. C., Buxton, R. B., and Frank, L. R. (1998) Correction of off-resonance related distortion in EPI using EPI based field maps. *Magn. Reson. Med.* **39,** 328–30.

Robson, M. W., Dorosz, J. L., and Gore, J. C. (1998) Measurements of the temporal fMRI response of the human auditory cortex to trains of tones. *NeuroImage* **7,** 185–98.

Sokoloff, L. (1991) Relationship between functional activity and energy metabolism in the nervous system: Whether, where and why? In: *Brain Work and Mental Activity: Quantitative Studies with Radioactive Tracers,* pp. 52–67. Eds. N. A. Lassen, D. H. Ingvar, M. E. Raichle, and L. Friberg. Munksgaard: Copenhagen.

Stefanacci, L., Reber, P., Costanza, J., Wong, E., Buxton, R., Zola, S., Squire, L., and Albright, T. (1998) fMRI of monkey visual cortex. *Neuron* **20,** 1051–7.

Turner, R., Jezzard, P., Wen, H., Kwong, K. K., Bihan, D. L., Zeffiro, T., and Balaban, R. S. (1993) Functional mapping of the human visual cortex at 4 and 1.5 tesla using deoxygenation contrast EPI. *Magn. Reson. Med.* **29,** 277–9.

Vasquez, A. L., and Noll, D. C. (1998) Nonlinear aspects of the BOLD response in functional MRI. *NeuroImage* **7,** 108–18.

Wong, E. C., Buxton, R. B., and Frank, L. R. (1997) Implementation of quantitative perfusion imaging techniques for functional brain mapping using pulsed arterial spin labeling. *NMR Biomed.* **10,** 237–49.

Woods, R. P., Dapretto, M., Sicotte, N. L., Toga, A. W., and Mazziota, J. C. (1999) Creation and use of a Talairach-compatible atlas for accurate, automated, nonlinear intersubject registration, and analysis of functional imaging data. *Human Brain Mapping* **8,** 73–9.

Woods, R. P., Mazziota, J. C., and Cherry, S. R. (1993) MRI-PET registration with automated algorithm. *J. Comput. Assist. Tomogr.* **17,** 536–46.

Yacoub, E., and Hu, X. (1999) Detection of the early negative response in fMRI at 1.5T. *Magn. Reson. Med.* **41,** 1088–92.

Yacoub, E., Le, T. H., Ugurbil, K., and Hu, X. (1999) Further evaluation of the initial negative response in functional magnetic resonance imaging. *Magn. Reson. Med.* **41,** 436–41.

Zijl, P. C. M. v., Eleff, S. E., Ulatowski, J. A., Oja, J. M. E., Ulug, A. J., Traystman, R. J., and Kauppinen, R. A. (1998) Quantitative assessment of blood flow, blood volume and blood oxygenation effects in functional magnetic resonance imaging. *Nature Med.* **4,** 159–67.

18

Statistical Analysis of BOLD Data

INTRODUCTION TO STATISTICAL ANALYSIS OF BOLD DATA

The statistical analysis of Blood Oxygenation Level Dependent (BOLD) data is a critical part of brain mapping with functional magnetic resonance imaging (fMRI). Many creative statistical methods have been proposed, and there has been considerable debate about which is the "correct" approach. Given the flexibility of fMRI and the range of experiments that is possible, it seems likely that a number of different statistical processing approaches can be applied to yield useful data. Indeed, a pluralistic analysis strategy applying several methods to the same data may be the best approach for pulling out and evaluating the full information content of the fMRI data (Lange et al., 1999). The goal of this chapter is to highlight some of the important aspects of statistical thinking about BOLD data analysis, rather than to provide a comprehensive review of different approaches. We will focus on the general linear model, which encompasses many of the techniques commonly used (Boynton et al., 1996; Friston et al., 1995; Friston, Jezzard, and Turner, 1994; Worsley et al., 1997). In the first section, we introduce the need for a statistical analysis and some of the basic ideas and strategies. In the second section, the general linear model is considered in more detail, emphasizing the geometrical view of the analysis. Chapter 19 focuses on how the statistical analysis sheds light on how to design an efficient experiment and provides a framework for comparing the relative merits of blocked and event-related stimulus paradigms.

Separating True Activations from Noise

The magnetic resonance (MR) signal change during activation due to the BOLD effect is quite small, on the order of 1% for a 50% change in cerebral blood flow (CBF) at 1.5 T. To use these weak signals for brain mapping, they must be reliably separated from the noise. With echo planar imaging (EPI), the intrinsic signal-to-noise ratio (SNR) in a single-shot image is often quite large, in the range of 100–200, but this is still not large enough to reliably detect a 1% signal change in a voxel from a single image in the stimulus state and a single image in the control state. For this reason, a large number of images is required to allow sufficient averaging to detect the small signal changes.

An example of data from a BOLD experiment was shown in Figure 6.3. The subject performed a simple finger-tapping task for 16 s, followed by an equal rest period, with a total of 8 cycles of this task/control cycle repeated in one run. EPI was performed throughout the run measuring 128 images/per slice, with TR = 2 s. The voxel resolution of the EPI images was $3.75 \times 3.75 \times 5$ mm. This experiment produced a four-dimensional (4D) data set (three spatial dimensions plus time). The analysis of these data is usually done slice by slice. Figure 6.3 shows one image plane and a grid of pixel time courses in the vicinity of the primary motor area. Because the motor BOLD response is large, a number of clearly activated voxels are detectable by eye. In general, however, we want to be able to detect activations that are not apparent to the eye but that are nevertheless statistically significant.

The most obvious processing strategy to identify activated voxels would be to simply subtract the average of all the images made during the control task from the average of all the images made during the stimulus task. If the signal variations due to noise are random with a normal distribution and independent for each time point, this averaging will improve the SNR and should provide a map of the activated areas. However, this naive approach to the data processing does not work well, and in practice the data processing can become quite a bit more involved.

The first problem with the simple averaging scheme is that the standard deviation of the noise is different in different voxels so that the noise is not uniform across the image plane. The noise that adds into the signal from a particular voxel has two sources: random thermal noise and physiological fluctuations. The random thermal noise arises primarily from stray currents in the body that induce random signals in the receiver coil. This thermal noise is spread throughout the raw acquired data, and when the image is reconstructed this noise is spread throughout the voxels of the image. The result is that this thermal noise can be accurately described as uniform random Gaussian noise, with the noise in each voxel having the same standard deviation and independent of the noise in the other voxels. If this thermal noise were the only source of fluctuations in the MR signal, the noise would have no spatial structure. But, in fact, the variance of the signal over time measured in a human brain is several times larger than would be expected from thermal noise alone, and it exhibits both temporal and spatial structure (Purdon and Weisskoff, 1998; Zarahn, Aguirre, and D'Esposito, 1997).

The additional variance of the MR signal in vivo is attributed to physiological fluctuations, which include several effects. Cardiac pulsations create a pressure wave that strongly affects the signal of flowing blood, but it also creates pulsations in CSF and in the brain parenchyma itself. Although these motions are small, they nevertheless can easily produce signal fluctuations on the order of 1%, and the magnitude of the fluctuations varies strongly across the image plane. Figure 18.1 shows the frequency spectrum for a voxel time course measured in the primary visual cortex with a simple block design, flashing checkerboard stimulus, showing a strong spike at the fundamental frequency of the stimulus. For simple Gaussian noise, the frequency spectrum should be flat except for this spike and its harmonics, but there are additional clear peaks that can be identified with cardiac and respiratory fluctuations. Note that the cardiac peak is easily identified in this study because the TR was unusually short in this experiment (250 ms). For a more typical TR of 2 s, the cardiac pulsations would be aliased in the data and could appear at lower frequencies associated with the stimulus presentation. In the spectrum, there are also true low-frequency variations that could result from drifts due to scanner hardware and that may also include additional slow physiological pulsations. A regular oscillation of blood flow and oxygenation called *vasomotion* has been observed in numerous optical studies at frequencies around 0.1 Hz (Mayhew et al., 1999). The source and physiological significance of these vasomotion oscillations are unknown, but because they involve slow oscillations in blood oxygenation, they can contribute to low-frequency oscillations of the BOLD signal, particularly at high magnetic fields.

This brings us to the central problem created by nonuniform noise. When two noisy images are subtracted to calculate a difference image, if there is no activation in a voxel, the signals should subtract out. But due to noise, there will be a residual difference, and the size of this random residual is on the order of the local noise standard deviation. In other words, the voxels with the largest signal fluctuations will show the largest random difference signal, and so we would expect that a simple difference map would be dominated by vessel and CSF artifacts. The maps of particular frequency components of the noise fluctuations shown in Figure 18.1 show substantial spatial structure. Therefore, the essential problem with a simple image difference approach is that there is no way to distinguish between a weak but true activation and a strong but false physiological fluctuation. To put it another way, a difference map alone carries no information on the statistical quality of the measured difference in a voxel. If the run were repeated, a true activation would show up with

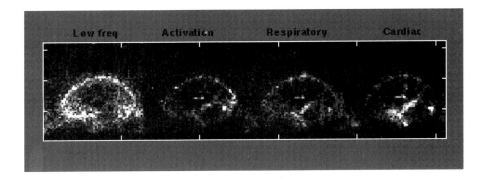

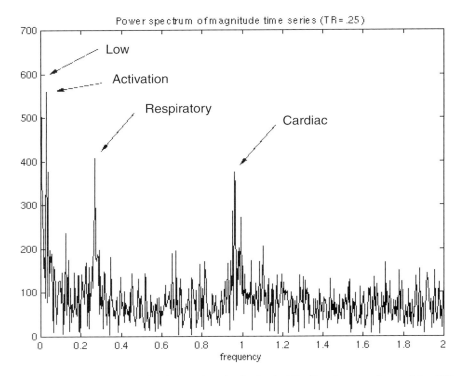

Figure 18.1. Spectrum of noise fluctuations in the brain. The Fourier transform of the MR signal measured during a simple block design, finger-tapping experiment with TR = 250 ms shows a strong peak at the fundamental period of the stimulus plus peaks due to cardiac and respiratory pulsations (bottom). There is also considerable noise power at low frequencies due to baseline drifts and possibly also physiological vasomotion. The images along the top show the amplitudes of different components in sagittal images, suggesting the strong spatial as well as temporal structure of the noise. (Data courtesy of L. Frank.)

approximately the same signal difference, whereas the difference signal from a voxel dominated by a blood vessel or CSF fluctuations might vary over a wide range.

To remove these artifacts due to voxels with highly variable signals, we can normalize each measured difference signal between task and control states by dividing by an estimate of the intrinsic variability of the signal from that voxel. In effect, this creates a map of the SNR of the difference measurement. Then voxels with a large signal difference due only to the fact that they have a large intrinsic variance will be suppressed, whereas true activations in which the signal change is much larger than the intrinsic variance will remain. The resulting map is thus a map of the statistical quality of the measurement, rather than a map of the effect itself (i.e., the fractional signal change). Such *statistical parametric maps* (SPMs) are the standard statistical tool used for evaluating fMRI data (Friston et al., 1995; Gold et al., 1998).

The *t*-Test

One of the standard statistical parameters used to quantify the quality of a measured activation is the *t*-statistic, which is closely related to the signal to noise of the difference measurement. In its simplest form, the signals measured from a particular voxel are treated as samples of two populations (active and rest); the *t*-test is used to assess whether there is a significant difference between the means of the two groups. The *t*-statistic is essentially a measure of how large the difference of the means is compared to the variability of the populations so that, as *t* gets larger, the probability that such data could have arisen from two populations with equal means becomes more and more unlikely. This measure is quantified with the *t*-distribution, from which one can calculate the probability that a particular value of *t* or larger could arise by chance if the means really are identical. Then the procedure for analyzing BOLD data begins with the calculation of the *t*-statistic for each voxel. One can then choose a threshold value of probability, such as $p < .01$, which corresponds to a particular threshold on *t,* and pick out all voxels whose *t*-value passes the threshold. These voxels are then displayed in color on an underlying map of the anatomy for ease of visualization.

The choice of a threshold on *t* for constructing the activation map involves consideration of the fact that the signals from many voxels are being measured simultaneously. For example, if we were considering the difference of means of only a single voxel, we could adopt the conventional criterion that if $p < .05$ the measured difference is considered to be significantly different from zero. But at this level of significance, the same or larger value of *t* will arise by chance 5% of the time. For a typical whole brain fMRI study, there may be on the order of 10,000 brain voxels that are analyzed, and so at this level of significance about 500 voxels should appear to be activated by chance alone! To account for these multiple measurements, a more conservative *p* value is chosen. For example, to reduce the probability of finding *any* false positive activations to the 5% level, the *p*-value chosen should be 5% divided by the number of voxels (Bonferroni correction), or $p = .000005$ for this example.

However, a second problem that must be dealt with when applying the *t*-test is that the hemodynamic response of the brain does not precisely match the stimulus. For example, consider a simple block design experiment in which the stimuli are presented in long blocks alternated with equal periods of rest. Then the stimulus as a function of time can be represented as a square wave equal to one during the stimulus task and zero during the control task. The simplest assumption we could make for the response of the BOLD function would be that it would follow the same curve, with the signal changing immediately at the start of each cycle of the square wave and returning cleanly to baseline at the end of each stimulus period. However, even if the neural activity closely follows the stimulus (e.g., within a few hundred milliseconds or so), the hemodynamic response is measurably delayed and broadened. A typical activated voxel will show a delay of about 2 s after the beginning of the stimulus period before the BOLD response begins, followed by a ramp of about 6 s duration before a new plateau of the signal is reached. After the end of the stimulus period, the BOLD signal ramps back down to the baseline over several seconds and often undershoots the baseline, with the undershoot lasting for 20 s or more (see Chapter 17).

Correlation Analysis

The statistical analysis can be enlarged to include the expected hemodynamic response with a correlation analysis (Bandettini et al., 1993). Instead of assuming that the hemodynamic response precisely matches the stimulus pattern, the delay and smoothing are incorporated by defining a *model response function.* A simple approximation for the model response to a block stimulus pattern is a trapezoid with 6-s ramps delayed by 2 s from the onset of the stimulus block. Having chosen a model response function, each measured voxel time course is analyzed by calculating the correlation coefficient r between the data and the model function. The correlation coefficient ranges from -1 to 1 and expresses the degree to which the measured signal follows the model function. The correlation coefficient is then used as the statistical parameter for mapping, and a threshold on r is chosen to select pixels that are reliably activated. Figure 6.4 shows an example of an activation map calculated from the correlation coefficient map.

In fact, a correlation analysis is closely related to the simple t-test comparison of means. The previously described test, in which the time course data are divided into two groups and the means compared, is equivalent to using a model reference function that precisely matches the square-wave stimulus pattern (instead of a delayed trapezoid). Then there is a one-to-one correspondence between the t-value calculated from the t-test and the r-value calculated from the correlation analysis. Any threshold based on t would precisely correspond to a particular threshold on r. The correlation analysis is more general, however, in that it allows one to use any model function, so the true response can be better approximated.

Correlation analysis, in turn, is a component of a more general linear regression analysis. In effect, what we are doing is trying to model the data as a linear combination of one or more model functions plus noise. With the single model function described earlier, we are trying to fit the data as well as we can by treating the data as a scaled version of the model function. That is, we try to determine the best value for a multiplicative parameter a, such that when the model function is multiplied by a the resulting time series best approximates the real data. Ideally, if we subtract this best-fit model curve from the data, the residuals should be only due to noise. The correlation coefficient r is then a measure of how much of the original variance of the data can be removed by subtracting the best-fit estimate of the model function. In this case, there is only one model function, but the analysis can be generalized to include any number of model functions. For example, it is not uncommon for the

MR signal from a voxel to drift slightly over the course of an experiment. One can try to take this into account by including an additional model function that is a linear function of time. Then the data are modeled as a linear combination of the hemodynamic response function and a linear drift. Quadratic and higher order drift terms also can be included as additional model functions. This basic multiple regression approach is referred to as the general linear model (Friston et al., 1995). It is important to remember here that "linear" refers to the fact that the data are modeled as a linear combination of model functions but that the model functions themselves need not be linear. The general linear model is described in more detail later in the chapter.

Fourier Analysis

Another closely related approach to analyzing BOLD data for block design experiments is to calculate the Fourier transform of the measured time course and examine the component at the fundamental frequency of the stimulus pattern (Engel et al., 1994; Sereno et al., 1995). For example, if four cycles of stimulus/control are performed, then the amplitude for the 4-cycle frequency in the Fourier spectrum should be a strong spike wherever there is activation. Figure 18.2 shows a blocked stimulus pattern, the expected hemodynamic response, and simulated data including noise. The Fourier spectrum of the stimulus pattern itself shows a prominent fundamental frequency, and a series of odd multiples of the fundamental frequency. (By symmetry, the even multiples of the fundamental frequency do not contribute to the stimulus waveform.) The smoothing effect of the hemodynamic response attenuates the high frequencies of the stimulus pattern, and in the data only one or two harmonics are apparent. Fourier analysis can be viewed as another variation on the general linear model. Calculating the Fourier component at the fundamental stimulus frequency is equivalent to a multiple regression analysis with a sine wave and a cosine wave, both at the fundamental frequency, as the two model functions.

A Fourier analysis has the added advantage for some applications that the delay of the response is easily calculated. There is accumulating evidence that the hemodynamic delay may vary from one part of the brain to another, and this can present a problem with a standard correlation analysis. If the delay used in the model for the hemodynamic response function does not match the true delay, the correlation coefficient will be reduced, and activated pixels, which should be identifiable, could be missed. To account for this problem, the correlation coefficient for the same model shape but different delays can be calculated, and the one giving the highest value of r chosen as the best fit to that voxel data. However, if the model response function is a sine wave, the best fit of the delay can be calculated directly from the Fourier transform (FT). For a sine wave model function, a hemodynamic delay is equivalent to a phase offset, and the FT directly provides the amplitude and phase at each frequency.

Another way of looking at an FT analysis in the context of a correlation analysis is to note that the comparison of a data time course with a model response function could also be done in the frequency domain as well as in the time domain. The FT of

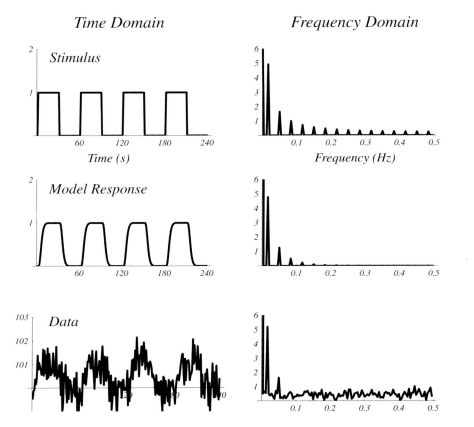

Figure 18.2. Fourier components of the BOLD signal. The spectral components of a blocked design stimulus pattern show a prominent fundamental frequency and a series of odd multiples of the fundamental frequency (top). The smoothed hemodynamic response attenuates the higher harmonics (middle). In the data with noise, only one harmonic is apparent.

the model response function shows spikes at multiples of the fundamental stimulus frequency, and the relative amplitudes and phases of these spikes depend on the shape of the response function in the time domain (Figure 18.2). The FT of an activated pixel should also show spikes at the same frequencies as the model response function; however, there will also be noise present in all the frequencies. The correlation analysis is then equivalent to comparing the amplitudes of the model and data frequency spectra at the fundamental frequency and each of its harmonics and determining whether these amplitudes in the data are sufficiently larger than the noise. For a general model response function, all the harmonics can contribute to the comparison and should be used to improve sensitivity. However, as the model function approaches a single sine wave at the fundamental frequency, the FT reduces to just a single spike at the fundamental frequency. For a sustained activation of 30 s or more, the response function is better approximated with a trapezoid than a sine wave, and so the more general correlation analysis that uses all the harmonics will give a more sensitive estimate of activation than just the amplitude of the fundamental frequency in the FT of the data. But when the stimulus is cycled more rapidly, a sine wave is a reasonable approximation to the response function, and a simple Fourier analysis should yield comparable results to a correlation with a trapezoid.

The Kolmogorov-Smirnov Test

Another statistical test used to evaluate the statistical significance of detected activations in block design experiments is the Kolmogorov-Smirnov (KS) test. Like the t-test, the KS test treats the signal values measured during the task and control periods as two populations and then tests whether the two populations are significantly different. With the t-test, the focus is on whether the means of the two populations are different. With the KS test, the focus is on whether the cumulative distributions of the two populations are significantly different. For each population (e.g., all signal values measured in the activated state), the measured values are sorted into ascending order. An estimate of the cumulative distribution is formed by calculating $P(x)$, the fraction of signal values greater than x for each x. From the two distributions $P_{act}(x)$ and $P_{rest}(x)$, the KS statistic is calculated as the maximum difference between the two cumulative distributions. Under the null hypothesis, the distribution of the KS statistic can be calculated, so the significance of any measured value can be estimated.

In general, the KS test is less sensitive (or more conservative) than the other approaches described. In other words, some weak activations could be missed with the KS test, but the ones that are deemed to be significant are likely to be highly reliable. One potential interesting aspect of the KS test is that in principle it could detect a difference between two populations which have the same mean but different standard deviations. If the variance of the MR signal changed with activation, even though the mean signal remained constant, the KS test could potentially detect this change. Such a physiological effect has not been observed, so whether this mathematical property has any significance for brain activation studies is not known.

Noise Correlations

The foregoing discussion has focused on identifying whether the expected signal response is present in the data. But a complete determination of the significance of a detected activation depends on a full understanding of the noise in the data, and the noise in BOLD measurements of the brain is still not understood in a quantitative way. To clarify the problem this creates, we can return to the simplest method of a t-test comparison of the mean signals during stimulus and rest conditions. To assess the significance of the measurement of a particular value of t, we need to know the degrees of freedom, which are essentially the number of independent measurements that went into the calculation. For example, with only two measurements each in the stimulus and control states, a value of $t > 3.0$ or larger is borderline significant ($p = 0.029$), but with 50 measurements in each state, $t > 3.0$ is highly significant ($p = .0017$). However, these estimates of the significance of t are based on two assumptions about the noise: the noise is normally distributed, and the noise in each measurement is independent of the noise in the other measurements. Although these assumptions are good for the thermal noise component, the physiological contribution is likely to violate both (Purdon and Weisskoff, 1998; Zarahn et al., 1997). For example, added low-frequency noise components due to respiration are likely to be quite structured and not normally distributed. Furthermore, because this noise has low frequencies, the noise added into a measurement at one time point is likely to be similar to the noise added in at the next time point, so the noise is not independent.

A similar question arises when we consider multiple voxels: is the noise in one voxel independent of the noise in a neighboring voxel? Again, random thermal noise is independent, but physiological noise is likely to have strong spatial correlations. For example, CSF pulsations are likely to affect nearby pixels in a similar way. The nature of these correlations will have a strong effect on calculating the significance of clusters of pixels. For example, any motion of the subject's head in synchrony with the stimulus will lead to a bulk shift in the MR images. At any edge in the image where there is a contrast difference, even small subpixel shifts will lead to a time-dependent signal that correlates strongly with the motion. Such stimulus-correlated motion artifacts are a common problem in fMRI, and the spurious correlations tend to occur in many contiguous pixels around the edge of the brain. As a result, clusters of false positive activations can occur much more frequently than would be expected for voxels with independent noise.

In short, structured noise remains a problem for the analysis of BOLD data, and further work is needed to understand these signal fluctuations so that they can be taken into account in the statistical analysis. For the remainder of this chapter, we will ignore these complications in order to clarify the basic ideas of the statistical analysis.

Interpreting BOLD Activation Maps

In the previous section some of the complexities of the statistical analysis were introduced. Although it often seems like many different approaches are used, in fact there is an underlying unity to these methods. In this section, we will step back from the details of the analysis to look at how the resulting maps can be interpreted. For this purpose, it is sufficient to return to the simple *t*-test comparing means, and forget complications such as the hemodynamic response function, systematic signal drift, and correlated noise. This basic approach is the simplest type of analysis of BOLD data; nevertheless, it captures the basic reasoning behind the analysis. The choice of the statistic and the justification for choosing a particular threshold may differ, but the basic structure is the same. It is important to be clear on the philosophy behind this approach. The goal is *not* to identify all voxels whose magnitude of change is greater than some threshold (e.g., all voxels with a fractional signal change greater than 1%). Instead, the goal is to identify all voxels whose signal change is sufficiently larger than what would be expected by chance alone, and the level of our statistical confidence depends on the threshold applied to the map of the statistical parameter.

But this makes the interpretation of activation maps such as Figure 6.4 somewhat subtle, and some of our natural impulses when viewing such maps need to be curbed. It is tempting to look at such a map and interpret it as a map of the activated regions. We can say with confidence, and we can specify exactly what level of confidence, that the voxels that are colored are "activated" (we will ignore for the moment various artifacts that might lead to false positive activations). But we cannot conclude that the pixels that are not colored are not activated. We can only say that the statistical quality of the measurements in those voxels is too low for us to be confident that there *is* an activation. In other words, strictly speaking, our failure to detect an activation in a particular voxel at a desired level of statistical quality cannot be taken as evidence of a lack of activation in that voxel. For example, one can imagine the simple, idealized case of two voxels with identical changes in CBF, which lead to identical 1% changes in the BOLD signal, but the intrinsic signal standard deviation in one voxel is 0.1% and in the other is 1%. The first would be detected and classified as an activated area, whereas the second would not, even though the CBF change is the same.

Another way of explaining this approach is that in analyzing BOLD data we are primarily concerned with eliminating false positives, such as vessels with high intrinsic signal variability. But we are not concerned with false negatives, in the sense that the analysis is not directed at eliminating false negatives. In fact, no negative finding is ever meaningful with this type of analysis alone. It is possible to carry the analysis further, for example to define confidence intervals for how much absolute activation (i.e., the signal change) might be present in a voxel (Frank, Buxton, and Wong, 1998), but this is not usually done. Similarly, the value of the statistic itself, such as t, should never be taken as a measure of the *degree* of activation: a larger value of t in one voxel than another does not imply that the level of activation is larger in the first. To draw such a conclusion, one must show that the difference in the t-values is due to a difference in the signal change, rather than a difference in the intrinsic variability of the signal.

THE GENERAL LINEAR MODEL

With these basic ideas in mind, we can consider in more detail how the general linear model works. This method provides a powerful and flexible tool for analyzing BOLD data and also for designing experiments to maximize the likelihood of detecting weak activations. As introduced earlier, this approach models the data as a linear combination of a set of model functions plus random noise. The model functions themselves have a known shape, but the amplitudes multiplying each model function are unknown. The analysis consists of finding the estimates of these amplitudes that provide the best fit of the model to the data in a least-squares sense. That is, the quality of a particular set of model parameters is gauged by calculating the sum of squares of the residuals after the model is subtracted from the data, and the best-fit set of parameters is the one that minimizes this sum. The general linear model is the framework for many commonly used statistical analysis techniques, including multiple regression analysis and analysis of variance (ANOVA). In thinking about the statistical analysis of BOLD data, a useful conceptual tool is to view the process as an exercise in multidimensional geometry, and throughout this chapter we will emphasize this geometric view (Frank et al., 1998). A useful introduction to this way of thinking is found in Saville and Wood (1991).

The Hemodynamic Response

The first step in applying a linear model analysis is to predict the shape of the BOLD response to a given stimulus pattern so that only the amplitude of this response is unknown. As discussed in Chapter 17, the hemodynamic response is not a simple function of the stimulus pattern, often including transient features such as a poststimulus undershoot. In addition, the response is not a linear function of the stimulus duration, in the sense that the response to a sustained stimulus is not as large as one would predict from the response to a brief stimulus (Boynton et al., 1996; Friston et al., 1998b; Glover, 1999; Vasquez and Noll, 1998). Furthermore, the hemodynamic response varies among individuals and regions of the brain (Aguirre et al., 1998). Nevertheless, a fruitful approach to the analysis of the data is to ignore the complications and use the simplified assumption that the hemodynamic response is linear with stimulus duration. Although not true, this assumption likely does not introduce large errors, but this question requires further attention.

To emphasize how the analysis works, we will assume that the response to a brief stimulus looks something like the curve shown in Figure 18.3. This model response is a gamma variate function described by

$$h(t) = \begin{cases} 0 & t < \Delta t \\ \dfrac{1}{\tau n!}\left(\dfrac{t}{\tau}\right)^n e^{-t/\tau} & \Delta t \le t \end{cases} \qquad [18.1]$$

The parameters for the curve in Figure 18.3 are $n = 3$, $\tau = 1.2$ s, and $\Delta t = 1$ s. The parameter Δt is a delay before the response begins. Assuming linearity, the response to a more sustained stimulus is the convolution of the stimulus pattern $X(t)$ and the hemodynamic response (or impulse response) function $h(t)$, written as $X(t)*h(t)$. The bottom panel of Figure 18.3 shows the model response for a sustained stimulus. The signal ramps up to a plateau level and then remains constant until the end of the stimulus. The ramp time is directly proportional to the width of $h(t)$, and the plateau level is proportional to the area under $h(t)$.

The hemodynamic response model shown in Figure 18.3 is a reasonable approximation to a typical response, but there is nothing special about the mathematical form used. Other forms have been suggested, but all are based just on the convenience of the mathematical shape, rather than a physiological model that would predict that particular form (Boynton et al., 1996; Friston et al., 1994). The balloon model predicts a similar shape when the flow change is a simple trapezoidal shape, but there exists no underlying mathematical theory of the blood flow response that would predict a particular flow response shape (Buxton, Wong, and Frank, 1998). For this reason, choosing a shape such as Equation [18.1] is simply an empirical convenience, and other shapes may work equally well.

Brief stimulus

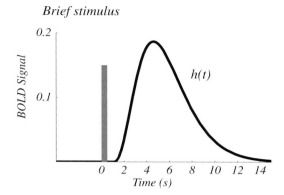

Sustained Stimulus

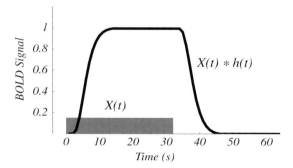

Figure 18.3. The hemodynamic response. A brief stimulus produces a BOLD hemodynamic response that is delayed and broadened, modeled in the top panel as a gamma variate function. Assuming that the BOLD response is linear, the response to a longer duration stimulus is the convolution of the impulse response *h(t)* with the stimulus pattern *X(t)*.

If *h(t)* is known, then we can predict the shape of the response to any stimulus pattern by defining the stimulus pattern *X(t)* as a function of time. The function *X* has a value of one at time *t* if the stimulus occurs, or zero if it does not. Then the model response function is *X(t)*h(t)*, as illustrated in Figure 18.3. If *h(t)* is unknown or variable across the brain, then more model functions can be used to describe a range of shapes. We will return to this later, but for now we consider the simple case of a known hemodynamic response.

Fitting the Data with a Known Model Response

To be specific, suppose that we are examining a BOLD time series from one voxel, consisting of *N* measurements of the signal, with a time separation TR between measurements. The stimulus pattern *X(t)* consists of two cycles of stimulus and control, as illustrated in the top left panel of Figure 18.4. The expected model response to this stimulus pattern is *X(t)*h(t)*, a smoothed and delayed version of the stimulus as shown in the second line. The activation signal is modeled as an

Statistical Analysis of BOLD Data

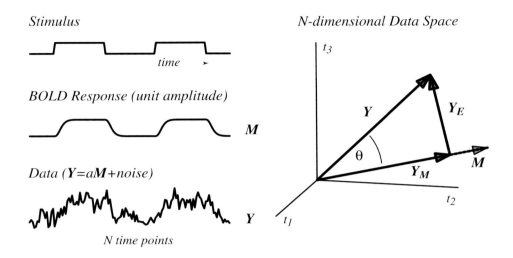

Stimulus

BOLD Response (unit amplitude)

Data (Y=aM+noise)

N-dimensional Data Space

Vectors in data space:

M = *model vector for unit amplitude response*
Y = *data vector*
Y_M = *projection onto model* = $\left(\dfrac{Y \cdot M}{M}\right)\left(\dfrac{M}{M}\right)$
Y_E = *error vector* = $Y - Y_M$

Parameter estimates:

a = *response amplitude* = $\dfrac{Y_M}{M}$

σ^2 = *noise variance* = $\dfrac{Y_E^2}{N-1}$

Statistics:
r = *correlation coefficient* = $\cos\theta = \dfrac{Y_M}{Y}$

t = *t-statistic* = $\left(\sqrt{N-1}\right)\cot\theta = \left(\sqrt{N-1}\right)\dfrac{Y_M}{Y_E}$

Figure 18.4. The basic linear model analysis of BOLD data. For a time series of N measurements, the data Y and the expected BOLD response M (upper left) are viewed as vectors in an N-dimensional data space. The data are modeled as an unknown amplitude a times M plus noise with standard deviation σ. The best-fit value of a is given by the projection of the data onto the model vector, Y_M, and σ is calculated from the remainder of the data, Y_E. The t-statistic and the correlation coefficient r are calculated from the triangle in the upper right. The mathematical relations are shown in the lower part of the figure.

unknown amplitude a times the model response, and this BOLD response is sampled at each of the measurement times. The full measured data include this sampled signal plus added noise at each of the measurement times. We assume that each noise value is independently drawn from a normal distribution with a mean of zero and a standard deviation σ.

For this analysis, we focus on the variance of the data. Part of the variance is due to the activation, and so depends on the magnitude of a, and the rest comes from the noise component. The goal of the analysis is to estimate a and σ and to assess the significance of the estimate of a. Because we are only interested in the variance, the first step is to remove the mean value of both the model function and the data itself, to create a vector of model response values M_i ($i = 1$ to N) and a vector of data values Y_i.

The essence of the geometric view of this analysis is to imagine an N-dimensional space in which each axis corresponds to one time point. Of course, we cannot picture more than three dimensions, but mathematically there is no problem in defining an N-dimensional space. Each of the measured data values Y_i is a coordinate along the ith axis, so the full measured time course corresponds to one point in this space. We can think of this point as defining a vector from the origin to the point, and the projection of this data vector Y onto the ith axis is simply the measured signal Y_i. We will use boldface symbols to denote a vector, and plain text to denote a scalar, or the magnitude of a vector. In other words, $\boldsymbol{Y}$ denotes the full data vector, whereas Y is the length of that vector.

In a similar fashion, the model response is also a vector ($\boldsymbol{M}$) in the N-dimensional data space, as illustrated in the upper right panel of Figure 18.4. It is important to be clear about the meaning of the magnitude M of this vector. As we will see, M is the key number that characterizes the sensitivity of an experimental design. The model response M is the unit amplitude response. For example, if the BOLD response is measured in image signal units, then $\boldsymbol{M}$ is the response for an activation-induced hemodynamic response of one signal unit. If the best-fit value of a is 2, this means that the signal change is twice as large as that described by $\boldsymbol{M}$.

If there was no noise, then we would expect that the vector $\boldsymbol{Y}$ would lie along the same direction as $\boldsymbol{M}$, and the estimate of a then would be simply Y/M. With noise, however, $\boldsymbol{Y}$ no longer lies along $\boldsymbol{M}$, and so the analysis is slightly more difficult. For any value of a, we could multiply the model function by a and subtract this prediction from the measured data to form the residuals. Our goal is to find the value of a that minimizes the sum of the squared residuals. But this process can be directly visualized with the geometric picture. Any value of a produces a vector with amplitude aM along the axis defined by $\boldsymbol{M}$. Subtracting this vector from $\boldsymbol{Y}$ creates a residual vector (or *error* vector) $\boldsymbol{Y_E}$. The sum of the squared residuals is the sum of the squares of each component of $\boldsymbol{Y_E}$, which is just Y_E^2, the length squared of the vector $\boldsymbol{Y_E}$. In other words, the sum of the squared residuals is simply the distance squared from the point defined by the model vector $a\boldsymbol{M}$ to the point defined by $\boldsymbol{Y}$ in the N-dimensional space. This is minimized by minimizing Y_E, so the best fit of a is calculated by finding the point along the direction defined by $\boldsymbol{M}$ that is closest to the data point defined by Y. It is this close connection of least squares with distance that makes the geometric picture a natural conceptual tool.

For this case of a single model function, the best-fit amplitude is calculated by taking the projection $\boldsymbol{Y_M}$ of the data onto the axis defined by $\boldsymbol{M}$. The best-fit value of a is given directly by the magnitude of Y_M, as $a = Y_M/M$. (Remember that the magnitude of M corresponds to a unit amplitude response, so M essentially calibrates the projection of the data in signal amplitude units.) Another way of looking at this is that we are breaking the data vector into two perpendicular components: the projection onto the model vector Y_M, and a remaining error component Y_E, with $Y^2 = Y_M^2 + Y_E^2$ (Figure 18.4). Because the mean of the data has been removed, Y^2 is the total variance of the signal. The decomposition of Y into Y_M and Y_E thus partitions the variance between the activation and the noise. The component of the variance due to the activation is Y_M^2, and the remaining variance due to noise is Y_E^2.

From the magnitude of Y_E, we can estimate the noise variance σ^2. The length squared Y^2_E is the sum of the squared values of each component of the vector, and each component corresponds to the random noise signal added in at a particular measurement time. For each of these noise signals, the expected squared value is σ^2. So in calculating the magnitude of Y_E^2, each dimension adds in a value of σ^2. This brings us to a critical question: how many dimensions contribute? At first glance, the answer appears to be N because that is the full dimensions of the data space. However, in the construction of Y_E, we have first removed the component along a single dimension in the direction of M, so Y_E is really a vector in an N–1 dimensional space. One can think of this as dividing the N-dimensional space into a model space and an error space. In this case, the model space is a single dimension, and the error space has N–1 dimensions. In a more general model with m model functions (discussed later), the model space has m dimensions, and the error space has N–m dimensions. The number of dimensions in the error space is usually called the degrees of freedom, $v = N - m$. Returning to our estimate of σ^2, if the error space has v dimensions, then the expected magnitude of Y_E^2, is $v\sigma^2$, so our estimate of the noise variance is $\sigma^2 = Y_E^2/v$.

The decomposition of the data vector into a model component and a noise component leads to direct estimates of the amplitude of the activation a and the noise variance σ^2. On average, the estimate of a should be the true value, but there will be some variance in the estimate due to the noise signal that falls along the direction of M. In other words, if we were to perform the experiment many times, with the same activation response but different noise samples, the estimates of a would have a variance we can call σ_a^2. The statistical significance of a measured value of a then depends directly on the magnitude of σ_a. For the current case of a single model vector, the variance of the estimate of a can be calculated in a direct way. Noise contributes to all dimensions of the data space equally, so there will be a noise component along M with variance σ^2. Scaling this variance to the units of the model function, the variance of a is $\sigma_a^2 = \sigma^2/M^2$.

A natural measure of the statistical quality of a measurement of a is the ratio of the measured value to the uncertainty of the measurement, the signal-to-noise ratio,

$$SNR = \frac{a}{\sigma_a} = \frac{aM}{\sigma} \tag{18.2}$$

This is an important relationship, and, as we will see, it provides a useful way of comparing the sensitivity of different experimental designs.

Statistical Significance

So far we have considered statistical significance in terms of the SNR of the estimate of the activation amplitude. A related and more common approach is to test how likely it is that a given measured model amplitude could have arisen by chance due to noise alone. In other words, this approach tests the significance of the null hypothesis that $a = 0$ (i.e., that there is no activation). This type of test can be done with either a t-test or a correlation coefficient, and both statistics have a natural geometric interpretation as shown in Figure 18.4.

Under the null hypothesis, the sum of squares of the data given by the magnitude Y^2 is due entirely to noise. The expected magnitude squared of each component of the N-dimensional data space is σ^2. If we isolate any one axis of the N-dimensional data space, the expected mean value of that component is zero with a variance σ^2. The t-statistic with v degrees of freedom (t_v) is the ratio of the amplitude measured along one axis to the noise standard deviation estimated from the remaining v dimensions of the data space. If the component along the model vector is due only to noise, then its amplitude should be on the order of σ, and t is about equal to one. As t grows larger, the probability of such a large noise amplitude appearing along the model vector becomes less and less likely. From the arguments in the previous sections, the estimate of σ is $Y_E/\sqrt{v}$, and the component along the model vector is Y_M, so $t = \sqrt{v}\, Y_M/Y_E$. In this way, t is proportional to the ratio of two legs of the triangle in Figure 18.4. Furthermore, this expression for t reduces precisely to the ratio of the estimate of a to the standard deviation of that estimate. In short, t is identical to our expression for the SNR (Equation [18.2]).

The correlation coefficient is the scalar product of Y and M, normalized by their respective magnitudes. In other words, the correlation coefficient is $r = \cos\theta$, where θ is the angle between Y and M in the data space. Because both t and r are calculated from the same triangle, there is a simple relation between them:

$$t = \sqrt{v}\,\cot\theta = \sqrt{v}\,\frac{r}{\sqrt{1 - r^2}} \qquad [18.3]$$

The test of significance then amounts to asking how often a value greater than a given value of t or r should occur due to noise. These distributions are calculated from the geometry shown in Figure 18.4 under the null hypothesis and are tabulated in standard statistics software packages. Given a measured value of t or r and the degrees of freedom v, the calculated probability of that result occurring by chance is the statistical significance. That is, the statistical significance reflects the confidence with which we can reject the null hypothesis that there is no activation.

Fitting the Data with a More General Linear Model

The preceding sections introduced the basic ideas of the general linear model, but in the limited context of a single model function. There are a number of experimental designs where more than one model function is desirable. Some examples follow.

1. *Removal of baseline trends.* In addition to the model response and noise, a real data time course often shows a drift over time. This can be taken into account by including other model functions (e.g., a linear drift term, a quadratic term) to account for this added variance.

2. *Two types of stimuli.* In more sophisticated BOLD experiments, multiple stimuli are used, and it is desirable to separate the responses to the different stimuli. Or, it may be useful to treat different aspects of the same stimulus as different events (e.g., in a simple motor task some areas may activate only at the beginning and end of the task, whereas other areas are activated throughout). Each type of stimulus can be modeled with a different response function.

3. *Unknown hemodynamic response.* The exact shape of the hemodynamic response is unknown and is likely to vary across the brain. Rather than using a single model function, a small set of model functions can be used to describe a range of shapes.

4. *Event-related fMRI.* The hemodynamic response itself can be estimated for each voxel by treating the response at each time point after an event as a separate model function.

To make the linear model more general by including these applications, we will consider the case of two model functions. The jump from one function to two may not sound like much of a generalization, but in fact this brings in all the new features of the general linear model that did not appear in the single model function case, and with only two model functions it is still possible to visualize the geometry.

The mathematical form of the general linear model is shown in Figure 18.5, and the geometry is illustrated in Figure 18.6. Instead of a single model vector, we now have a matrix of model vectors, with the first column representing M_1 and the second column representing M_2, the two model vectors. We will denote the matrix with the symbol M, and continue to use the symbol M for individual vectors that make up the design matrix. For example, if two types of stimulus are intermixed during an experimental run, then M_1 and M_2 could represent the separate responses to the two stimuli. That is, M_1 is calculated by convolving the first stimulus pattern $X_1(t)$ with a hemodynamic response function, and M_2 is the convolution of the other stimulus pattern $X_2(t)$ with the hemodynamic response. (More explicitly, M_1 is the magnitude of $X_1(t)*h(t)$ with the mean removed.) The implicit assumption here is that the responses simply add, so that the response to both stimuli is the sum of the responses to each separate stimulus.

There are now two amplitudes to be estimated, so the single amplitude a is replaced with a vector a consisting of two amplitudes, a_1 and a_2. We can think of a as a vector in a parameter space that defines the amplitudes of the model functions (i.e., the vector a defines a point in a two-dimensional parameter space in which one axis corresponds to a_1 and the other corresponds to a_2). But the basic form of the model is the same. The data are modeled as a sum of two model vectors with a known shape but with unknown amplitudes a_1 and a_2, plus noise with variance σ^2. From the geometric viewpoint (Figure 18.6), the model space now has two dimen-

General Linear Model

$$Y = M \cdot a + e$$

Y = *data vector*
M = *matrix of model functions*
a = *amplitude vector*
e = *noise vector*

2 model functions

$$
\begin{pmatrix} Y(t_1) \\ Y(t_2) \\ ... \\ Y(t_N) \end{pmatrix}
=
\begin{pmatrix} M_1(t_1) & M_2(t_1) \\ M_1(t_2) & M_2(t_2) \\ ... & ... \\ M_1(t_N) & M_2(t_N) \end{pmatrix}
\begin{pmatrix} a_1 \\ a_2 \end{pmatrix}
+
\begin{pmatrix} e_1(t_1) \\ e_2(t_2) \\ ... \\ e_N(t_N) \end{pmatrix}
$$

N time points

Amplitudes

Data   **Design Matrix**   **Noise**

$$a = (M^T M)^{-1} M^T Y$$

$$C = (M^T M)^{-1} = covariance\ matrix$$

Figure 18.5. The mathematical structure of the general linear model. The data are modeled as a linear combination of a set of model functions with unknown amplitudes plus noise. The design matrix M contains one column for each model function, and the amplitudes form a vector a. The best-fit estimates of the amplitudes are calculated from the design matrix as shown in the lower part of the figure, and the variances of the estimated amplitudes are calculated from the covariance matrix (see Box 18 for mathematical details).

sions, defined as the plane that includes both M_1 and M_2, and the dimension of the error space is $v = N - 2$.

The procedure for fitting the data is similar to the earlier case of a single model function. The goal is to find the point in the model space that is closest to the data point defined by Y, and this point is the projection Y_M onto the model plane. Although conceptually similar to the single model function case, the mathematics is now more complicated because the projection onto the model space does not fall on either of the model vectors, but rather the plane formed by those vectors, and so Y_M cannot be calculated as readily. For the ideal case in which M_1 and M_2 are perpendicular, the analysis is simple, and the projection of Y separately onto M_1 and M_2 works just like it did for the single model function case. If we call the magnitudes of these two projections Y_{M_1} and Y_{M_2}, then the amplitudes are simply the appropriately scaled versions: $a_1 = Y_{M_1}/M_1$ and $a_2 = Y_{M_2}/M_2$.

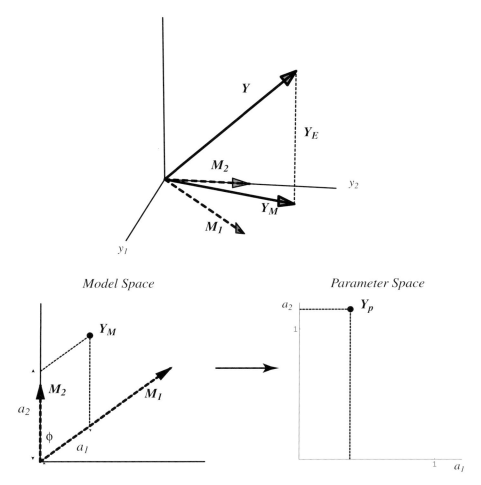

Figure 18.6. The geometric structure of the general linear model. The illustration shows two model functions that define a two-dimensional model space. The projection Y_M of the data onto the model space (top) is modeled as a linear combination of the two model functions, and the remaining component Y_E provides a measure of the noise. The point Y_M in the model space is transformed to a parameter space in which the axes correspond to the amplitudes a_1 and a_2. This transformation accounts for the different amplitudes of the model functions and the fact that they may not be orthogonal (the mathematical details are in Box 18).

The complication comes in when the two model functions are not perpendicular, as illustrated in the lower left panel of Figure 18.6. Our goal is to find amplitudes a_1 and a_2 such that $a_1 M_1 + a_2 M_2 = Y_M$, the full projection of the data onto the model space. But the correct amplitudes are not given by the separate projections Y_{M_1} and Y_{M_2} onto M_1 and M_2. The correct values come from the parallelogram shown because this represents the vector sum that produces Y_M. Mathematically, we can think of representing the projection Y_M in two spaces: the model space (the subspace of the full data space that is spanned by the model functions) and the parameter space in which one axis corresponds to a_1 and the other to a_2. The goal is to transform the coordinates of Y_M in the model space into the coordinates of the parameter space. The essential problem is that in the general case the parameter space is defined by two vectors that are not orthogonal to each other and that, in addition, have unequal lengths M_1 and M_2. Both these factors are taken into account in the coordinate transformation shown graphically in Figure 18.6, and the mathematical details are described in Box 18.

The Variance of the Parameter Estimates

With any statistical analysis, a critical question is whether the estimated amplitudes are statistically significant. As we found earlier in considering a single model function, there are two related ways to address this question. The first is to estimate the SNR of the measurement, the ratio of the measured amplitude to the expected variance in that measurement. The second approach is to define a t-statistic and ask how likely it would be for that value of t or larger to occur just due to random noise even though the true amplitude of the model function is zero (i.e., there is no activation). We found that these two dimensionless numbers, the SNR and the t-statistic, were identical for the case of a single model function. We now want to consider the same question for the more general linear model.

Random noise occurs along all the axes of the data space, and so noise components also fall in the model space and are transformed into variance of the model parameter estimates. Figure 18.6 illustrates the transformation from the model space to the parameter space defined by the amplitudes a_1 and a_2. To begin with, suppose that there is no activation, so that the true values of a_1 and a_2 are zero. In the model space, noise is isotropic, in the sense that the random component along any axis has the same variance σ^2. If the experiment were performed many times, the random data points that fall in the model space would form a symmetric cloud centered on the origin. We can represent this by drawing a circular set of points in the model space with each point a distance σ from the origin and then ask how this ring of points is transformed into the parameter space (i.e., transformed into values of a_1 and a_2).

Figure 18.7 illustrates this transformation into the parameter space for several examples. If M_1 and M_2 have the same amplitude and are perpendicular to each other, the ring of noise points transforms into another ring. But if M_1 and M_2 are not perpendicular, the noise points are spread into an ellipse oriented at 45° to the a_1- and a_2-axes in the parameter space. As the angle between M_1 and M_2 decreases, the ellipse becomes more elongated but remains at the same orientation as long as the magnitudes M_1 and M_2 are equal. When M_1 and M_2 have different magnitudes the axes are scaled differently, changing the orientation of the ellipse.

We can now return to the more general case in which the values of a_1 and a_2 are not necessarily zero. If we performed the same experiment many times with the same stimuli and the same true responses, the projections into the model space would transform into a cloud of points in the parameter space centered on the correct values of a_1 and a_2 (shown as a contour map in Figure 18.8). If the model functions are not orthogonal, the cloud is elongated as discussed above. The variance of the estimate of a particular parameter or a linear combination of parameters is cal-

BOX 18. ESTIMATING THE MODEL FUNCTION AMPLITUDES AND THEIR VARIANCE

The calculation of the best-fit amplitudes a is done in terms of the matrices and vectors defined in Figure 18.7. The total data vector is $Y = Y_M + Y_E$, with $Y_M = M\,a$, where M is the design matrix formed from the model vectors M_1 and M_2. Now consider the scalar products of Y with each of the model vectors M_1 and M_2. In matrix terms, these components are given as a vector by multiplying Y by the transpose of M:

$$M^T Y = M^T Y_M + M^T Y_E = M^T M\,a \qquad\qquad [B18.1]$$

Because we have constructed Y_E to be perpendicular to M_1 and M_2, the second term is zero, and we have used the relation $Y_M = M\,a$. The vector of best-fit amplitudes is then:

$$a = (M^T M)^{-1}\,M^T Y \equiv LY \qquad\qquad [B18.2]$$

where the superscript -1 indicates matrix inverse, and L is defined as the combined linear transformation matrix that converts the data to best-fit amplitude estimates.

If the model vectors are not perpendicular, then there will be some covariance in the errors of each of the amplitude estimates. In some cases, we are interested only in the error of a particular amplitude, such as when one model function is a known hemodynamic response and the second model function is a linear drift of the signal. In this case, we do not care what the drift slope actually is; we simply want to account for it and remove it in order to improve the estimate of a_1, the activation response. On the other hand, if the two model functions represent the responses to two different stimuli, the errors in each amplitude and different linear combinations are important. For example, $a_1 - a_2$ is a measure of the differential response to the two stimuli, and so the uncertainty in the estimate of $a_1 - a_2$ is of interest.

Now we can consider how noise in the data space propagates into uncertainties of the parameter estimates. In general, any linear combination of the model amplitudes can be thought of as a contrast of the form $c = w_1 a_1 + w_2 a_2$ and the weights w_1 and w_2 are treated as the components of a vector in the parameter space (Friston et al., 1999). In matrix form, this contrast can be written as $c = a^T \mathbf{w}$. For example, if the contrast of interest is simply the amplitude $c = a_1$, then $w_1 = 1$ and $w_2 = 0$, whereas if the contrast of interest is the differential response to the two stimuli $c = a_1 - a_2$, then $w_1 = 1$ and $w_2 = -1$. The variance of the chosen contrast, σ_w^2, is calculated from the expected value of c^2:

$$\begin{aligned} c^2 &= (a^T w)^T\,(a^T w) = w^T\,(aa^T)w \\ \langle c^2 \rangle &= w^T\,\langle aa^T \rangle\,w \end{aligned} \qquad\qquad [B18.3]$$

where we have used the matrix relation $(AB)^T = B^T A^T$ for matrices A and B, and the notation $\langle b \rangle$ indicates the expected value of a scalar b. Because only the projection of the data into the model space determines the amplitudes, we can rewrite Equation [B 18.2] as $a = LY_M$ and substitute this in Equation [B 18.3]:

$$\begin{aligned} aa^T &= (LY_M)\,(LY_M)^T = L(Y_M Y_M{}^T)\,L^T \\ \langle aa^T \rangle &= L\,\langle Y_M Y_M{}^T \rangle\,L^T \end{aligned} \qquad\qquad [B18.4]$$

If each component is independent Gaussian noise, then $<Y_M Y_M{}^T> = \sigma^2 I$, where I is the identity matrix with ones down the diagonal and zeroes everywhere else. Then

$$\langle aa^T \rangle = \sigma^2 \, \textbf{\textit{LL}}^T = [(M^T M)^{-1} \, M^T] \, [M \, (M^T M)^{-1}]$$
$$\langle aa^T \rangle = \sigma^2 (M^T M)^{-1}$$

[B18.5]

So for any contrast of interest defined by a vector of weights w, the variance is

$$\sigma_w^2 = \sigma^2 w^T \, (M^T M)^{-1} \, w$$

[B18.6]

This is a very useful equation for evaluating the sensitivity of an fMRI experiment. As one would expect, the variance of any combination of estimated amplitudes is proportional to the intrinsic noise variance σ^2, but there is an additional scaling factor determined by the design of the experiment through the matrix of model functions M (the design matrix). Combining this equation with the estimated value of the contrast $c = a^T w$, we can write a general expression for the SNR of this contrast as

$$SNR \, (w) = \frac{a^T w}{\sigma \sqrt{w^T \, (M^T M)^{-1} w}}$$

[B18.7]

This expression is the generalization of Equation [18.2]. Under the null hypothesis that the contrast is zero, this quantity should follow a t-distribution with v degrees of freedom.

culated from this distribution by projecting the two dimensional distribution onto an appropriate axis (Figure 18.8). For example, to find the variance of the estimate of a_1 independent of the estimate of a_2, we project all the points onto the a_1-axis and calculate the variance of this distribution. The same procedure applies to any linear combination of the amplitudes. For example, suppose that M_1 and M_2 represent model functions for the responses to two different stimuli. Then we would certainly be interested in the separate responses to the two stimuli (a_1 or a_2), but we might also be interested in the combined response ($a_1 + a_2$) or the differential response ($a_1 - a_2$) to the two stimuli. Any linear combination of a_1 and a_2 corresponds to a line in the a_1-a_2 plane, and the variance of the estimate of that linear combination is the variance of the projection of the points onto that line. Figure 18.8 shows examples of projections for $a_1, a_1 + a_2$, and $a_1 - a_2$ for two model functions with equal amplitudes oriented 45° apart (the example from the third row of Figure 18.7). Note that for this case the variance of the estimate of $a_1 + a_2$ is much smaller than the variance of the estimate of $a_1 - a_2$, and the variance of a_1 alone (or a_2 alone) is intermediate between these two.

These illustrations are meant to show graphically how the noise is amplified when the model functions are not perpendicular to each other, increasing the variances of the estimates of both a_1 and a_2. Furthermore, the sensitivity of the experimental design to different linear combinations of the amplitudes clearly depends strongly on the geometry of the model functions. For example, the pattern of two stimuli that yielded the model vectors M_1 and M_2 of Figure 18.8 would be a poor design for measuring the differential response to the two stimuli because the variance of such a measurement is so high. In practice, the calculation of the variance of any linear combination of the model functions can be done in a straightforward way

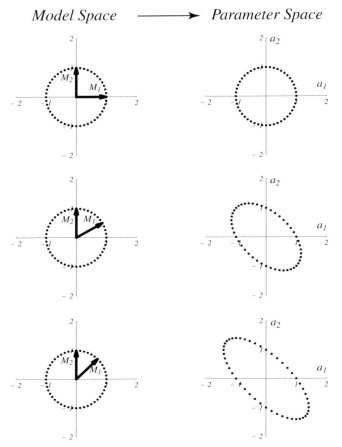

Figure 18.7. Noise transformations from the model space to the parameter space. Noise contributes to all dimensions of the data space, including the model space. The noise is assumed to be isotropic and is illustrated as a ring of points with a radius σ to represent the uncertainty of the projected data point in the model space (left column). When transformed to the parameter space, the ring is distorted into an ellipse at an angle of 45° (for equal amplitudes M_1 and M_2 when the model functions are not orthogonal (right), and this distortion increases the variance of the estimated parameters.

with the covariance matrix of the model functions, as described in Box 18. From the matrix calculations, a more general expression for the SNR can be derived (Equation [B18.7]), analogous to Equation [18.2] for the single model function case.

Another equivalent way to look at the uncertainties of the parameter estimates is to interpret the distribution shown in Figure 18.8 as a two-dimensional (2D) probability distribution for particular amplitudes of a_1 and a_2 given the measured data, called the *a posteriori* (or simply posterior) probability (Frank et al., 1998). The posterior probability distribution has the elliptical shape shown in Figure 18.8 and peaks at the best-fit values of a_1 and a_2. This is a 2D probability distribution, and the one-dimensional (1D) probability distribution for a particular amplitude is a projection onto the appropriate axis. For example, projecting the 2D distribution onto the

Variance of the Model Amplitude Estimates

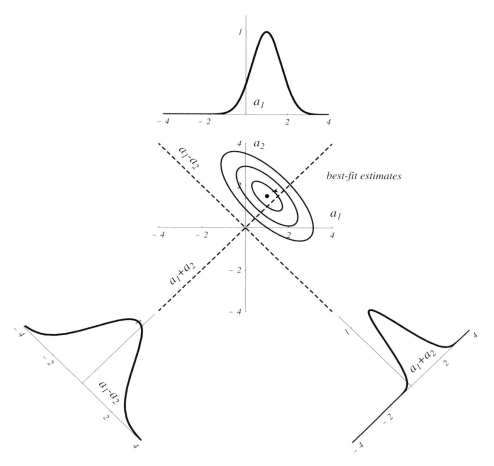

Figure 18.8. Variance of the estimated parameters. The variance of any parameter, or linear combination of parameters, is calculated by projecting the two-dimension distribution of noise points onto the appropriate axis. In this example, the model functions form an angle of 45°, and this nonorthogonality makes some projections have a lower variance than others. For example, the estimate of $a_1 + a_2$ has a much lower variance (the narrower distribution on the lower right) than the estimate of $a_1 - a_2$ (lower left).

a_1-axis is equivalent to integrating over all possible values of a_2 and gives the 1D probability distribution of a_1 independent of the estimate of a_2. The significance of the estimate can be calculated from the degree to which these 1D projected probability distributions overlap zero. Specifically, the probability that the data could have arisen just from noise alone is the area under the curve on the opposite side of zero from the peak. This is equivalent to sliding the 1D distribution until it is centered on zero (the null hypothesis) and calculating the area from the estimated parameter value to infinity (or negative infinity, if the amplitude estimate is negative), which is the probability of obtaining that value or greater by chance alone. For example, in

Figure 18.8 the estimate of $a_1 + a_2$ is reasonably significant because there is very little area under the curve to the left of zero. The estimate of a_1 is somewhat less significant, and the estimate of $a_1 - a_2$ is not significant at all.

Statistical Significance Revisited

In the previous section (and in Box 18), we discussed the variance of the parameter estimates with a view toward deriving a more general expression for the SNR of the measurement of any combination of the model function amplitudes. As with the single model function case, we can also approach the question of statistical significance by constructing a statistic whose distribution is well known under the null hypothesis that there is no activation. However, the appropriate statistic depends on what the model functions actually represent. We can illustrate the basic reasoning with two examples.

For the first example, suppose that we are dealing with a single stimulus type and that we know the hemodynamic response quite well but, in addition, that we want to account for a linear drift of the signal. The activation response is modeled as M_1, and M_2 is the linear drift. Both a_1 and a_2 are calculated from Equation [B18.2], but we are primarily interested in just the amplitude a_1. In other words, we include a second model function to better model the data, but we do not really care about the value of a_2. In mathematical terms, we simply want to project the 2D probability distribution onto the a_1-axis. The ratio of the estimate of a_1 to the expected variance of a_1 is calculated from Equation [B18.7], and just as with the single model function case, this SNR estimate follows a t-distribution under the null hypothesis. However, the degrees of freedom is now $v = N - 2$, because the model space has two dimensions. So the SNR of the measurement of a_1 can be taken as t_v, and the significance can be assessed just as for the case of a single model function.

For the second example, we consider the case where both model functions are necessary to describe the hemodynamic response to a single stimulus. Suppose that the shape of the response is well known but that the delay after stimulus onset and the amplitude of the response are unknown. This can be cast in the form of a linear model by the clever trick of defining $h(t) = h_1(t) + h_2(t)$, where $h_1(t)$ is the hemodynamic response for a fixed delay and $h_2(t)$ is the first time derivative of $h_1(t)$ (Friston et al., 1998a). To first order, a linear combination of a function and its first derivative simply shifts the same function shape along the time axis. Then if $X(t)$ is the stimulus pattern, the model function M_1 is $X(t)*h_1(t)$ with the mean removed, and M_2 is $X(t)*h_2(t)$ with the mean removed. The amplitude a_1 then describes the magnitude of the response, and the amplitude a_2 is proportional to the delay after stimulus onset.

The important difference with the first example is that now both amplitudes are necessary to describe the activation response. In geometric terms, there is no longer a single axis in the model space that is of interest. Instead, we are interested in the significance of the full model estimate, including a_1 and a_2. To test the significance of the model fit, we use an F-statistic, which is essentially a generalization of the t-statistic to model spaces with more than one dimension (Friston et al., 1998a). By the null hypothesis, if there is no activation, then any projection of the data into the model space is entirely due to noise. For any subspace of the data space, we can estimate the noise variance by dividing the length squared of the projection onto that space by n, the dimensions of the space. (Again, this is just the argument that, with independent Gaussian noise, each dimension of a subspace contributes a component σ^2 to the net length squared of the vector in that subspace.) Now consider dividing the data space into a model space with m dimensions and an error space with $v = N - m$ dimensions. In each space, we can calculate an estimate of σ^2, and the ratio of these two estimates is F. Under the null hypothesis, F should be about equal to one, and the question is whether F is sufficiently larger than one to justify rejection of the null hypothesis. The distribution of F depends on the dimensions of the two spaces, and so is usually written as $F_{m,v}$.

Using our earlier notation in which Y_M is the projection onto the model space and Y_E is the length of the component remaining in the error space, we have for our example:

$$F_{2,v} = \frac{Y_M^2/2}{Y_E^2/v} \qquad [18.4]$$

The connection between F and t is clear when the model space has only one dimension, so that $F_{1,v} = t^2_v$. From the value of F, the probability that such a large projection in the model space could have arisen by chance alone can be calculated to determine the statistical significance. Note that this test of significance does not depend on how we decompose Y_M into a set of model amplitudes, and so does not depend on the orthogonality of the model functions (Friston et al., 1998a). The model vectors define the model space, but F depends only on the length of the projection in that space. This point will be important in Chapter 19 when we consider event-related fMRI experimental paradigms.

REFERENCES

Aguirre, G. K., Zarahn, E., and D'Esposito, M. (1998) The variability of human, BOLD hemodynamic responses. *NeuroImage* **8,** 360–76.

Bandettini, P. A., Jesmanowicz, A., Wong, E. C., and Hyde, J. S. (1993) Processing strategies for time-course data sets in functional MRI of the human brain. *Magn. Reson. Med.* **30,** 161–173.

Boynton, G. M., Engel, S. A., Glover, G. H., and Heeger, D. J. (1996) Linear systems analysis of functional magnetic resonance imaging in human V1. *J. Neurosci.* **16,** 4207–21.

Buxton, R. B., Wong, E. C., and Frank, L. R. (1998) Dynamics of blood flow and oxygenation changes during brain activation: The balloon model. *Magn. Reson. Med.* **39,** 855–64.

Engel, S. A., Rumelhart, D. E., Wandell, B. A., Lee, A. T., Glover, G. H., Chichilnisky, E.-J., and Shadlen, M. N. (1994) fMRI of human visual cortex. *Nature* **369, 370 [erratum],** 525, 106 [erratum].

Frank, L. R., Buxton, R. B., and Wong, E. C. (1998) Probabilistic analysis of functional magnetic resonance imaging data. *Magn. Reson. Med.* **39,** 132–48.

Friston, K. J., Fletcher, P., Josephs, O., Holmes, A., Rugg, M. D., and Turner, R. (1998a) Event-related fMRI: Characterizing differential responses. *NeuroImage* **7,** 30–40.

Friston, K. J., Holmes, A. P., Worsley, K. J., Poline, J.-B., Frith, C. D., and Frackowiak, R. S. J. (1995) Statistical parametric maps in functional imaging: A general linear approach. *Human Brain Mapping* **2,** 189–210.

Friston, K. J., Jezzard, P., and Turner, R. (1994) Analysis of functional MRI time-series. *Human Brain Mapping* **1,** 153–71.

Friston, K. J., Josephs, O., Rees, G., and Turner, R. (1998b) Non-linear event related responses in fMRI. *Magn. Reson. Med.* **39,** 41–52.

Friston, K. J., Zarahn, E., Josephs, O., Henson, R. N. A., and Dale, A. M. (1999) Stochastic designs in event-related fMRI. *NeuroImage* **10,** 607–19.

Glover, G. H. (1999) Deconvolution of impulse response in event-related fMRI. *Neuroimage* **9,** 416–29.

Gold, S., Christian, B., Arndt, S., Zeien, G., Cizadlo, T., Johnson, D. L., Flaum, M., and Andreasen, N. C. (1998) Functional MRI statistical software packages: a comparative analysis. *Human Brain Mapping* **6,** 73–84.

Lange, N., Strother, S. C., Anderson, J. R., Nielsen, F. A., Holmes, A. P., Kolenda, T., Savoy, R., and Hansen, L. K. (1999) Plurality and resemblance in fMRI data analysis. *Neuroimage* **10,** 182–303.

Mayhew, J., Zheng, Y., Hou, Y., Vuksanovic, B., Berwick, J., Askew, S., and Coffey, P. (1999) Spectroscopic analysis of changes in remitted illumination: The response to increased neural activity in brain. *Neuroimage* **10,** 304–26.

Purdon, P. L., and Weisskoff, R. M. (1998) Effect of temporal autocorrelation due to physiological noise and stimulus paradigm on voxel-level false-positive rates in fMRI. *Human Brain Mapping* **6,** 239–49.

Saville, D. J., and Wood, G. R. (1991) *Statistical Methods: The Geometric Approach.* Springer-Verlag: New York.

Sereno, M. I., Dale, A. M., Reppas, J. R., Kwong, K. K., Belliveau, J. W., Brady, T. J., Rosen, B. R., and Tootell, R. B. H. (1995) Functional MRI reveals borders of multiple visual areas in humans. *Science* **268,** 889–93.

Vasquez, A. L., and Noll, D. C. (1998) Nonlinear aspects of the BOLD response in functional MRI. *Neuroimage* **7,** 108–18.

Worsley, K. J., Poline, J. B., Friston, K. J., and Evans, A. C. (1997) Characterizing the response of PET and fMRI data using multivariate linear models. *Neuroimage* **6,** 305–19.

Zarahn, E., Aguirre, G. K., and D'Esposito, M. (1997) Empirical analysis of BOLD fMRI statistics: I. Spatially unsmoothed data collected under null-hypothesis conditions. *Neuroimage* **5,** 179–97.

19

Efficient Design of BOLD Experiments

Implications of the General Linear Model for the Design of fMRI Experiments
The Sensitivity for Detection of Weak Activations
The Cost of Multiple Model Functions
Comparing the Responses to Two Different Stimuli
Modeling the Hemodynamic Response

BOX 19. VARIANCE ESTIMATES FOR TWO MODEL
FUNCTIONS

Event-Related fMRI
Trial-Based Experimental Designs
Estimating an Unknown Hemodynamic Response
Detecting an Unknown Hemodynamic Response

IMPLICATIONS OF THE GENERAL LINEAR MODEL FOR THE DESIGN OF fMRI EXPERIMENTS

The Sensitivity for Detection of Weak Activations

The general linear model discussed in Chapter 18 is a powerful and highly flexible technique for analyzing Blood Oxygenation Level Dependent (BOLD) data to estimate the strength and significance of activations. In addition, it provides a useful framework for designing functional magnetic resonance imaging (fMRI) experiments and comparing the sensitivity of different experimental paradigms. For most fMRI applications, the goal is to detect a weak signal change associated with the stimulus, and a direct measure of the sensitivity is the signal-to-noise ratio (SNR) of the measured activation amplitude. Much of the discussion of the general linear model in Chapter 18 was geared toward deriving expressions for the SNR and for the associated statistical measures such as t and F. This chapter focuses on the implications of these SNR considerations for the design of fMRI experiments.

From the arguments made in Chapter 18 for the case of a known hemodynamic response represented by a single model function M, the SNR is given by the simple expression aM/σ. The vector M is the unit amplitude response to the stimulus pattern with the mean removed, and M is the amplitude of M. The true amplitude of the response in the data is a, and σ is the standard deviation of the noise added in to each measurement. The intrinsic activation amplitude a is set by brain physiology, and the noise standard deviation σ is set by the imaging hardware and the pulse sequence used for image acquisition, so we can think of these as being fixed aspects of the experiment. But M, which is proportional to the standard deviation of the data produced by a unit amplitude hemodynamic response, depends on how the stimuli are presented and the shape of the hemodynamic response function. To focus this point, consider a simple experiment with the goal of identifying areas of the brain that respond to a brief stimulus, an *event*. For example, the stimulus could be a single finger tap or a brief flash of light. Suppose that a single run of the experiment consists of a fixed number of events. How should the timing of the events be designed to maximize the sensitivity of the experiment for detecting weak activations? At first glance, it might appear that the timing of the stimuli does not really matter because it will always be the responses to the same number of events that are averaged. However, the somewhat surprising result is that the sensitivity depends strongly on the design of the stimulus presentation.

To be concrete, suppose that we divide the time axis into steps of duration δt smaller than any of the other time intervals of interest in the experiment. For any pattern of identical events, we can describe the stimulus pattern by a function X_i, where X_i, has a value of one if an event occurs at the ith time step and zero if there is no event. The unit amplitude hemodynamic response is h_i, where h_i is the amplitude of the signal change at i time steps after an event. The terminology "unit amplitude" means that this is the amplitude of response corresponding to $a = 1$ in our analysis. Then the unit amplitude BOLD response to the stimulus pattern is the convolution of the stimulus pattern with the hemodynamic response, $X_i * h_i$. This response is then sampled at intervals of TR, the repetition time, and the vector M consists of these sampled values with the mean subtracted. If there are N images in the experimental run, then M is a vector in an N-dimensional data space. The magnitude of M directly reflects the variance in the data due to a unit amplitude response. Specifically, the variance is $M^2/(N - 1)$. The sensitivity for detection of a response depends on how large this variance is compared with the noise variance σ^2, so the magnitude of M is a useful index of the sensitivity of an experiment.

Figure 19.1 shows three types of timing pattern for an fMRI experiment: evenly spaced single trials, randomized single trials, and blocked stimuli, with examples for 8 stimuli and 16 stimuli presented in a 1-min run. For each example, the hemodynamic response to each stimulus (modeled as Equation [18.1]) is the same. However, the magnitude of M for these different experimental designs differs by more than a factor of 2 for the example with 8 stimuli and by nearly a factor of 4 for the example with 16 stimuli! For the case of 16 stimuli, the hemodynamic response smooths out the individual responses in the periodic single trial paradigm, creating little variance in the net response and a corresponding low value of M. In contrast,

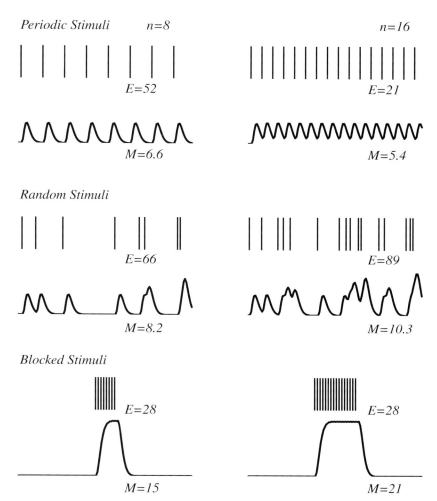

Periodic Stimuli $n=8$ $n=16$

$E=52$ $E=21$

$M=6.6$ $M=5.4$

Random Stimuli

$E=66$ $E=89$

$M=8.2$ $M=10.3$

Blocked Stimuli

$E=28$ $E=28$

$M=15$ $M=21$

Figure 19.1. The sensitivity of different experimental designs. Timing patterns of stimuli and the expected hemodynamic response are shown for periodic single trials (top row), randomized single trials (middle row), and blocked stimuli (bottom row). Examples for 8 trials (left) and 16 trials (right) within a 1-min time frame are shown. The sensitivity of each pattern (the expected SNR) for *detecting* an activation is proportional to the standard deviation of the response vector measured by M. The efficiency of each pattern for *estimating* the shape of the hemodynamic response E is calculated from Equation [19.3]. Note that the blocked design is best for detecting an activation, the randomized pattern is best for estimating the shape of the hemodynamic response, and the periodic single trial pattern is poor for both tasks.

with the blocked design, the combination of long off periods without a response and overlapping responses from different events when they are bunched together creates a large variance. Because M is four times larger with the blocked design, the SNR also is four times larger for the same response. To match the sensitivity of the blocked design, by repeating the single trial paradigm and averaging, would require 16 times as many stimuli because SNR increases only with the square root of the number of averages.

The sensitivity of the SNR to the exact stimulus pattern comes about because the hemodynamic response is broad compared to the minimum interval between the onsets of repeated events. In this analysis, we assume that each event produces the same, stereotypical BOLD response. In particular, this assumes that overlapping responses to different events simply add. There is a limit to how close together two events can be such that the neural activity evoked by each event is the same. But this limiting interval typically is on the order of 1 s or less (Friston et al., 1999). If we take this as a practical lower limit for event spacing to maintain approximate linearity of the response, this minimum interval is still much less than the width of the hemodynamic response. If the hemodynamic response had a comparable width of about 1 s, then the response to each event would be essentially finished before the next event occurs. In this case, the exact timing of the events would not make any difference. Each event would elicit a brief response, and the SNR of the average response would just depend on the total number of events presented.

But with a broader hemodynamic response, there is much more opportunity for responses to overlap. Interestingly, this overlap can either increase or decrease M. In the block design, the signal difference between the control and activated states is maximized because of the constructive build-up of overlapping responses during the activation; thus, M is maximized with a block design for any given number of stimuli. However, for periodic single trials, the regularity of the overlap of responses tends to smooth out the intrinsic variance of the stimulus pattern and produces a minimum value for M for any given number of stimuli. For a periodic single trial design, the dependence of M on the number of stimuli is a bit subtle. Suppose that we start with a single stimulus, and each time we add another we rearrange them into a periodic pattern. When the stimuli are widely separated, each new stimulus adds to the variance and so increases M. However, once the responses from different stimuli begin to overlap, the smoothing effect of the hemodynamic response reduces the variance, so M decreases with any further increase in the number of stimuli (e.g., in going from 8 to 16 stimuli in Figure 19.1). For this reason there is an optimal spacing of about 12–15 s between stimuli that maximizes M for a periodic design. However, even at this optimal spacing, the sensitivity of the periodic single trial design is much less than a block design with the same number of stimuli.

Randomized events allow for longer off periods and some constructive bunching of the stimuli, creating a value of M intermediate between the optimal block design and a periodic single trial design. Increasing the number of events in a randomized design produces a rather counterintuitive effect. Naively, we might expect that the overlap of responses would decrease the sensitivity just as it does for periodic single trials. However, the result is just the opposite (Figure 19.1). Increasing the number of stimuli in a randomized pattern continues to increase the variance of the response, creating a larger M and improved sensitivity.

One way to understand these effects of experimental design is to look at the frequency content of the stimulus pattern (Figure 19.2). For a fixed number of stimuli, the variance of the stimulus pattern itself is always the same, but the distribution of that variance among different frequency components depends strongly on the exact timing of the stimuli. The hemodynamic response is essentially a smoothing function

Time Domain   *Frequency Domain*

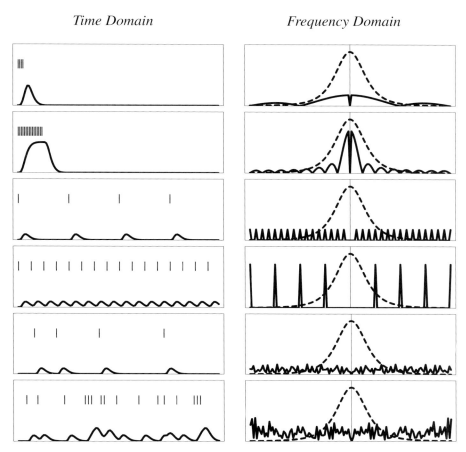

Figure 19.2. Frequency domain analysis of the sensitivity of different experimental designs. Panels show examples of blocked (top two rows), periodic single trial (middle two rows), and randomized (bottom two rows) stimulus events. Time domain plots (left) show the stimulus events and the expected BOLD signal changes calculated by convolving the stimulus pattern with the hemodynamic response. In the frequency domain (right), the convolution multiplies the hemodynamic response (dashed curve) with the frequency spectrum of the stimulus pattern, attenuating the high frequencies. The sensitivity is roughly proportional to the area of the stimulus spectrum under the envelope of the hemodynamic response. Sensitivity of a block design or a random design is improved by increasing the number of events, but for a periodic single trial design, as the time between events is reduced, the fundamental frequency moves out from under the hemodynamic response envelope, and sensitivity is reduced.

that attenuates the higher frequencies of the stimulus pattern. For stimulus patterns dominated by low frequencies, such as the block design, more of the intrinsic variance of the stimulus pattern is preserved after the smoothing, producing a larger M. For the periodic single trial design, the lowest frequency component corresponds to the fundamental stimulus frequency, and the rest of the energy is in higher harmonics of the fundamental frequency. The fundamental frequency of the stimulus pattern continues to grow as more stimuli are added and the spacing between stimuli is reduced, so more of the intrinsic variance of the stimulus pattern is attenuated due to the smoothing by the hemodynamic response function. For the randomized design, the frequency spectrum is essentially flat, and as more stimuli are added, all frequency components increase, including the low frequencies. Because of this, the remaining variance after smoothing with the hemodynamic response continues to grow as more randomized events are added.

The Cost of Multiple Model Functions

The same design arguments carry over to the more general case of multiple model functions. The question of how many model functions to include in the general linear model is critical for the analysis, yet this is probably the most difficult question to answer in a general way. Clearly, if we use insufficient model functions to describe the data, we run the risk of systematic errors in the estimates of the parameters. On the other hand, using more model functions than necessary decreases the sensitivity. To see how these conflicting considerations come into play, we can examine a simple example of a single cycle of a block design stimulus presentation in the presence of a potential linear drift of the baseline signal. This is illustrated with two examples in Figure 19.3, one with the stimulus block at the beginning of the run and one with the block centered in the run. The important difference in these two scenarios is that the response to the stimulus and a linear drift are nearly orthogonal when the stimulus is centered but that they are strongly nonorthogonal when the stimulus is offset to one end of the run. For each example, the simulated data were analyzed with only a single model function M_1 representing the response to the stimulus or with two model functions with the second model function M_2 representing the linear drift. The resulting best-fit model curve in each case is shown as a dashed line superimposed on the data. The activation amplitude a and the noise standard deviation σ are the same for all the variations of the experiment.

These examples illustrate the trade-offs between systematic errors due to a failure to account for part of the data (e.g., the linear drift) and the reduction in sensitivity that comes with including model functions that are not required (e.g., accounting for the drift when none is present). Consider first the systematic errors that occur if only a single model function is used (left column in Figure 19.3). If the magnitude of the drift is negligible (middle row in each panel), the analysis with a single model function provides a good fit to the data and an accurate estimate of the response amplitude as indicated by the best-fit model curve. Furthermore, the statistical significance is quite high as measured by t.

Now suppose that a linear drift *is* present, as shown in the bottom row of each panel. If we only use a single model function, the response amplitude is greatly underestimated when the stimulus is off-center in the run. This systematic error in the estimate of a comes about because the model function M_1 is not perpendicular to a linear drift. If instead we had carefully centered the stimulus in the middle of the run, as shown in the lower panels of Figure 19.3, the estimate of a would still be correct even in the presence of a linear drift because M_1 is nearly orthogonal to the linear drift. However, the significance of the detection (t) is substantially reduced because the additional variance due to the linear drift adds to the variance due to noise, effectively causing us to overestimate the noise magnitude and thus underes-

Stimulus Response Not Orthogonal to Drift

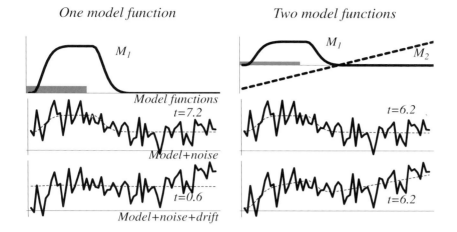

Stimulus Response Orthogonal to Drift

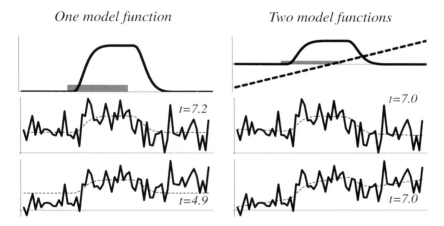

Figure 19.3. Accounting for signal drift. The costs and benefits of analyzing a BOLD pixel time course with a single model function M_1 (left) and with two model functions where M_2 is a linear drift are illustrated. The effects of a linear drift depend on whether the stimulus response is orthogonal to the drift (bottom) or nonorthogonal (top). If no drift is present (middle row of each panel), the cost of analyzing the data with two model functions is a reduction of significance (lower t) when the two model functions are not orthogonal. When a drift is present (third row of each panel), analysis with M_1 alone yields an incorrect estimate of the amplitude when the stimulus response is not orthogonal to the drift, but it yields a correct estimate with reduced t when they are orthogonal.

timate the significance of the measured response. In short, the minimum damage caused by neglecting a baseline drift is that the statistical significance is underestimated, and in the worst case both the estimated activation amplitude and the statistical significance are grossly misestimated.

Now consider what happens when we include a linear drift as a second model function M_2 in the analysis, as illustrated in the right column of Figure 19.3. The general linear model provides an accurate estimate of a, even if M_1 and M_2 are not orthogonal, so systematic errors are no longer a problem. However, the sensitivity is reduced, and the cost in sensitivity of including a drift term in the analysis depends strongly on the geometrical relationship of M_1 to M_2. If they are perpendicular to each other, as in the bottom of Figure 19.3, the cost is minimal. The degrees of freedom v is reduced by one because the model space now has two dimensions, but this is a negligible change when the number of images is on the order of 100. But if the two model functions are not orthogonal, the resulting t-statistic is reduced further (upper right panel of Figure 19.3).

The loss in sensitivity is directly related to the angle ϕ between M_1 and M_2. If one follows through the calculations outlined in Box 18 for the case of two model functions (see Box 19), the SNR of the estimate of a_1 for the case of two model functions turns out to be $SNR_0 \sin \phi$, where SNR_0 is the SNR that would be measured if the data were analyzed with only a single correct model function. The factor of $\sin \phi$ is the mathematical result of the spreading of noise points into an ellipse, as illustrated in Figure 18.8. Note that the reduction in SNR is independent of whether or not a linear drift is actually present in the data. It comes about simply because we have included the possibility in the analysis. The resulting degradation in fact is completely independent of the actual magnitude of the slope in the data.

In summary, the failure to include systematic effects such as a baseline drift in the analysis can severely degrade the sensitivity of the experiment. Including additional model functions that are orthogonal to the model function of interest exacts a negligible cost in sensitivity, but including model functions that are not orthogonal can severely decrease the sensitivity. For this reason it is important to choose a stimulus pattern that is as orthogonal as possible to simple systematic drift patterns. A single block of activity centered in the run is orthogonal to a linear drift, as in the foregoing example. However, it is not orthogonal to a quadratic drift. In general, for block designs, it is better to use several cycles to make M_1 approximately orthogonal to slow variations of the baseline. Another way of looking at this is that the Fourier spectrum of the signal often has large components at low frequencies due to baseline drift, and choosing the fundamental stimulus frequency to be higher moves the desired signal to a less noisy part of the spectrum (Zarahn, Aguirre, and D'Esposito, 1997b).

Unfortunately, however, this prescription is in direct conflict with the arguments of the preceding section: to maximize SNR, the smoothing effect of the hemodynamic response should be minimized by concentrating the energy of the stimulus pattern at the lowest frequencies, as in the single block design. There is thus a trade-off between two factors that affect the SNR: the magnitude of M_1 and the orthogonality of M_1 with low-frequency signal drifts. In practice, blocked design experimental runs usually contain four to eight cycles of stimulus/control as a compromise between these two effects.

Comparing the Responses to Two Different Stimuli

Another example of the use of two model functions is the task of detecting a differential response to two stimuli. Suppose that our goal is to detect areas that are

BOX 19. VARIANCE ESTIMATES FOR TWO MODEL FUNCTIONS

In Box 18 the mathematical formalism for the general linear model was developed. We now want to examine the specific case of two model functions to derive expressions for evaluating the sensitivity of different experimental designs. The two model functions M_1 and M_2 describe vectors in an N-dimensional data space, where N is the number of measured time samples in the data. The two vectors M_1 and M_2 form the two columns of the design matrix M. If M_1 and M_2 are the magnitudes of these vectors, and ϕ is the angle between them in the data space, then

$$M^T M = \begin{pmatrix} M_1^2 & M_1 M_2 \cos(\phi) \\ M_1 M_2 \cos(\phi) & M_2^2 \end{pmatrix} \qquad \text{[B19.1]}$$

And the covariance matrix is

$$(M^T M)^{-1} = \frac{1}{M_1^2 M_2^2 (1 - \cos^2(\phi))} \begin{pmatrix} M_2^2 & -M_1 M_2 \cos(\phi) \\ -M_1 M_2 \cos(\phi) & M_1^2 \end{pmatrix} \qquad \text{[B19.2]}$$

The parameters a_1 and a_2 are estimated from Equation [B18.2]. The variance of the estimate of any linear combination of the parameters a_1 and a_2 is calculated from the covariance matrix by defining an appropriate contrast w and using Equation [B18.6]. We can now use this to estimate the sensitivity of two example experiments. The first is the case where the hemodynamic response is known and is modeled with M_1, but in addition we include a linear drift of the signal modeled with M_2. Then the contrast of interest is just a_1, so with $w = \{1,0\}$, we find from Equation [B18.6]:

$$\sigma_1 = \sigma \frac{1}{M_1 \sin(\phi)} \qquad \text{[B19.3]}$$

The variance of the estimated amplitude depends inversely on the magnitude of M_1, as expected but also on the angle ϕ. If the stimulus response is not orthogonal to the signal drift, the sensitivity is reduced.

As a second example, suppose that M_1 and M_2 model the responses to two different stimuli. If the goal is to measure the differential response, we can construct an expression for the variance of the estimate of $a_1 - a_2$ by using the contrast $w = \{1, -1\}$ and Equation [B18.6]:

$$\sigma_{1-2} = \sigma \frac{\sqrt{M_1^2 + M_2^2 + 2 M_1 M_2 \cos(\phi)}}{M_1 M_2 \sin(\phi)} \qquad \text{[B19.4]}$$

Note that this variance depends on the magnitudes M_1 and M_2 and also on the angle between them. If M_1 and M_2 have equal magnitudes, then the variance for $a_1 - a_2$ reduces to

$$\sigma_{1-2} = \sigma \frac{1}{M_1 \sin\left(\frac{\phi}{2}\right)} \qquad \text{[B19.5]}$$

(continued)

BOX 12, continued

From this we can see that it is not possible to maximize simultaneously the sensitivity for
detecting a response to one of the stimuli (e.g., a_1) and for detecting the differential
response to the two stimuli ($a_1 - a_2$). The former is maximized when $\phi = 90°$, while the
latter is maximized when $\phi = 180°$. For example, a block of stimulus 1 alternated with a
block of stimulus 2 creates an angle ϕ of about $180°$ (the response to one stimulus is
approximately minus one times the response to the other). This is excellent for detecting
the differential response but poor for detecting the response to either stimulus alone.

---

activated by stimulus 1, areas that are activated by stimulus 2, and areas that
respond differentially to the two stimuli. For example, in one of the original demonstrations of the use of randomized stimuli, Clark and co-workers used a more
sophisticated version of this paradigm to compare responses to a memorized target
face, novel faces, and scrambled nonsense faces (Clark, Maisog, and Haxby, 1998).
For our simplified thought experiment we can imagine that the two stimuli are novel
faces and scrambled faces. Stimuli are presented on a time grid with one second
intervals, so that in each second either stimulus 1, stimulus 2, or no stimulus is presented.

Again we model the data as a linear combination of two model functions M_1 and
M_2 with unknown amplitudes a_1 and a_2. However, unlike the previous example in
which M_2 represented a nuisance function (signal drift), M_2 now models the
response to stimulus 2. We would like to optimize the experiment to allow precise
estimates of a_1 and a_2 as well as the differential response $a_1 - a_2$. The mathematical
formalism for analyzing such data with the general linear model was developed in
Box 18, and specific equations for the case of two model functions are derived in
Box 19. The general approach is to form unit amplitude response models M_1 and M_2
by convolving the hemodynamic response function separately with each of the stimulus patterns $X_1(t)$ and $X_2(t)$. The design matrix M is constructed from the vectors
M_1 and M_2, and the covariance matrix is calculated from M. With the covariance
matrix, the variance of the estimate of any linear combination of the model amplitudes can be calculated.

In Box 19 the general result for two model functions is calculated. For simplicity,
consider the case in which the magnitudes M_1 and M_2 are equal (this is usually
approximately true if equal numbers of each stimulus type are presented). Then if
the intrinsic noise standard deviation is σ, the standard deviation σ_1 of the estimate
of a_1 is

$$\sigma_1 = \sigma \, \frac{1}{M_1 \sin (\phi)} \qquad\qquad [19.1]$$

and the standard deviation for a_2 is the same. The standard deviation σ_{1-2} of the estimate of $a_1 - a_2$ is

$$SNR \propto \frac{1}{\sqrt{T_1}} \left[\sqrt{\frac{T_1}{TR}} \ s \right.$$ [19.2]

In these equations ϕ is the angle formed between the vectors $\mathbf{M_1}$ and $\mathbf{M_2}$. Because our goal is to estimate both a_1 and $a_1 - a_2$ with high precision, we can take $1/\sigma_1$ and $1/\sigma_{1-2}$ as measures of the sensitivity of the experiment. Figure 19.4 shows examples of several stimulus patterns and the corresponding sensitivities. From Equations [19.1] and [19.2], it is clear that it is not possible to optimize the experiment simultaneously for measuring both the separate response to stimulus 1 and the differential response $a_1 - a_2$. Both sensitivities are improved with larger values of M_1, but the optimum angle ϕ is 90° for sensitivity to a_1 and 180° for sensitivity to $a_1 - a_2$. For example, the top row of Figure 19.4 shows the case of one block of stimulus 1 alternated with one block of stimulus 2. In this case, $\mathbf{M_1}$ is approximately equal to $-\mathbf{M_2}$, so ϕ is near 180°. This produces good contrast for the differential response, but because there is essentially no period without one of the stimuli, the estimate of a_1 (or a_2) alone is poor. Shorter blocks produce a better estimate of a_1, but at the expense of the estimate of $a_1 - a_2$. Randomized patterns often produce orthogonal response patterns, but because the magnitudes of M_1 and M_2 are smaller for the same number of stimuli with random designs than with blocked presentations, the sensitivity is reduced.

Modeling the Hemodynamic Response

In the preceding examples, additional model functions were used to describe systematic effects in the data in addition to the activation response itself or to model the responses to different stimuli. But another potential source of systematic error is that the hemodynamic response varies from person to person and from one brain region to another (Aguirre, Zarahn, and D'Esposito, 1998). Assuming the wrong shape for the hemodynamic response will reduce the sensitivity because the response is not adequately described. Using several model functions to model a range of hemodynamic responses to a single stimulus is a useful approach for dealing with this problem.

The most likely source of error in this regard is using the wrong delay for the hemodynamic response, and in general a block design is less sensitive to systematic errors due to an unknown delay than a single trial paradigm. To deal with this problem, suppose that we model the effects of a delay in an approximate way by including a second model function proportional to the time derivative of the hemodynamic response, as introduced in Chapter 18 (Friston et al., 1998a). That is, instead of modeling the full hemodynamic response as $ah(t)$, we model it as $a_1h_1(t) + a_2h_2(t)$, with $h_2(t)$ proportional to the derivative of $h_1(t)$. Then the model vectors $\mathbf{M_1}$ and $\mathbf{M_2}$ are derived from the convolutions of $h_1(t)$ and $h_2(t)$, respectively, with the stimulus pattern $X(t)$. Figure 19.5 illustrates an example of the two hemodynamic response functions and also shows how different values of the amplitude of the second function shift the curve along the time axis. Note that it is not a clean time shift because there is some change of shape as well, but this approach never-

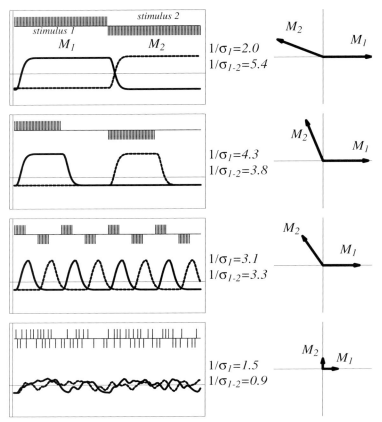

Figure 19.4. Comparing the responses to two different stimuli. Data measured with two different stimuli can be analyzed with two model functions M_1 and M_2 calculated by convolving the separate stimulus patterns with the hemodynamic response. The sensitivity for detecting the response to a single stimulus (e.g., a_1) or the differential response ($a_1 - a_2$) depends on the geometry of the two vectors M_1 and M_2 (illustrated on the right). For each pattern of stimulus presentation, the figure of merit for the sensitivity is the inverse of the expected standard deviation (i.e., $1/\sigma_1$ is the sensitivity for measuring a_1 and $1/\sigma_{1-2}$ is the sensitivity for measuring $a_1 - a_2$). The two sensitivities are different: a single block of stimulus 1 alternated with a single block of stimulus 2 is sensitive to the differential response but poor for estimating the response to either stimulus alone. The sensitivity depends both on the magnitudes of M_1 and M_2 and on the angle between them.

theless provides a way to model a range of hemodynamic responses with only two model functions.

To avoid systematic errors, it is important to include a sufficiently flexible model for the hemodynamic response that can provide a reasonable description of any response that could occur. But as the number of model functions grows, there is a cost in sensitivity that is directly related to the number of dimensions of the model space. To estimate this cost, we can make the following comparison for the case of an unknown delay but a known shape of the response. Imagine that we analyze a data set naively with a single model function that happens to have the right delay, so there is no systematic error, and also with our two previously described model func-

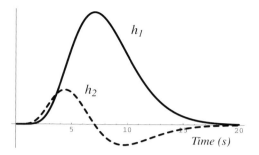

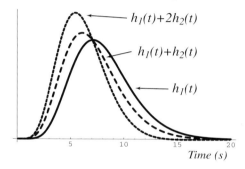

Figure 19.5. Modeling a range of hemodynamic response shapes. The effect of an unknown delay to peak after activation can be modeled by including a second model function M_2 that is proportional to the time derivative of the assumed hemodynamic response modeled with M_1 (top) (Friston et al., 1998a). A linear combination of the two functions then approximates a shift of the response along the time axis (bottom).

tions, which allow for variations of the delay. Because we have imagined that M_1 is constructed with the correct delay, the true amplitude of M_2 is $a_2 = 0$.

From the geometric viewpoint, the correct model function is M_1. Then the difference in the two analysis approaches is whether we treat the model space as simply the axis M_1 or whether we also include a second axis M_2. For each approach, we construct an expected F-statistic from Equation [18.4] to gauge the sensitivity. That is, we calculate the typical magnitude of F that we would expect to find for a true amplitude a_1 and then evaluate the significance of that value for the appropriate degrees of freedom. To calculate F, we take the squared length of the component of the data in the model space divided by the dimensionality of the model space and divide this by the estimate of σ^2 from the error space. For both modeling schemes, the magnitude of the component along M_1 is $a_1 M_1$. For the single model function case, this is the full projection onto the model space, so the expected value of the F-statistic is $F_{1,N-1} = a_1^2 M_1^2/\sigma^2$. For the case with two model functions, the full length of the model space component is $a_1 M_1$ plus a noise component along the other axis of the model space (i.e., the axis perpendicular to M_1 but lying in the plane formed by M_1 and M_2). This noise component is expected to add a factor σ^2 to the total length squared of the projection of the data onto the model space. Our estimate of the magnitude of the F-statistic is then $F_{2,N-2} = (a_1^2 M_1^2 + \sigma^2)/2\sigma^2$. As an example of the difference in sensitivity this creates, suppose that $a_1 M_1$ is two times larger than σ and that $N = 100$. Then the associated p-values for these two F-statistics are 0.048 for the single model case and 0.087 for the two model case. Including even more model functions to describe the hemodynamic response further decreases the sensitivity. Essentially, the source of this effect is that the probability of finding a vector of length M_1 in an m-dimensional space by chance continues to grow as m increases, so the significance for any fixed magnitude of response continues to diminish as more model functions are added.

In summary, the choice of the number of model functions required to model the hemodynamic response is a balancing act between too few functions and the resulting potential systematic errors and too many functions and the resulting loss in sensitivity. As our understanding of the hemodynamic response improves, it should be possible to define a minimal set of basis functions that strikes an efficient compromise.

EVENT-RELATED fMRI

Trial-Based Experimental Designs

Early fMRI studies used a block design of stimulus presentation, with individual trials or events tightly clustered into "on" periods of activation alternated with equally long "off" control periods. However, for many applications, a block design is not feasible, or at the very least introduces an artificial quality into the stimulus that makes the results difficult to interpret. A trial-based (or event-related) design significantly broadens the types of neural processes that can be investigated (Buckner et al., 1996, 1998; Burock et al., 1998; Dale, 1999; Dale and Buckner, 1997; Friston et al., 1998a, 1998b, 1999; Josephs, Turner, and Friston 1997; Zarahn, Aguirre, and D'Esposito, 1997a). A block design by definition presents similar stimuli together, which makes it difficult to study processes where predictability of the stimulus is an important consideration. For example, studies of recognition using familiar stimuli and novel stimuli are hampered if all the familiar stimuli are presented together. A trial-based design allows randomization of different stimuli and a more sophisticated experimental design.

Event-related experiments often involve a second feature distinct from the single trial presentation aspect: no assumptions are made about the shape of the hemodynamic response. This second feature is motivated by concerns about the variability of the shape of the hemodynamic response in different brain regions. In the simplest form of this approach, one can do an fMRI experiment analogous to an evoked potential experiment. Single trials of a particular stimulus are presented, and the responses are averaged time-locked to the stimulus presentation. That is, the images are rearranged into time order following a stimulus and appropriately averaged. If the separation between trials is sufficiently long so that there is no overlap of responses, this selective averaging approach directly provides a measure of the hemodynamic response on a voxel-by-voxel basis.

Event-related paradigms make possible a broader range of experiments with fMRI, and these techniques are now being applied in many studies. However, there is still some controversy in the literature over the sensitivity of different patterns of stimulus presentation, and whether the hemodynamic response is important in determining this sensitivity (Dale, 1999; Friston et al., 1999). In this section, we will try to clarify these issues and argue that the controversy arises primarily because there are two distinct types of sensitivity that can be addressed by the statistical analysis. The crux of the argument of this section is that there are really two questions one could ask: (1) which stimulus pattern provides the most sensitive *estimate* of the local hemodynamic response when the shape is unknown?, and (2) which stimulus pattern provides the most sensitive *detection* of activation when the shape of the hemodynamic response is unknown? These two questions are distinct, and as we will see next the answers are different.

For many applications, the choice of experimental design is dictated by the cognitive processes under investigation, and the experimenter may have little flexibility about when events occur. For example, to correlate neural activity separately with correct and incorrect identifications of target stimuli, the pattern of correct responses is not known until after the experiment is completed. For such an experiment, there may be little room for optimizing the stimulus presentation. However, it is important to consider the efficiency of different designs in a more general way so that the potential costs of one design over another can be compared. In this section, we will focus on this more general question of sensitivity, as if we have complete control over when stimuli occur. We consider an idealized stimulus that could be presented in either a block design, periodic single trials, or randomized single trials. In either case, we assume that each trial (or event) elicits the same hemodynamic response. As we put events closer together, this assumption will break down, so we assume that there is a minimum interval between events t_{min}. Specifically, we assume that the neural activity induced by an event occurring at time t_{min} or greater after another event is identical to the neural activity produced by the first event and that these two bursts of neural activity create identical hemodynamic responses that add linearly. With this simple model, we can address the two questions posed earlier: which design is best for estimating the hemodynamic response?, and which is best for detecting an activation?

Estimating an Unknown Hemodynamic Response

The framework for understanding these experiments is still the general linear model. To model the hemodynamic response on a voxel-by-voxel basis, we treat the response at each time lag t_i as a separate model function. For example, if we assume that the hemodynamic response to an event lasts for 10 s, and we want to measure this response at 1-s intervals, then we need ten model functions. It is easiest to visualize this in the simplified case in which stimuli are presented and images are acquired on an evenly spaced grid of 1-s time intervals. That is, the stimulus pattern X_i is a series of ones and zeros at regular time intervals of 1 s, describing whether an event does or does not occur at that time point. Images also are acquired with a regular interval of 1 s. (In fact, these assumptions can be substantially relaxed, but this simple case illustrates the basic ideas.)

The most direct way to estimate the hemodynamic response is to average all the images that are made 1 s after an event, all images that are measured 2 s after an event, and so on until we have estimated the response at 10 s after an event. This selective averaging approach is much like the approach used in evoked potential recordings, in which many stimuli are presented and the responses averaged time-locked to the stimuli (Dale and Buckner, 1997). However, the problem with the naive version of this approach is that overlap of responses is not taken into account. For example, a particular image could be both 2 s after an event and 5 s after another event, and the two responses are thus combined in that image.

We can analyze event-related data directly in terms of the general linear model using the formalism developed in Box 18 by defining a design matrix M consisting of ten model functions. The model function corresponding to a lag of 0 s is simply the stimulus pattern X_i itself, and the model function for a lag of n s is simply the pattern X_i shifted n steps to the right. Each successive column of the design matrix is then X_i shifted down by one from the previous column. (More completely, each column is a shifted version of X_i with zeroes added at the beginning and with the mean removed.) The estimated hemodynamic response to a single event then consists of a vector of amplitudes a, which is calculated with Equation [B18.2]. Note that if the model functions were all orthogonal to each other, the covariance matrix $(M^T M)^{-1}$ would simply reduce to a diagonal matrix, and the remaining term $M^T Y$ in Equation [B18.2] is equivalent to a simple time-locked averaging of the response to individual stimuli. In other words, the correction for response overlap that is missing from the naive reordering approach is taken into account by the covariance matrix in Equation [B18.2].

The result of the model fitting is a set of ten amplitudes defining the local hemodynamic response. How precise is this estimate? As described in Box 18, the variance of any parameter or combination of parameters can be calculated with the covariance matrix. However, in the current formulation, each parameter is the amplitude of one time point of the hemodynamic response, and we are really interested in the error of the whole estimated response. A useful way to think about this is to consider the parameter space defined by the set of amplitudes a_i (i.e., each axis corresponds to one of the a_i). The true hemodynamic response then corresponds to a point in this ten-dimensional parameter space, and our estimated hemodynamic response is another point displaced from the true point. The two points do not coincide because noise produces some variance in each of the estimates of a_i, and the distance between the estimated point and the true point is a measure of the error in the estimate of the hemodynamic response. The expected distance measured in the parameter space is simply the sum of the variances for each of the a_i, and this in turn is proportional to the sum of the diagonal terms of the covariance matrix, called the *trace* of the matrix (symbolized by "Tr"). So a useful measure of the efficiency of our experimental design for estimating the hemodynamic response is the inverse of the expected error measured in the parameter space (Dale, 1999):

$$E = \frac{1}{\sigma \sqrt{\mathrm{Tr}\left\{(M^T M)^{-1}\right\}}}$$

[19.3]

Maximizing E is equivalent to minimizing the sum of the squared errors at each time point of the hemodynamic response. In practical terms, if the efficiency E of one experimental design is only half that of another, then the less efficient design would have to be repeated and averaged four times to achieve the same statistical quality of the estimated hemodynamic response. The efficiency is, of course, inversely proportional to the noise standard deviation but also depends on a geometric factor through the covariance matrix. Note that the actual hemodynamic response does not enter into the expression for E. That is, the design matrix M is constructed directly from the stimulus pattern, not the stimulus pattern convolved with a hemodynamic response function. Or to put it another way, for any shape of the hemodynamic response, the efficiency for estimating that response depends only on the stimulus pattern itself.

The efficiency E can be used to rank the sensitivity of any pattern of stimuli. For example, one can compare different random sequences generated with different mean interstimulus intervals. The remarkable result is that the efficiency E continues to improve as the interstimulus interval is decreased (i.e., as more stimuli are included in a run of the same total duration) (Dale, 1999). In other words, even though the interstimulus interval is significantly less than the width of the hemodynamic response, the efficiency is improved. However, even for a fixed average interstimulus interval, there is a wide variation in E for different random patterns. We can understand both of these effects from the arguments developed earlier. In general, the larger the variance of the expected model response (i.e., the magnitude of the vector M in our earlier analysis), the better the SNR will be. For this case, each model function is essentially a shifted version of the stimulus pattern X_i, so the variance of the data due to the response at each time point after an event (and thus the magnitudes of M_1, M_2, M_3, etc.) increases as more stimuli are added in and the interstimulus interval decreases. On the other hand, we found earlier that nonorthogonality of the model functions can severely degrade the SNR of the amplitude estimates. So the variability of E for different random patterns with the same number of stimuli (and thus the same intrinsic variance of the model vectors) is due to different degrees of nonorthogonality of the model functions. In practice, typically many stimulus patterns are generated and their efficiency calculated to find a pattern with desirable properties (Dale, 1999).

Detecting an Unknown Hemodynamic Response

The preceding arguments answer the first question posed earlier: the best pattern of stimuli for estimating the hemodynamic response is found by maximizing the efficiency E. However, to answer the second question and determine the best design for *detecting* an activation, we need to reason a bit differently. We return to our original geometric view of the general linear model, in which Y_M is the projection of the data into a defined model space and Y_E is the remaining error component perpendicular to the model space. In the current case, the model space has ten dimensions and completely describes any hemodynamic response that could occur within 10 s of an event. In other words, the only assumptions we are making about the form of the hemodynamic response is that it varies slowly enough that it is fully captured by describing its value at 1-s intervals, and it does not last more than 10 s. Either of these assumptions could be relaxed by increasing the number of time points defining the hemodynamic response, which would simply increase the number of dimensions of the model space.

The important factor in determining the sensitivity for detecting activation is the magnitude of the projection Y_M compared to Y_E. As described earlier, this ratio defines an F-statistic that can be used to test whether the magnitude of the component of the data lying in the model space can be attributed to chance alone. The important point is that we do not care how the projection Y_M is modeled in terms of individual amplitude estimates; F is based just on the magnitude of Y_M. In contrast, for estimating the hemodynamic response, we are specifically interested in the amplitudes a_i and the errors in the estimates of each of the a_i. In both cases, we are looking at the point Y_M, but the distinction is that F is evaluated in the model space and E is evaluated in the parameter space. And the added feature of the parameter space is that noise is amplified in the transformation from the model space to the parameter space if the model vectors are not perpendicular to each other in the model space. Then it is possible for two stimulus patterns to produce identical expected values of F but have radically different values of E because one pattern creates a more regular pattern of overlap of the responses and a correspondingly more severe case of nonorthogonality of the model functions.

We can further explore this distinction by estimating the magnitude we should expect for F, as we did earlier. For any brain region, there is a true hemodynamic response, even if we do not know its shape, and when this true response is convolved with the stimulus pattern, it produces a vector M. Then, for a true activation with amplitude a, the expected magnitude of the projection of the data into the model space is aM, and so the magnitude of F is directly determined by M. To put it another way, the true model response corresponds to a particular direction in the data space. We do not know what direction this is, but by using ten model functions to describe a general response, we are confident that the true model vector falls within our model space. The F-statistic depends on the magnitude of the component of the data vector in the model space and so depends directly on M (plus noise contributions from the remaining dimensions of the model space). Because F is calculated just from the magnitude of the projection into a well-defined model subspace, it is independent of whether the model vectors that originally defined that space are orthogonal to each other.

We can thus consider two figures of merit for evaluating the sensitivity of a particular experimental design, as illustrated in Figure 19.1. As before, the factor M is a measure of the sensitivity for detecting an activation and depends strongly on the hemodynamic response. The factor E is a measure of the efficiency for estimating the shape of the hemodynamic response and depends only on the stimulus pattern and not on the hemodynamic response. Both F and E are affected by overlapping responses, but in different ways. The expected value of F primarily depends on the magnitude of M, the variance of the expected response. With a block design, the addition of overlapping responses produces a large variance, but for a rapidly cycled periodic single trial paradigm, the variability of the response is damped out by the hemodynamic response, producing a low value of M. In a similar way, the measure E depends on the intrinsic variance of the stimulus pattern, which continues to increase as the number of stimuli increases. But in addition, E depends on overlap through the nonorthogonality of the model functions.

Periodic single trials perform poorly by both measures of sensitivity. The smoothing of the hemodynamic response reduces M, as described earlier. These designs also have a low value of E because the regular overlap makes the model functions severely nonorthogonal so that noise is strongly amplified when transformed into the parameter space. Also, for this reason, a blocked design has a poor efficiency for estimating the hemodynamic response (low E) even though it has a high sensitivity for detecting a response (high F). Randomized trials are generally more efficient for estimating the hemodynamic response than either periodic single trials or blocked trials, but a block design is more sensitive for detecting activations. This distinction is critical for the optimal design of event-related experiments, emphasizing that the design criteria depend on which question is being asked.

Finally, the three types of stimulus patterns described here are really three points on a continuum, and mixtures of these patterns may provide a more optimal balance. For example, one goal would be to satisfy the combined needs of making the stimulus presentation sufficiently random so that the subject cannot predict the next stimulus and also produce a sensitivity for detecting an activation that approaches that of a single block design. This can be done by defining a probability for occurrence of a stimulus that varies through the duration of the run and constructing a random pattern from this probability model (Friston et al., 1999). For example, if the probability varies like a sine wave with one cycle through the duration of the run, the stimuli will occur randomly but roughly clustered in a loose block, producing a better SNR than a uniformly random sequence of events.

In summary, the sensitivity of an fMRI experiment is remarkably dependent on exactly how the stimuli are presented. In this chapter, we made simple assumptions about the shape and linearity of the hemodynamic response to emphasize ideas of how the approach to analyzing the data also provides a useful tool for optimizing the design of experiments. In fact, though, the hemodynamic response is more complicated than what we have assumed and is still poorly understood (see Chapters 16 and 17). As our understanding of the BOLD response improves, the analysis of the data will become more sophisticated, but the basic ideas of the general linear model will still apply. It is clear that event-related paradigms will continue to be a fruitful area of research, and future developments are likely to broaden significantly the range of applications of fMRI.

REFERENCES

Aguirre, G. K., Zarahn, E. and D'Esposito, M. (1998) The variability of human, BOLD hemodynamic responses. *NeuroImage* **8,** 360–76.

Buckner, R. L., Bandettini, P. A., O'Craven, K. M., Savoy, R. L., Peterson, S. E., Raichle, M. E., and Rosen, B. R. (1996) Detection of cortical activation during averaged single trials of a cognitive task using functional magnetic resonance imaging. *Porc. Natl. Acad. Sci. USA* **93,** 14878–83.

Buckner, R. L., Goodman, J., Burock, M., Rotte, M., Koutstaal, W., Schacter, D., Rosen, B. R., and Dale, A. M. (1998) Functional-anatomic correlates of object priming in humans revealed by rapid presentation event-related fMRI. *Neuron* **20,** 285–96.

Burock, M. A., Buckner, R. L., Woldorff, M. G., Rosen, B. R., and Dale, A. M. (1998) Randomized event-related experimental designs allow for extremely rapid presentation rates using functional MRI. *NeuroReport* **9,** 3735–9.

Clark, V. P., Maisog, J. M., and Haxby, J. V. (1998) fMRI study of face perception and memory using random stimulus sequences. *J. Neurophysiol.* **76,** 3257–65.

Dale, A. M. (1999) Optimal experimental design for event-related fMRI. *Human Brain Mapping* **8,** 109–14.

Dale, A. M., and Buckner, R. L. (1997) Selective averaging of rapidly presented individual trials using fMRI. *Human Brain Mapping* **5,** 329–40.

Friston, K. J., Fletcher, P., Josephs, O., Holmes, A., Rugg, M. D., and Turner, R. (1998a) Event-related fMRI: Characterizing differential responses. *NeuroImage* **7,** 30–40.

Friston, K. J., Josephs, O., Rees, G., and Turner, R. (1998b) Non-linear event related responses in fMRI. *Magn. Reson. Med.* **39,** 41–52.

Friston, K. J., Zarahn, E., Josephs, O., Henson, R. N. A., and Dale, A. M. (1999) Stochastic designs in event-related fMRI. *NeuroImage* **10,** 607–19.

Josephs, O., Turner, R., and Friston, K. J. (1997) Event related fMRI. *Human Brain Mapping* **5,** 243–8.

Zarahn, E., Aguirre, G., and D'Esposito, M. (1997a) A trial based experimental design for fMRI. *NeuroImage* **5,** 179–97.

Zarahn, E., Aguirre, G. K., and D'Esposito, M. (1997b) Empirical analysis of BOLD fMRI statistics: I. Spatially unsmoothed data collected under null-hypothesis conditions. *NeuroImage* **5,** 179–97.

Appendix

The Physics of NMR

The dynamics of nuclear magnetic resonance (NMR) is primarily due to the interplay of the physical processes of precession and relaxation. The sources of relaxation were discussed in Chapter 8, but precession has been treated more or less as a given physical fact. Precession is at the heart of NMR, and in this appendix the physical origins of precession are developed in more detail for the interested reader. The physical description of NMR presented in the earlier chapters is the classical physics view, but in fact the interaction of a particle possessing spin with a magnetic field is a hallmark example of quantum physics. The reader with NMR experience from chemistry may well be wondering how this classical view of NMR relates to the more fundamental quantum viewpoint. This appendix attempts to bridge that gap by describing how precession arises from both the classical and the quantum physics viewpoints.

THE CLASSICAL PHYSICS VIEW OF NMR

The Field of a Magnetic Dipole

The physics of NMR is essentially the physics of a magnetic dipole interacting with a magnetic field. There are two basic models for a magnetic dipole that we will use: a small circular current loop and a rotating charged sphere. The dipole moment

$\boldsymbol{\mu}$ has both a magnitude and an associated direction and so is described as a vector. For the current loop, μ is proportional to the product of the current and the area of the loop and points in the direction perpendicular to the plane of the loop. A rotating charged sphere can be thought of as a stack of current loops, produced as the charge on the sphere is carried around by the rotation. Adding up the fields produced by all the current loops that comprise the sphere yields outside the sphere a net field that is identical to the field of a single current loop at the center. The spinning sphere is an easily visualized classical model for a proton and so is useful in thinking about NMR. The dipole moment of the sphere is proportional to three terms: the volume V of the sphere, the charge Q, and the angular frequency ω. The direction of $\boldsymbol{\mu}$ is the spin axis of the sphere, defined by a right-hand rule (with the fingers of your right hand curling in the direction of rotation, your thumb points along the direction of $\boldsymbol{\mu}$).

The field produced by a magnetic dipole was illustrated in Figure 7.2. Often in magnetic resonance (MR) applications, we are interested only in the z-component of the dipole field produced by a dipole aligned along z. The form of this field is

$$B_z = \frac{\mu(3\cos^2\theta - 1)}{r^3} \qquad\qquad\qquad [A.1]$$

This field pattern recurs frequently in magnetic resonance imaging (MRI) applications (compare, for example, with Figures 5.10 and 5.11) because it is the prototype field distortion created by a magnetized body. For example, consider a sphere of material, composed of many dipole moments, sitting in an external magnetic field along z. The action of the field on the dipoles is to cause them to align partly with the field. This creates a net dipole moment density within the sphere, and the result is that the entire sphere creates a net field that is itself a dipole field. That is, a uniformly magnetized sphere creates a dipole field outside, and the dipole moment that describes this field is proportional to the volume of the sphere and the dipole density inside. For a less symmetrical body, the field produced is more complicated, but for many shapes a good first approximation is a dipole field. For example, a sinus cavity produces a dipole-like field distortion throughout the head (Figure 5.10) due to the different magnetic susceptibilities of air and water.

Interactions of a Dipole with an External Field

In the preceding discussion, we focused on the field produced by a magnetic dipole, but to understand how NMR works, we also need to know how a dipole moment $\boldsymbol{\mu}$ behaves when placed in an external field $\boldsymbol{B}$. There are three interrelated effects. First, the energy of the dipole depends on its orientation:

$$E = -\boldsymbol{\mu} \cdot \boldsymbol{B} = -\mu B \cos\theta \qquad\qquad\qquad [A.2]$$

where θ is the angle between the dipole moment vector and the magnetic field. The energy of a dipole in a magnetic field is lowest (most negative) when the dipole is aligned with the field ($\theta = 0$). Second, the natural effect of this orientation dependence is that the field creates on the dipole a torque that would tend to align it with the magnetic field, just as a compass needle is twisted into alignment with the earth's magnetic field because that is its lowest energy state. The torque W is the vector cross product of the dipole moment and the field:

$$W = \mu \times B \qquad [A.3]$$

This torque acts to twist the dipole, but there is no net force if the magnetic field is uniform. But if B varies with position, there will be a net force F tending to draw the dipole toward a region of stronger field:

$$F = \mu \frac{dB}{dz} \qquad [A.4]$$

These physical interactions can be understood from the basic forces exerted on a current loop placed in an external magnetic field. The force F (called the Lorentz force) on a particle with charge q moving with velocity v through a magnetic field B is

$$F \propto q\, v \times B \qquad [A.5]$$

Because F is proportional to the vector cross product of v and B, it is perpendicular to both. Picturing a magnetic dipole as a small loop of current (electrons in motion), the forces on opposite sides are not balanced unless μ is aligned with B (Figure A.1). The energy then depends on the orientation of the dipole with respect to the field, and the moment arm between the unbalanced forces creates a torque. In a non-uniform field, the forces are not balanced even when the dipole is aligned with the field because of the curving field lines, creating a net force toward the region of stronger field.

Equilibrium Magnetization

Both the torque produced by the field and the force produced by a nonuniform field can be understood in terms of the energy of a dipole. In both cases, the effect of the external field is to push the dipole toward a lower energy state, either by aligning it with the field or moving it to a region of stronger field or both. Based on these energy arguments, we expect that the long-term behavior of a collection of dipoles will be to align with a uniform magnetic field because this is the lowest energy state. However, in any thermodynamic system, energy is constantly exchanged between different forms. For example, in a sample of pure water, the energy of the molecules is distributed between translational motions, rotational motions, and vibrational motions. If the water is also in a magnetic field, there is additional energy in the orientations of the magnetic dipole moments. At equilibrium, the net energy is distributed among these different forms, and this prevents the dipoles from reaching their lowest energy state of complete alignment with the field. The total energy of the water molecules is reflected in the temperature, and as temperature is increased, the energy in each form increases. This means that alignment of the dipoles will be most complete at very low temperatures, but as the temperature increases, the alignment will become less pronounced.

We can quantify this dependence with a thermodynamic argument by assuming that each dipole in the magnetic field B_0 is either aligned with the field or opposite

Magnetic Forces

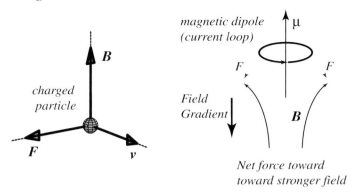

Torque on a Dipole

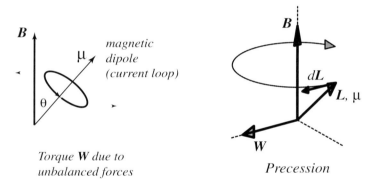

Figure A.1. Classical physics view of precession. A magnetic field *B* exerts a force *F* on a positive charge moving with velocity *v* that is proportional to *v*×*B* and, thus, is always perpendicular to both *v* and *B* (top left). A magnetic dipole **μ** can be viewed as a small loop of current (moving charges), with the direction of **μ** perpendicular to the plane of the current loop. In a nonuniform field, there is a net force on a dipole in the direction of the stronger field (top right). When **μ** is at an angle to the magnetic field, unbalanced forces on opposite sides of the loop create a torque *W* on the dipole (bottom). For a nuclear magnetic dipole, the angular momentum *L* is proportional to **μ**. The change in angular momentum *dL* in a short time *dt* is in the direction of *W*, so the change *dL* creates precession, a rotation of *L* around *B* without changing its magnitude or the angle it makes with *B* (lower right).

to the field, defining these two states as + and –. This is a very nonclassical assumption, but is in accord with the quantum view described later. In any system in thermodynamic equilibrium, the ratio of the populations of two states is given by

$$\frac{n_+}{n_-} = e^{-\Delta E/kT} \qquad\qquad [A.6]$$

where ΔE is the difference in energy between the two states, k is Boltzmann's constant, and T is temperature. At room temperature the alignment of spins in a 1.5-T field is quite small, with a difference of only about one in 10^5 between those spins aligned with the field and those aligned opposite to the field. Nevertheless, this small difference creates a small magnetization M_0 in the sample. This magnetization is simply the net dipole moment density of the sample, proportional to the difference between n_+ and n_-, and we can derive an expression for it from the thermodynamic equilibrium condition. For the two states of the dipole, $\Delta E = -2\mu B_0$ (it is negative because the energy of the + state is lower than the energy of the – state). Because this energy difference is much smaller than kT at room temperature, we can expand the exponential in Equation [A.6] to give

$$M_0 = \mu(n_+ - n_-) \approx \frac{n\mu^2 B_0}{kT} \qquad [A.7]$$

where n is the total spin density ($n_+ + n_-$). Thus, the equilibrium magnetization, which ultimately sets the scale for the magnitude of the NMR signal, increases in proportion to the main magnetic field B_0. This is a primary motivation for doing MRI at increasing field strengths, and human imaging systems with B_0 as high as 8 T have been constructed.

Precession

The arguments so far indicate that a collection of magnetic dipoles will eventually reach a thermal equilibrium state in which they are partially aligned with the magnetic field, and this creates a uniform magnetization M_0 of the body containing the dipoles. The time required to reach this state of equilibrium is T_1, the longitudinal relaxation time. But if this alignment of the spins was the only effect of a magnetic field acting on a dipole, there would be no NMR phenomenon and no MRI. What we have described is the final state of the spins. The additional interesting physics is what happens along the way toward this equilibrium state. The additional effect, which gives rise to the resonance of NMR, is precession of the dipole.

The source of precession is that nuclear dipoles possess angular momentum in addition to a magnetic moment. The association of a magnetic dipole moment with angular momentum is clearly seen in the prototype example of a spinning charged sphere. Both the angular momentum and the dipole moment are proportional to how fast the sphere is spinning, the angular frequency ω. Because of this, we can define a proportionality constant between the two called the *gyromagnetic ratio, γ*:

$$\gamma = \frac{\mu}{L} \qquad [A.8]$$

where $\mathbf{L}$ is the angular momentum vector (and L is the magnitude of that vector). Because μ is also proportional to the charge Q, and angular momentum is also proportional to the mass of the particle, m, we would expect that the gyromagnetic ratio would vary with the ratio Q/m. For nuclei, the largest ratio of Q/m is for hydrogen because it consists of just a single proton. For any other nucleus, the neutrons add to *m* without contributing to *Q*, so the gyromagnetic ratio is smaller. The hydrogen nucleus thus has a higher resonant frequency in a magnetic field than any other nucleus. For electrons, *Q* is the same as for the proton, but the mass is much smaller, so the gyromagnetic ratio is about three orders of magnitude larger.

The significance of the gyromagnetic ratio becomes clear when we consider the immediate behavior of a dipole when acted on by a torque and the resulting phenomenon of precession. Imagine placing a dipole **μ** at an angle to a magnetic field *B*$_0$. The angular momentum *L* is in the direction of **μ,** with a magnitude μ/γ. The torque *W* is the rate of change of angular momentum, and with γ*L* substituted for **μ** in Equation [A3], we have

$$W = \frac{dL}{dt} = \gamma L \times B_0 \qquad\qquad [A.9]$$

Precession results because the *change* in angular momentum, *dL,* acquired in any brief interval *dt,* is always perpendicular to the current direction of *L*. The new angular momentum is then *L* + *dL*, but this is simply a rotation of *L* rather than a change in magnitude. In short, the dipole precesses around the field *B*$_0$ without changing the angle that it makes with the field. The rate of change of the phase angle in the transverse plane is the precessional frequency. In a time *dt*, the precession angle is $d\phi = dL/L = \gamma B_0 dt$. The fundamental relation of NMR is then that a magnetic dipole precesses in a magnetic field with a frequency, called the Larmor frequency, of

$$\omega_0 = \gamma B_0 \qquad\qquad [A.10]$$

Precession makes it possible to tip the net magnetization into the transverse plane and generate a detectable NMR signal. If all the dipoles are tipped, then the net magnetization *M*$_0$ also tips, and as the dipoles precess so does the net magnetization. Thus the net magnetization mimics the behavior of an individual dipole.

The two important processes in NMR are thus precession and relaxation. Precession does not change the angle between the dipole and the field, and so does not lead to alignment, but over time relaxation does lead to a gradual alignment. The time scales for these two processes are enormously different. The precessional period for a proton in a 1.5-T field is about 10^{-8} s, whereas the relaxation time T_1 required to reach thermal equilibrium is about 1 s.

THE QUANTUM PHYSICS VIEW OF NMR

The previous section described a physical picture of the NMR phenomenon based on a classical physics viewpoint. With the development of quantum mechanics in the last century, we know that this classical view is wrong. The correct view is much stranger, and unfortunately quantum mechanics does not offer an easily visualized physical picture of the phenomenon in the same way that the classical view does. So important questions are: in precisely what way is the classical view wrong? and what kind of errors will we make if we adopt the classical view in thinking about NMR? These questions are important because the behavior of a particle with spin in a magnetic field is a quintessential example of quantum mechanics. Based on the quantum view, one encounters statements suggesting that the proton's spin can only be up or down in a magnetic field. But if this is strictly true, it would seem that a transverse, precessing magnetization can never arise, and yet this is the crux of the classical view of NMR.

The answer to the questions posed here is that the classical view is wrong in terms of describing the behavior of a single spin but gives an accurate description of the *average* behavior of many spins. This brings out a disturbing feature of quantum mechanics that violates our intuitive sense of logic, that the average behavior of many identical particles in precisely the same state can be so different from the behavior of any one of them. However, in a sense, it is somewhat reassuring, in that it points toward the reasons why our experience with the world on the macroscopic scale leads us to a view of physics that is so different from the fundamental picture provided by quantum mechanics. The following is a sketch of how the classical view of a precessing magnetization vector emerges from a quantum mechanical description. A much more complete description can be found in Feynman, Leighton, and Sands (1965).

Quantum Effects

To illustrate the fundamental strangeness of quantum mechanics, we begin with a thought experiment that is an idealization of one of the key physics experiments of the twentieth century, originally performed by Stern and Gerlach in the early 1920s. The experiment involves a simple device for measuring the component of a particle's magnetic moment along a particular spatial axis. The device is a box with an entry opening on one end and a wide exit opening on the other, and in the experiment particles are sent in one end and then observed to see whether they are deflected from their original path as they emerge from the exit (Figure A.2). Inside the box, magnets are arranged to create a magnetic field that points primarily perpendicular to the path of the particle. From our classical ideas about the behavior of a magnetic dipole moment in a magnetic field, we would expect that the magnetic moment would precess a little while it is in the field but that, if the field is uniform, it would not be deflected. This precession is, of course, the phenomenon we are interested in for NMR, but this is not what we are after in this experiment. Here we want to explore the more fundamental concept of the spin state of a particle. The precession is a secondary effect that we will try to minimize by using a weak field and fast-moving particles that spend only a short time inside the box. We will return to precession after illustrating how different quantum effects are from our classical physics intuitions.

Our goal with this experiment is to deflect the particles by making the magnetic field nonuniform, with a strong gradient running perpendicular to the path of the particle. When a magnetic moment is placed in a nonuniform magnetic field, it feels a force in the direction of the field gradient, and the magnitude of the force is proportional to the component of the magnetic moment that lies along the gradient

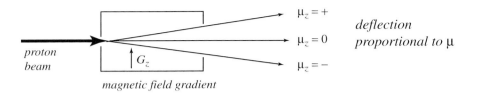

magnetic field gradient

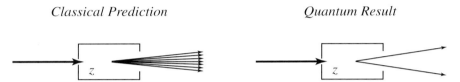

Figure A.2. The Stern-Gerlach experiment to measure the magnetic dipole moment of a proton. Protons pass through a box containing a magnetic field gradient that deflects the proton in proportion to the z-component of its magnetic dipole moment, μ_z. Classical physics predicts a continuous range of μ_z, but experiment shows that μ_z can take on only one of two values, corresponding to spin up or spin down relative to the field.

direction (Equation [A.4]). The magnetic force thus deflects the particle from its initial path as it passes through the box, and the amount of deflection will be proportional to the component of the magnetic moment in the direction of the field gradient. This box can then be used to measure one component of the magnetic moment from the magnitude of the deflection, and the component along any axis can be measured by rotating the box. The original experiment measured the electron magnetic moment, but for our thought experiment we can as easily imagine doing the experiment with protons.

From a classical viewpoint, the physical picture of this experiment is clear. The magnetic moment of the proton is simply a vector in three-dimensional space, and so it has a well-defined projection onto any spatial axis. We could measure the full vector by passing the proton through three successive boxes appropriately arranged to measure the vector's components along three orthogonal directions, such as x, y, and z. Having measured a set of three projections, we have complete information about the orientation and magnitude of the magnetic moment, and we could then predict precisely what any other experiment would yield if we measured the projection along an arbitrary axis. This classical view is so simple that it seems intuitively obvious, and yet this is not the way nature works at all, as we can see from a few experiments.

In the first experiment, we send a large number of protons through the box with the box aligned so that the field gradient is along the z-axis. Each proton is then deflected by an angle proportional to the z-component of its magnetic moment, so what would we expect to see emerging from the box? If we have done nothing to prepare the protons (i.e., nothing to align them initially), then the magnetic moment is equally likely to be pointing in any direction, and if the magnitude of the vector is M, we would expect that the z-component is equally likely to be anywhere between $-M$ and $+M$. From the classical physics viewpoint, we would thus expect the beam of protons to spread into a uniform fan, with the maximum deflections corresponding to those protons whose magnetic moment is perfectly aligned or antialigned with z and thus have the largest z-component.

Furthermore, from a classical view, we would expect that the angular momentum would vary among the protons. That is, if we think of the angular momentum as just another form of motion of the particle (rotational rather than translational), then we would expect for thermodynamic reasons that the total energy would divide up among the various possible forms. Then just as there would be a distribution of translational velocities, with some particles moving rapidly and some nearly still, there would be a distribution of rotational velocities and thus a distribution of magnetic moments. A proton with weak spin would have a weak magnetic moment and so would suffer only a small deflection. The full classical prediction then would be that the beam of protons is spread into a fan distribution peaked at the center (no deflection).

However, when we carry out this experiment, we see the first surprise of quantum mechanics (Figure A.2). Instead of a fan of particle paths, the beam is split cleanly into two precise beams, one deflected up and the other deflected down. By measuring the amount of deflection, the z-component of the magnetic moment is measured, and because the magnetic moment is proportional to the angular momentum, this provides a measurement of the proton's spin. The experimental result is that the spin of the proton is either $+\hbar/2$ or $-\hbar/2$, where $\hbar$ (h-bar) is Planck's constant h divided by 2π. This result is not at all consistent with viewing the angular momentum as a randomly oriented vector. Instead of taking on any value from the minimum to the maximum, the z-component takes on only one of two particular values, and *every* particle is deflected. We can refer to these two values as spin up and spin down, indicating whether the z-component is positive or negative. Suppose that we now repeat the experiment, but first we heat up the gas of protons before sending them through the box. From a classical viewpoint, each proton carries more energy; in particular, there should be more energy in rotational motions, so more large angular momenta and magnetic moments should be present. When we pass these heated protons through the box, the results are precisely as before: the beam is split in two, with angular momenta of $+\hbar/2$ or $-\hbar/2$. The angular momentum is independent of the energy of the protons.

From these results, we must conclude that *spin*, despite the familiar sounding name, is unlike anything in classical physics. Rather than viewing it as a result of the state of the proton (i.e., how fast it is rotating), we must instead look at it as an intrinsic property of the proton, on an equal standing with the proton's mass and charge as irreducible properties. All protons carry an angular momentum and a magnetic moment whose magnitude cannot be changed. Furthermore, there is nothing special about the particular axis we used in our experiment. If we had instead oriented our box to measure the x-component of the magnetic moment, we would have measured the same result: the x-component also takes on only the values $+ \hbar/2$ or $- \hbar/2$. At this basic level of fundamental particles, nature allows only discrete values for the outcomes of measurements of some physical quantities. Whatever state a proton is in, if the component of the angular momentum along *any* axis is measured, the measurement will yield either $+ \hbar/2$ or $- \hbar/2$. Angular momentum is quantized, and the measure of this quantization is $\hbar$. On the macroscopic scale, we are unaware of the quantized nature of angular momentum because $\hbar$ is in fact quite small. For example, a spinning curveball in a baseball game carries more than 10^{31} of these basic quanta of angular momentum, so angular momentum on the terrestrial scale appears to be a continuously varying quantity. The laws of classical physics thus provide an approximate, but extremely accurate, description of macroscopic phenomena. It is only when we look closely at the behavior of individual particles that the quantum nature of the world becomes clear.

The experimental result so far is that the component of the angular momentum along any spatial axis is quantized. What happens if we try to measure several components in succession? That is, what happens when we take the output of our z-box and send it into another box? To begin with, suppose we simply measure the z-component a second time by passing the spin down beam from the first box through a second z-box (Figure A.3). The result is that all the protons are deflected down. In other words, all the protons that had spin down after the first box still have spin down after the second box, and the spin up protons after the first box also would still show spin up in a second z-box. This is not surprising; it is completely consistent with our classical idea that the spin has a definite z-component. The first box sorted the spins into the two states, and the second simply confirmed that the spins are still in those states. Carrying this idea further, we might naively expect that the same holds true for the other axes as well so that, although the component along any axis is

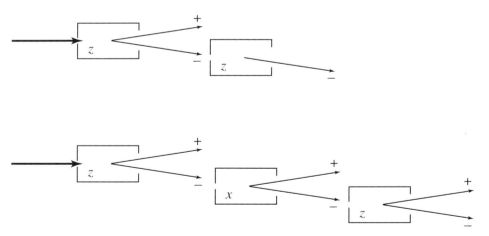

Figure A.3. Quantum uncertainty. After measuring the z-component of the spin with one box, sending the spin down beam through a second z-box shows that all the protons are still in the spin down state (top). But if another box is inserted between these two to measure the x-component of the spin, the z-component becomes unpredictable and can be either up or down with equal probability (bottom).

quantized and takes on only one of two values, these components nevertheless have definite values determined by the state of the particle. That is, we can imagine that it might be possible to describe the spin state of the proton in terms of the spin components of the three axes, something like {+,+,–} to indicate spin up along x and y and spin down along z. However, this idea is wrong, and the behavior of the spins is even stranger.

We can show this second surprising feature of quantum mechanics by extending our experiment. Now we replace the second box with an x-box to measure the x-component of the magnetic moment (Figure A.3). Specifically, we let the spin down beam from the z-box pass through the x-box. The result is that the beam is split into two beams corresponding to spin up and spin down relative to the x-axis. This result is still highly nonclassical, but it is at least consistent with our earlier finding of quantization. But now we take it one step further and add a third box to remeasure the z-component of the magnetization. Based on our naive interpretation that the component of spin along any axis has a definite value, we should expect that all the protons emerging from the second z-box should be deflected into the spin down beam. Instead, the protons are split equally into the spin up and spin down beams. Somehow the measurement of the x-component of the magnetization has changed the state of the z-component. The initial z-box sorted the spins into up and down z-components, and this was confirmed by another z-box. But when an x-box is inserted between the two z-measurements, the state of the spin is jumbled so that the z-component becomes indefinite: it is equally likely to be up or down after another measurement.

The Rules of Quantum Mechanics

In the 1920s, physicists developed a mathematical framework for describing quantum phenomena such as those already sketched out. This framework can be expressed in a few rules and has proven to be highly accurate in describing the physical world. However, in the process, several ideas that were so entrenched in classical physics as to seem obviously true had to be abandoned. For example, the picture of the angular momentum as a vector with three well-defined components along the x-, y-, and z-axes must be replaced by a view in which these quantities cannot all have definite values. This introduces an uncertainty into the workings of nature that is entirely different from the classical view. The most complete description of the spin state of a proton only tells us the *probabilities* for measuring spin up or down along an axis. And indeed the role of dynamical laws of physics is not to describe how the components of the magnetic moment evolve in time but rather to describe how the probabilities evolve in time.

This indeterminacy is not because of ignorance on our part. Even with a classical picture, if we measured only one component of spin, there would be uncertainty about what another measurement along a different axis would yield, but this uncertainty is due to our ignorance of the full state of the spin, the three-dimensional (3D) vector. The uncertainty of quantum mechanics is wholly different and more fundamental. If we measure the component of the spin along one axis, the component along a perpendicular axis is indefinite. That is, if a spin has a definite component along z, which is how the spin is left after our initial measurement of the z-component, then it is in a state in which there is no definite value for the x-component. If we then measure the x-component, the spin will be left in a state with a definite x-component (either up or down), but now the z-component is completely indefinite.

This strange behavior can be described within the mathematical framework of quantum mechanics. For the spin state of the proton, we have the following rules of quantum mechanics.

1. A measurement of the component of the spin along any axis will yield a measurement of either $+\hbar/2$ or $-\hbar/2$. The result of any one measurement is usually unpredictable, but a full description of the spin state allows us to calculate probabilities for finding spin up or down along any axis. After a measurement, the spin is left in a state such that a subsequent identical measurement will yield the same value.

2. The spin state can always be described as a mixture of two states, corresponding to spin up or spin down along any chosen spatial axis. The spin state is then completely described by specifying two complex numbers, the amplitudes a_+ and a_-, which underlie the probabilities for measuring the spin component to be up or down. Specifically, the probability for finding the component up is $|a_+|^2$, the square of the magnitude of a_+, which we will write simply as a_+^2. And similarly, the probability for finding it down is a_-^2. In practice, we will call the chosen axis z, and the corresponding amplitudes a_{z+} and a_{z-}. Specifying these two complex numbers for one axis completely specifies the spin state.

3. For any other axis, there are also two associated amplitudes. For example, for the x-axis the amplitudes are a_{x+} and a_{x-}, and from these amplitudes the probabilities for the results of a measurement of the x-component of the spin are calculated using rule 2. The amplitudes for finding the spin up or down along any other axis can be expressed as a linear combination of the amplitudes for z. The transformation rules for x and y follow:

$$a_{x+} = \frac{1}{\sqrt{2}}(a_{z+} + a_{z-})$$

$$a_{x-} = \frac{1}{\sqrt{2}}(-a_{z+} + a_{z-})$$

$$a_{y+} = \frac{1}{\sqrt{2}}(a_{z+} + ia_{z-})$$

$$a_{y-} = \frac{1}{\sqrt{2}}(ia_{z+} + a_{z-})$$

4. The amplitudes evolve over time depending on the energy associated with the two states. Each amplitude must be multiplied by a factor $e^{i\omega t}$, where the angular frequency ω is directly proportional to the energy E of the corre-

sponding state, $\omega = E/\hbar$. This quantum mechanical time evolution is the source of the precession observed in NMR, as we will see shortly.

These rules were presented baldly, without any supporting argument. Each requires some amplification in order to deal with more complicated situations, but these bare rules are sufficient to describe the behavior of the spin state of a proton. However, the rules involve some subtlety. The first is the fact that the most complete specification of the spin state still does not allow one to predict the outcome of a measurement, only the probabilities for different outcomes. The only situation in which an experimental outcome *is* predictable is when one of the probabilities is one (e.g., when passing a beam of protons through two successive *z*-boxes, as in the foregoing experiment, the result of the second box is determined with a probability of one).

An important feature of these rules is that the amplitudes from which the probabilities are calculated are complex numbers. In other words, each amplitude can be represented in the form $ae^{i\phi}$, where a is the magnitude and ϕ is the phase. The squared magnitude is then calculated by multiplying $ae^{i\phi}$ by $ae^{-i\phi}$. For the probabilities for the *z*-axis, the phase does not matter because it cancels out in the calculation of the probabilities. But when amplitudes are added, as in the calculation of a_{x+}, the phases of the individual amplitudes will make a difference in the calculated probabilities. Because the state of the system is described by two complex numbers, and each complex number is composed of two real numbers (a magnitude and a phase), it appears that the specification of the spin state requires four numbers. But, in fact, only two numbers are required, for two reasons. First, a measurement of the *z*-component must yield either spin up or spin down, so the probabilities of the two outcomes must sum to one: $a_{z+}^2 + a_{z-}^2 = 1$. Thus the magnitude of one amplitude fixes the magnitude of the other. The second reason is that the absolute phase of each amplitude does not matter, only the phase *difference* between the two amplitudes. For example, if the phase of a_{z+} is ϕ_+ and the phase of a_{z-} is ϕ_-, one could always factor out a phase $e^{i\phi_+}$ in the expressions for the *x* and *y* amplitudes, leaving a_{z-} with a phase $\phi_- - \phi_+$. Then the factor involving ϕ_+ alone would disappear from the calculation of any of the probabilities. It is only the probabilities that are physically measurable, and these depend on the magnitude squared of the net amplitude. So, the spin state of the proton can be represented by just two numbers: one describing the magnitudes of the amplitudes and the other describing the relative phase angle. Because the sum of the squares of the magnitudes must be one, a natural choice is to describe the magnitudes in terms of the sine and cosine of an angle. A convenient form to choose is

$$a_{z+} = \cos\left(\frac{\theta}{2}\right) e^{i\omega_+ t}$$

$$a_{z-} = \sin\left(\frac{\theta}{2}\right) e^{i(\omega_- t + \phi)}$$

[A.12]

These equations for the *z* amplitudes, combined with the preceding transformation rules for calculating the *x* and *y* probabilities, completely describe the proton spin state. The two numbers θ and ϕ can be thought of as angles, and we will see below how this choice of representation of the spin state leads to a natural physical interpretation of these angles.

Note that the time dependence of the spin system depends entirely on the energy of the two states. If there is no magnetic field, then the frequencies ω_+ and ω_- are both zero because there is no energy difference between the two states. The amplitudes are then constant, and the spin state does not change over time. Now suppose that a uniform magnetic field with magnitude B_0 is turned on pointing along the z-axis. From Equation [A.2], the energy of a magnetic dipole moment μ in a magnetic field is $-\mu B_0$ for the spin up state and $+\mu B_0$ for the spin down state (the lowest energy configuration occurs when μ is aligned with B_0). The angular momentum of the proton is $\hbar/2$, and the dipole moment is proportional to the angular momentum: $\mu = \gamma\hbar/2$. By our rule 4, the angular frequency ω associated with an energy E is $\omega = E/\hbar$, so the frequencies associated with the spin up and spin down states, respectively, are $\omega_+ = -\gamma B_0/2$ and $\omega_- = +\gamma B_0/2$. Thus, over time the relative phases of the two amplitudes steadily change at a rate $\omega_0 = \omega_- - \omega_+ = \gamma B_0$, which is precisely the Larmor precession frequency we found in the classical view of precession (Equation [A.10]). Because only the relative phase of the amplitudes matters to the physics of the state, we can write the spin state amplitudes as

$$a_{z+} = \cos\left(\frac{\theta}{2}\right)$$

$$a_{z-} = \sin\left(\frac{\theta}{2}\right) e^{i(\omega_0 t + \phi)} \quad\quad\quad\quad [A.13]$$

From these expressions for the z-amplitudes, we can now calculate the probabilities for measuring spin up along the x-, y-, or z-axes for an arbitrary spin state specified by the numbers θ and ϕ:

$$p_{x+} = \frac{1}{2}\{1 + \sin\theta\cos(\omega_0 t + \phi)\}$$

$$p_{y+} = \frac{1}{2}\{1 + \sin\theta\cos(\omega_0 t + \phi)\} \quad\quad [A.14]$$

$$p_{z+} = \cos^2\left(\frac{\theta}{2}\right)$$

Figure A.4 illustrates the spin state of a proton by plotting a surface such that the length of a line drawn in any direction from the origin to this surface is the probability p_+ of measuring spin up along that direction. This tomato-shaped surface comes directly from the expression above for p_{z+}, because for any chosen direction we can choose a coordinate system with the z-axis along that direction, and the probability of measuring spin up is then p_{z+}. In other words, the spin state of the proton is defined by a particular direction in space, and the probability of measuring spin up along any axis is then $\cos^2(\theta'/2)$, where θ' is the angle between the measurement axis and the direction defining the spin state.

We can now describe the basic interactions of a spin in a magnetic field in terms of this quantum picture. The spin state is described by a direction defined by two

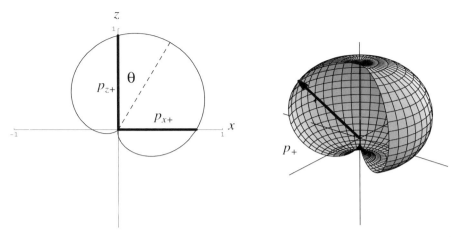

Figure A.4. The spin state of the proton. The spin state of the proton describes the probability that a measurement of the spin component along a particular axis will yield spin up or spin down, the only two possible results allowed by quantum theory. This state can be visualized by plotting the surface shown on the right, such that the distance from the origin to the surface along a particular direction is the probability for measuring spin up along that axis. A two-dimensional cut through this surface is shown on the left. The spin state is described by angles θ and ϕ, which are 30° and 0° in this example. The time evolution of the spin state is a steady precession of this surface such that $\phi = \phi_0 + \omega_0 t$, where ω_0 is the classical Larmor frequency.

angles θ and ϕ. Over time, the evolution of the spin state is a steady increase of the angle ϕ with the Larmor frequency ω_0. Only one spatial axis, the orientation direction of the spin state, has a definite component of the spin. For all other axes, we can think of the state as being a mixture of spin up and spin down states. If a component of the spin is measured along any axis, the probability for measuring spin up is defined by the surface in Figure A.4. Furthermore, the act of measurement causes the spin state to jump to a new orientation defined by the outcome of the measurement. If the spin is measured to be up along a particular axis, the direction defining the new spin state will be the positive direction of the measured axis, or the negative direction if the spin is down. In other words, the spin state evolves in two ways: a continuous precession described by the steady increase of the phase ϕ and a discrete jump each time a measurement is made. For example, suppose that the spin state is defined by an angle θ of 30° with the z-axis. In the absence of a measurement, we can picture the tomato-shaped surface as precessing around the z-axis (the magnetic field direction). If we then measure the z-component of the spin, the spin state will jump to either pointing along $+z$ (with probability 0.933) or pointing along $-z$ (with probability .067). (Remember that our experiment with successive z-boxes showed that, when the spin down beam from the first box is passed through the second z-box, the probability of measuring spin down again is one, so the new spin state after the first box must be oriented along $-z$.) The spin state then continues to evolve from this new starting point until the next measurement. This dual pattern of change, combining both smooth continuous evolution and discrete jumps, is one of the deep mysteries of quantum mechanics. Nevertheless, this picture of how the world works is highly accurate.

Macroscopic Measurements

The foregoing probabilities are for the results of a measurement of one spin. But in an NMR experiment, we are measuring the net effect of many spins, the net magnetization M. If the material contains identical spins, all prepared in the same state, then the net magnetization along a particular axis is simply proportional to the average value of the spin that would be measured along that axis if we measured each spin individually. And the average measured value of the spin component along the axes x, y, and z is calculated from the probabilities for finding spin up along each of these axes: the expected value of a measurement along a particular axis is $\hbar/2$ $(p_+ - p_-)$ and $p_- = 1 - p_+$. When the probabilities for spin up and spin down are equal, we expect to find a zero average spin component, and when the spin is in a definite state along a particular axis, we expect to find $\hbar/2$ along that axis. For intermediate probabilities, the average for each spin lies between zero and $\hbar/2$. From the expressions for the probabilities, the components of the net average magnetization are

$$M_x \propto \sin\theta \cos(\omega_0 t + \phi)$$

$$M_y \propto \sin\theta \sin(\omega_0 t + \phi)$$

$$M_z \propto \cos\theta \qquad\qquad\qquad [A.15]$$

With these three equations, we have arrived at our goal of relating the phenomenon of NMR to the quantum behavior of a spin in a magnetic field. These three equations for the average components of the spin describe a vector tipped at an angle θ to the z-axis, with the transverse component in the x-y plane precessing with an angular frequency ω_0. In other words, we have reached a crucial connection between the quantum view and the classical view: the *average* behavior of many quantum spins is precisely described by a classical, precessing magnetization vector M. The two numbers that specify the quantum state, θ and ϕ, translate into the angle between M and the z-axis and the angle between the transverse component of M and the x-axis at $t = 0$, respectively. The precession itself arises from the time-dependent phase of the quantum amplitudes for the spin up and spin down states, with the phase changing cyclically with an angular frequency that is proportional to the energy difference of the two states.

The result of this long argument is that, despite the quantum nature of spin interactions with a magnetic field, the average behavior of many spins is accurately described by classical physics concepts. Except for the existence of spin itself, which is indeed a quantum phenomenon, the behavior of the net magnetization due to protons in water is purely classical. For this reason, classical reasoning is perfectly adequate for understanding most of the NMR physics associated with MRI. However, in spectroscopy studies, and virtually all applications of NMR in chemistry, the quantum nature of NMR is critical for understanding the experimental phenomena. The reason for this is that liquid water, with only a single proton resonance, is a very simple system. In more complex molecules, protons in different chemical forms will have different resonant frequencies (chemical shift effect), and often protons will interact with one another and other nuclei. In such cases, the quantum nature of spin is evident even in a macroscopic experiment involving averaging over many spins. For example, in many molecules, the orientation of the spin at one location affects the magnetic field in the vicinity of another spin in the same molecule, an effect called *J*-coupling. In the interaction of the two spins, the first spin is either up or down and so causes the local field at the second spin to be shifted either up or down by a discrete amount. As a result, the resonant frequency is shifted up or down. Averaging over many spins, the NMR signal will sample some spins whose resonance was shifted up, and some whose resonance was shifted down in frequency. In the resulting NMR spectrum, the resonance line is split into two slightly shifted lines, a direct reflection of the fact that the first spin has only two possible states. In this example, the quantum nature of spin passes through to macroscopic measurements because the precession frequency of the second spin depends on its interaction with the state of *one* other spin, not with the average behavior of many spins. If the sample is irradiated at the resonant frequency of the first spin to randomize its spin state, then the second spin effectively interacts with an average spin state of the first, and the line splitting disappears.

In conclusion, quantum mechanics is the most complete and accurate description of how the physical world works that we have, and yet the description of observable phenomena is often rather subtle and counterintuitive. One of the most profound implications of quantum mechanics is that a physical system can exist in a kind of mixture of two states, a phenomenon called *superposition*. We encountered this phenomenon in our simple example of a spin in a magnetic field, where the spin can be in a state that is neither purely a spin up nor a spin down state, despite the fact that a measurement of the spin orientation will yield either spin up or spin down. In this case, we describe the spin state as a mixture of the spin up and spin down states, with associated amplitudes that give the probabilities for the measured orientation to be up or down. Superposition brings an intrinsic indeterminacy into the description of the world, and this is the source of the uncertainty principles of quantum mechanics. In our spin example, this uncertainty principle takes the form that, if the spin state is definite along one axis (e.g., spin up along *z*), it is indefinite along all other axes. For these other axes, only probabilities can be given for what a measurement of the spin will yield. There are classical examples of physical systems, such as a compound pendulum, whose state can be described as a mixture of two more fundamental normal modes. But in a classical mixed system, any measured quantity will be found to be *between* the two values associated with the normal modes, *not* one or the other. The phenomenon of superposition has no analog in classical physics. Fortunately, for understanding MRI, we can visualize the NMR phenomenon as a classical precessing magnetization vector, and virtually all the mathematical reasoning that goes into the design of imaging pulse sequences is based on this classical view.

REFERENCES

Feynman, R. P., Leighton, R. B., and Sands, M. (1965) *The Feynman Lectures on Physics.* Addison-Wesley: New York.

Index

acidosis, 36

acoustic noise, 263–6, 270. *See also* noise

action potential, and neural activity, 6, 7f, 8, 422–3

activation, brain: and arterial spin labeling (ASL), 381–4; and BOLD effect, 116–18, 409–12, 446–9, 454–5, 473–8; contrast agents and measurement of, 110–11; and glucose metabolism, 18–19; and magnetic resonance, 104–108; and MR signal increase, 391; and perfusion, 55–7; physiological changes during, 41–4, 55–7; size of CBF increase during, 44–54

adenosine, 36

adenosine diphosphate (ADP), 9, 10, 13

adenosine monophosphate (AMP), 9

adenosine triphosphate (ATP), 9–10, 13, 48

adiabatic inversion, and continuous arterial spin labeling, 358–60, 380

adiabatic radiofrequency (RF) pulse, 144, 146

age range, and variance in CBF measurements, 342–3

aliasing, and signal processing, 234

alkalosis, 36

amplitude, and Gibbs artifact, 245

analysis of variance (ANOVA), and statistical analysis of BOLD data, 455. *See also* variance

anatomy, MRI and fine details of, 66–7

anesthesia, and BOLD experiments, 412

angular momentum: and magnetic dipole, 136–7; and physics of NMR, 501, 502; and spin, 69, 125

animal studies: and association of glucose metabolism and functional activity, 18–19; and blood oxygenation, 115; and BOLD effect, 409, 432; and continuous arterial spin labeling (ASL), 361; and contrast agents, 345; and perfusion studies, 346

anistropic diffusion: definition of, 186; and diffusion imaging, 196–208; and measurement issues, 205

apparent diffusion coefficient (ADC) map, 191, 195, 346

arterial concentration, and tracer kinetics, 312

arterial pressure, 34

arterial spin labeling (ASL): applications of, 379–84; basic approaches to, 353; and BOLD effect, 412, 420, 421, 425; definition of, 311; and functional activity, 111–13; and measurement of CBF, 107, 351–3, 398; and relaxation time, 354–8; and radiofrequency (RF) pulse, 146; and systematic errors, 372–9; techniques of, 358–72

arterioles, and CBF, 34–5

artifacts: and data acquisition window, 226; and diffusion imaging in human brain, 193; and image distortions in MRI, 288–305; trade-offs between signal-to-noise ratio and, 440; and variations in magnetic field, 66. *See also* Gibbs artifact; motion artifacts

astrocytes, 10, 19, 20f, 36

asymmetric spin echo (ASE) pulse sequence: and data acquisition, 83, 250–3; and localization, 421; and mapping of brain activation, 118; and SE-BOLD experiment, 407

attenuation, and diffusion imaging, 210–12

auditory cortex, and BOLD signal change, 410

autoradiography, 14

autoregulation, of CBF, 35

average: and behavior of quantum spins, 508; and statistical analysis of BOLD data, 446–7. *See also* signal averages

axis of spin, 69–70